AF669849

Pathology Reviews • 1989

Pathology Reviews • 1989

Edited by

Emanuel Rubin, MD

Gonzalo Aponte Professor and Chairman
Department of Pathology and Cell Biology
Jefferson Medical College
Thomas Jefferson University
Philadelphia, Pennsylvania

and

Ivan Damjanov, MD

Professor
Department of Pathology and Cell Biology
Jefferson Medical College
Thomas Jefferson University
Philadelphia, Pennsylvania

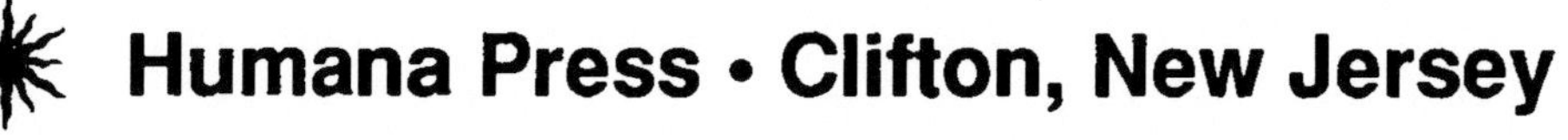

Humana Press • Clifton, New Jersey

U.S.-Canadian Division
International Academy of Pathology
1003 Chafee Ave.
Augusta, Georgia 30904

Made in the United States of America

ISBN: 0-89603-162-4

Preface

The concept that human disease is a specialized branch of biology is universally accepted today, but in historical perspective, is actually of recent origin. At one time, the heliocentric theories of astronomy and the metallurgic transmutations of alchemy had their counterparts in magical and vitalistic approaches to human disease. Any relation between disease of humans and that of animals was not only unacceptable intellectually, but abhorrent theologically. Humans (and their diseases) were unique, and biology was the domain of those who studied animals and plants.

The unification of biology and the study of human disease, though begun some centuries ago, was conspicuously stimulated by the work of Darwin, and reached its full flower in this century. For example, the recognition that spontaneous diseases in animals often were similar to human disease led to the use of animal models in experiments with agents as diverse as bacteria and chemical carcinogens, and to the manipulation of cells in tissue culture. The trend toward accepting the importance of basic biological phenomena to elucidate the etiology and pathogenesis of disease became irreversible, and the visionary goal of interpreting morphologic observations on the basis of biochemical and physical events is being realized today. The change in emphasis in the study of disease was not revolutionary, as was, for example, the replacement of Newtonian mechanics by concepts based on the theories of Planck and Einstein. Rather, until the mid-20th century, the accretion of individual examples of the biological nature of disease processes provided the framework for an evolutionary change in thinking. The new psychological and philosophical milieu provided the basis for an unprecedented acceleration in the pace of biomedical research. It is clear that the biological revolution of the last 35 years was made possible not only by technological advances and innovative analytical methods, but also by an intellectual emphasis on the unity of biological processes. High school students are now aware that there is much to be learned about the human condition by studying bacterial DNA, the chloroplasts of green leaves, or the kinetics of enzymes in vitro.

This volume, to be followed by others on an annual basis, is derived from material published in Laboratory Investigation, and is devoted to exploring this interface of biology and disease. Techniques and experimental models, once considered esoteric or exotic, are now in the forefront of research directed toward a fuller understanding of human disease. The presentations of the various authors in this volume are not only expositions of scientific data, but also represent contributions to the continuing trend toward unifying all of science.

Emanuel Rubin
Ivan Damjanov

Contents

Section I

Cell and Metabolic Disorders

Biology of Disease

Mammalian Glucocerebrosidase: Implications for Gaucher's Disease

ROBERT H. GLEW, ALAKANANDA BASU, KAREN L. LAMARCO, AND ELIZABETH M. PRENCE

Department of Microbiology, Biochemistry and Molecular Biology, The University of Pittsburgh School of Medicine, Pittsburgh, Pennsylvania

INTRODUCTION

More than 20 years ago Brady, Kanfer, and Shapiro and coworkers (13) and Patrick (49) identified the deficiency of glucocerebroside: β-glucosidase (glucocerebrosidase) as the cause of Gaucher's disease, the first sphingolipidosis for which the biochemical-enzymatic basis was established. In the intervening years, many investigators working in laboratories around the world have made important contributions to the fund of knowledge which has allowed us to construct the current picture we have of mammalian glucocerebrosidase.

Between 1965 and the early 1970s, research efforts were oriented primarily towards establishing reliable enzymatic methods for the diagnosis of Gaucher's disease and carrier detection. Beutler and Kuhl (9) were the first to demonstrate the usefulness of nonphysiologic aryl-β-D-glucosides as substrates for estimating relative glucocerebrosidase activity, thereby facilitating the development of β-glucosidase assays that could be used for diagnostic purposes, for monitoring glucocerebrosidase purifications and for investigating the physical-chemical and kinetic properties of the enzyme. These water-soluble arylglucosides have permitted kinetic studies that would otherwise be difficult, if not impossible, to conduct or interpret because of the extreme water-insolubility of the natural substrate, glucocerebroside.

The emphasis during the 1970s was on identifying isolation schemes that would yield pure preparations of glucocerebrosidase in quantities sufficient to permit therapy through replacement of the deficient enzyme, and which could be used in structure-function studies. During that decade, the heat-stable glucocerebrosidase activator protein was discovered by Ho and O'Brien (39).

In the mid 1970s, models of Gaucher's disease were created by administering inhibitors of glucocerebrosidase (*e.g.*, conduritol B-epoxide) to animals and cultured cells. Toward the end of that decade, as it became clear that our knowledge of glucocerebrosidase was inadequate to explain the clinical, biochemical, and genetic heterogeneity that forms the spectrum of Gaucher's disease, efforts were made to identify biochemical distinctions between the subgroups. Specifically, investigators sought to explain in biochemical and molecular terms, why some patients with a profound glucocerebrosidase deficiency lived into their eighth decade without brain involvement while others with apparently the same degree of glucocerebrosidase deficit died of extensive central nervous system disease before their first birthday. Especially useful in this regard, were the insights provided by Ho and Light (38) in their studies on the phospholipid requirement of glucocerebrosidase and the effects of a heat-stable factor (isolated from the spleen of patients with Gaucher's disease) on the enzyme. Parallel efforts along this same track by Glew *et al.* (32) and Wenger and Roth (71) led to the finding that most Gaucher's disease cases fall into only two major biochemical categories: those who are mildly-afflicted (type 1 patients) and whose residual mutant glucocerebrosidase can be reconstituted markedly by acidic membrane lipids, and the more severe cases (type 2 patients) that have extensive central nervous system pathology and whose residual glucocerebrosidase cannot be reconstituted to any significant extent by natural acidic lipids.

At the present time, investigators at a number of centers are working to improve our understanding of the mechanism of action of the glucocerebrosidase activators; these studies are aimed specifically at providing insight into: the structure of the heat-stable factor; the structure and composition of complexes formed between glucocerebrosidase, acidic membrane phospholipids and the heat-stable factor; and the mechanism of activation of glucocerebrosidase by these physiologically relevant substances.

In parallel with these aforementioned studies, a major effort by molecular biologists is now underway to determine the primary structure of the glucocerebrosidase gene itself, and to define the steps and intermediates involved in the biosynthesis and processing of the enzyme, from the initial mRNA transcript to insertion of the completed protein into or attachment to the lysosomal membrane.

In preparing this review, we invited about a dozen investigators from around the world who have made significant contributions to our understanding of the biochemistry of Gaucher's disease to submit several of their most important publications that deal with the enzymology of this particular lysosomal storage disease. In addition, we asked these same individuals to cite two publications, other than their own, which they thought had provided significant insight about the enzymology of Gaucher's disease. By focusing our attention on these 50 or so key publications, our goal was to provide the reader with the same insights that might otherwise have required days of intense library work to obtain.

This review is intended not only for those with a special interest in Gaucher's disease; it should also be of interest to medical students and residents, especially to those specializing in internal medicine, pediatric neurology, and pathology. In addition, it should be helpful to new investigators whose research projects may have led them to a consideration of lysosomal hydrolases, and who want to become familiar with the general principles that pertain to this class of enzymes. Although this article addresses only one of the more than two dozen different lysosomal enzymes that have been extensively investigated, in most cases, the principles and concepts derived from the study of one particular lysosomal enzyme or storage disease also hold for many other enzymes of the lysosomal hydrolase family. Finally, we hope that our review, by concentrating on the glucocerebrosidase enzyme, and leaving the treatment of the more clinical aspects of Gaucher's disease to others, might provide even the Gaucher's disease afficionado with a more complete, integrated picture of the chemistry, kinetics, and biosynthesis of glucocerebrosidase that can be absorbed in one sitting.

WHAT IS GAUCHER'S DISEASE?

Gaucher's disease is an autosomal recessive lysosomal storage disease, and the most common of the sphingolipidoses, that group of genetic diseases that result from deficiencies of the lysosomal enzymes which degrade glycosphingolipids and sphingomyelin. Although the first case was reported in the literature in 1882 by Philippe C. E. Gaucher, a French physician, it was not until 1965 that Brady, Kanfer and Shapiro (13) and Patrick (49) identified the precise enzyme deficiency that causes Gaucher's disease.

Glucocerebrosidase, the deficient enzyme in people with Gaucher's disease, catalyzes the hydrolysis of glucocerebroside to yield ceramide and glucose (Fig. 1). As a result of insufficient glucocerebrosidase activity (<20% of control), the substrate for the deficient enzyme, namely glucocerebroside (glucosylceramide), accumulates in phagocytic cells mainly in liver, spleen, and bone marrow (*i.e.*, the macrophage or reticuloendothelial system).

Glucocerebroside arises primarily from the degradation of glucosphingolipids from membranes of white blood cells and senescent red blood cells. The highly hydrophobic glucocerebroside molecules self-associate to form bilayers that stack up as membranous sheets (Fig. 2). These structures give the cytoplasm of the Gaucher

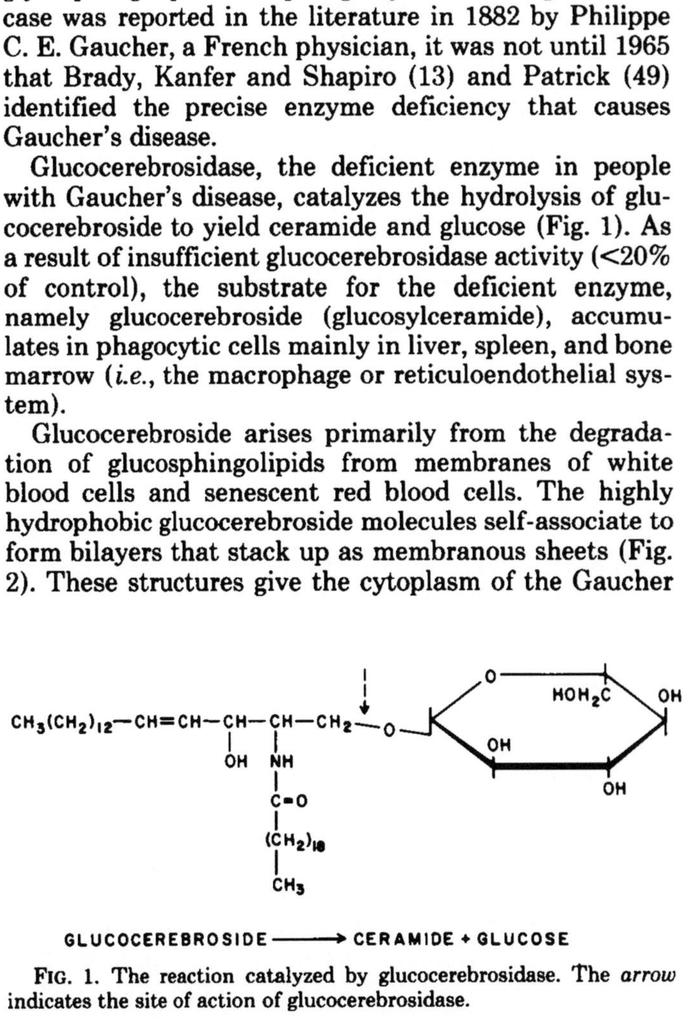

GLUCOCEREBROSIDE ⟶ CERAMIDE + GLUCOSE

FIG. 1. The reaction catalyzed by glucocerebrosidase. The *arrow* indicates the site of action of glucocerebrosidase.

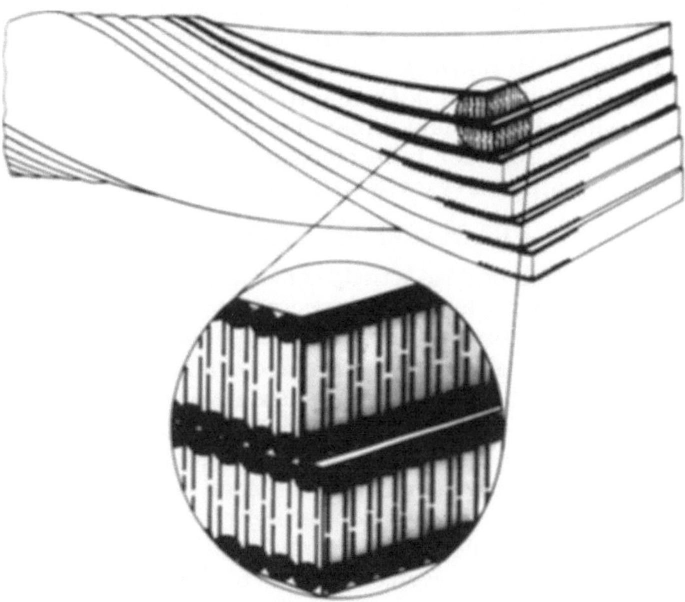

FIG. 2. The bilayer structure of the glucocerebroside-rich storage deposits in the Gaucher cell.

storage cell its characteristic striated appearance which was first appreciated in the 19th century by Dr. Gaucher.

Because glucocerebroside is insoluble in body fluids, the glycolipid cannot be excreted in the urine. Thus, glucocerebroside molecules deposit in the cells where they are generated, and in the cases of spleen and liver, give rise to splenomegaly and hepatomegaly, respectively. The storage cells in the bone marrow crowd out the hematopoetic tissues; in addition, the enlarged spleen and liver prematurely destroy red cells, white cells, and platelets, thereby contributing to the anemia, leukopenia, and thrombocytopenia that are common in individuals with Gaucher's disease.

Accumulation of Gaucher cells in the bone marrow can lead to skeletal afflictions, including frequent fractures, bone and joint pain, and swelling of the tender surrounding tissues. Osteonecrosis and collapse of the femoral head is often severe enough to require hip replacement surgery; the so-called "Erlenmeyer flask" deformity is observed frequently in younger patients undergoing rapid bone growth and arises from expansion of the cortex of the distal femur (12).

Because the phagocytic cells of the macrophage system are lysosome-rich, one secondary effect which results from glucocerebroside storage is the elevation of serum acid phosphatase activity in patients with Gaucher's disease. Progressive engorgement of lysosomes with glucocerebroside leads to their eventual lysis and release of their contents into the blood; therefore, since macrophages contain predominantly type 5 acid phosphatase, it is this isoenzyme that is elevated in serum from Gaucher patients. Using high concentrations of the reducing agent, β-mercaptoethanol, several years ago Chambers *et al.* (14) devised an acid phosphatase assay protocol that specifically detects the elevation of the type 5 acid phosphatase isoenzyme in the serum from Gaucher patients. However, because an occasional (approximately 1/20) Gaucher patient will have normal serum acid phosphatase value, one should not attempt to diagnose the disease using this test.

Patients with Gaucher's disease generally fit into one of three clinical subtypes. Those with the type 1 or "adult" form of Gaucher's disease present with an incidence of 1/2,500 within the Ashkenazi Jewish population. Patients with the type 1 form of the disease follow a chronic, progressive course characterized by hepatosplenomegaly, pancytopenia, and erosion of the cortices of the long bones. Also referred to as "chronic, non-neuronopathic" Gaucher's disease, type 1 is distinguished from types 2 and 3 by the absence of neurologic involvement. The range of clinical severity within this group is great, and it is not yet understood why some patients suffer clinical manifestations of the disease early in life (age 3 to 4 years), while others remain undiagnosed into their sixth or seventh decade (12).

Infants suffering from the type 2 ("infantile," "acute neuronopathic") form of Gaucher's disease usually die before the age of 2, and the brains of these patients contain typical Gaucher cells. Characteristic clinical symptoms of type 2 Gaucher's disease include: neurologic involvement, mental retardation, failure to thrive, strabismus, retroflexion of the head, and muscle hypertonicity.

A "juvenile" or "subacute neuronopathic" form (type 3) of Gaucher's disease has also been observed, predominantly in patients of Scandinavian origin; although these patients usually live longer than type 2 patients, they, too, suffer from neurologic dysfunction and their symptoms are similar to those observed in type 2 patients. Factors which biochemically distinguish the neuronopathic and non-neuronopathic forms of Gaucher's disease will be considered in subsequent sections of this review.

THE DISCOVERY OF THE GLUCOCEREBROSIDASE DEFICIENCY IN PATIENTS WITH GAUCHER'S DISEASE

Brady, Kanfer, and Shapiro (13) at the National Institutes of Health in Bethesda, Maryland in the United States and Patrick (49) at the Institute of Child Health at the Hospital for Sick Children in London discovered the deficiency of glucocerebrosidase, the glucocerebroside, cleaving enzyme, in Gaucher's disease. Since the manuscripts of Brady's group and Patrick documenting the glucocerebrosidase deficiency in Gaucher's disease were submitted for publication within months of each other, it is appropriate to consider that this important discovery was made virtually simultaneously and independently by the investigators in the two countries; the authors of those two key papers exhibited originality and deserve to be acknowledged equally for their scientific achievement.

It is interesting to contrast the experimental techniques these two groups used in arriving at this common conclusion. While Brady, Kanfer, and Shapiro (13) and Patrick (49) both used authentic glucocerebroside as the substrate, and spleen as their source of enzyme, the tissue preparation and the composition of the incubation medium used to determine glucocerebrosidase activity differed significantly between the investigators. First, in their initial study, Brady, Kanfer, and Shapiro used the high-speed supernatant fraction (100,000 × *g*, 1 hour) from an aqueous extract of freeze-thawed spleen homogenate prepared in 0.1 M potassium phosphate buffer, pH 7.0 as their source of glucocerebrosidase. Subsequent studies by many investigators have shown that under these conditions of homogenization, very little of the glucocerebrosidase (less than 10% of the total) that is firmly bound to the lysosomal membranes is released in a form that would allow it to be recovered in the 100,000 × *g* supernatant fraction; efficient extraction and solubilization of glucocerebrosidase from membranes requires strong ionic detergents. Secondly, the National Institutes of Health group carried out their glucocerebrosidase incubations at pH 7.0, a hydrogen ion concentration nearly 2 pH units above the pH optimum of the enzyme. In retrospect, considering the extraction procedure they used to prepare the enzyme, and the assay conditions they employed to estimate glucocerebrosidase activity, it seems that the documentation of the enzyme deficiency in Gaucher's disease was made using spleen extracts that contained only a small fraction of the tissue's glucocerebrosidase, and grossly suboptimal assay conditions.

In contrast, Patrick (49) used a crude, unfractionated "water homogenate" of spleen as the enzyme source in his experiments, thereby making no assumptions about the subcellular localization of glucocerebrosidase and ensuring that he had not discarded any fraction that might contain a significant fraction of the enzyme activity in question. In addition, he performed the glucocerebrosidase assay at pH 5.6, a hydrogen ion concentration close to the enzyme's pH optimum. It is not surprising, then, to find that the glucocerebrosidase specific activities obtained by the two groups differed by nearly 20-fold, with Patrick (49) reporting the higher values.

Thus, it was established, for the first time, "that there is a pronounced diminution of the activity of the glucocerebroside-cleaving enzyme in patients with Gaucher's disease" (13). Specifically, Patrick (49) reported that spleen homogenates at 4/4 Gaucher's disease cases had undetectable glucocerebrosidase activity. In contrast, Brady, Kanfer, and Shapiro (13) found a significant amount of residual glucocerebrosidase activity (approximately 10% of control), in all 11 of the Gaucher's disease cases they analyzed, a finding that would be confirmed subsequently by many other investigators around the world who together have biochemically analyzed hundreds of different cases of Gaucher's disease.

PRACTICAL ENZYMOLOGY

Glucocerebrosidase activity can be estimated unambiguously by using authentic glucocerebroside as the substrate. Unfortunately, difficulty in synthesizing radiolabeled glucocerebroside, its restricted availability, and the relatively tedious assay procedure involved in its use make it inconvenient for routine use. Furthermore, the extreme water-insolubility of glucocerebroside compels one to use some detergent in the assay medium which sometimes complicates the interpretation of results (see the "Non-physiologic Detergents" section). This difficulty can be partly overcome by use of the water-soluble, non-physiologic aryl glucoside, 4-methylumbelliferyl-β-D-glucopyranoside (MUGlc) as the substrate.

In 1970, Beutler and Kuhl (9) measured leukocyte β-glucosidase activity across a wide pH range utilizing this readily available, highly fluorogenic substrate. They discovered that white blood cell β-glucosidase activity exhibited two pH optima, one at pH 4.0, and another at pH 5.5, suggesting the existence of two distinct β-glucosidases with different pH optima. In patients with Gaucher's disease, activity was decreased at both pH levels; however, the enzyme deficiency was much more pronounced at pH 4.0 (Fig. 3*A*), prompting Beutler and Kuhl (9) to remark "the relatively simple explanation that two isozymes exist, each under a separate genetic control, does not explain all of our findings." Thus was made the first tenuous link between glucocerebrosidase and a second β-glucosidase of unknown origin and function which is present in most mammalian tissues.

Although Beutler and Kuhl's (9) leukocyte "acid β-glucosidase" (pH 4.0) assay effectively distinguished patients with Gaucher's disease from controls, there was considerable overlap of heterozygote (carrier) and control glucocerebrosidase levels; furthermore, to achieve maximum distinction between patients and controls, it was

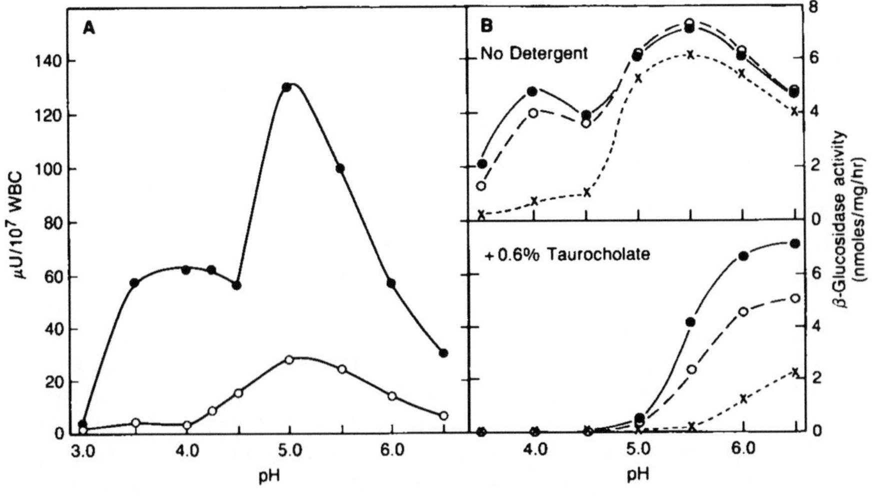

FIG. 3. The effect of pH on β-glucosidase activity from control and Gaucher's leukocytes. *A*, β-Glucosidase activity was measured using 0.1 M sodium citrate buffer. Controls (●), Gaucher's disease (○) (modified from Ref. 9). *B*, β-Glucosidase activity was measured in the absence and presence of 0.6% sodium taurocholate using 0.2 M sodium acetate buffer. Controls (●), Gaucher heterozygote (○), and Gaucher homozygote (×) (taken from Ref. 53).

necessary to perform the β-glucosidase assay at a suboptimal pH (pH 4.0). Clearly, there was need at that time for a more suitable diagnostic test which would identify not only Gaucher patients but carriers as well.

In 1976, Peters, Coyle, and Glew (53) developed a β-glucosidase assay that differentiated between glucocerebrosidase and the broad-specificity β-glucosidase which hydrolyzes MUGlc but not glucocerebroside. The broad specificity β-glucosidase is inhibited by sodium taurocholate, while lysosomal glucocerebrosidase is stimulated by the bile salt. To minimize the contribution of the broad specificity β-glucosidase to the hydrolysis of MUGlc, they included 0.6% sodium taurocholate in the assay medium to inhibit this nonspecific β-glucosidase, while simultaneously activating glucocerebrosidase; by using white cell preparations from Gaucher patients, heterozygotes, and controls, the greatest distinction among the three groups was observed when the assay was performed at pH 5.5 to 6.0 (Fig. 3*B*). In that particular study, there was no overlap of heterozygote β-glucosidase levels with those of either the controls or Gaucher patients. However, when many more heterozygotes were analyzed for leukocyte β-glucosidase, they found that this method did not completely eliminate misdiagnosis of the heterozygote condition. Nevertheless, it continues to be the most reliable and widely utilized diagnostic procedure for the detection of Gaucher patients and carriers.

ENZYMOLOGY

Isolation and Purification of Glucocerebrosidase

Glucocerebrosidase has been isolated from a variety of tissues, including human placenta, spleen and liver, bovine brain, and rat liver. Detergents are required to extract the enzyme from the lysosomal membrane (50), and the one most often used for this purpose is sodium cholate (22).

Many investigators have purified glucocerebrosidase to apparent homogeneity using affinity columns (2, 22, 60, 68). A high recovery (30% yield) purification scheme for human placental glucocerebrosidase, resulting in an apparently homogeneous enzyme preparation that was suitable for use in enzyme replacement therapy, was reported in 1977 by Furbish *et al.* (22). Their procedure involves decyl-agarose chromatography of butanol-extracted, partially purified glucocerebrosidase, followed by octyl-Sepharose chromatography and finally concentration by ethanol precipitation. A linear (30 to 80%) ethylene glycol gradient was applied to both columns and glucocerebrosidase was eluted from each when the ethylene glycol concentration reached approximately 60%. The enzyme exhibited a final specific activity of 1.11×10^6 nmol/hour/mg (using [^{14}C]glucocerebroside as the substrate), and yielded a single 67 kilodalton (kd) band on sodium dodecyl sulfate-polyacrylamide gel electrophoresis (SDS-PAGE).

Another high yield purification scheme was recently described by Grabowski and Dagan (33). Using affinity chromatography, they purified human placental glucocerebrosidase to a specific activity of 4.5×10^6 nmol/hour/mg with an overall yield of 27%. The enzyme was sequentially chromatographed on columns consisting of Sepharose-bound substrate analogs: first, 6′-aminohexanoyl-(2-*N*-sphingosyl-1-0-β-D-glucoside) and then, 6′-aminohexyl-dodecanedioyl-1-(2-*N*-sphingosyl-1-0-β-D-glucoside). Glucocerebrosidase was eluted from the first column with a linear ethylene glycol gradient (20 to 90%) and from the second column with 90% ethylene glycol. The final glucocerebrosidase preparation yielded a single 67 kd band on SDS-PAGE. Glucocerebrosidase purified in this manner is stable for at least 1 year when stored at −20° C in 90% ethylene glycol.

While the two purification schemes just described resulted in similar yields, the specific activity of the glucocerebrosidase purified by Grabowski and Dagan (33) was much higher than that of the enzyme obtained by Furbish *et al.* (22). An explanation for this difference in the specific activities of two apparently homogeneous enzyme preparations was offered by Grabowski and Dagan (33). Using immunoelectrophoresis, these researchers found that whereas glucocerebrosidase purified by hydrophobic chromatography was contaminated with human serum albumin (which comigrates with glucocerebrosidase on SDS-PAGE) no albumin was detected in their affinity-chromatography purified enzyme. Therefore, although the recoveries of the two purification schemes were similar, the substrate-analogue affinity chromatography method apparently provides a more homogeneous enzyme preparation.

More recently, Murray *et al.* (46) reported that gel-permeation high performance liquid chromatography (HPLC) on Spherogel TSK 3000SW (Beckman/Altex, Berkeley, California) was an effective way to remove very hydrophobic contaminants from glucocerebrosidase prepared by chromatography on hydrophobic columns (*e.g.*, phenyl-Sepharose, octyl-Sepharose), provided the elution buffer (0.1 M sodium citrate, pH 5.0) contained 50% ethylene glycol; the specific activity of the final preparation was 1.6×10^6 nmol/hour/mg of protein.

Physical Chemical Properties of Glucocerebrosidase

Carbohydrate Content

Glucocerebrosidase is a glycoprotein that contains approximately 7% carbohydrate. Studies performed on glucocerebrosidase isolated from human placenta (66), human fibroblasts, and porcine kidney (20) have provided information regarding the structure, number, and steps involved in the processing of its oligosaccharide side chains.

Erickson *et al.* (20) showed that porcine kidney glucocerebrosidase contains four *N*-linked oligosaccharide chains which are synthesized as high-mannose forms and then processed to complex carbohydrate structures. The oligosaccharide side-chains (66) consist mainly of biantennary and triantennary complex structures; less than one-fourth of the isolated sugar chains are of the high-mannose type. Figure 4 shows the structure of the major triantennary oligosaccharide of placental glucocerebrosidase.

An interesting characteristic of the structure is that all of the sialic acid residues occur in a NeuAcα2→3Gal linkage. Although this type of linkage is found in other glycoproteins, it is usually present together with the

```
NeuAcα2→3Galβ1→4GlcNAcβ1
                        \
                         6
                          Manα1
                         2      \
                        /        6
NeuAcα2→3Galβ1→4GlcNAcβ1          Manβ1→4GlcNAcβ1→4GlcNAc
                                 3
                                /
NeuAcα2→3Galβ1→4GlcNAcβ1→2 Manα1
```

FIG. 4. Structure of the *N*-asparagine-linked oligosaccharide units of human placental B-glucocerebrosidase (taken from Ref. 66).

NeuAcα2→6Gal linkage. According to Takasaki *et al.* (66), the presence of exclusively the α2→3 sialic acid linkage has been found in only one other glycoprotein, namely human chorionic gonadotropin. It remains to be seen if this rare sialic acid linkage is important for glucocerebrosidase function, or if it is simply a common property of placental glycoproteins.

It is not known if the oligosaccharide chains on glucocerebrosidase are required for enzymatic activity or structural stability. However, the carbohydrate moieties have been shown to play a role in the uptake of infused glucocerebrosidase by various rat tissues (23) and in the targeting of the enzyme to lysosomes (1).

MOLECULAR WEIGHT

Glucocerebrosidase has been isolated from a number of sources and its molecular weight has been determined by a variety of methods. The subunit size of placental glucocerebrosidase, as determined by SDS-PAGE, is approximately 60 kd, while aggregates representing two and four subunits have been detected by molecular sieve chromatography in the absence of SDS.

Differences in the size of glucocerebrosidase isolated from tissues of patients with various forms of Gaucher's disease have been noted. Using sucrose gradients (25) and radiation inactivation (43), native spleen glucocerebrosidase of patients with type 1 Gaucher's disease appears to have a native molecular weight in the 100 to 125 kd range, indicating it may be a dimer. However, using SDS-PAGE, normal subunit sizes were observed for glucocerebrosidase derived from fibroblasts and brains of type 1 cases, although the relative abundance of the different processed forms of the subunit appeared to be abnormal in fibroblasts (post-translational processing is discussed in the "Biosynthesis of Glucocerebrosidase" section of this review).

The native glucocerebrosidase of patients with type 2 Gaucher's disease appears to be much larger than that of healthy controls. Using sucrose gradient centrifugation, Garrett, Prence, and Glew (25) observed a very large size for type 2 glucocerebrosidase (>200 kd) that could not be dispersed by chaotropic salts (*e.g.*, sodium thiocyanate). In another study (30), with brain from type 2 Gaucher's disease patients, only the high molecular weight forms of glucocerebrosidase were detected using SDS-PAGE; none of the processed (56 kd) form found in normal cells was present. Therefore, it seems that mutations causing the above mentioned types of Gaucher's disease produce larger than normal glucocerebrosidase proteins.

Although the subunit size of normal human glucocerebrosidase is approximately 60 kd, in order to express optimum catalytic activity it seems the enzyme must be in the form of larger "active complex." Sucrose density gradient analysis of mixtures of glucocerebrosidase and phosphatidylserine (25, 54) or the ganglioside G_{M1} (5) have shown that reconstitution of glucocerebrosidase activity is accompanied by an increase in the size of the enzyme. For the G_{M1}-activated rat liver glucocerebrosidase, the active complex appears to consist of 2 glucocerebrosidase subunits plus enough lipid activator to yield a molecular weight of 178 kd (5). When phosphatidylserine and heat-stable factor were used to activate either rat liver (54) or normal human spleen (25) glucocerebrosidase, the size of the active enzyme complex was 190 to 230 kd. Glucocerebrosidase isolated from the spleens of patients with type 1 Gaucher's disease behaved similarly to the control enzyme when incubated with phosphatidylserine and heat-stable factor (25). However, these activators had no apparent effect on the glucocerebrosidase of a case of type 2 Gaucher's disease.

KINETIC PROPERTIES

SUBSTRATE SPECIFICITY

Glucocerebroside is composed of a hydrophilic glucose molecule attached through a β-linkage to ceramide, a lipophilic moiety (Fig. 1). The enzyme has strict specificity with regard to the sugar moiety: it hydrolyzes glucosides, but no other glycosides (*e.g.*, β-D galactosides, α-L-arabinosides, β-D-fucosides) to any significant extent. However, there is a report which shows that glucocerebrosidase possesses low but detectable β-xylosidase activity (71).

Glucocerebrosidase is less stringent with regard to the aglycon portion of the molecule, and when the ceramide moiety is replaced with *p*-nitrophenol or 4-methylumbelliferone, the enzyme retains its ability to hydrolyze the β-glucoside bond. In fact, water-soluble aryl glucosides like 4-methylumbelliferyl-β-D-glucoside and *p*-nitrophenyl-β-D-glucoside are excellent glucocerebrosidase substrates. When glucocerebroside is deacylated or if the long chain fatty acyl group is substituted with an *N*-hexyl group, the resulting derivatives, glucosylsphingosine and *N*-hexyl-*O*-glucosylsphingosine, respectively, are hydrolyzed by glucocerebrosidase but at much reduced rates (50, 71).

INHIBITORS

Inhibitors have provided useful information about the structure, function, and kinetic properties of glucocerebrosidase. In addition, inhibitors have been used to create chemical models of Gaucher's disease in animals and cultured cells. The glucocerebrosidase inhibitors can be divided into two major classes: (a) reversible inhibitors and (b) irreversible inhibitors.

a. Reversible Inhibitors. Sphingosine-based structural analogs of glucocerebroside are potent inhibitors of glucocerebrosidase. Glucosylsphingosine (glucocerebroside minus the long chain fatty acid residue) is one of the most effective inhibitors in this class of compounds. Galactosylsphingosine, which differs from glucosylsphingosine only in the orientation of the 4-hydroxyl group of the sugar moiety, does not inhibit glucocerebrosidase (21) thereby indicating that: (a) the inhibitor is highly specific, and (b) the inhibition by glucosylsphingosine (GS) is probably not the result of the detergent property of these amphipathic, glycosylated sphingosines.

Since naturally occurring glucocerebroside has a lipoidal substituent, namely a long chain (C_{18} to C_{26}) fatty acid, attached to the nitrogen atom of the sphingosine moiety, one might expect that *N*-alkyl derivatives of GS would be effective inhibitors of glucocerebrosidase. Substitution of the fatty acid amide group of glucocerebroside with an alkyl group generates a secondary amine that possesses a positive charge on the nitrogen atom. Erickson and Radin (21) showed that the *N*-alkylglucosylsphingosines are more effective than glucosylsphingosine in inhibiting glucocerebrosidase. In light of the fact that the naturally occurring glucosphingolipids are comprised of a very long carbon chain ($\geq C_{18}$) attached to the nitrogen atom, it is puzzling that the most effective inhibitors in the *N*-alkyl glucosylsphingosine series are ones that contain relatively short (C_6 to C_{10}) alkyl chains; for example, *N*-hexylglucosylsphingosine (HGS), the best inhibitor in the series, inhibits glucocerebrosidase activity to a greater extent (85%) than does *N*-octadecylglucosylsphingosine (56%) (21).

Because of structural similarity to glucocerebroside, GS and HGS would be expected to inhibit glucocerebrosidase activity in a competitive manner. However, for unexplained reasons, the pattern and extent of inhibition seems to depend on the source of enzyme, and the particular assay conditions one uses. For example, using a crude rat spleen preparation, Erickson and Radin (21) found HGS to be a competitive inhibitor of glucocerebrosidase. In contrast, using either a partially purified or purified and delipidated (sodium cholate-, butanol-extracted) glucocerebrosidase preparation from rat liver, human placenta or human spleen, Basu and Glew (4), Grabowski *et al.* (34), and Gatt *et al.* (26) all observed noncompetitive or mixed type inhibition with both GS and HGS. The presence of different endogenous lipids in these enzyme preparations or the use of detergents (*e.g.*, bile salts, Triton X-100), or other activator lipids (*e.g.*, phosphatidylserine) in the assay media might explain these discrepant results.

The mixed type inhibition caused by GS and HGS indicates the presence of a second binding site for hydrophobic glycosides on glucocerebrosidase that accommodates these sphingolipid inhibitors, and which is distinct from the site where substrates bind. Radin (58) hypothesized that: "glucocerebrosidase is an enzyme which originally mutated by gene duplication to a protein with two active sites. In due time it mutated further to render one of the sites enzymatically inactive but still able to bind compounds resembling the substrate."

Natural activators of glucocerebrosidase, such as phosphatidylserine and heat-stable factor, markedly influence the degree of inhibition of glucocerebrosidase achieved with HGS and GS (4). For example, the K_i of HGS decreased from 2.2 μM to 0.11 μM when a mixture of phosphatidylserine and the heat-stable factor was included in the assay medium. The addition of these activator substances to the assay medium did not alter the mixed type character of the inhibition. Taken together, these observations suggest the presence of a third binding site on glucocerebrosidase, one that is distinct from the substrate binding site and the inhibitor binding site where GS and HGS bind. We suggest that this third site is where glucocerebrosidase interacts with activator substances such as acidic lipids and heat-stable factor.

Radin (57) postulated that "HGS and related lipoidal amines exert their effects by forming a strong salt linkage with an essential carboxyl group at the active site of the enzyme." Our own observation that HGS obliterates ionizable groups with pK values of 4.5 and 5.1 that play an important catalytic function (4) supports Radin's hypothesis.

Attempts to create an animal model of Gaucher's disease by injecting rats with HGS intraperitoneally were unsuccessful (58).

b. Conduritol B-Epoxide, an Irreversible Inhibitor. Conduritol B-epoxide (CBE), first synthesized by Legler (42) in Koln, Germany, is an active site-specific inhibitor of certain β-glucosidases (Fig. 5). It is a low molecular weight, water-soluble derivative of myoinositol and it inactivates β-glucosidases by reacting with an essential carboxyl group (presumably aspartate) at the enzyme's active center (Fig. 5).

CBE inhibits only the lysosomal glucocerebrosidase; it has little effect on the broad specificity β-glucosidase isoenzyme that is present along with glucocerebrosidase in most mammalian tissues. This differential sensitivity of the two β-glucosidases to inactivation by CBE permitted us to devise a useful assay for glucocerebrosidase using the fluorogenic substrate MUGlc (17). The CBE-dependent β-glucosidase assay is so effective in discriminating glucocerebrosidase from the broad specificity β-glucosidase that one can use the assay to diagnose Gaucher's disease even when liver serves as the source of enzyme. Before the study by Daniels *et al.* (17), it was not possible to confirm a diagnosis of Gaucher's disease using MUGlc as the substrate and liver as the source of enzyme because this tissue contained so much of the nonlysosomal β-glucosidase.

β-Glucosidases generally catalyze the hydrolysis of glucosides in two discrete steps: (1) the enzyme interacts with the substrate to form a covalent glucosyl-enzyme complex, which is followed by (2) hydrolysis of the complex and release of glucose. CBE is a reactant in the first step of this reaction sequence. Negatively charged acidic activator lipids (*e.g.*, phosphatidylserine, phosphatidylglycerol), alone or in combination with heat-stable factor (HSF), increase the rate of inactivation of the enzyme by CBE (4, 6). This finding suggests that these activators

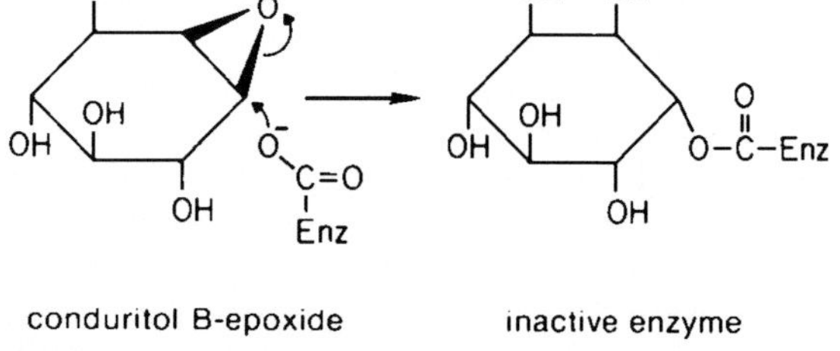

FIG. 5. Reaction of conduritol β-epoxide with a carboxyl group of glucocerebrosidase.

influence the substrate binding step apparently by interacting with glucocerebrosidase. Bromo conduritol B-epoxide (Br CBE) is an even more effective inhibitor of glucocerebrosidase than CBE.

^{3}H-Labeled bromo conduritol B-epoxide (^{3}H-Br CBE) was used as an affinity label to identify the amino acid sequence around the active site of human placental glucocerebrosidase (19). Under optimal conditions, 1 mole of glucocerebrosidase bound 1 mole of ^{3}H-Br CBE indicating a single catalytic center/molecule of enzyme. Amino acid sequencing of one of the radiolabeled peptides isolated from a F_8 protease digest of the derivatized protein provided the primary structure of the catalytic site; however, the instability of the ester linkage between the inhibitor and the peptide prevented Dinur *et al.* (19) from identifying the amino acid to which ^{3}H-Br CBE was bound. The 37 amino acid sequence at the active site was consistent with a sequence predicted for residues 429-465 from the cDNA of glucocerebrosidase. Based on the amino acid sequence encoded by a full-length (496 amino acids) cDNA, it was concluded that the active site of the enzyme is located near its carboxyl terminus.

The first really useful chemically induced animal model of Gaucher's disease was created by administering CBE to young mice (41). To maintain the enzyme activity in tissues at a very low level, animals received daily intraperitoneal injections of the inhibitor. Young animals are preferred for two reasons: (a) the amount of CBE required to produce an effect is less compared with older, larger animals, and (b) glycolipid metabolism in general, and glucocerebroside turnover specifically, are more rapid in the brains of younger animals.

Injection of CBE into mice resulted in nearly complete inactivation of glucocerebrosidase but did not alter the activities of five other lysosomal hydrolases including α-mannosidase, β-hexosaminidase, β-galactosidase, α-glucosidase, and β-glucuronidase (41). By measuring tissue glucocerebrosidase activity at various times after the last CBE injection, the half-life of glucocerebrosidase was estimated to be 6 to 9 days. The glucocerebroside content in peripheral tissues (liver and spleen) was increased 50% and 3- to 5-fold in brain. Some signs of neurologic dysfunction were also evident. As observed in humans with Gaucher's disease, in addition to glucocerebroside accumulation, several complex glycosphingolipids (*e.g.*, lactosylceramide, trihexosylceramide, globoside, hematoside) were also found to be elevated in the visceral organs (65) of CBE-treated animals; however, no such accumulation occurred in the brains of these animals.

Fifty percent of the β-glucosidase activity in brain was CBE-resistant if the assay was performed at pH 5.5 to 5.8 by using MUGlc as the substrate. However, at a lower pH (pH 4.1 to 4.8) there was no detectable β-glucosidase activity in homogenates of brain from CBE-treated animals, indicating that brain tissue contains at least two β-glucosidases with different pH optima (37).

A puzzling observation in the CBE-mice studies of Radin and coworkers was the rapid decrease in β-glucuronidase activity in liver, spleen, and kidney and an increase in brain β-glucuronidase after CBE administration (58). Radin (57) postulated that newly synthesized β-glucuronidase contains a glucose moiety and "the enzyme must lose part of its glucose in order to enter lysosomes; if this cannot be done, the enzyme leaks out, or is expelled, into the extracellular fluid." In fact, the increase in β-glucuronidase activity in the CBE-treated animals appears in the cytosolic fraction of the brain. Radin's hypothesis implies that glucocerebrosidase participates in the biosynthesis of some lysosomal enzymes, including β-glucuronidase, and that the action of glucocerebrosidase on these enzymes influences their targeting to lysosomes. It remains to be seen if β-glucuronidase, at some point in its lifetime in the cell, possesses terminal, nonreducing, β-linked glucose residues that are removed by glucocerebrosidase. One problem with this hypothesis is that glucocerebrosidase has a lysosomal location, and Radin's postulation envisions the removal of glucose units from β-glucuronidase before it reaches the lysosome.

Activators

Glucocerebrosidase, an integral membrane protein, can be solubilized, and at the same time delipidated, by sequential extraction with either sodium cholate and 1-butanol, or by extraction with acetone. These procedures dissociate the enzyme from endogenous membrane lipids and cause extensive, but reversible, inactivation of glucocerebrosidase; enzyme activity can be restored *in vitro* by inclusion of exogenous lipids in the assay medium.

a. Nonphysiologic Detergents. The conventional method for obtaining high glucocerebrosidase activity *in vitro* is to incorporate some detergent into the assay medium. Nonionic detergents like Triton X-100 or Cutscum are only weak activators of the enzyme. Effective reconstitution of enzyme activity requires strong ionic detergents that carry a net negative charge (*e.g.*, bile salts). Raghavan, Topol, and Kolodny (59) compared the effects of various detergents as activators of human leukocyte glucocerebrosidase, and found that at the level of 0.2% (w/v) detergent, sodium taurodeoxycholate > sodium glycodeoxycholate > sodium taurocholate and sodium glycocholate > Triton X-100. However, at higher concentrations (>0.6%, w/v), sodium taurocholate was almost as effective as sodium taurodeoxycholate in stimulating glucocerebrosidase activity.

Bile salts like sodium taurocholate and sodium taurodeoxycholate stimulate glucocerebrosidase primarily by raising the V_{max} without having a significant effect on the K_m. Sodium taurodeoxycholate significantly increases the rate of heat inactivation (45° C) of the enzyme, suggesting that bile salts interact directly with glucocerebrosidase.

From a practical standpoint, bile salts have proven extremely useful in glucocerebrosidase studies because: (a) they facilitate interaction between the enzyme and authentic substrate by dispersing highly water-insoluble glucocerebroside; (b) they are potent activators of glucocerebrosidase, accelerating the hydrolysis of both glucocerebroside and water-soluble aryl glucosides (*e.g.*, MUGlc, PNPGlc); (c) while markedly activating glucocerebrosidase, they inhibit the broad specificity, cytosolic

β-glucosidase, thereby providing a useful assay for glucocerebrosidase when the aryl glucoside (*e.g.*, MUGlc) is employed as the substrate; and (d) they do not depend on any other effectors, such as the heat-stable factor.

Despite these attributes, bile salts are regarded as nonphysiologic activators of glucocerebrosidase for, although they are components of the enterohepatic circulation, they are not normal constituents of the lysosomal membrane, and therefore cannot serve to activate glucocerebrosidase *in vivo*. Furthermore, when residual tissue glucocerebrosidase activity of patients with Gaucher's disease is measured in the presence of bile salts, it is impossible to distinguish between neurologic and nonneurologic forms of the disease on enzymatic grounds (32). Finally, bile salts obscure the effects of any other activators like acidic membrane lipids (*e.g.*, phosphatidylserine) and heat-stable factor (6, 38, 45).

b. Heat-stable factor. The first potential physiologic activator of glucocerebrosidase was discovered fortuitously by Ho and O'Brien (39) in 1971. In their search for a soluble glucocerebrosidase inhibitor in the spleen of patients with Gaucher's disease that might account for reduced enzyme activity, they performed a mixing experiment using homogenates from a control spleen and a spleen from a patient with Gaucher's disease and observed an unexpected 2- to 3-fold increase in glucocerebrosidase activity. They designated the glucocerebrosidase from control spleen as 'factor C' and the activator substance from the patient's spleen as 'factor P'. The activator was tentatively identified as a glycoprotein, which itself was devoid of β-glucosidase activity.

The activator protein, variously referred to as heat-stable factor (HSF) (due to its resistance to boiling), cohydrolase (in analogy with colipase, the proteinaceous activator of pancreatic lipase), or sphingolipid activator protein (SAP), was first isolated from Gaucher spleen (39) and later purified to homogeneity from both control and Gaucher spleen (52). The Gaucher spleen HSF corresponds to SAP-II, as defined by Fujibayashi and Wenger (24); it is present in approximately the same concentration in all three forms of Gaucher's disease (51).

The heat-stable factor of control spleen is distinct in several respects from that derived from the spleen of patients with Gaucher's disease: (1) it is only 6% as active as Gaucher spleen HSF, (2) it has a molecular weight of 8,800 as compared to 11,000, which is the molecular weight of the Gaucher spleen HSF, (3) it is devoid of carbohydrate, whereas the HSF from Gaucher spleen consists of 17% carbohydrate, (4) the amino acid compositions of the two HSFs are different. Based on these observations, Peters et al. (52) concluded that HSFs from control and Gaucher spleen are not closely related structurally. However, Iyer, Berent, and Radin (40) suggested that "Gaucher's cohydrolase is formed from normal cohydrolase by the nonenzymatic action of cellular glucose over a period of many years due to slowed catabolism of the cofactor." The presence of glucose in cohydrolase from Gaucher spleen and the lack of carbohydrate in the HSF from control spleen provide the only basis for this hypothesis. Unless mentioned otherwise, in subsequent discussions of HSF it should be assumed we are referring to the factor isolated from Gaucher spleen.

The glucocerebrosidase-stimulating potential of HSF resists extraction with organic solvents, boiling, and exposure to proteolytic enzymes (*e.g.*, pronase, chymotrypsin, trypsin), or 2% trichloroacetic acid (39). It has been suggested that its small size and a random-coil tertiary structure might account for the above mentioned properties (58). The HSF is rich in hydrophobic amino acids and nuclear magnetic resonance studies performed over a range of temperatures (20 to 100° C) (62) revealed the presence of a conformationally rigid hydrophobic pocket in the activator protein, and a relatively compact tertiary structure.

The interaction between glucocerebrosidase and HSF seems to be relatively specific. The activator protein from Gaucher spleen has no effect on several other lysosomal and nonlysosomal enzymes including arylsulfatase, acid phosphatase, α-glucosidase, β-galactosidase, β-hexosaminidase, catalase, and cytochrome *c* oxidase (52). Furthermore, it has no effect on the activity of the broad specificity, cytosolic β-glucosidase isolated from human or rat liver. However, HSF does enhance the hydrolysis of sphingomyelin and G_{M1} ganglioside by sphingomyelinase and G_{M1} ganglioside:β-galactosidase, respectively. On the other hand, several other glycoproteins including ovalbumin, thyroglobulin, and fetuin, do not activate glucocerebrosidase. However, two other heat-stable, low molecular weight, acidic proteins that are not glycoproteins, namely, calmodulin and parvalbumin, are modest activators of glucocerebrosidase (31). The presence of ethyleneglycoltetraacetic acid, a calcium chelator, is required to augment the effect of these calcium-binding proteins in stimulating glucocerebrosidase. Interestingly, another calcium-binding protein, namely troponin-C, and one which is structurally very similar to calmodulin, has little effect on glucocerebrosidase activity.

The association of HSF with its membrane-bound catalytic counterpart, glucocerebrosidase ('factor C'), is time- and temperature-dependent (39). The role of HSF in activating glucocerebrosidase will be discussed more extensively below.

Aerts *et al.* (3) obtained evidence that the heat-stable factor (*i.e.*, SAP-2) may influence the physical state of glucocerebrosidase in various mammalian tissues. It had been known for some time that multiple forms of glucocerebrosidase exist in extracts of cells and tissues of normal persons and patients with Gaucher's disease; these forms could be separated by electrophoresis (44), or sedimentation (25), and detected by radiation inactivation analysis (43). Using immunologic techniques, Aerts et al. (3) distinguished two forms of glucocerebrosidase in extracts of human spleen; form I has a molecular mass of 60 kd and is precipitable by polyclonal or monoclonal anti-glucocerebrosidase antibodies, whereas form II is larger (200 kd) and not precipitable by the same antibodies. Form II reacts with SAP-2 antibodies but form I does not. Furthermore, incubation of form I of glucocerebrosidase with SAP-2 resulted in masking of the epitope on form I which otherwise would have reacted with one of the monoclonal antibody preparations. It was concluded that form I glucocerebrosidase is a monomer and that form II is a high molecular weight complex of the enzyme and SAP-2.

c. Natural Membrane Lipids. Another important contribution of Ho and O'Brien (39) was their observation that "although membrane-bound factor C (glucocerebrosidase) reacted optimally with factor P, solubilized factor C was preferentially activated by sodium taurocholate." This finding led them to consider that physiologic components of lysosomes, namely membrane lipids might be required for the reconstitution of glucocerebrosidase activity. They reported that factor P (heat-stable factor) had a nearly absolute requirement for acidic phospholipids. All of the acidic phospholipids they tested were effective in stimulating glucocerebrosidase activity in the presence of factor P, including phosphatidic acid, phosphatidylserine, and phosphatidylinositol; all three lipids have a net charge of −1 between pH 4.5 to 5.5, the pH range in which glucocerebrosidase exhibits optimum activity. Neutral phospholipids like phosphatidylcholine or phosphatidylethanolamine could not reconstitute glucocerebrosidase activity.

However, Ho and Light (38) could not demonstrate any significant stimulation of glucocerebrosidase by acidic phospholipids in the absence of the HSF. This discrepancy with subsequent studies (4–6) could be explained by the following: (1) incomplete and variable delipidation of their glucocerebrosidase preparation (the presence of endogenous lipids might compete or interfere with the exogenous acidic lipid and block further stimulation); (2) use of a suboptimal pH (pH 4.5) in their β-glucosidase assay. In the absence of HSF, the pH at which optimal activation by phospholipids is obtained might be different from that at which HSF activates glucocerebrosidase; (3) inadequate solubilization of the glucocerebroside substrate by 0.05% (v/v) Triton X-100, (4) the presence of a low concentration of Triton X-100, while not sufficient to support a high level of glucocerebrosidase activity, might still obscure the effects of exogenous acidic phospholipids.

Dale, Villacorte, and Beutler (16) were the first to describe a procedure for making a detergent-free, soluble preparation of glucocerebrosidase. They subjected sodium taurocholate-solubilized placental glucocerebrosidase to acetone precipitation; when the acetone powder was rehydrated, they found that glucocerebrosidase remained in solution, even when detergent was excluded from the buffer. Using this enzyme preparation, they showed that acidic phospholipids, by themselves, were capable of activating glucocerebrosidase significantly; the order of effectiveness of the phospholipids was: phosphatidylserine > phosphatidylinositol ≫ phosphatidic acid. Neutral phospholipids (phosphatidylcholine, phosphatidylethanolamine) were ineffective in reconstituting glucocerebrosidase.

The phospholipid requirement of glucocerebrosidase was investigated further by Basu and Glew (4, 6) using butanol-delipidated glucocerebrosidase preparation from rat liver and human spleen as their enzyme source and MUGlc as substrate. Use of water-soluble MUGlc is advantageous for it obviates the need for some detergent in the assay medium; as stated previously, most detergents desensitize glucocerebrosidase to exogenous physiologic lipid activators like phosphatidylserine and gangliosides. They demonstrated that, in addition to the polar head group, the nature of the fatty acids in the sn-1 and sn-2 positions of the phospholipid influences its glucocerebrosidase activator potency. Within a particular phospholipid family, the glucocerebrosidase-stimulating power increases with decreasing chain length and increasing degree of unsaturation of the fatty acids.

The importance of the acidic nature of a phospholipid in promoting glucocerebrosidase reconstitution was reinforced by the finding that conversion of an ineffective neutral phospholipid (*e.g.*, phosphatidylethanolamine) to a negatively charged structure by *N*-acylation of the polar head group (thereby generating *N*-acyl phosphatidylethanolamine), confers upon the lipid the ability to activate glucocerebrosidase (7).

In addition to phospholipids, other negatively charged natural membrane lipids, including gangliosides (*e.g.*, G_{M1}, G_{D1}, G_{T1}) and galactocerebroside-3-sulfate are also effective activators of glucocerebrosidase (5, 45, 55). The presence of negatively charged sialic acid in the ganglioside is critical since asialo-G_{M1} and asialo-G_{M2} have little effect on enzyme activity (45). However, the effectiveness of a ganglioside does not increase with increasing negative charge; for example, with rat liver glucocerebrosidase, singly charged G_{M1} is a better activator than G_{D1} or G_{T1}, the latter two containing two and three negative charges, respectively (5). The oligosaccharide chain length of a ganglioside also seems to be important; the glucocerebrosidase activator potency of monosialogangliosides increases with the number of carbohydrate residues such that $G_{M1} > G_{M2} > G_{M3}$ (45).

The search for *in situ* lipid activators of glucocerebrosidase was also pursued by Basu *et al.* (8). They fractionated phospholipids isolated from extensively purified rat liver lysosomes by thin layer chromatography and determined their ability to activate glucocerebrosidase. The results of this study were consistent with those of *in vitro* reconstitution experiments and supported the view that phosphatidylserine and phosphatidylinositol are the likely physiologic activators of glucocerebrosidase. Another unique acidic phospholipid, bis-(monoacylglyceryl) phosphate (BMP), which is present exclusively in lysosomes and known to accumulate in some lysosomal storage disorders, also activates glucocerebrosidase *in vitro.* However, its relatively low abundance in lysosomes, compared with phosphatidylserine or phosphatidylinositol, makes it unlikely that it is an important natural activator of glucocerebrosidase, unless it is somehow concentrated near the enzyme in the lysosomal membrane.

d. How do the Acidic Lipids and Heat-Stable Factor Reconstitute Glucocerebrosidase? Although the list of acidic lipids of natural origin which can reconstitute normal glucocerebrosidase is long, emphasis will be given to those that have yielded the most insight and information about the lipid requirement of the enzyme; these lipids include phosphatidylserine, galactocerebroside-3-sulfate (sulfolipid) and the ganglioside G_{M1}.

Kinetically, the principal results of the efficient reconstitution of normal glucocerebrosidase are the marked reduction in the K_m value of the substrate and increase in the specific activity or V_{max}. Because the natural substrate of glucocerebrosidase, namely glucocerebroside, is so insoluble in dilute aqueous buffers, and because strong detergents like sodium taurocholate that are required to solubilize or disperse glucocerebroside render the enzyme insensitive to phosphatidylserine, G_{M1}, sulfolipid and other natural membrane lipids, it is difficult to characterize the reconstituted glucocerebrosidase using assays that utilize glucocerebroside as the substrate. Consequently, most investigators interested in characterizing the interaction between glucocerebrosidase and physiologically relevant lipid activators utilize one of the water-soluble β-glucosidase substrates in their studies. The substrate most widely used to measure the β-glucosidase activity of glucocerebrosidase is MUGlc which is soluble in water over a wide range of pH, and at concentrations that are 10 to 100 times greater than the K_m of glucocerebrosidase.

As shown in Table 1, acidic lipids like sulfolipid and phosphatidylserine (PS) all decrease the K_m for MUGlc from 8 mM to less than 2 mM. These same activator lipids markedly increase the V_{max}.

HSF, by itself, is a poor activator of human spleen glucocerebrosidase; as shown in Table 1, in the absence of acidic lipid, the inclusion of HSF in the assay medium does not increase the V_{max} (77 *versus* 67 units/ mg of protein). The principal effect of HSF is to increase the specific activity of glucocerebrosidase expressed at suboptimal concentrations of activator lipids. In Figure 6, for example, note how the activity *versus* lipid activator concentration curves are shifted to the left by including a small amount (approximately 1 μg/0.1 ml of assay) of HSF in the assay medium. At low concentrations of PS or G_{M1}, the fold-stimulation of the reaction rate is 3 to 5, whereas at relatively high concentrations of these acidic lipids, HSF enhances β-glucosidase activity only moderately.

It should be noted in Table 1, that although the HSF does not affect the V_{max} of glucocerebrosidase, it does significantly decrease the K_m of the enzyme for MUGlc, thereby providing kinetic evidence that the factor does, indeed, bind to the enzyme, even in the absence of exogenous acidic phospholipid.

With regard to the effect of activators on the activity *versus* hydrogen ion concentration curve of glucocerebrosidase acting on MUGlc, the inclusion of a mixture of HSF and PS in the assay medium shifts the pH optimum from 5.5–6.0 to 4.5–5.2. In their kinetic study of log (V_{max}/K_m) *versus* pH, Basu and Glew (4) found that PS affects catalysis by recruiting two ionizable groups with pK values of 4.5 and 5.1 into the catalytic center of glucocerebrosidase (Fig. 7); inclusion of HSF together with PS makes apparent an additional ionizable group with a pK value of 4.5. These activators, therefore, appear to influence catalysis by inducing a conformational change in the enzyme which causes ionizable groups that participate in catalysis to come into close proximity with one another.

It has been shown convincingly that certain enzymes which utilize amphipathic lipids as substrates (*e.g.*, phospholipases) or depend upon them for activity (*e.g.*, pro-

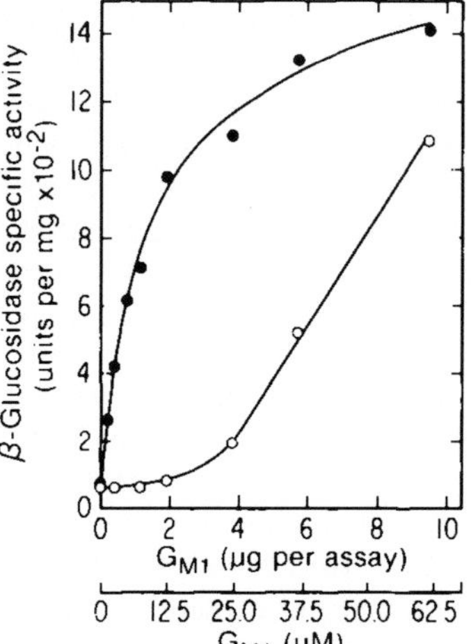

FIG. 6. The effect of heat-stable factor on the activation of β-glucosidase by G_{M1}. β-Glucosidase activity was determined in the absence (○) or presence (●) of 0.81 μg of heat-stable factor/assay over the indicated concentration range of G_{M1} (taken from Ref. 5).

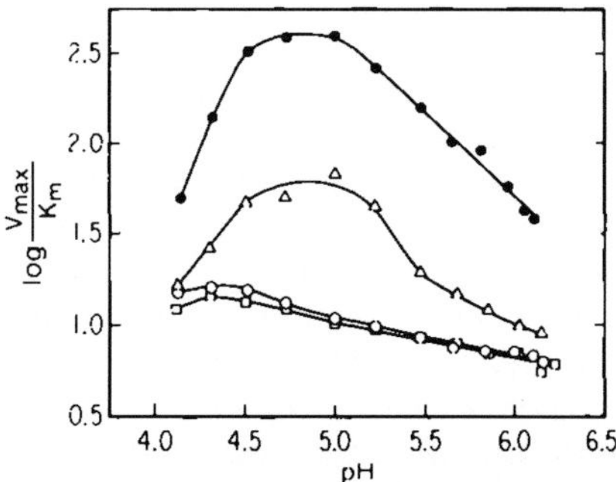

FIG. 7. The effects of phosphatidylserine and heat-stable factor on the pH dependence of the hydrolysis of 4-methylumbelliferyl-β-D-glycopyranoside by β-glucosidase. β-Glucosidase activity was determined as a function of MUGlc concentration either in the absence of any effector (○), or in the presence of 1.1 μg of HSF (□), 10 μg of PS (△), or 1.1 μg of HSF plus 10 μg of PS (●) using 0.2 M sodium acetate buffer at the indicated pH. The kinetic constants, K_m and V_{max} were determined using double-reciprocal plots. The log V_{max}/K_m values were plotted as a function of pH (taken from Ref. 4).

TABLE 1. THE EFFECTS OF ACIDIC MEMBRANE LIPIDS AND HEAT-STABLE FACTOR ON K_m AND V_{max} OF HUMAN SPLEEN GLUCOCEREBROSIDASE[a]

Experiment	Addition	K_m		V_{max}		Reference
		−HSF	+HSF	−HSF	+HSF	
	μg/assay	*mM*		*units/mg protein*		
1	None	8.0	4.9	77	67	6
	Phosphatidylserine (1.0)	4.6	1.6	357	769	
	Phosphatidylserine (1.0)	1.9	ND	870	ND[b]	
2	None	11.0	3.0	84.4	26.0	55
	Sulfatide (0.08)	4.6	2.6	46.5	35.6	
	Sulfatide (8.0)	1.6	1.9	239	357	

[a] Glucocerebrosidase was extracted with *n*-butanol.
[b] ND, not determined.

tein kinase C) undergo aggregation when incubated with appropriate lipid. Pancreatic phospholipase A_2, for example, is activated markedly by phosphocholine-containing lipids (*e.g.*, sphingomyelin, phosphatidylcholine) and activation is accompanied by an obligatory aggregation of the enzyme from a monomer to a hexamer (69). Hannun and Bell (36) have shown that diacylglycerol (diglyceride) and PS, the physiologic activators of protein kinase C, activate the kinase by binding to it and promoting dimerization.

Basu and Glew (5), using a partially purified enzyme preparation from rat liver and a combination of gel permeation chromatography and sucrose density gradient ultracentrifugation in D_2O and H_2O, investigated the effect of G_{M1} on the size of glucocerebrosidase. The Stokes radii of the inactive and reconstituted enzyme were determined from the chromatographic behavior of the glucocerebrosidase on a Sephadex G-200 column, after preincubation in the presence and absence of G_{M1}. The sucrose density gradient experiments in D_2O and H_2O yielded the enzymes' sedimentation coefficients and partial specific volumes. From all of these data, they estimated the sizes of the nonreconstituted enzyme and the G_{M1}-activated glucocerebrosidase to be 45,800 and 178,500 daltons, respectively. Based on a comparison of the partial specific volumes of the two forms of the enzyme, they concluded that the reconstituted glucocerebrosidase consists of 50% protein (*i.e.*, two monomers) and 50% ganglioside (56 moles of G_{M1}/178,500 gm of complex).

At low concentrations, amphipathic lipids like G_{M1}, PS, and sulfolipid exist in aqueous solutions as monomers; as the concentration is increased, the lipids self-associate, forming aggregates called micelles. The concentration of total lipid at which aggregation occurs is referred to as the critical micellar concentration (CMC). The CMC for a particular lipid is not invariant; it depends, among other things, upon the pH, ionic strength, temperature, and composition of the medium. Further compounding the problem is the fact that many amphipathic lipids often exhibit more than one CMC. For example, bile salts like sodium taurocholate can exist in a variety of micellar states (dimers, tetramers, octamers), depending upon the concentration of the lipid and the composition of the medium. The same is true for the acidic lipids which activate glucocerebrosidase.

A convenient way to estimate micellar transitions is to use a dye whose fluorescent properties change when it moves out of the bulk water phase and intercalates in a micellar structure; for example, in the case of *n*-phenylnaphthylamine, the intrinsic fluorescence of the dye increases markedly when it interacts with micelles. With G_{M1}, a moderately effective activator of glucocerebrosidase, Basu and Glew (5) observed two CMC values (Fig. 8) in the concentration range 0.5 to 50 μM. Phosphatidylserine and sulfolipid exhibit even more CMCs (55). Thus, in interpreting the results of lipid-glucocerebrosidase reconstitution studies, one must be aware of the problems of lipid insolubility and the tendency for amphipathic lipids to form micelles of varying sizes and shapes.

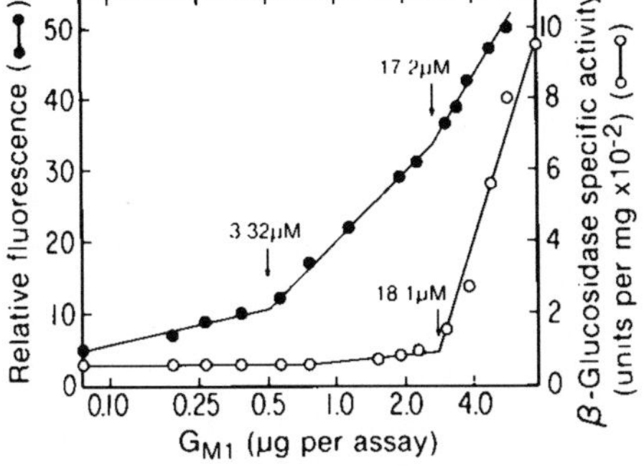

FIG. 8. Correlation of β-glucosidase activation by G_{M1} with the critical micellar concentration (CMC) of the ganglioside. β-Glucosidase activity (O) was determined at 37° C in the presence of various concentrations of G_{M1}. The solid symbols (●) indicate how the CMC was determined using *N*-phenylnaphthylamine in 0.2 M sodium acetate buffer, pH 5.25 at 37° C. The relative fluorescence of the dye was measured at 350 nm. Note that the concentration of ganglioside is plotted on a logarithmic scale. The CMC values are indicated by the *arrows* (taken from Ref. 5).

With regard to the question of whether monomers or micellar aggregates of the acidic lipids are the form of the acidic lipid preferred by glucocerebrosidase, we have examined this issue in detail with G_{M1} (Fig. 8), PS, and sulfolipid. In each case, as the concentration of activator lipid is raised, each time a CMC is passed, one sees a large increase in specific activity. Furthermore, the highest specific activity is obtained in the higher acidic lipid concentration range. Assuming the micelles formed at the higher concentration of lipid are larger than those that predominate at low lipid concentrations, it seems that glucocerebrosidase interacts best with the large, acidic lipid micelles. If this assumption turns out to be correct, it would appear that glucocerebrosidase has a lipid-binding site on its surface which conforms best to a micellar surface that has a minimum curvature.

e. Physiologic Significance of the Heat-Stable Factor. To this day, the physiologic significance of HSF in the metabolism of glucocerebroside is still a matter of debate; furthermore, its accumulation in Gaucher's disease remains an enigma. Is it involved in the degradation of glucocerebroside, or is it a consequence of glucocerebroside storage? Since HSF from control spleen is less than 10% as active as the Gaucher spleen HSF, it is unlikely that the normal physiologic function of the activator protein is to enhance glucocerebroside hydrolysis. In addition, significant differences in kinetic properties, amino acid composition and carbohydrate content between HSF isolated from both normal and Gaucher's tissues argue against their physiologic relevance. However, one implicit assumption that has been made regarding the isolation of control HSF is that, like the HSF from Gaucher spleen, it occurs in a soluble form. If the HSF in normal tissues is membrane-associated, purification schemes like the ones that have been used to purify the HSF from Gaucher spleen would have caused HSF in non-Gaucher tissue to escape isolation. It is conceivable that when the defective membrane-bound glucocerebrosidase in Gaucher's disease is incapable of binding to the activator protein the latter then accumulates in a soluble form.

Recently, Iyer, Berent, and Radin (40) isolated HSF from control and Gaucher tissues and compared their properties. They concluded that the cohydrolases were closely related since their immunologic properties, specific activities, and electrophoretic mobilities were similar. The only major difference they noted between the two cohydrolases was in their carbohydrate content. They postulated that HSF contains a polysaccharide chain terminated with a β-linked glucose and that the degradation of the glycoproteinaceous HSF is initiated by the action of glucocerebrosidase. The possibility cannot be excluded that the reduced level of glucocerebrosidase activity in Gaucher's disease somehow enhances the cell's production of HSF in an effort to increase the catalytic potential of the defective enzyme. However, no correlation has been demonstrated between the tissue content of HSF and the severity of the disease. An alternate possibility is that the increase in the glucocerebroside content of Gaucher cells induces them to synthesize HSF.

A second piece of evidence indicating that the HSF may be physiologically relevant is its partial deficiency in patients with I-cell disease. An interesting aspect of I-cell disease is that, whereas most of the lysosomal enzymes are deficient in cultured fibroblasts derived from these patients, β-glucosidase activity is nearly normal when it is estimated in the presence of exogenous activator lipid. However, it was recently shown that a reduction in β-glucosidase activity can be demonstrated in I-cell fibroblast extracts when glucocerebrosidase activity is estimated in the absence of nonphysiologic activators like sodium taurocholate or Triton X-100 (70). The fact that glucocerebrosidase in I-cell patients exhibits normal activity in the presence of detergents, suggests that the enzyme is present in normal amounts but that some physiologic activator of the enzyme is deficient. In fact, a partial deficiency of HSF in I-cell disease was actually demonstrated using rocket immunoelectrophoresis; in addition, glucocerebrosidase activity could be restored by co-cultivation or fusion of cultured fibroblasts from patients with I-cell disease and those from patients with Gaucher's disease. Fujibayashi and Wenger (24) concluded that this observation provides evidence that "the activator has an important role in regulating β-glucosidase activity *in vivo* and a complete deficiency of HSF might lead to severe deficiency of β-glucosidase."

Finally, on this issue of the pathophysiologic significance of HSF (called cohydrolase), Datta, Snider, and Radin (18) reported some interesting observations on the effect of the heat-stable activator protein on the uptake of glucocerebrosidase by neuroblastoma cells cultured in serum-free medium. Although uptake of the enzyme was augmented by phosphatidylserine, glucocerebrosidase uptake was most rapid if the enzyme-phosphatidylserine complex was offered to cells together with cohydrolase. In order to determine if glucocerebrosidase taken up by the neuroblastoma cells had reached a subcellular location where glucocerebroside hydrolysis occurs (presumably lysosomes), Datta, Snider, and Radin (18) had to first produce a version of Gaucher's disease in the cultured cells. This was done by incorporating large amounts of glucocerebroside in the culture medium. They then showed that degradation of glucocerebroside occurred only when the medium was supplemented with phosphatidylserine and glucocerebrosidase and that the maximum rate of disappearance of stored lipid took place when the ternary mixture of enzyme and activator protein plus phosphatidylserine was present. Apart from shedding light on the question of the role of the activator protein in glucocerebroside catabolism, the results of this study may provide insights regarding the treatment of Gaucher's disease.

MOLECULAR BASIS OF CLINICAL HETEROGENEITY IN GAUCHER'S DISEASE

An Enzymologic Basis for the Differentiation of the Various Subtypes of Gaucher's Disease

For many years, the molecular basis that distinguishes individuals with different types of Gaucher's disease was obscure. Why was it, given the assays which were available at the time (principally bile salt-supplemented assays), that the level of residual glucocerebrosidase activity in the various forms of Gaucher's disease did not correlate with the clinical severity of the cases? The *in vitro* assay conditions used for many years to estimate residual glucocerebrosidase activity in Gaucher's disease invariably employed one of the conjugated bile salts to stimulate glucocerebrosidase activity and to disperse the water-insoluble authentic substrate, glucocerebroside. However, since bile salts are not normal constituents of the lysosomal membrane, it is clear, in retrospect, that the composition of the *in vitro* assays did not reflect the *in vivo* environment of glucocerebrosidase.

Wenger and Roth (71) were the first to develop a diagnostic β-glucosidase assay that utilized physiologically relevant activators. Substitution of the activator protein (HSF) for bile salt in the glucocerebrosidase assay medium provided the first clue that one could distinguish the two major types of Gaucher's disease on enzymologic grounds. Using a mixture of phosphatidylserine and partially purified activator protein and crude extracts of leukocytes and fibroblasts as their enzyme source, they noted that "the cells from type 2 patients were barely stimulated by activator protein, as opposed to type 1 patients which were stimulated more than controls." Although Wenger and Roth (71) included PS in the assay medium to achieve maximum stimulation of glucocerebrosidase by HSF, they did not assess the relative contribution of PS and HSF to the enzymic differentiation of Gaucher subtypes.

The importance of natural membrane lipids in the successful enzymic differentiation of neurologic and nonneurologic forms of Gaucher's disease was first documented by Glew *et al.* (32). Using the procedure devised by Furbish *et al.* (22), they delipidated glucocerebrosidase by extraction of tissue homogenates sequentially with sodium cholate and 1-butanol thereby rendering the enzyme dependent upon exogenous lipid activators (Fig. 9). Using glucocerebrosidase preparations from both spleen and brain tissue, they showed that incorporation of an acidic phospholipid-like phosphatidylserine into the β-glucosidase assay medium (in the absence of any other activators) permitted differentiation of type 1 and type 2 forms of Gaucher's disease. In the presence of an optimal amount of phosphatidylserine (20 to 30 μg/100 μl of assay), the maximum β-glucosidase specific activity expressed by glucocerebrosidase isolated from tissues of non-neuronopathic (type 1) cases was 5 to 10 times higher than that exhibited by the mutant glucocerebrosidase of neuronopathic (type 2 and type 3) Gaucher's disease cases.

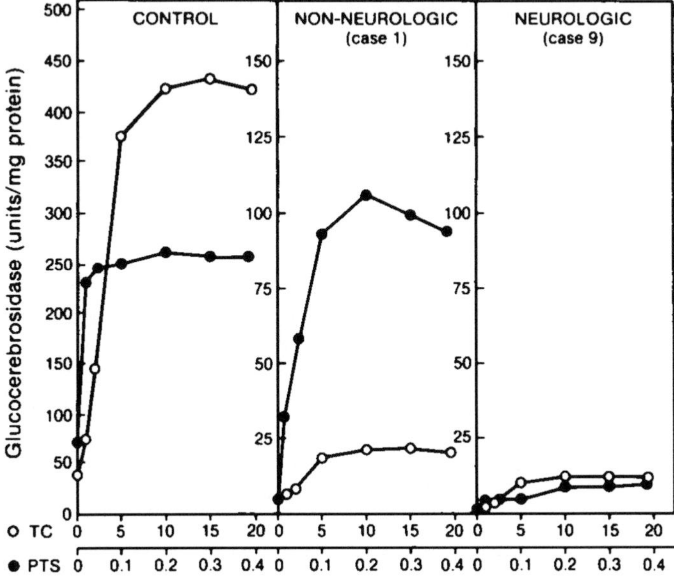

FIG. 9. Effect of sodium taurocholate (*TC*) and phosphatidylserine (*PTS*) on β-glucosidase activity in butanol-extracted membranes from spleens of controls and patients with non-neurologic and neurologic Gaucher's disease. Partially purified glucocerebrosidase preparations from human spleens were assayed for β-glucosidase activity using 4-methylumbelliferyl-β-D-glucopyranoside as the substrate in the presence of varying amounts of sodium taurocholate (○) or phosphatidylserine (●). Note the change in scale of β-glucosidase activity for the enzyme from Gaucher's disease spleen (taken from Ref. 32).

With regard to the specific activity of glucocerebrosidase supported by sodium taurocholate *versus* phosphatidylserine, the major distinction was that whereas glucocerebrosidase from control or neurologic cases was activated comparably by either phosphatidylserine or bile salt (Table 2, experiment 1), the glucocerebrosidase from type 1 patients was stimulated only moderately by the bile salt; furthermore, in a bile salt-supplemented β-glucosidase assay, the maximum glucocerebrosidase specific activities exhibited by extracts of tissues from neurologic and non-neurologic cases were not significantly different (20.9 *versus* 14.0 units/mg). The differential responsiveness of glucocerebrosidases from cases of type 1 and type 2 Gaucher's disease to phosphatidylserine is especially apparent when water-soluble MUGlc is used as the β-glucosidase substrate.

That particular study (32) was significant not only because it defined assay conditions that distinguished the mutant glucocerebrosidases of Gaucher's disease cases with profound brain disease from those without central nervous system involvement, but also because it demonstrated that the active site of the glucocerebrosidase of patients with type 1 Gaucher's disease was relatively intact and that the enzyme was capable of supporting rates of catalysis approximately 50 to 60% (Table 2, experiment 3) of those exhibited by control glucocerebrosidase, provided it was supplied with the proper acidic phospholipid activator (*e.g.*, phosphatidylserine) and not a bile salt.

The relative importance of acidic lipids (*e.g.*, phosphatidylserine) and the activator protein (HSF) in determining the basis of the genetic diversity of Gaucher's disease

TABLE 2. COMPARISON OF THE ABILITY OF VARIOUS LIPIDS AND HEAT-STABLE FACTOR TO DIFFERENTIATE GLUCOCEREBROSIDASES OF NONNEUROLOGIC AND NEUROLOGIC FORMS OF GAUCHER'S DISEASE

Experiment	Activators	Final conc.	β-Glucosidase specific activity[a]							
			Control		Type 1		Type 2			
			−HSF	+HSF	−HSF	+HSF	−HSF	+HSF	+HSF	Ref.
		µg/assay	*units/mg protein*							
	None		62.5		11.3		2.2			32
1	Sodium taurocholate	1200	607		20.9		14.0			
	Phosphatidylserine	30	431		82.3		13.9			
2	None		27.3	36.7	4.7	4.8	0.2	1.1		6
	Phosphatidylserine	10	136	581	12.5	23.8	2.5	4.3		
	Phosphatidylserine	25	596	ND[b]	66.7	ND[b]	1-.7	ND[b]		
3	None		35.5	38.1	1.0	2.3	0.1	2.1		E. M. Prence and R.H. Glew, unpublished data
	Sulfatide	10	68	119	31	34	1.8	5.6		
	Sulfatide	20	168	284	87	96	4.2	6.3		

[a] Glucocerebrosidase was prepared from human spleen and extracted with butanol; activity is expressed in terms of nanomoles/hour/milligrams of protein. The substrate was MUGlc.

[b] ND, not determined.

was explored further by Basu et al. (6). Again, using butanol-delipidated human spleen glucocerebrosidase as their enzyme source, they demonstrated that the primary effect of HSF was to markedly decrease the amount of phosphatidylserine needed for optimal reconstitution of glucocerebrosidase. However, especially noteworthy was the observation that the residual glucocerebrosidase from non-neuronopathic type 1 cases was much less responsive to HSF when compared with the control enzyme; for example, the combination of a relatively small amount of phosphatidylserine (1 μg/assay) and HSF, or a much higher amount of phosphatidylserine alone (25 μg/assay) were equally effective in reconstituting control enzyme activity *in vitro*. In contrast, glucocerebrosidase from type 1 patients exhibited a much higher specific activity in the presence of high concentrations (25 to 30 μg/assay) of phosphatidylserine alone (Table 2, experiment 2).

To investigate whether the ability of the phosphatidylserine-supplemented β-glucosidase assay system to distinguish different forms of Gaucher's disease was dependent on the acidic nature of the phospholipid, other negatively charged lipids were tested for their ability to differentially reconstitute glucocerebrosidase from neurologic and non-neurologic cases of Gaucher's disease. A series of gangliosides (G_{M1}, G_{D1}, G_{T1}) comprised of a common core structure (CerβGlcβGalβGalNAcβGal) and different numbers of sialic acid residues were tested for their ability to reconstitute various glucocerebrosidase preparations (6). Unlike phosphatidylserine, all three gangliosides activated the residual glucocerebrosidase from either type 1 or type 2 Gaucher's patients to the same extent, thereby obscuring differences between the two major classes of Gaucher's disease. However, a prominent acidic brain glycosphingolipid, namely, galactocerebroside-3-sulfate (sulfatide), was even more effective than phosphatidylserine in terms of its ability to distinguish glucocerebrosidase from non-neurologic and neurologic cases of Gaucher's disease (56). As observed with phosphatidylserine, the sulfatide-reconstituted glucocerebrosidase from type 1 cases did not respond to HSF (Table 2, experiment 3).

A model we have proposed to account for most of the published observations regarding the reconstitution of glucocerebrosidase is built on the assumption that there are two acidic lipid binding sites, designated as L_1 and L_2, on the normal enzyme and that maximum catalytic activity is expressed only when both L_1 and L_2 are occupied by activator lipids. We further postulate that acidic lipids like phosphatidylserine and sulfatide which are capable of distinguishing glucocerebrosidases of patients with type 1 and type 2 Gaucher's disease interact with both L_1 and L_2. We envision that a particular activator lipid, when it exists in solution as a monomer, or in the form of primary micelles, is capable of binding to the L_1 site. However, the impact of the conformational change invoked by such an interaction of acidic lipid at the L_1 site influences primarily substrate binding (as evidenced by the lowering of the K_m for MUGlc by sulfatide) without increasing the rate of catalysis (*i.e.*, V_{max} is not increased) (Table 3). As the concentration of the lipid activator is increased to the point where, presumably larger (*e.g.*, secondary or tertiary) micelles predominate, these lipid aggregates bind to the second site (L_2), favorably affecting the catalytic domain, and thereby causing a significant increase in V_{max}.

Any valid model of the glucocerebrosidase:acidic lipid activator interaction should consider the role of HSF. Since HSF, in the absence of any exogenously added acidic lipid, lowers the K_m of control glucocerebrosidase for both glucocerebroside and MUGlc without altering V_{max} (Table 2), we postulate that HSF can also bind at L_1, the site which regulates K_m. In addition, since HSF by itself does not influence the rate of inactivation of the enzyme by CBE or heat, it seems that, in the absence of lipid activators, it has little or no effect on the enzyme's catalytic site. However, when both HSF and acidic lipids are present, two things can occur: either HSF binds to L_1 and allows acidic lipids to interact at L_2 at low lipid concentrations (*i.e.*, where monomers and primary micelles predominate), or both HSF and acidic lipids interact at L_1, inducing a conformational change which not only enhances substrate binding but also increases the reaction velocity.

Finally, we propose that those acidic lipids (*e.g.*, bile salts, gangliosides, bis-(monoacylglyceryl) phosphate (BMP), monoacylglycol sulfates, diacylglycerol sulfate) which do not permit differentiation of the two major forms of Gaucher's disease, enhance glucocerebrosidase activity primarily by interacting with the enzyme at L_1. The basis of this speculation will be discussed later in this section.

The model presented in the preceding paragraphs fits with our ideas of how control glucocerebrosidase and the corresponding mutant glucocerebrosidase respond to activator lipids and HSF. We envision that, in the case of control enzyme, acidic lipids, either alone or coupled with HSF, interact with both L_1 and L_2 on glucocerebrosidase to support maximal rates of substrate hydrolysis. We speculate that in type 1 patients, the L_1 lipid

Table 3. Effects of the State of Aggregation of Sulfatide on the Kinetic Parameters of Human Spleen Glucocerebrosidase from a Control and Patients with Type 1 and Type 2 Gaucher's Disease[a]

Concentration of sulfatide	State of aggregation of sulfatide	K_m			V_{max}		
		Control	Type 1	Type 2	Control	Type 1	Type 2
μg/assay			*mM*			*units/mg protein*	
0		11	2.8	9.2	84.4	2.47	2.03
0.08	Monomer	4.6	1.9	ND[b]	46.5	2.12	ND[b]
0.8	Primary micelles	2.5	1.1	1.6	67.3	9.84	2.60
8.0	Tertiary micelles	1.6	1.2	1.5	239	148	6.48

[a] Adapted from Ref. 55.

[b] ND, not determined.

binding site of glucocerebrosidase is defective. The evidence supporting this view is based on the following observations: (1) the residual glucocerebrosidase of type 1 cases is much less responsive than the control enzyme to stimulation by anionic detergents, gangliosides, monoacylglycol sulfates, diacylglycerol sulfates, or BMP than it is to phosphatidylserine or sulfatide, (2) glucocerebrosidase of type 1 patients is resistant to further stimulation by HSF when phosphatidylserine or sulfatide is present, and (3) acidic lipids like sulfatide are incapable of lowering the K_m of the mutant type 1 enzyme for MUGlc (Table 3). However, noteworthy is the finding that the K_m of the type 1 enzyme, even in the absence of exogenous activators, is low when compared with the K_m values of control and type 2 glucocerebrosidase (Table 3).

The radiation inactivation experiments of Maret *et al.* (43) and the sucrose density gradient ultracentrifugation studies of Garrett, Prence, and Glew (25) both suggest that the native glucocerebrosidase of type 1 Gaucher's disease cases is about twice as large as the corresponding control enzyme (125,000 *versus* 60,000 daltons). It is conceivable that the genetic defect in the type 1 enzyme promotes subunit interactions, possibly through the L_1 site, which yields dimers that have an increased affinity for substrate (*i.e.*, lower K_m). We propose that when glucocerebrosidase is in the dimeric form, only L_2 is available for interaction with acidic lipids; therefore, only the large micellar forms of acidic lipids like phosphatidylserine and sulfatide, which according to our model interact at L_2, are capable of stimulating type 1 glucocerebrosidase. However, assuming the above model, since L_1 is non-functional or inaccessible in type 1 glucocerebrosidase, the maximum catalytic activity exhibited by the type 1 enzyme in the presence of phosphatidylserine or sulfatide is still less than the control enzyme which has two functional lipid activator binding sites that promote catalysis.

A recent report by Grabowski *et al.* (35) provided kinetic evidence that the catalytic site of glucocerebrosidase is functional in patients with type 1 Gaucher's disease. Using the active site-directed inhibitor Br CBE, they were able to estimate the concentration of the catalytically active enzyme in tissues. They demonstrated that the actual turnover rate of type 1 enzyme is comparable to that of the normal enzyme. This observation is in accordance with our model that postulates that the L_2 lipid-binding site that regulates the reaction velocity as well as the enzyme's catalytic center are unimpaired in type 1 glucocerebrosidase.

In the case of type 2 patients, we speculate that the active site of their glucocerebrosidase is so profoundly compromised that, even though acidic lipids and HSF can interact with the enzyme, they are incapable of overcoming the fundamental defect at the enzyme's active site and thus incapable of stimulating catalysis.

A Possible Chemical Basis for the Different Forms of Gaucher's Disease

It has been suggested (48) that differences in tissue GS levels in patients with Gaucher's disease provides a chemical basis for the different pathophysiology of the three clinical subtypes of the disease.

GS has never been detected in normal tissue; however, it is present in spleen, liver, and brain from all three forms of Gaucher's disease. Nilsson *et al.* (48) observed that although there was no clear-cut difference in the level of tissue glucocerebroside among various phenotypes of Gaucher's disease, the concentration of GS did correlate with the clinical severity of the disease; specifically, the GS level was much higher in neurologic (type 2 and type 3) cases than in non-neurologic cases, and within a single subtype, a type 1 patient with a more severe clinical course had a higher level of GS than a patient with a milder form of non-neurologic Gaucher's disease.

GS could arise biosynthetically from UDP-glucose and sphingosine, or it may be produced by the deacylation of glucocerebroside. Although this second pathway has not been demonstrated, it may operate in patients with Gaucher's disease, thereby providing a means for disposal of the excessive amount of accumulated glucocerebroside. In normal tissues, any small amount of glucosylsphingosine that might be generated would presumably be degraded by glucocerebrosidase. Thus, the defect in glucocerebrosidase in Gaucher's disease could ultimately lead to the accumulation of GS. A hypothesis brought forth by the Swedish group (48) postulates that in severe cases of Gaucher's disease (*e.g.*, type 2 and type 3) the GS content of the brain reaches such high levels that nerve cells are destroyed.

As discussed above, studies with natural glucocerebrosidase activators (*e.g.*, phosphatidylserine, HSF) have shown that the residual activity in tissues of patients with various forms of Gaucher's disease correlates well with the severity of phenotypic manifestations between subtypes. Therefore, the higher enzyme activity in the tissues of type 1 patients may prevent the excessive accumulation of GS *in vivo* assuming, of course, that GS is degraded by glucocerebrosidase. However, differences in the GS concentrations reported in two type 1 patients (48) with different clinical courses suggest genetic heterogeneity within a subtype (26, 34). This implies that the mutation in two different type 1 patients affects the catalytic activity or specificity of the residual enzymes differently so that the glucocerebrosidase of a more severely affected patient might not be capable of degrading GS as efficiently as the enzyme of a milder case. This hypothesis could be tested directly by measuring glucocerebrosidase activity in the two type 1 cases simultaneously using glucocerebroside and GS as the substrates. However, since the assignment of different subtypes is strictly based on the presence or absence of central nervous system involvement, and since the more severely afflicted type 1 patient studied by Nilsson *et al.* (48) died at an early age (3 years), the possibility remains that neurologic dysfunction would have developed later, if the child had lived longer. In fact, the authors mentioned that the more severely affected patient, although clinically and neuropathologically classified as a type 1 homozygote, possibly had an "acid β-glucosidase" (glucocerebrosidase) mutation which was similar to that of Norbottnian (type 3) patients.

Another conspicuous distinction which correlated primarily with the clinical severity classes of Gaucher's disease lies in the fatty acid composition of glucocerebroside which accumulates in their brains. Nilsson *et al.* (48) found that in severe cases of Gaucher's disease (*e.g.*, type 2, several type 3 and one severely affected type 1 patient), the ceramide portion of the accumulated glucocerebroside contained predominantly stearic acid (C18:1) as the fatty acyl group and eicosasphingenine (d20:1) as the sphingosine base. Since this fatty acid composition of ceramide is characteristic of brain gangliosides, this observation indicates that a significant portion of the glucocerebroside in the brains of severe cases is the result of incomplete turnover of gangliosides. In contrast, the glucocerebroside isolated from the brains of milder cases (type 1 and a few type 3) were rich in behenic (C22:0) and lignoceric (C24:0) acid and d18:1 sphingosine, implying that glucocerebroside was primarily derived from glucocerebroside-laden macrophages which migrated to the brain from the blood.

This interesting observation raises several questions: first, does the specific mutation in the severe and mild forms of Gaucher's disease affect the specificity of the residual enzymes differently, such that glucocerebrosidase from a severe case cannot efficiently degrade glucocerebroside which is the metabolic remnant of ganglioside catabolism, whereas the enzyme from less severe cases can hydrolyze these complex glycolipid-derived glucocerebrosides but not glucocerebrosides of extracerebral origin? Second, are there two distinct glucocerebrosidase isoenzymes in the brain, with each one being specific for glucocerebrosides originating from two different metabolic pools?

BIOSYNTHESIS OF GLUCOCEREBROSIDASE

The pathway for the biosynthesis of glucocerebrosidase was investigated by Erickson, Ginns, and Barranger (20); using the approach of *in vivo* cell free translation of glucocerebrosidase mRNA, they demonstrated that the enzyme undergoes extensive post-translational processing. They concluded that, in both porcine kidney cells and human fibroblasts, glucocerebrosidase is synthesized initially as a 60 kd glycoprotein containing four asparagine-linked, high-mannose carbohydrate chains. They postulated that: (a) the initial translation product is a 52 kd peptide which contains a 1 kd NH_2-terminal signal sequence similar to that of many secretory proteins and which is cleaved as the enzyme is translocated across the endoplasmic reticulum membrane; (b) the high-mannose carbohydrate chains are added in the endoplasmic reticulum to yield the initial 60 kd glycosylated form of the enzyme; (c) within 2 hours after it has been synthesized, the 60 kd form is then converted to a 59 kd form which still possesses the high-mannose carbohydrate chains; (d) the carbohydrate side chains are processed from the high-mannose type to the complex type, so that by 24 hours, glucocerebrosidase exists as a 56 kd species devoid of high-mannose oligosaccharide side-chains; and (e) finally, after 72 hours, all of the 56 kd form has been converted to a 55-kd form. Erickson, Ginns, and Barranger (20) suggested that this last processing step may be involved in initiating turnover of the enzyme since it occurs so long after biosynthesis has taken place. The nature of each of the processing steps (*i.e.*, glycolytic, proteolytic, or both) has not yet been elucidated.

Defects in the processing of newly synthesized glucocerebrosidase have been implicated by Ginns *et al.* (27) in differentiating the various clinical forms of Gaucher's disease. Using radiolabeled polyclonal glucocerebrosidase antibody, they showed that normal human fibroblasts contained two major forms of glucocerebrosidase, with molecular weights of 63 kd and 56 kd (27). Glucocerebrosidase in fibroblasts from persons with type 1 Gaucher disease (no neurologic involvement) occurred mostly in a 56 kd form with only a small amount of the 63 kd form being present. In contrast, fibroblasts from type 2 and type 3 Gaucher patients (with neurologic disease) contained only the 63 kd form. Essentially the same results were obtained when extracts of brain were used as the source of glucocerebrosidase. Based on these results, the authors speculated that processing of glucocerebrosidase occurs in type 1 Gaucher's disease, but at a reduced rate as compared with the normal condition, whereas in types 2 and 3 Gaucher's disease, processing either does not occur at all, or is incomplete.

In another study, Ginns *et al.* (30) detected differences in the reactivity of a glucocerebrosidase monoclonal antibody with extracts of fibroblasts from controls and patients with Gaucher's disease. Their monoclonal antibody detected three forms of glucocerebrosidase in control cells, corresponding to 63 kd, 61 kd, and 56 kd species. Components of the same molecular sizes, but in different proportions, were observed with fibroblast extracts from type 1 patients. However, fibroblasts from a patient with type 2 Gaucher's disease lacked material that cross-reacted with this monoclonal antibody. In contrast, fibroblasts from a person with type 3 Gaucher's disease contained only a 63 kd glucocerebrosidase antigen detectable with the same monoclonal antibody. These results suggest that three distinct mutations are responsible for the three major clinical subtypes of Gaucher disease, and that these mutations apparently affect glucocerebrosidase processing.

Beutler and Kuhl (10) performed a similar study but arrived at somewhat different conclusions. First of all, Beutler and Kuhl (10) found that the 56 kd band was probably not related to glucocerebrosidase since that band was present even when the radiolabeled extracts of fibroblasts were treated with preimmune serum. These workers found that the earliest detectable glucocerebrosidase species synthesized by control fibroblasts had a molecular weight of 60 kd. This form of the enzyme is gradually converted to a 63 kd form, whose position corresponds to that of native, purified placental glucocerebrosidase, presumably the mature enzyme. It was concluded that glucocerebrosidase biosynthesis in normal cells proceeds from a 60 kd nonglycosylated form to a 63 kd glycosylated form. They acknowledged that the conversion might also involve removal, by proteolysis, of a 19 or 39 amino acid leader sequence.

With regard to Gaucher's disease fibroblasts, Beutler and Kuhl (10) found that processing of glucocerebrosidase in patients with the type 1 form of the disease was exactly the same as normal. This conclusion conflicts with that of Erickson, Ginns, and Barranger (20). In contrast, Butler and Kuhl (10) seem to agree with the conclusion of Erickson, Ginns, and Barranger (20) that patients with type 2 Gaucher's disease produce a very unstable 60 kd glucocerebrosidase precursor which is not converted to the mature 60 kd form. Thus, while the processing of glucocerebrosidase in type 1 cases seems to be entirely normal, in type 2 Gaucher's disease there appears to be a defect in the post-translational processing of glucocerebrosidase.

Willemsen *et al.* (72) performed a very interesting comparative study of the ultrastructural localization of glucocerebrosidase in normal fibroblasts and cells of patients with non-neuronopathic and neuronopathic Gaucher's disease. Glucocerebrosidase antigen was visualized under the electron microscope using polyclonal rabbit antibodies against the placental enzyme and a second goat antibody coupled to colloidal gold. In control cells and cells of three of four type 1 cases, the glucocerebrosidase antigen was concentrated in lysosomes. In contrast, cells from neuronopathic type 2 and 3 cases had very little glucocerebrosidase cross-reactive material in their lysosomes. It appears that the defective processing of glucocerebrosidase in type 2 and type 3 Gaucher's disease results in rapid destruction of the enzyme and failure to deliver the protein to the lysosome.

Another interesting aspect of the biosynthesis of glucocerebrosidase which has not yet been adequately investigated is the mechanism by which this enzyme is targeted to the lysosome. Whereas most hydrolases are targeted to lysosomes via the mannose-6-phosphate receptor (47), glucocerebrosidase does not seem to follow this pathway. In I-cell disease, where the mannose-6-phosphate marker is not formed and multiple lysosomal enzyme deficiencies result, glucocerebrosidase and acid phosphatase are present in normal amounts (47). Therefore, these two enzymes must reach the lysosome through some targeting mechanism other than the mannose-6-phosphate receptor pathway. The fact that both of these enzymes are firmly membrane-bound, whereas other lysosomal hydrolases are soluble, or easily released in soluble form from the organelle, suggests a reason for the existence of a second targeting mechanism. Perhaps one pathway exists for delivery of the soluble hydrolases to lysosomes, while another is responsible for delivery of the membrane-bound lysosomal hydrolases. Thus far, this alternate mode of lysosomal targeting has not been described.

Aerts *et al.* (1, 2) investigated the role of the oligosaccharide chains of glucocerebrosidase in the routing of the enzyme to lysosomes. Using cultured human monoblasts and inhibitors of the glycosidases involved in the pathway of "complex"-type oligosaccharide chain biosynthesis (swainsonine, deoxymannonojirimycin), they concluded that the oligosaccharides of glucocerebrosidase are essential for the efficient routing of the enzyme to lysosomes. They postulated that the oligosaccharide chains may serve as specific recognition markers for transport to the lysosome or, alternatively, that the targeting determinant may include some domain of the polypeptide chain that is expressed only when complex-type oligosaccharide chains are present.

MOLECULAR BIOLOGY OF GLUCOCEREBROSIDASE

Several groups have embarked upon the characterization of glucocerebrosidase at the level of the gene. Ginns *et al.* (28), at the National Institutes of Health (Bethesda, Maryland) have used a λgt 11 expression vector to isolate two complementary DNA (cDNA) clones (λGC-1, λGC-2) for human glucocerebrosidase from a human hepatoma cDNA library; based on restriction mapping data, both clones contained approximately 1900 base pair inserts and gave rise to a 165 kd fusion protein. Evidence which supports the identification of the cDNAs as encoding the glucocerebrosidase protein include cross-reaction of the fusion protein with anti-human placental glucocerebrosidase antibody, and identification of a region of the amino acid sequence deduced from the nucleotide sequence of the cDNA clone which was perfectly homologous with a peptide fragment of the glucocerebrosidase protein isolated from placenta. Additionally, the two glucocerebrosidase cDNAs hydribized to each other, and to four different synthetic oligonucleotides constructed from the amino acid sequence of a homogeneous preparation of human placental glucocerebrosidase. Subcloning of the 1900 base pair insert into pBR322 yielded a 50-kd polypeptide which cross-reacts with anti-glucocerebrosidase antibody; however, the insert is large enough to encode a polypeptide greater than 50 kd and must, therefore, contain untranslated sequences. The estimated molecular size of the cDNA-encoded protein agrees well with the size (52 kd) of nascent glucocerebrosidase synthesized in *in vitro* translation systems in the absence of added microsomal membranes.

On the opposite coast, at the Scripps Clinic (La Jolla, California), Sorge *et al.* (64) also utilized the λgt 11 expression vector to identify a glucocerebrosidase cDNA clone (GCS 2Kb) that displays amino acid sequence homology with fragments of purified glucocerebrosidase and hybridizes with human chromosome 1, which contains the glucocerebrosidase gene. This cDNA, when expressed in bacteria, gives rise to a polypeptide that is recognized by affinity purified, highly specific anti-glucocerebrosidase antibody. GCS-2kb contains the entire coding region of the human glucocerebrosidase gene, and 2227 nucleotides have been sequenced; the sequence data, which has been disclosed, suggests that the initiator ATG codon resides at nucleotides 154-156, and would yield a proglucocerebrosidase protein consisting of 515 amino acids (approximately 57 kd). Comparison of the deduced amino acid sequence with protein sequencing data compiled for a purified preparation of glucocerebrosidase supports the conclusion that the first 19 amino acids are removed to generate the mature form of glucocerebrosidase. Especially illuminating is the finding that the first 19 amino acids, determined from the nucleotide sequence, constitute the most hydrophobic portion of the glucocerebrosidase protein. This hydrophobic domain could serve as a leader sequence, which is commonly found in secreted and membrane proteins, and which is cleaved to yield the mature form of these proteins. The deduced amino acid sequence of the portion of the cDNA corresponding to the C-terminus of glucocerebrosidase, is also highly hydrophobic, as expected, since the carboxyl terminal segment of the mature protein is known to contain the enzyme's active site. Using their own cDNA clones, Ginns *et al.* (29) have independently identified a putative hydrophobic leader sequence 19 amino acids in length at the amino terminus, as well as a hydrophobic C-terminal core.

Sorge *et al.* (63) have utilized their cloned fragment of the glucocerebrosidase gene as a probe to unmask restriction site polymorphisms in glucocerebrosidase genes from Jewish and non-Jewish type I Gaucher patients; restriction analysis revealed two genetic variants: (a) a common polymorphism apparent when the DNA is digested with the restriction endonuclease, *Pvu*II, and (b) a rare variant surfacing after *Kpn*I digestion.

The *Pvu*II variant revealed itself through the appearance of a 1.1 kb band (Pv 1.1+), with the simultaneous loss of a normally present 1.0 kb band; the heterogeneity is presumably the result of the loss of a *Pvu*II restriction site formerly located approximately 100 base pairs from the end of the 1.1 kb fragment generated by the polymorphism. Using the Hardy-Weinberg equation, the authors predicted that the *Pvu*II polymorphism is an ancient one, whereas the Gaucher mutations probably occurred more recently. The present study revealed that 5 Jewish Gaucher's disease patients were heterozygous for the *Pvu*II polymorphism, indicating that the Gaucher genes are linked to the Pv 1.1+ variant as well as the Pv 1.1− variant which is lacking the Pvu restriction site, and therefore, the 1.1 kb band. Considering that the Gaucher's disease mutations are believed to be more recent than the ancient *Pvu*II polymorphisms, and realizing that the Gaucher phenotype is linked to both the Pv 1.1+ and Pv 1.1−alleles, it appears that mutations giving rise to the Gaucher phenotype have occurred on more than one occasion in the Jewish population. Sorge *et al.* (63) commented that "to be repeatedly amplified in one population, mutations producing glucocerebrosidase deficiency must have provided a selective advantage." Recognizing that a second β-glucosidase exists in mammalian tissues which is related to glucocerebrosidase, and is of unknown function, we speculate that perhaps mutation of one allele of the glucocerebrosidase gene does not perturb the organism, because a related enzyme can be recruited to replace in part the lost glucocerebrosidase activity.

The second restriction polymorphism at a *Kpn*I site, which was observed in a non-Jewish, type 1 Gaucher's disease patient, argues that the Gaucher's disease mutation which arose in association with the *Kpn*I polymorphism occurred as a separate, independent genetic event. The exact base pair alterations which gave rise to the restriction polymorphisms and the Gaucher's disease phenotypes have not yet been identified; however, the information presented by Sorge *et al.* (63) regarding linkage of the Gaucher mutations to restriction polymorphisms suggests that the glucocerebrosidase genes of Gaucher variants house mutations at different locations. Supporting this hypothesis is the observation that the clinical severity of Gaucher's disease varies greatly, even within the Jewish population.

Tsuji *et al.* (67) cloned the glucocerebrosidase gene from a patient with type 2 Gaucher's disease and compared the sequence to that of wild type glucocerebrosidase. A single base substitution (T→C) was detected in exon X which replaces leucine with proline at amino acid position 444 of the glucocerebrosidase protein. This missense mutation fortuitously produced a new cleavage site for the restriction endonuclease, *Nci*I. Restriction digests of genomic DNA from controls and various Gaucher patients revealed that 4 of 5 type 2 patients and 11 of 11 type 3 patients bore this base substitution in at least 1 allele, whereas 2 of 5 and 7 of 11 type 2 and type 3 patients, respectively, were homozygous for the mutation. The mutant allele was detected in only 4 of 20 type 1 patients, and in none of the 29 controls tested. Insertion of a proline, known to disrupt α-helices, into the primary sequence of glucocerebrosidase can have profound effects on the protein's 3-dimensional conformation; structural studies of the mutant glucocerebrosidase should shed light on the mechanism by which this particular amino acid substitution impairs hydrolysis of glucocerebroside in Gaucher patients.

The detection of restriction polymorphism made possible by isolation of the cDNA for the glucocerebrosidase gene, may prove useful in the identification of Gaucher's disease heterozygotes and in the prenatal diagnosis of Gaucher's disease. The cloned glucocerebrosidase gene can also be used to acquire large quantities of protein for physical studies, or possibly enzyme replacement therapy, although previous attempts to infuse Gaucher patients with purified glucocerebrosidase have not been successful. Additionally, investigators can use the cloned genes to aid in identifying, at the molecular level, the precise defects which give rise to the three clinical subtypes of Gaucher's disease.

After subcloning gGc-1 into a pBR322 vector (pGC-1), Choudary, Ginns, and Barranger (15) utilized this fragment to screen two human genomic libraries, one constructed from fetal DNA, and the second from adult liver DNA. Two positive clones were identified from each library; the fetal clone, γTM4, measured approximately 4000 base pairs in length, whereas the adult liver clone, γPCN9, was larger (approximately 5100 base pairs). Heteroduplex mapping of γTM4 and γPCN9, performed using nick-translated pGC-1, revealed that each contained 10 exons and 9 introns.

With respect to chromosomal location, original studies employing somatic cell hybridization techniques (61) mapped the glucocerebrosidase gene to human chromosome 1, specifically to the region 1pII to 1gter. Later, again using somatic cell hybrids, the location of the gene was further narrowed to the region q21-q31 of chromosome 1. Recently, Ginns *et al.* (28) utilized a nick-translated glucocerebrosidase cDNA to more precisely localize the gene by *in situ* hybridization to human metaphase chromosomes, followed first by autoradiography and finally, by G-banding. The results of *in situ* hybridization argue strongly that the glucocerebrosidase structural gene resides at a single locus, specifically at region q21 of human chromosome 1, which lies adjacent to a region (1 qh) that contains structural heteromorphisms. This region may serve as an identifiable linkage marker in the study of variant Gaucher genotypes.

Note added in proof: A juvenile atypic patient with Gaucher's disease was recently described whose excessive glucocerebroside storage was caused not by a deficiency of glucocerebrosidase, but by the lack of the heat-stable activator protein. (Christomanou H, Aigensberger A, Linke RP: Immunochemical characterization of two activator proteins stimulating enzymatic sphingomyelin degradation *in vitro*: absence of one of them in a human Gaucher disease variant. Biol Chem Hoppe-Seyler 367:879, 1986).

This work was supported by National Institutes of Health Grant AM31357.

REFERENCES

1. Aerts JMFG, Brul S, Donker-Koopman WE, van Weely S, Murray GJ, Barranger JA, Tager JM, Schram AW: Efficient routing of glucocerebrosidase to lysosomes requires complex oligosaccharide chain formation. Biochem Biophys Res Commun 141:452, 1986
2. Aerts JMFG, Donker-Koopman WE, Barranger JA, Tager JM, Schram AW: A procedure for the rapid purification in high yield of human glucocerebrosidase using immunoaffinity chromatography with monoclonal antibodies. Anal Biochem 154:655, 1986
3. Aerts JMFG, Donker-Koopman WE, van Laar C, Brul S, Murray G, Wenger DA, Barranger JA, Tager JM, Schram AW: Relationship between the two immunologically distinguishable forms of glucocerebrosidase in tissue extracts. Eur J Biochem 163:583, 1987
4. Basu A, Glew RH: Characterization of the phospholipid requirement of a rat liver β-glucosidase. Biochem J 224:515, 1984
5. Basu A, Glew RH: Characterization of the activation of rat liver β-glucosidase by sialosylgangliotetraosylceramide. J Biol Chem 260:13067, 1985
6. Basu A, Glew RH, Daniels LB, Clark LS: Activators of spleen glucocerebrosidase from controls and patients with various forms of Gaucher's disease. J Biol Chem 259:1714, 1984
7. Basu A, Prence E, Garrett K, Glew RH, Ellingson JS: Comparison of *N*-acyl phosphatidylethanolamines with different *N*-acyl groups as activators of glucocerebrosidase in various forms of Gaucher's disease. Arch Biochem Biophys 243:28, 1985
8. Basu A, Glew RH, Wherrett JR, Huterer S: Comparison of the ability of phospholipids from rat liver lysosomes to reconstitute glucocerebrosidase. Arch Biochem Biophys 245:464, 1986
9. Beutler E, Kuhl W: The diagnosis of the adult type of Gaucher's disease and its carrier state by demonstration of deficiency of β-glucosidase activity in peripheral blood leukocytes. J Lab Clin Med 76:747, 1970
10. Beutler E, Kuhl W: Glucocerebrosidase processing in normal fibroblasts and in fibroblasts from patients with type I, type II and type III Gaucher disease. Proc Natl Acad Sci USA 83:7472, 1986
11. Beutler E, Kuhl W, Sorge J: Cross-reacting material in Gaucher disease fibroblasts. Proc Natl Acad Sci USA 81:6506, 1984
12. Brady RO, Barranger JA: Glucosylceramide lipidosis: Gaucher's disease. In The Metabolic Basis of Inherited Disease. edited by Stanbury, JB, Wyngaarden JB, Fredrickson DS, Goldstein JL, Brown MS, p 842. New York, McGraw-Hill, 1983
13. Brady RO, Kanfer JN, Shapiro D: Metabolism of glucocerebrosides II. Evidence of an enzymatic deficiency in Gaucher's disease. Biochem Biophys Res Commun 18:221, 1965
14. Chambers JP, Aquino L, Glew RH, Lee RE, McCafferty LR: Determination of serum acid phosphatase in Gaucher's disease using 4-methylumbelliferyl phosphate. Clin Chim Acta 80:67, 1977
15. Choudary PV, Ginns EI, Barranger JA: Molecular cloning and analysis of the human β-glucosidase gene. DNA 4:74, 1984
16. Dale GL, Villacorte DG, Beutler E: Solubilization of glucocerebrosidase from human placenta and demonstration of a phospholipid requirement for its catalytic activity. Biochem Biophys Res Commun 71:1048, 1976
17. Daniels LB, Glew RH, Diven WF, Lee RE, Radin NS: An improved fluorometric leukocyte β-glucosidase assay for Gaucher's disease. Clin Chim Acta 115:369, 1981
18. Datta SC, Snider RM, Radin NS: Uptake by neuroblastoma cells of glucosylceramide, glucosylceramide glucosidase, its stimulator protein, and phosphatidylserine. Biochem Biophys Acta 877:387, 1986
19. Dinur T, Osiecki KM, Legler G, Gatt S, Desnick RJ, Grabowski GA: Human acid β-glucosidase: isolation and amino acid sequence of a peptide containing the catalytic site. Proc Natl Acad Sci USA 83:1660, 1986
20. Erickson AH, Ginns EI, Barranger JA: Biosynthesis of the lysosomal enzyme, glucocerebrosidase. J Biol Chem 260:14319, 1985
21. Erickson JS, Radin NS: *N*-hexyl-*O*-glucosylsphingosine, an inhibitor of glucosyl ceramide β-glucosidase. J Lipid Res 14:133, 1973
22. Furbish FS, Blair HE, Shiloach J, Pentchev PG, Brady RO: Enzyme replacement therapy in Gaucher's disease: large-scale purification of glucocerebrosidase suitable for human administration. Proc Natl Acad Sci USA 74:3560, 1977
23. Furbish FS, Steer CT, Krett NL, Barranger JA: Uptake and distribution of placental glucocerebrosidase in rat hepatic cells and effects of sequential deglycosylation. Biochim Biophys Acta 673:425, 1981
24. Fujibayashi S, Wenger DA: Studies on a sphingolipid activator protein (SAP-2) in fibroblasts from patients with lysosomal storage diseases, including Niemann-Pick disease Type C. Clin Chim Acta 146:147, 1985
25. Garrett KO, Prence EM, Glew RH: Sucrose gradient analysis of phospholipid activated β-glucosidase in type 1 and type 2 Gaucher's disease. Arch Biochem Biophys 238:344, 1985
26. Gatt S, Dinur T, Osiecki K, Desnick RJ, Grabowski GA: Use of activators and inhibitors to define the properties of the active site of normal and Gaucher disease lysosomal β-glucosidase. Enzyme 33:109, 1985
27. Ginns EI, Brady RO, Pirruccello S, Moore C, Sorrell S, Furbish FC, Murray GJ, Tager JM, Barranger JA: Mutations of glucocerebrosidase: discrimination of neurologic and non-neurologic phenotypes of Gaucher's disease. Proc Natl Acad Sci USA 79:5607, 1982
28. Ginns EI, Choudary PV, Martin BM, Winfield S, Stubblefield B, Mayor J, Merkle-Lehman D, Murray GJ, Bowers LA, Barranger JA: Isolation of cDNA clones for human β-glucocerebrosidase using the λgt11 expression system. Biochem Biophys Res Commun 123:574, 1984
29. Ginns EI, Choudary PV, Tsuji S, Martin B, Stubblefield B, Sawyer J, Hozier J, Barranger JA: Gene mapping and leader polypeptide sequence of human glucocerebrosidase: implications for Gaucher's disease. Proc Natl Acad Sci USA 82:7101, 1985
30. Ginns EI, Tegelaers FPW, Barneveld R, Galjaard H, Reuser AJJ, Brady RO, Tager JM, Barranger JA: Determination of Gaucher's disease phenotypes with monoclonal antibody. Clin Chim Acta 131:283, 1983
31. Glew RH, Coffee CJ: Calmodulin and parvalbumin: activators of human liver glucocerebrosidase. Arch Biochem Biophys 229:55, 1984
32. Glew RH, Daniels LB, Clark LS, Hoyer SW: Enzymic differentiation of neurologic and non-neurologic forms of Gaucher disease. J Neuropathol Exp Neurol 41:630, 1982
33. Grabowski GA, Dagan A: Human lysosomal β-glucosidase: purification by affinity chromatography. Anal Biochem 141:267, 1984
34. Grabowski GA, Gatt S, Kruse J, Desnick RJ: Human lysosomal β-glucosidase: kinetic characterization of the catalytic, aglycon, and hydrophobic binding sites. Arch Biochem Biophys 231:144, 1984
35. Grabowski GA, Osiecki-Newman K, Dinur T, Fabbro D, Legler G, Gatt S, Desnick RJ: Human acid β-glucosidase: use of conduritol B epoxide derivatives to investigate the catalytically active normal and Gaucher disease enzymes. J Biol Chem 261:8263, 1986
36. Hannun YA, Bell RM: Phorbol ester binding and activation of protein kinase C on Triton X-100 mixed micelles containing phosphatidylserine. J Biol Chem 261:9342, 1986
37. Hara A, Radin NS: Destruction and resynthesis of mouse β-glucosidases. Biochim Biophys Acta 582:412, 1979.
38. Ho MW, Light D: Glucocerebrosidase: reconstitution from macro-

molecular components depends on acidic phospholipids. Biochem J 136:821, 1973
39. Ho MW, O'Brien JS: Gaucher's disease: deficiency of "acid" β-glucosidase and reconstitution of enzyme activity *in vitro.* Proc Natl Acad Sci USA 68:2810, 1971
40. Iyer SS, Berent SL, Radin NS: The cohydrolases in human spleen that stimulate glucosylceramide β-glucosidase. Biochim Biophys Acta 748:1, 1983
41. Kanfer JN, Legler G, Sullivan J, Raghavan SS, Mumford RA: The Gaucher mouse. Biochem Biophys Res Commun 67:85, 1975
42. Legler G: Untersuchungen zum wirkungsmechanisms glykosidspaltender enzyme, I darstellung und eigenschaften spezifischen inaktivation. Hoppe Seyler's Z Physiol Chem 345:197, 1966
43. Maret A, Potier M, Salvayre R, Douste-Blazy L: Modification of subunit interaction in membrane-bound acid β-glucosidase from Gaucher disease. FEBS Letters 160:93, 1983
44. Maret A, Salvayre R, Negre A, Douste-Blazy L: Proprietes des formes molecularies de la β-glucosidase et de la glucocerebrosidase de rate humaine normale et de maladie de Gaucher. Eur J Biochem 115:455, 1981
45. Mueller OT, Rosenberg A: Activation of membrane-bound glucosylceramide:β-glucosidase in fibroblasts cultured from normal and glucosylceramidotic human skin. J Biol Chem 254:3521, 1979
46. Murray GJ, Youle RJ, Gandy SE, Zirzow GC, Barranger JA: Purification of β-glucocerebrosidase by preparative-scale high performance liquid chromatography: the use of ethylene glycol-containing buffers for chromatography of hydrophobic glycoprotein enzymes. Anal Biochem 147:301, 1985
47. Neufeld EF, McKusick VA: Disorders of lysosomal enzyme synthesis and location in I-cell disease and pseudo-Hurler polydystrophy. In The Metabolic Basis of Inherited Disease, edited by Stanbury JB, Wyngaarden JB, Fredrickson DS, Goldstein JL, p 778. New York, McGraw-Hill 1983
48. Nilsson O, Grabowski GA, Ludman MD, Desnick RJ, Svennerholm L: Glycosphingolipid studies of viscera tissues and brain from type 1 Gaucher disease variants. Clin Genet 27:443, 1985
49. Patrick AD: A deficiency of glucocerebrosidase in Gaucher's disease. Biochem J 97:17, 1965
50. Pentchev PG, Brady RO, Hibbert SR, Gal AE, Shapiro P: Isolation and characterization of glucocerebrosidase from human placental tissue. J Biol Chem 248:5256, 1973
51. Peters SP, Coffee CJ, Glew RH, Lee RE, Wenger DA, Li SC, Li YT: Isolation of heat-stable glucocerebrosidase activators from the spleen of three variants of Gaucher's disease. Arch Biochem Biophys 183:290, 1977
52. Peters SP, Coyle P, Coffee CJ, Glew RH, Kuhlenschmidt MS, Rosenfeld L, Lee YC: Purification and characterization of a heat-stable glucocerebrosidase activating factor from control and Gaucher spleen. J Biol Chem 252:563, 1977
53. Peters SP, Coyle P, Glew RH: Differentiation of β-glucocerebrosidase from β-glucosidase in human tissues using sodium taurocholate. Arch Biochem Biophys 175:569, 1976
54. Prence E, Chakravorti S, Basu A, Clark LS, Glew RH, Chambers JA: Further studies on the activation of glucocerebrosidase by a heat-stable factor from Gaucher spleen. Arch Biochem Biophys 236:98, 1985
55. Prence EM, Garrett KO, Glew RH: A kinetic study of the effects of galactocerebroside-3-sulphate on human spleen glucocerebrosidase: evidence for two activator-binding sites. Biochem J 237:655, 1986
56. Prence RM, Garrett KO, Panitch H, Basu A, Glew RH, Wherrett, JR, Huterer S: Sulfogalactocerebroside and bis-(monacylglyceryl)-phosphate as activators of spleen glucocerebrosidase. Clin Chim Acta 156:179, 1986
57. Radin NS: Inhibitors of β-glucosidases of animal tissues. Adv Exp Med Biol 101:589, 1978
58. Radin NS: Inhibitors and stimulators of glucocerebrosidase metabolism. In Progress in Clinical and Biological Research, Vol 95, edited by Desnick RJ, Gatt S, Grabowski GA, pp 357–383. New York, Alan R Liss, Inc., 1982
59. Raghavan SS, Topol J, Kolodny EH: Leukocyte β-glucosidase in homozygotes and heterozygotes for Gaucher's disease. Am J Hum Genet 32:158, 1980
60. Reddy PUM, Murray GJ, Barranger JA: Purification and characterization of bovine brain glucocerebrosidase. Biochem Med 33:200, 1985
61. Shafit-Zagardo B, Devine EA, Smith M, Arrandondo-Vega F, Desnick RJ: Assignment of the gene for acid β-glucosidase to human chromosome 1. Am J Hum Genet 33:564, 1981
62. Sheh L, Glew RH, Bothner-By AA, Mishra PK: High-resolution proton nuclear magnetic resonance studies of the glucocerebrosidase activator protein from Gaucher spleen. Biochemistry 24:6645, 1985
63. Sorge J, Gelbart T, West C, Westwood B, Beutler E: Heterogeneity in type 1 Gaucher disease demonstrated by restriction mapping of the gene. Proc Natl Acad Sci USA 82:5442, 1985
64. Sorge J, West C, Westwood B, Beutler E: Molecular cloning and nucleotide sequence of the human glucocerebrosidase cDNA. Proc Natl Acad Sci USA 82:7289, 1985
65. Stephens MC, Bernatsky A, Burachinsky V, Legler G, Kanfer JN: The Gaucher mouse: differential action of conduritol β epoxide, a reversibility of its effects. J Neurochem 30:1023, 1978
66. Takasaki S, Murray GJ, Furbish FS, Brady RO, Barranger JA, Kobata A: Structure of the N-asparagine-linked oligosaccharide units of human placental β-glucocerebrosidase. J Biol Chem 259:10112, 1984
67. Tsuji S, Choudary PV, Martin BM, Stubblefield BK, Mayer JA, Barranger JA, Ginns EI: A mutation in the human glucocerebrosidase gene in neuronopathic Gaucher's disease. N Engl J Med 316:570, 1987
68. Uchida T, Filburn CR: Affinity-chromatography of protein kinase C-phorbol ester receptor on polyacrylamide-immobilized phosphatidylserine. J Biol Chem 259:12311, 1984
69. van Oort MG, Dijkman R, Hille JDR, de Haas GH: Kinetic behavior of porcine pancreatic phospholipase A_2 on zwitterionic and negatively charged single-chain substrates. Biochemistry 24:7987, 1985
70. Varon R, Kleijer WJ, Thompson EJ, d'Azzo A: Evidence for the deficiency of β-glucosidase-activating factor in fibroblasts of patients with I-cell disease. Hum Genet 62:66, 1982
71. Wenger DA, Roth S: Homozygote and heterozygote identification. In Progress in Clinical and Biological Research Vol 95, edited by Desnick RJ, Gatt S, Grabowski GA, pp 551–572. New York, Alan R Liss, Inc., 1982
72. Willemsen R, van Dongen JM, Ginns EI, Sips HJ, Schram AW, Tager JM, Barranger JA, Reuser AJJ: Ultrastructural localization of glucocerebrosidase in cultured Gaucher's disease fibroblasts by immunocytochemistry. J Neurol 234:44, 1987

Biology of Disease

Human Amyloidosis, Alzheimer Disease and Related Disorders

EDUARDO M. CASTAÑO AND BLAS FRANGIONE

Department of Pathology and Kaplan Cancer Center, New York University Medical Center, New York, New York

INTRODUCTION

The term amyloidosis describes a group of diseases characterized by the deposition of abnormal fibrillar proteins in the extracellular and intracellular spaces. These proteins are assembled forming amyloid fibrils, that accumulate leading to cellular dysfunction and death. Regardless of their biochemical composition, all the types of amyloid fibrils share the following properties: (a) β-pleated sheet secondary structure; (b) green birefringence under polarized light after Congo red staining, and (c) a fibrillar quaternary structure with a typical electron microscopic appearance (11, 37, 38). Moreover, they all share the physical property of being highly insoluble under physiologic conditions and this is probably one of the most important features that precludes their complete degradation *in vivo* by cellular proteases.

TYPES OF HUMAN AMYLOIDOSIS

The deposition of amyloid fibrils can affect several organs in the systemic forms of the disorder or can be restricted to one organ in the localized forms, the latter condition stressing the importance of tissue-specific factors involved in amyloidogenesis.

Amyloidosis is the result of many pathologic conditions of diverse etiology (Table 1). Primary amyloidosis (AL) presents in 90% of the cases an M component that can be identified in serum, urine, or cerebrospinal fluid and in 20% of the patients with AL, an association with multiple myeloma can be found (54, 60, 68,). The amyloid subunit of AL was the first amyloid protein biochemically characterized. The amino terminal sequence showed homology with immunoglobulin light chains (41). This and subsequent studies have shown that amyloid fibrils in AL are composed of the amino terminal fragment of monoclonal immunoglobulin light chains with a molecular weight ranging from 5 to 23 kilodalton (kd) (41, 112). Furthermore, it has been shown that certain subgroups of light chains have a highly amyloidogenic primary structure as shown by the preferential association of λVI with AL and the *in vitro* formation of amyloid fibrils by some, but not all of the Bence-Jones proteins studied (39, 74, 118).

Secondary or reactive amyloidosis (AA) is a rare complication of common chronic inflammatory conditions such as rheumatoid arthritis, tuberculosis, bronchiectasia, leprosy, or osteomyelitis. Several malignancies have been associated with AA including Hodgkin lymphoma and renal cell carcinoma (31, 98). By contrast, amyloidosis AA is a common feature and cause of early death due to renal failure in the autosomal recessive familial Mediterranean fever, particularly in the ethnic group of North African Sephardic Jews (117). This disease deserves special consideration since it has been demonstrated that the long-term treatment with colchicine can prevent the development of amyloidosis in the high risk population and may prevent additional impairment of renal function in familial Mediterranean fever patients with proteinuria that have not reached the stage of nephrotic syndrome (140). Therefore, familial Mediterranean fever represents the only type of human amyloidosis that can be effectively treated at the present time,

Table 1. Clinical and Biochemical Classification of Systemic Amyloidosis

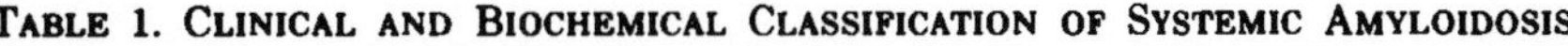

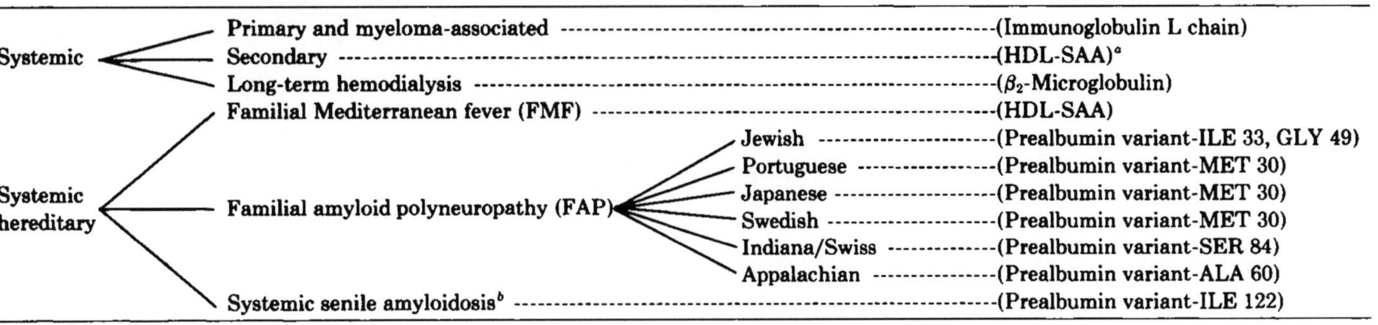

Group	Form	Subtype	Amyloid subunit
Systemic	Primary and myeloma-associated		(Immunoglobulin L chain)
Systemic	Secondary		(HDL-SAA)[a]
Systemic	Long-term hemodialysis		(β_2-Microglobulin)
Systemic hereditary	Familial Mediterranean fever (FMF)		(HDL-SAA)
Systemic hereditary	Familial amyloid polyneuropathy (FAP)	Jewish	(Prealbumin variant-ILE 33, GLY 49)
		Portuguese	(Prealbumin variant-MET 30)
		Japanese	(Prealbumin variant-MET 30)
		Swedish	(Prealbumin variant-MET 30)
		Indiana/Swiss	(Prealbumin variant-SER 84)
		Appalachian	(Prealbumin variant-ALA 60)
Systemic hereditary	Systemic senile amyloidosis[b]		(Prealbumin variant-ILE 122)

[a] High density lipoprotein-serum amyloid A.

[b] The presence of a prealbumin variant in this disease suggests that it can be genetically determined (47a).

although, the mechanisms by which colchicine controls amyloid deposition are not fully understood. The amyloid fibrils in secondary amyloidosis, regardless of the etiology, are made up of a protein called AA. This protein has been shown in most of the cases, to be the amino terminal fragment of 76 residues of a serum precursor, protein SAA (10, 71, 72). SAA is an acute phase reactant with a molecular weight of 12 kd, is synthesized in the liver, and circulates as part of the HDL3 complex (9, 106). Serum levels of SAA are dramatically increased by inflammatory insults and it has been reported that interleukin 1 can enhance the production of this protein by the hepatocyte (103, 105). Yet, the physiologic role of SAA remains unknown. In contrast to what occurs in AL, there is no evidence so far of a preferential association of any of the SAA isotypes described in humans and the development of amyloidosis AA.

In these two groups of amyloidosis (AL and AA), abnormal proteolytic cleavage of the serum precursors by the reticuloendothelial system has been suggested as a mechanism of amyloidogenesis (37). Furthermore, it has been shown *in vitro* that monocytes of patients with amyloidosis AA were unable to degrade completely SAA releasing fragments with the molecular weight of protein AA (69). The unusual cleavage of SAA found in the thyroid amyloid deposits of some patients with AA suggests that the degradation of this serum precursor may be tissue-specific (100).

Another group of systemic amyloidosis includes the familial amyloidotic polyneuropathies, senile cardiac or systemic amyloidosis (47a, 114) and familial cardiomyopathy of Danish origin (56). These diseases share the same serum precursor, prealbumin or transthyretin as the amyloid subunit. Familial amyloidotic polyneuropathies (FAP) present an autosomal dominant mode of transmission and several variant prealbumin genes have been described. FAP type 1, or lower limbs polyneuropathy in families of Portuguese, Japanese, and Swedish origin, presents a prealbumin variant with a substitution of methionine for valine at position 30 (29, 108, 123). In the Jewish kindred (patient S.K.O.), substitution of glycine for threonine at position 49 and isoleucine for phenylalanine at position 33 have been observed (99). In FAP type 2, or upper limbs polyneuropathy described in patients of Swiss-German origin, a substitution of serine for isoleucine at position 84 has been found (30). Recently, a distinct type of FAP with predominant cardiac involvement (Appalachian type) has been reported to present a variant prealbumin with Ala for Thr at position 60 (128). It has been proposed that these genetic variants of prealbumin are prone to an abnormal aggregation and/or proteolytic cleavage which may in turn account for the amyloid fibril formation and deposition in the systemic vessel walls and peripheral nerves (97). The early detection of these abnormal prealbumin variants in family members will provide an important tool for genetic counseling (128).

The amyloid subunit of the systemic form of amyloidosis that complicates the course of patients on long-term hemodialysis, (hemodialysis-related amyloidosis) has been recently identified: β_2-microglobulin is an 11.8 kd part of the class I histocompatibility complex in cell membranes and is also normally present in the circulation (48). High serum levels of β_2-microglobulin are found in renal diseases and cannot be eliminated by conventional cuprophan dialysis membranes (47). In some series, more than 70% of the patients on long-term dialysis with carpal tunnel syndrome presented amyloid deposits in bone and synovium (8). The amyloid deposits have been shown to be composed of the intact normal β_2-microglobulin, emphasizing the notion that tissue-related factors play a major role in hemodialysis-related amyloidosis (33, 47). The periodic use of dialysis membranes with a higher permeability or hemofiltration needs to be considered in order to prevent this common complication of long-term hemodialysis.

In the group of non-cerebral localized amyloidosis (Table 2), the amyloid subunits that have been characterized thus far include procalcitonin in the amyloid deposits of the medullary carcinoma of the thyroid (113) and the insulinoma amyloid polypeptide in pancreatic islet amyloidosis associated with type 2 diabetes mellitus and insulinoma. Insulinoma amyloid polypeptide shows homology with the neuropeptide calcitonin gene-related peptide (132).

Regardless of the etiology and biochemical diversity of amyloid proteins, it appears evident that some common factors interact in the mechanisms of amyloidogenesis in most of the types of amyloidosis considered so far:

(a) The existence of a circulating soluble precursor protein that includes an amyloidogenic primary structure. In most of the cases, a proteolytic fragment of the precursor adopts a β-pleated sheet secondary structure and assembles into a fibrillar quaternary structure that

TABLE 2. CLINICAL AND BIOCHEMICAL CLASSIFICATION OF LOCALIZED AMYLOIDOSIS

	Clinical type	Familial	Amyloid protein
Cerebral	Hereditary cerebral hemorrhage with amyloidosis (Icelandic type)	Autosomal-dominant	Cystatin C
Cerebral	Hereditary cerebral hemorrhage with amyloidosis (Dutch type)	Autosomal-dominant	β-Protein
Cerebral	Alzheimer disease and Down's syndrome	[a]	β-Protein
Cerebral	Sporadic cerebral amyloid angiopathy		β-Protein
Cerebral	Transmissible spongiform encephalopathies[b]		Protease-resistant protein 27–30 kd
Endocrine	Medullar carcinoma of the thyroid		Procalcitonin
Endocrine	Pancreatic (diabetes mellitus—type II insulinoma)		Insulinoma amyloid polypeptide (homologous to calcitonin gene-related peptide)

[a] Familial cases of Alzheimer disease have been described with an autosomal-dominant mode of transmission.
[b] Creutzfeldt-Jakob disease, kuru, Gerstmann-Straussler syndrome, and scrapie in animals.

is resistant to further enzymatic digestion. However, in some cases, the intact precursor molecule itself forms the amyloid fibril as in the case of β_2-microglobulin in hemodialysis-related amyloidosis or prealbumin monomers in FAP.

(b) Increased serum levels of the precursor, reflecting overproduction, impaired clearance or both. Nevertheless, only a small percentage of patients with high serum levels of amyloid precursors develop amyloidosis. Therefore, an individual abnormal processing of the precursor should be considered.

(c) This abnormal processing can be determined, in some instances by the primary structure of the precursor itself as it has been proposed for the prealbumin variants or some subgroups of immunoglobulin light chains. In other cases, incomplete degradation of the precursor has been attributed to an impaired cellular function as it has been shown with the *in vitro* degradation of SAA by monocytes and macrophages. In addition, several amyloid-related substances of diverse chemical nature may be involved in the processes of amyloid deposition. These include the glycoprotein P component (see below), glycosaminoglycans, particularly heparin sulfate-chondroitin sulfate (115, 116) inorganic components (19) and the amyloid enhancing factor in experimentally-induced amyloidosis in rodents (6, 7,55). Yet unidentified tissue-specific enzymes and/or enzymatic inhibitors may also play a role in amyloidogenesis.

AMYLOID P COMPONENT

Amyloid P component (AP) is a glycoprotein formed by 10 subunits of 25 kd that has been found associated with nearly all types of amyloid deposits (22, 111, 131). AP has been localized in the normal glomerular basement membrane and elastic tissue and is present in serum (serum amyloid P) (16, 28). Serum amyloid and AP are encoded by one gene located on chromosome 1 (80, 89) and belong to a family of pentameric proteins (pentraxins) that includes the acute phase-reactant C-reactive protein and the female hamster protein (24, 92). Although AP also behaves as an acute phase reactant in rodents, its physiologic role in humans has not been determined.

AP has the property of Ca^{++}-dependent binding to different ligands including amyloid fibrils, fibronectin, and C_4 binding protein (27, 93). Whether this binding is important in the process of amyloidogenesis is not well understood. The significance of AP in the pathogenesis of amyloid fibrils formation and deposition has been challenged considering its nonspecific binding capacity and the lack of AP in some particular amyloid deposits, *i.e.*, neurofibrillary tangles (131). Nevertheless, it has been shown that this serum protein has elastase inhibitor activity *in vitro* (73). If this is the case *in vivo*, the presence of amyloid-bound AP may enhance the resistance of amyloid fibrils to proteolytic cleavage.

CEREBRAL AMYLOIDOSIS

The amyloid fibril deposition restricted to the central nervous system is probably the most frequent form of localized amyloidosis. Congophilic lesions in the brain have been described in a large number of diseases of diverse etiology including hereditary conditions, chronic trauma, chromosomal abnormalities, mineral imbalance and viral infections (51, 59, 79, 107, 134). A list of some of these diseases is summarized in Table 3. The pattern of distribution of amyloid deposits in the brain is restricted to three basic types of pathological changes: (a) intraneuronal deposits (neurofibrillary tangles, NFT), (b) extracellular amyloid cores of neuritic plaques, and (c) cerebrovascular amyloidosis affecting small vessels of the leptomeninges and cerebral cortex.

HEREDITARY CEREBRAL HEMORRHAGE WITH AMYLOIDOSIS OF ICELANDIC TYPE (HCHWA-I)

The first cerebral amyloid protein biochemically characterized was a variant of cystatin C, an inhibitor of cysteine proteases, in HCHWA-I (25). HCHWA-I is an autosomal dominant form of cerebral amyloidosis identified in 128 affected individuals within 8 families from 1 geographical area in Iceland. The pathologic findings show cerebrovascular involvement due to amyloid fibril infiltration of the walls of small arteries and arterioles in the cerebral cortex and leptomeninges. HCHWA-I patients usually die before the age of 40 years, of massive intracerebral hemorrhages (51). The amyloid protein isolated from the leptomeninges starts at position 11 of the normal urinary cystatin C (or γ-trace) and presents

TABLE 3. DISEASES WITH CONGOPHILIC LESIONS IN THE CENTRAL NERVOUS SYSTEM

Disease	Neurofibrillary tangles	Neuritic plaques	Cerebrovascular amyloid	Amyloid-related proteins
Alzheimer	+++	+++	+++	β-Protein
Down's syndrome	+++	+++	+++	β-Protein
Creutzfeldt-Jakob	+	++	+	PrP
Kuru	−	++	+	PrP
Gerstmann-Straussler	−	++	+	PrP
Scrapie (animals)	−	++	−	PrP
Dementia pugilistica	+++	−	+	[a]
Subacute sclerosing panencephalitis	+++	−	−	[a]
Guam Parkinson-Dementia complex	+++	−	−	β-Protein
Postencephalitic Parkinson's	+++	−	−	[a]
Hereditary cerebral hemorrhage with amyloidosis (Icelandic)	−	−	+++	Cystatin C
Hereditary cerebral hemorrhage with amyloidosis (Dutch)	−	++	+++	β-Protein
Sporadic cerebral amyloid angiopathy	±	++	+++	β-Protein
Asymptomatic age-related amyloidosis	++	++	+	β-Protein

[a] Unknown.

an amino acid substitution, glutamine for leucine at position 68. Cystatin C is a 13-kd basic protein related to kininogens and stefins that is present in body fluids and has been immunocytochemically localized in human brain, pancreas, thyroid and adrenal gland (34, 49, 75). Recently, the gene coding the human cystatin C has been cloned and sequenced, confirming the amino acid sequence of the normal urinary cystatin C and that a single base substitution can explain the presence of Gln instead of Leu at position 68 (1). This substitution may reflect a point mutation in these families leading to the production of an abnormal protein that cannot be normally processed. Nevertheless, the possibility that the cystatin C variant represents a normal genetic polymorphism cannot be excluded (34, 35).

TRANSMISSIBLE SPONGIFORM ENCEPHALOPATHIES

The human transmissible spongiform encephalopathies is a group of diseases pathologically characterized by neuronal spongiform degeneration, astrocytic gliosis and parenchymal amyloid deposition in the form of amyloid plaques. This group includes Creutzfeld-Jakob Disease, Gerstmann-Strassler syndrome and Kuru (32). Plaques are located mainly in the cerebellar cortex but have been also described in other regions of the central nervous system (53, 66). The animal model of the disease, Scrapie, has provided most of the biochemical information about this type of amyloidosis (13, 65). The amyloid subunit in these diseases has a molecular weight of 27 to 30 kd and is called Protease resistant Protein (PrP) (14, 84, 101). This type of cerebral amyloidosis represents an example of amyloid formation in direct relationship with an infectious agent (36). Scrapie infectivity has been related to PrP 27-30 and it has been postulated that this protein is the major component of an infectious particle called prion although, the possibility that a small nucleic acid molecule is included in these particles cannot be ruled out (102). Cloning of the PrP gene has shown that it encodes a precursor of 35 kd that is expressed in both normal and infected brains (23, 88). The mechanisms by which PrP behaves in an abnormal way in Scrapie-infected tissues aggregating to form amyloid fibrils remains to be determined.

ALZHEIMER DISEASE

Alzheimer Disease (AD) is the most common form of human amyloidosis and the major cause of dementia. It has been estimated that more than 5% of the population above the age of 65 years are affected by the disease. AD accounts for more than 50% of all the cases of dementia representing a major public health problem in the United States where more than two million people suffer from this devastating illness (63). The disease was defined by Alois Alzheimer in 1907 when he described the hallmark lesions in the brain of a pre-senile demented patient, the senile plaques and the neurofibrillary tangles (4).

Senile plaques are spherical lesions of variable size ranging from 10 to 200 μm found in the cerebral cortex. There are some regions of the brain that are preferentially affected such as the associative areas of neocortex and limbic structures. The primary sensory and motor areas are relatively spared (17). The typical mature plaque is formed of three elements: (a) a central amyloid core, (b) degenerated neuronal processes, and (c) glial cells. Under the electron microscope, the amyloid core appears composed of typical straight 10 nm non-branching fibrils (85, 124). Blessed, Tumlinson, and Roth (12) have demonstrated a significant correlation between the number of senile plaques in the cerebral cortex and the appearance and degree of cognitive impairment. Moreover, a correlation has been established between the number of plaques, cognitive function and deficit of cortical cholinergic innervation assessed by the levels of acetylcholinetransferase, the biosynthetic enzyme of neurotransmitter acethycholine (15, 94).

NFT are intraneuronal deposits found mainly in pyramidal neurons of the neocortex, hippocampus, amygdala and basal nuclei (109). NFT are hairpin-like structures that can be seen with argentic impregnation techniques, thioflavin-S, or Congo red staining showing the typical green birefringence. Electron microscopic examination reveals that NFT are bundles of twisted fibrils called paired helical filaments (PHF) (Fig. 1*A*). PHF

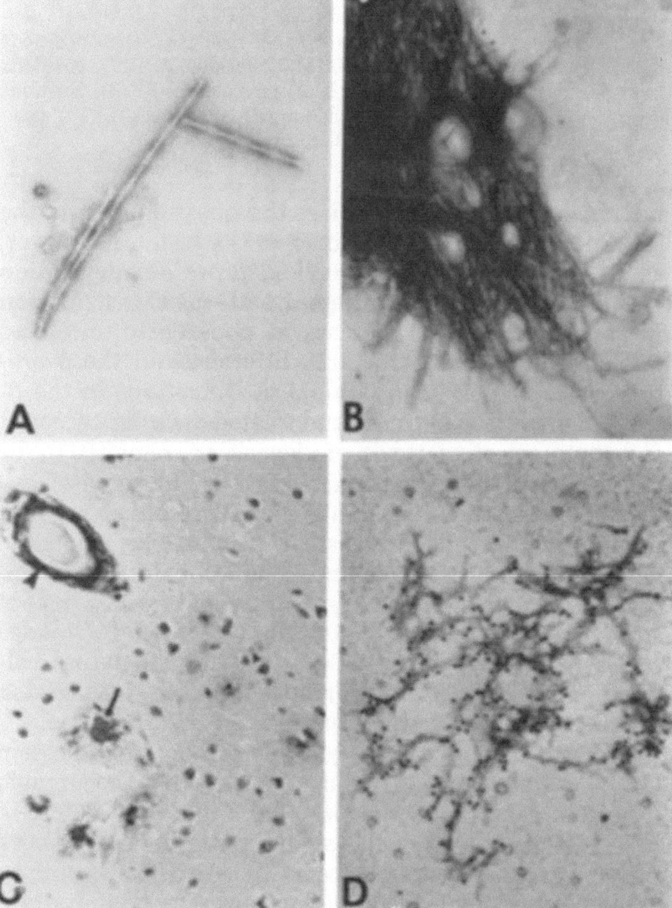

FIG. 1. *A*, Electron micrograph of isolated paired helical filaments of AD. *B*, Electron micrograph of amyloid fibrils extracted from the leptomeninges of a case of AD. *C*, Immunoperoxidase of AD brain section. A polyclonal antibody against a synthetic peptide homologous to the amino terminal 28 residues of β-protein (SP28) labels the cerebrovascular amyloid (*arrowhead*) and the amyloid cores of senile plaques (*arrows*). *D*, Electron micrograph of *in vitro* formed amyloid fibrils using SP28 and immunogold labeling with anti-SP28 Figure 1*A*, ×50,000; *B*, ×50,000; *C*, ×100; D, ×38,000.

show a typical crossing-over of 60 to 100 nm with a maximal width of 20 nm and a minimal width of 10 nm at the crossing points (64, 135). Ultrastructural studies have shown that each strand of PHF is formed of globular subunits of 3 to 5 nm arranged in a helical fashion (133, 136). PHF similar to those found in the neuronal perikaria are also present in the degenerated neurites that surround the amyloid cores of the senile plaques (124).

More than 90% of the cases of AD present amyloid deposition within the vessel walls of the leptomeninges and cerebral cortex (cerebrovascular amyloidosis, CVA) (40, 58, 70, 77, 81). This deposition affects mainly the media and adventitia of small arteries and veins. Electron microscopic evidence has been provided for the close relationship between small cortical vessels and senile plaques (86). In spite of the high incidence of CVA in AD, the frequency of massive cerebral hemorrhage in these patients is very low, probably related to the number and/or severity of the vascular involvement (26). Electron microscopically, CVA amyloid fibrils also show the typical appearance of straight 10 nm non-branching fibrils as other types of amyloids (Fig. 1*B*).

Biochemical Aspects. Since the isolation and characterization of the amyloid protein from the leptomeninges of AD (42), several biochemical and immunologic studies have demonstrated that CVA and amyloid cores of senile plaques in AD and aged Down's Syndrome (DS) share the same amyloid subunit (3, 21, 43, 83, 137) (Fig. 1*C*). This protein has a molecular weight of 4 kd, and it has been called β-protein (or A4) (42, 83). The initial amino acid sequence of β-protein yielded 28 amino acids that showed no homology to any known sequence (42, 137). *In vitro* studies have been conducted using synthetic peptides of different lengths homologous to the β-protein and demonstrated that synthetic peptides of 28 residues (positions 1–28), 17 residues (positions 12–28) and 14 residues (15–28) spontaneously formed amyloid fibrils *in vitro* in water and saline solutions without any further treatment. Synthetic fibrils displayed a typical electron microscopic appearance (Fig. 1*D*) and Congo red staining with green birefringence although, they differed from the native β-protein in the solubility pattern. Moreover, we predicted that a hydrophobic carboxy terminal was responsible for its insolubility. This has been recently confirmed, showing that the actual length of the β-protein has 42 amino acids with a highly hydrophobic tail of 14 residues (62). We also concluded that a sequence included in a 14 residue peptide (positions 15–28) is essential for the fibrillar configuration and that a 10-residue sequence (19–28) is sufficient for the typical x-ray diffraction pattern, providing an *in vitro* model system for further studies on amyloid fibril formation (21, 45) (Fig. 2).

Relationship Between PHF and Amyloid. Although it seems clear that amyloid fibrils of the senile plaques and vascular deposits share the same β-protein, the issue whether PHF are made up of the same subunit remains controversial. Several groups have reported that the amino acid composition of NFT is similar to vascular/plaque amyloids (2, 46, 82). Nevertheless, the strikingly different morphology between PHF and the typical amyloid fibril together with the lack of cross-reactivity between plaque/vascular amyloid and NFT using antibodies against β-protein or homologous synthetic peptides, are the major arguments held against the notion that PHF and vascular plaque amyloid are made up of the same protein. The isolation of β-protein or A4 from fractions enriched in PHF from AD brains after formic acid treatment has been reported (79). This finding has been challenged based on the usual cross-contamination between amyloid cores and NFT during the extraction procedure and the relative insolubility of PHF under the conditions for protein characterization, namely gel electrophoresis and chromatography (110).

A different approach for the characterization of PHF has been used by several groups based on immunologic cross-reactivity. In this way PHF have been shown to cross-react with normal constituents of the neuronal cytoskeleton including the 200-kd component of neurofilaments, microtubule-associated proteins (MAP_2) and MAP-τ (5, 50, 67, 96, 138, 139). τ includes a group of

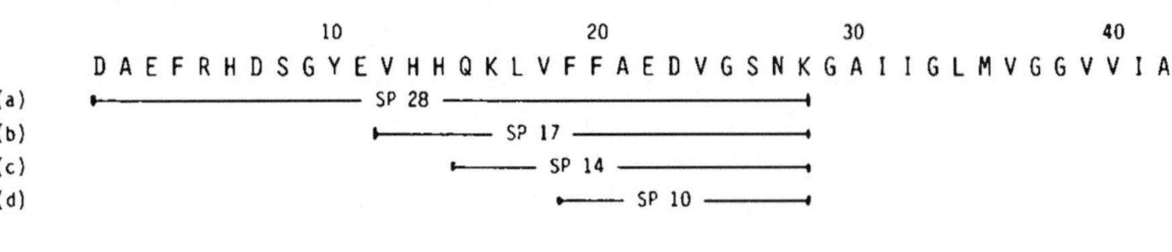

FIG. 2. The amino acid sequence of amyloid β-protein (or A4 protein) deduced from a cDNA (62). Synthetic peptides of: (*a*) 28 residues (SP28), positions 1–28; (*b*) 17 residues (SP17), positions 12–28; (*c*) 14 residues (SP14), positions 14–28; and (*d*) 10 residues (SP10), positions 19–28.

phosphoproteins that can promote the *in vitro* assembly of α-β-tubulin dimers to form microtubules (130). Furthermore, some investigators have suggested that abnormally phosphorylated τ proteins are structural components of PHF (57). The biochemical composition of PHF in AD will remain unclear until complete solubilization of these fibrils is achieved for protein analysis and amino acid sequencing. Alternatively, experiments using synthetic peptides homologous to the β-protein under diverse conditions could lead to the *in vitro* formation of PHF. In this regard, fibrils with a similar morphology of PHF have been obtained from purified τ protein after deamination with 6M urea and from amyloid AA after guanidine-treatment and prolonged dialysis to remove the denaturing agent (87, 100). It was suggested that amino terminal heterogeneity of β-protein interacting with cytoskeletal proteins (*i.e.*, τ) or ubiquitin (95), in a unique environment as it is the intraneuronal space may account for the peculiar assembly of this amyloid subunit to form PHF in AD (20). The recent report of the isolation of β-protein from the NFT present in Parkinson-dementia of Guam (PDG) supports this concept and provides indirect evidence that β-protein is a structural component of PHF (52). The lack of cross-reactivity between PHF and vascular/plaque amyloid possibly reflects that β-protein epitopes are hidden in the former structures due to conformational changes (21).

β-Protein Gene. The complementary DNA encoding the β-protein has been recently isolated and sequenced by several groups (44, 62, 104). This cDNA was obtained from normal human brain libraries using oligonucleotides corresponding to different portions of the amino terminal 28-residue sequence of β-protein. An open-reading frame of cDNA encodes for a protein of 695 residues with the β-protein starting at position 597 within the carboxy terminal of the molecule. This putative precursor has a molecular weight of 78 kd and presents features that resemble glycosylated cell-surface receptors (62). In this model, the 42-residue amyloid β-protein or A4 (Fig. 2) is included in the transmembrane domain of the precursor. Northern blot hybridization using cDNA fragments as probes has been used to detect the expression of the gene in human and animal tissues. A single 3.5 kd mRNA has been identified in several organs. The strongest signals have been obtained from normal human brain, kidney, heart and spleen (121). Lower levels of β-protein mRNA have been found in AD brains and it has been suggested that this finding may represent a nonspecific degradation of RNA in these patients. In addition, β-protein mRNA of the same size has been detected in mouse, rat, and bovine brains (44), indicating that the β-protein gene has been largely conserved through evolution. The finding of significant amounts of β-protein mRNA in several organs raises the question of why the amyloid deposition is restricted to the brain. Moreover, as we will discuss later, amyloid β-protein deposition within the brain adopts different patterns of distribution in several neurologic diseases of apparently unrelated etiologies. Whether structural differences in the β-protein genes or post-translational modifications in the β-protein precursor(s) in AD and related disorders account for these selective types of deposition remains to be clarified. By the examination of DNA of somatic cell hybrids, the gene encoding the β-protein has been mapped to human chromosome 21 (44, 62, 104, 121). This finding can provide an explanation for the development of typical AD changes in patients with DS that survive beyond the age of 40 years (18). Genetic linkage to DNA markers in four families with an autosomal-dominant form of AD (FAD), have led to the localization of the genetic abnormality also on chromosome 21, within the region as the gene encoding the β-protein (120). However, recent findings indicate that the amyloid β-protein gene is not the site of the inherited defect in FAD (122, 125). Although a significant progress has been made regarding genetic aspects in AD, little is known about environmental factors that may play an important role in triggering the abnormal mechanisms that lead to amyloid deposition. Nevertheless, the cloning of the β-protein gene have provided powerful tools for a systematic study of the biology of the amyloid β-protein and its precursor in health and disease.

Hereditary Cerebral Hemorrhage with Amyloidosis of Dutch Type (HCHWA-D)

HCHWA-D is an autosomal-dominant form of amyloidosis restricted to the brain. This disease has been described in four families in two coastal villages in The Netherlands (Katwjik and Schveningen) comprising 150 affected family members (76, 126, 129). Clinically, HCHWA-D is characterized by recurrent cerebral hemorrhage leading to death in the fifth and sixth decades of life. The pathologic findings include amyloid deposition within the walls of small arteries and arterioles of the leptomeninges and cerebral cortex. In some cases, parenchymal amyloid deposits resembling early or immature senile plaques have been identified. The peculiarity of these senile plaques is their fibrillar appearance lacking the dense amyloid core of the typical AD senile plaques. The absence of neurofibrillary tangles appears to be a characteristic feature of this disease.

We have recently demonstrated that the amyloid subunit in HCHWA-D is similar to the β-protein of AD and DS (126). Immunocytochemical studies carried out on five typical HCHWA-D patients showed that the amyloid deposits in the vessel walls and early plaques were specifically labeled by an antibody raised against a synthetic peptide homologous to the amino terminal 28-residues of β-protein (anti-SP28). Moreover, amyloid fibrils were extracted from the leptomeninges of one patient and the amyloid protein was sequenced to position 21, showing homology with the amyloid β-protein of AD, DS and PDG. The lack of neurofibrillary tangles suggests that the neuronal population is not involved in the process of amyloidogenesis in HCHWA-D. Furthermore, the type of amyloid distribution may indicate that β-protein is primarily deposited in the vessel walls and that parenchymal involvement is a secondary event.

The complete amino acid sequence of the β-protein and the cloning and sequencing of its gene in Dutch patients with HCHWA will clarify whether structural differences in this locus account for the particular type of amyloid distribution and clinical manifestations in these patients.

Sporadic Cerebral Amyloid Angiopathy and Asymptomatic Age-Related Amyloidosis

In addition to the inherited forms of cerebrovascular amyloidosis (HCHWA-D and HCHWA-I), the nonfamilial or sporadic type of cerebrovascular amyloidosis represents an important cause of nontraumatic intracerebral hemorrhage in hormotensive elderly patients. It has been estimated that sporadic cerebral amyloid angiopathy (SCAA) accounts for 5 to 10% of all strokes (61, 78, 90, 91). This clinico-pathological entity has also gained significance because it is closely related to the commonest forms of cerebral amyloidosis: AD and normal aging of the brain. In effect, most of the reported series of SCAA include patients that in addition to the cerebrovascular-related clinical manifestations, presented dementia and pathologic features indistinguishable from AD including senile plaques and NFT. This overlapping has been estimated to be present in 40% of the cases of SCAA (127). Nevertheless, there is a small group of SCAA patients without AD typical changes in which the clinical manifestation is brain hemorrhage related to an exclusive vascular amyloid deposition. The cerebrovascular involvement is usually severe with extensive amyloid infiltration of the small vessels of the leptomeninges and cerebral cortex. In some cases, atypical or early senile plaques are also present, as described in HCHWA-D. Recently, we have conducted immunocytochemical studies on SCAA patients with the latter conditions in order to characterize the amyloid subunit (26). The results using our immunological probe, anti-SP28, indicated that the amyloid protein in SCAA is antigenically related to the β-protein of AD, DS, PDG, and HCHWA-D. Yet, biochemical studies are needed to establish the degree of homology between the β-protein of SCAA and other diseases. Moreover, immunoperoxidase staining of brain sections of asymptomatic elderly persons presenting senile plaques and cerebrovascular amyloidosis showed that these amyloid deposits were specifically labeled by anti-SP28 indicating that age-related brain amyloid is also made of β-protein.

β-AMYLOID DISEASES (TABLE 4)

Our results strongly suggest that at least one type of familial cerebrovascular amyloidosis (HCHWA-D), sporadic cerebral amyloid angiopathy and the cerebral amyloid related to aging share a similar amyloid subunit. These findings together with the characterization of β-protein from AD, DS, and PDG indicate that amyloid β-protein deposition in the brain comprises a spectrum of clinico-pathologic entities that we designate "β-amyloid diseases." This group of diseases includes a variety of etiologies, patterns of amyloid distribution and clinical manifestations. The differences in the anatomical distribution of amyloid fibrils are clearly delineated: an exclusive neuronal involvement in PDG, and at the other extreme, the exclusive or predominant vascular lesions of HCHWA-D, and SCAA. AD and DS display a multiple distribution presenting the three types of cerebral amyloids, vascular, extracellular and intraneuronal. It appears evident that a diversity of etiological factors may promote a common pathogenic mechanism leading to the amyloid β-protein deposition. In the same way that amyloidosis AA is inherited in familial Mediterranean fever or results from a complication of many inflammatory diseases or malignancies (100), cerebral β-protein deposition is related to genetic defects (HCHWA-D, FAD) (126); chromosomal abnormalities (DS) (43), or environmental factors (PDG) (119). The list might be enlarged

TABLE 4. CEREBRAL β-AMYLOID DISEASES

	Disease	Amyloid Distribution	Clinical manifestations
Familial	Familial Alzheimer Disease (autosomal-dominant)	Multiple[a]	Dementia
	Hereditary cerebral hemorrhage with amyloidosis—Dutch type (autosomal-dominant)	Vascular[b]	Intracerebral hemorrhage
Nonfamilial	Alzheimer Disease	Multiple	Dementia
	Down's Syndrome	Multiple	Dementia
	Sporadic cerebral amyloid angiopathy	Vascular	Intracerebral hemorrhage
	Parkinson-Dementia of Guam	Neuronal	Dementia, Parkinsonism, and motor neuron disease
	Asymptomatic age-related amyloidosis	Multiple	Asymptomatic

[a] Multiple refers to the presence of the three types of lesions: cerebrovascular amyloid, senile plaques, and neurofibrillary tangles.
[b] Vascular refers to an exclusive or predominant cerebrovascular amyloid deposition.

with the biochemical characterization of amyloid fibrils from the brains of patients with dementia pugilistica, subacute sclerosing panencephalitis, or vascular malformations. Genetic differences may account for the diversity of clinical and pathologic manifestations in some of these diseases, either at the β-protein locus and/or other related genetic loci. Alternatively, if no genetic defects are found, abnormal processing of a normally expressed β-protein precursor determined by different etiologic factors, may lead to anomalous cleavage and deposition of the highly insoluble 4 kd β-protein. Altered expression and/or processing in different cell types, *i.e.*, neurons, glial cells, cellular components of vessel walls, could provide the explanation for the heterogeneity of the amyloid localization. The experimental data available at the present time are insufficient to raise satisfactory theories regarding the pathogenesis of amyloid formation and deposition in this group of diseases and its relationship with the process of normal aging of the brain. Nevertheless, the availability of immunological and cDNA probes will make possible a systematic study of cerebral amyloidogenesis in the near future.

This work was supported by National Institutes of Health Grants AG 05891, AM 01431, and AM 02594.

Address reprint requests to: Dr. Blas Frangione, New York University Medical Center, 550 First Avenue, New York, NY 10016.

REFERENCES

1. Abrahamson M, Grubb A, Olafsson I, Lundwall A: Molecular cloning and sequence analysis of cDNA coding for the precursor of the human cysteine proteinase inhibitor Cystatin C. FEBS Lett 216:229, 1987
2. Allsop D: Biochemistry of cerebral amyloid in Alzheimer's disease, the unconventional flow virus diseases and Icelandic cerebrovascular amyloidosis. In Amyloidosis, edited by Marrink J, Van Rijswijk MH, p 243. Dordrecht, Martinus Nijhoff, 1986
3. Allsop D, Landon M, Kidd M, Lowe JS, Reynolds GP, Gardner A: Monoclonal antibodies raised against a subsequence of senile plaque core protein react with plaque cores, plaque periphery and cerebrovascular amyloid in Alzheimer's disease. Neurosci Lett 68:252, 1986
4. Alzheimer A: Uberline eigenartige erkrangkung der hirnrinde. Allg Z Psychiat 64:146, 1907
5. Anderton BH, Breinberg D, Downes MJ, Green PJ, Tomlinson BE, Ulrich J, Wood JN, Kahn J: Monoclonal antibodies show that neurofibrillary tangles and neurofilaments share antigenic determinants. Nature 298:84, 1982
6. Axelrad MA, Kisilewsky R: Biological characterization of amyloid enhancing factor. In Amyloid and Amyloidosis, edited by Glenner GG, Costa PP, Freitas AF, p 527. Amsterdam, Excerpta Medica, 1980
7. Axelrad MA, Kisilewsky R, Willmer J, Chen SJ, Skinner M: Further characterization of amyloid-enhancing factor. Lab Invest 47:139, 1982
8. Bardin T, Kuntz D, Zingraff J, Voisin MC, Zelmar A, Lansanuan J: Synovial amyloidosis in patients undergoing long-term hemodialysis. Arthritis Rheum 28:1052, 1985
9. Benditt EP, Erikssen N: Amyloid protein SAA is associated with high density lipoprotein from human serum. Proc Natl Acad Sci USA 74:4025, 1977
10. Benditt EP, Erikssen N, Hermodson NA, Ericsson LH: The major proteins of human and monkey amyloid substance: common properties including unusual *N*-terminal amino acid sequences. FEBS Lett 19:169, 1971
11. Bladen HA, Nylen MU, Glenner GG: The ultrastructure of human amyloid as revealed by the negative staining technique. J Ultrastruct Res 14:449, 1966
12. Blessed G, Tomlinson BE, Roth M: The association between quantitative measures of dementia and of senile change in the cerebral grey matter of elderly subjects. Br J Psychiatry 114:797, 1968
13. Bockman JM, Kingsbury DT, McKinley MP, Bendheim PE, Prusiner SB: Creutzfeldt Jakob disease prion proteins in human brains. N Engl J Med 312:73, 1985
14. Bolton DC, McKinley MP, Prusiner SB: Molecular characteristics of the major scrapie prion protein. Biochemistry 23:5898, 1984
15. Bowen DM, Benton JS, Spillane JA, Smith CCT, Allen SJ: Choline acetyltransferase activity and histopathology of frontal neocortex from biopsies of demented patients. J Neurol Sci 57:191, 1982
16. Breathreach SM, Melrose SM, Bhogal B, deBeer FC, Dyck RF, Tennent G, Black MM, Pepys MB: Amyloid P component is located on elastic fibre microfibrils in normal human tissue. Nature 293:652, 1981
17. Brun A, Gustafson L: Distribution of cerebral degeneration in Alzheimer's disease. A clinical pathological study. Arch Psychiatr Nervenkr 223:15, 1976
18. Burger PC, Vogel FS: The development of the pathological changes of Alzheimer's disease and senile dementia in patients with Down's syndrome. Am J Pathol 73:457, 1973
19. Candy JM, Oakley AE, Klinowski J, Carpenter TA, Perry RH, Atack JR, Perry EK, Blessed G, Fairbairn A, Edwardson JA: Aluminum silicates and senile plaque formation in Alzheimer's disease. Lancet 1:354, 1986
20. Castaño EM, Frangione B: Human amyloidosis and *in vitro* formation of Alzheimer amyloid fibrils. In Alteration of the Neuronal Cytoskeleton in Aging and Dementia, edited by Perry G, New York, Plenum Press, in press 1988
21. Castaño EM, Ghiso J, Prelli F, Gorevic PD, Migheli A, Frangione B: *In vitro* formation of amyloid fibrils from two synthetic peptides of different lengths homologous to Alzheimer's disease β-protein. Biochem Biophys Res Commun 141:782, 1986
22. Cathcart ES, Comerford FR, Cohen AS: Immunologic studies on a protein extracted from human secondary amyloid. N Engl J Med 273:143, 1965
23. Chesebro B, Race R, Wehrly K, Nishio J, Bloom M, Lechner D, Bergstrom S, Robbins K, Mayer L, Keith JM, Garon C, Haase A: Identification of scrapie prion protein—specific mRNA in scrapie—infected and uninfected brain. Nature 315:331, 1985
24. Coe JE, Margossian SS, Slayter HS, Sogn JA: Hamster female protein. A new pentrax in structurally and functionally similar to C-reactive protein and amyloid P component. J Exp Med 153:977, 1981
25. Cohen DH, Feiner H, Jensson O, Frangione B: Amyloid fibril in hereditary cerebral hemorrhage with amyloidosis (HCHWA) is related to the gastroenteropancreatic neuroendocrine protein, gamma trace. J Exp Med 158:623, 1983
26. Coria F, Castaño EM, Frangione B: Brain amyloid in normal aging and cerebral amyloid angiopathy is antigenically related to Alzheimer's disease β-protein. Am J Pathol 129:422, 1987
27. de Beer FC, Baltz ML, Holford S, Feinstein A, Pepys MB: Fibronectin and C_4-binding protein are selectively bound by aggregated amyloid P component. J Exp Med 154:1134, 1981
28. Dyck RF, Lockwood CM, Kershaw M, McHugh N, Duance VC, Baltz ML, Pepys MB: Amyloid P component is a constituent of normal human glomerular basement membrane. J Exp Med 152:1162, 1980
29. Dwulet FE, Benson MD: Primary structure of an amyloid prealbumin and its plasma precursor in a heredofamilial polyneuropathy of Swedish origin. Proc Natl Acad Sci USA 81:694, 1984
30. Dwulet FE, Benson MD: Characterization of a transthyretin (prealbumin) variant associated with familial amyloidotic polyneuropathy type II (Indiana/Swiss). J Clin Invest 78:880, 1986
31. Franklin EC, Pras M, Levin M, Frangione B: The partial amino acid sequence of the major low molecular weight component of two human amyloid fibrils. FEBS Lett 22:121, 1972
32. Gajdusek DC: Unconventional viruses and the origin and disappearance of Kuru. Science 197:943, 1977
33. Gejyo F, Yamada T, Odani S, Nakagawa Y, Arakawa M, Kunimoto T, Kataoka H, Sujuki M, Hirasawa Y, Shirahama T, Cohen AS, Schmid K: A new form of amyloid protein associated with chronic hemodialysis was identified as β_2-microglobulin. Biochem Biophys Res Commun 129:701, 1985
34. Ghiso J, Jensson O, Frangione B: Amyloid fibrils in hereditary cerebral hemorrhage with amyloidosis of Icelandic type is a variant

of gamma-trace basic protein (Cystatin C). Proc Natl Acad Sci USA 83:2974, 1986
35. Ghiso J, Pons-Estel B, Frangione B: Hereditary cerebral amyloid angiopathy: the amyloid fibrils contain a protein which is a variant of Cystatin C, an inhibitor of lysosomal cysteine proteases. Biochem Biophys Res Commun 136:548, 1986
36. Gibbs CJ Jr, Gajdusek DC: Infection as the etiology of spongiform encephalopathy/Creutzfeldt-Jakob disease. Science 165:1023, 1969
37. Glenner GG: Amyloid deposits and amyloidosis: the β-fibrilloses. N Engl J Med 302:1283, 1980
38. Glenner GG, Eanes ED, Page DL: The relation of the properties of Congo red stained amyloid fibrils to the β-conformation. J Histochem Cytochem 20:821, 1972
39. Glenner GG, Ein D, Eanes ED, Bladen HA, Terry W, Page D: Creation of amyloid fibrils from Bence Jones proteins *in vitro.* Science 174:712, 1971
40. Glenner GG, Henry JH, Fujihara S: Congophilic angiopathy in the pathogenesis of alzheimer's degeneration. Ann Pathol 1:120, 1981
41. Glenner GG, Terry W, Harada M, Isersky C, Page C: Amyloid fibril proteins: proof of homology with immunoglobulin light chains by sequence analysis. Science 172:1150, 1971
42. Glenner GG, Wong CW: Alzheimer's disease: initial report of the purification and characterization of a novel cerebrovascular amyloid protein. Biochem Biophys Res Commun 120:885, 1984
43. Glenner GG, Wong CW: Alzheimer's disease and Down's syndrome: sharing of a unique cerebrovascular amyloid fibril protein. Biochem Biophys Res Commun 122:1131, 1984
44. Goldgaber D, Lerman MJ, McBride OW, Saffiotti V, Gajdusek DC: Characterization and chromosomal localization of a cDNA encoding brain amyloid of Alzheimer's disease. Science 235:877, 1987
45. Gorevic PD, Castaño EM, Sarma R, Frangione B: Ten to fourteen residue peptides of Alzheimer's disease β-protein are sufficient for amyloid fibril formation and its characteristic X-ray diffraction pattern. Biochem Biophys Res Commun 147:854, 1987
46. Gorevic PD, Goñi F, Pons-Estel B, Alvarez F, Peress NS, Frangione B: Isolation and partial characterization of neurofibrillary tangles and amyloid plaque core in Alzheimer's disease: immunohistological studies. J Neuropathol Exp Neurol 45:647, 1986
47. Gorevic PD, Munoz PC, Casey TT, DiRaimondo CR, Stone WJ, Prelli FC, Rodrigues MM, Poulik MD, Frangione B: Polymerization of intact β_2-microglobulin in tissue cases amyloidosis in patients on chronic hemodialysis. Proc Natl Acad Sci USA 83:7908, 1986
47a. Gorevic PD, Prelli FC, Wright J, Pras M, Frangione B: Systemic senile amyloidosis: identification of a new prealbumin (transthyretin) variant in cardiac tissue: structural similarity to one form of familial amyloidotic polyneuropathy. J Clin Invest, in press 1988
48. Grey HM, Kubo RT, Colon SM, Poulik MD, Cresswell P, Springer T, Turner M, Strominger JL: The small subunit of HLA-antigens in β_2-microglobulin. J Exp Med 138:1608, 1973
49. Grubb A, Löfberg H: Human γ-trace, a basic microprotein: amino acid sequences and presence in the adenohypophysis. Proc Natl Acad Sci USA 79:3024, 1984
50. Grundke-Iqbal I, Iqbal K, Quinlan M, Tung YC, Zaidi MD, Wisnieswski HM: Microtubule-associated protein tau, a component of Alzheimer paired helical filaments. J Biol Chem 261:6084, 1986
51. Gudmundsson G, Hallgrimsson J, Jonasson TA, Bjarnason O: Hereditary cerebral hemorrhage with amyloidosis. Brain 95:387, 1972
52. Guiroy DC, Miyazaki M, Multhaup G, Fischer P, Garruto RM, Beyreuther K, Masters CL, Simms G, Gibbs CJ, Gajdusek DC: Amyloid of neurofibrillary tangles of Guamanian Parkinson-dementia and Alzheimer disease share identical amino acid sequence. Proc Natl Acad Sci USA 84:2073, 1987
53. Hadlow WJ: Scrapie and Kuru. Lancet 2:289, 1959
54. Hansotia P, Ganik K, Friedenberg W: Cerebrospinal fluid monoclonal gammopathy in multiple myeloma and Waldenstrom's macroglobulinemia. Neurology 33:1411, 1983
55. Hol PR, Snel FWJJ, Niewold ThA, Gruys E: Amyloid enhancing factor (AEF) in the pathogenesis of AA amyloidosis in the hamster. Virchows Arch 52:273, 1986
56. Husby G, Ranlow PJ, Sletten K: The amyloid in familial amyloid cardiomyopathy of Danish origin is related to prealbumin. Clin Exp Immunol 60:207, 1985
57. Iqbal K, Grundke-Iqbal I, Zaidi T, Merz PA, Wen GY, Shaikh SS, Wisniewski HM: Defective brain microtubule assembly in Alzheimer's disease. Lancet 2:421, 1986
58. Ishii N, Nishihara Y, Horie A: Amyloid angiopathy and lobar cerebral hemorrhage. J. Neurol Neurosurg Psychiatry 47:1703, 1984
59. Ishii T, Nakamura Y: Distribution and ultrastructure of Alzheimer's neurofibrillary tangles in postencephalitic Parkinsonism of economo type. Acta Neuropathol (Berl) 55:59, 1981
60. Isobe T, Osserman EF: Patterns of amyloidosis and their association with plasma cell dyscrasia, monoclonal immunoglobulins and Bence Jones proteins. N Engl J Med 290:473, 1984
61. Kalyan-Raman UP, Kalyan-Raman K: Cerebral amyloid angiopathy causing intracranial hemorrhage. Ann Neurol 16:321, 1984
62. Kang J, Lemaire HG, Unterbeck A, Salbaum JM, Masters CL, Grezeschik KH, Multhaup G, Beyreuther K, Muller-Hill B: The precursor of Alzheimer disease amyloid A4 protein resembles a cell-surface receptor. Nature 325:733, 1987
63. Katzman R: Alzheimer's disease. N Engl J Med 314:964, 1986
64. Kidd M: Paired helical filaments in electron microscopy of Alzheimer's disease. Nature 197:192, 1963
65. Kitamoto T, Tateishi J, Tashirua T, Takeshita I, Barry RA, DeArmond SJ, Prusiner SB: Amyloid plaques in Creutzfeldt-Jakob disease stain with prion protein antibodies. Ann Neurol 20:204, 1986
66. Klatzo I, Gajdusek DC, Zigas V: Pathology of Kuru. Lab Invest 8:799, 1959
67. Kosik KS, Joachim CL, Selkoe DJ: Microtubule associated protein tau (τ) is a major antigenic component of paired helical filaments in Alzheimer's disease. Proc Natl Acad Sci USA 83:4044, 1986
68. Kyle RA, Greipp PR: Amyloidosis (AL) clinical and laboratory features in 229 cases. Mayo Clinic Proc 58:665, 1983
69. Lavie G, Zucker-Franklin D, Franklin EC: Degradation of serum amyloid A protein by surface-associated enzymes of human blood monocytes. J Exp Med 148:1020, 1978
70. Lee SS, Stemmerman GN: Congophilic angiopathy and cerebral hemorrhage. Arch Pathol Lab Med 102:317, 1978
71. Levin M, Franklin EC, Frangione B, Pras M: The amino acid sequence of a major non-immunoglobulin component of some amyloid fibrils. J Clin Invest 51:2773, 1972
72. Levin M, Pras M, Franklin EC: Immunologic studies of the major non-immunoglobulin protein of amyloid. Identification and partial characterization of a related serum component. J Exp Med 138:373, 1973
73. Li JJ, McAdam KPWJ: Human amyloid P component: an elastase inhibitor. Scand J Immunol 20:219, 1984
74. Linke RP, Tischendorf FW, Zucker-Franklin D, Franklin EC: The formation of amyloid-like fibrils in vitro from Bence Jones proteins of the λ_1 subclass. J Immunol 111:24, 1973
75. Löfberg H, Stromblad LG, Grubb AO, Olsson O: Demonstration of γ-trace in normal and neoplastic endocrine A cells of the pancreatic islets: an immunohistochemical study in monkey, rat and man. Biomed Res 2:527, 1981
76. Luyendijk W, Bots GThAM: Vegter-vander Vlis M, Went LN: Familiaire Hersenbloedingen als gevolg van crebrale amyloide angiopathie. Ned Tijdschr Geneekd 130:1935, 1986
77. Mandybur TI: The incidence of cerebral amyloid angiopathy in Alzheimer's disease. Neurology 25:120, 1975
78. Mandybur TI, Bates SRD: Fatal massive intracerebral hemorrhage complicating cerebral amyloid angiopathy. Arch Neurol 35:246, 1978
79. Mandybur TI, Gore I: Amyloid in late postiradiation necrosis of brain. Neurology 19:983, 1969
80. Mantzouranis EC, Dowton BS, Whitehead AS, Edge MD, Bruns GAP, Colten HR: Human serum amyloid P component. cDNA isolation, complete sequence of pre-serum amyloid P component and localization of the gene to chromosome 1. J Biol Chem 260:7752, 1985
81. Masters CL, Gajdusek DC, Gibbs CJ Jr: Creutzfeldt-Jakob disease virus isolation from the Gerstmann-Straussler syndrome. Brain

104:559, 1981

82. Masters CL, Multhaup G, Simms G, Pottgieser J, Martins RN, Beyreuther K: Neuronal origin of a cerebral amyloid: neurofibrillary tangles of Alzheimer's disease contain the same protein as the amyloid of plaque cores and blood vessels. EMBO J 4:2757, 1985
83. Masters CL, Simms G, Weinman NA, Multhaup G, McDonald BL, Beyreuther K: Amyloid plaque core protein in Alzheimer disease and Down Syndrome. Proc Natl Acad Sci USA 82:4245, 1985
84. McKinley MP, Bolton DC, Prusiner SB: A protease-resistant protein is a structural component of the scrapie prion. Cell 35:57, 1983
85. Merz PA, Wisniewski HM, Somerville RA, Bobin SA, Masters CL, Iqbal K: Ultrastructural morphology of amyloid fibrils from neuritic and amyloid plaques. Acta Neuropathol (Berl) 60:113, 1983
86. Miyakawa T, Shimoji A, Kuramoto R, Higuchi Y: The relationship between senile plaques and cerebral blood vessels in Alzheimer's disease and senile dementia. Virchows Arch [B] 40:121, 1982
87. Montejo de Garcini E, Serrano L, Avila J: Self assembly of microtubule associated protein tau into filaments resembling those found in Alzheimer's disease. Biochem Biophys Res Commun 141:790, 1986
88. Oesch B, Westaway D, Walchli M, McKinley MP, Kent SBH, Aebersold R, Barry RA, Tempst P, Teplow DB, Hood LE, Prusiner SB, Weissman C: A cellular gene encodes scrapie Prp 27-30 protein. Cell 40:735, 1985
89. Ohnishi S, Maeda S, Himada K, Arar T: Isolation and characterization of the complete complementary and genomic DNA sequences of human serum amyloid P component. J Biochem 100:849, 1986
90. Ojenmann RG, Heros RC: Spontaneous brain hemorrhage. Stroke 14:468, 1983
91. Okazaki H, Reagan TJ, Campbell RJ: Clinico-pathological studies of primary cerebral amyloid angiopathy. Mayo Clin Proc 54:22, 1979
92. Osmand AP, Friedenson B, Gewurz H, Painter RH, Hofmann T, Shelton E: Characterization of C-reactive protein and the complement subcomponent C1t as homologous proteins displaying cyclic pentameric symmetry (Pentraxins). Proc Natl Acad Sci USA 74:739, 1977
93. Pepys MB, Dyck RF, de Beer FC, Skinner M, Cohen AS: Binding of serum amyloid P component (SAP) by amyloid fibrils. Clin Exp Immunol 38:284, 1979
94. Perry EK, Tomlinson BE, Blessed G, Bergmann K, Gibson PH, Perry RH: Correlation of cholinergic abnormalities with senile plaques and mental test scores in senile dementia. Br Med J 2:1457, 1978
95. Perry G, Friedman R, Shaw G, Chau V: Ubiquitin is detected in neurofibrillary tangles and senile plaque neurites of Alzheimer disease brains. Proc Natl Acad Sci USA 84:3033, 1987
96. Perry G, Rizzuto N, Autilio-Gambetti L, Gambetti P: Paired helical filaments from Alzheimer disease patients contain cytoskeletal components. Proc Natl Acad Sci USA 82:3916, 1985
97. Pras M, Franklin EC, Prelli F, Frangione B: A variant of prealbumin from amyloid fibrils in familial polyneuropathies of Jewish type. J Exp Med 154:989, 1981
98. Pras M, Franklin EC, Shibolet S, Frangione B: Amyloidosis associated with renal cell carcinoma is of the AA type. Am J Med 73:426, 1982
99. Pras M, Prelli F, Gafni J: Genetic heterogeneity of familial amyloid polyneuropathies of Jewish type. In Amyloidosis, edited by Glenner GG, Osserman EF, Benditt EP, Calkins E, Cohen AS, Zucker-Franklin D, p 385. New York, Plenum Press, 1986
100. Prelli F, Pras M, Frangione B: The degradation and deposition of amyloid AA fibril is tissue specific. Biochemistry 26:8251, 1987
101. Prusiner SB: Novel proteinaceous infectious particles cause scrapie. Science 216:136, 1982
102. Prusiner SB, De Armond SJ: Prions causing nervous system degeneration. Lab Invest 56:349, 1987
103. Ramadori G, Sipe JD, Dinarello CA, Mizel B, Colten HR: Pretranslational modulation of acute phase hepatic protein synthesis by murine recombinant interleuken I (IL1) and purified human IL-1. J Exp Med 162:930, 1985
104. Robakis NK, Ramkrishna N, Wolfe G, Wisniewski HM: Molecular cloning and characterization of a cDNA encoding the cerebrovascular and the neuritic plaque amyloid peptides. Proc Natl Acad Sci USA 84:4190, 1987
105. Rosenthal CJ, Franklin EC: Variation with age and diseases of an amyloid A protein-related serum component. J Clin Invest 55:746, 1975
106. Rosenthal CJ, Franklin EC, Frangione, B: Isolation and partial characterization of SAA. An amyloid related protein from human serum. J Immunol 116:1415, 1976
107. Rudelli R, Strom JO, Welch PT, Ambler MW: Post-traumatic premature Alzheimer's disease: neuropathologic findings and pathogenetic considerations. Arch Neurol 39:570, 1982
108. Saraiva MJM, Birken S, Costa PP, Goodman DS: Amyloid fibril protein in familial amyloidotic polyneuropathy Portuguese type. J Clin Invest 74:104, 1984
109. Selkoe DJ, Ihara Y, Abraham C, Rasool CG, McCluskey AA: Biochemical and immunocytochemical studies of Alzheimer paired helical filaments. In Biological Aspects of Alzheimer's Disease. Banbury Report 15. edited by Katzman R, New York, Cold Spring Harbor, 1983
110. Selkoe DJ, Ihara Y, Salazar FJ: Alzheimer's disease: insolubility of partially purified paired helical filaments in sodium dodecyl sulfate and urea. Science 215:1243, 1982
111. Skinner M, Cohen AS, Shirahama T, Cathcart ES: P-component (pentagonal unit) of amyloid: isolation, characterization and sequence analysis. J Lab Clin Med 84:604, 1974
112. Sletten K, Husby G, Natvig JB: *N*-terminal amino acid sequence of amyloid fibril protein AR, prototype of a new lambda-variable subgroup V_{VI}. Scand J Immunol 3:833, 1974
113. Sletten K, Westermark P, Natvig JB: Characterization of amyloid fibrils proteins from medullary carcinoma of the thyroid. J Exp Med 143:993, 1976
114. Sletten K, Westermark P, Natvig JB: Senile cardiac amyloid related to prealbumin. Scan J Immunol 12:503, 1980
115. Snow AD, Kisilevsky R: Temporal relationship between glyaminoglycan accumulation and amyloid position during experimental amyloidosis: a histochemical study. Lab Invest 53:37, 1985
116. Snow AD, Willmer J, Kisilevsky R: Sulfated glycosaminoglycans: A common constituent of all amyloids? Lab Invest 56:120, 1987
117. Sohar E, Gafni J, Pras M, Heller H: Familial Mediterranean fever: a survey of 470 cases and review of the literature. Am J Med 43:227, 1967
118. Solomon A, Frangione B, Franklin EC: Bence Jones proteins and light chains of immunoglobulins: preferential association of the $V\lambda_{VI}$ subgroup of human light chains with amyloidosis AL (λ). J Clin Invest 70:453, 1982
119. Spencer PS, Nunn PB, Hugon J, Ludolph AC, Ross SM, Roy DN, Robertson RC: Guam amyotrophic lateral sclerosis-parkinsonism-dementia linked to a plant excitant neurotoxin. Science 237:517, 1987
120. St. George-Hyslop PH, Tanzi RE, Pilinsky RJ, Haines JL, Nee L, Watkins PC, Myers RH, Feldman RG, Pollen D, Drachman D, Growdon J, Bruni A, Foncin JF, Salmon D, Frommelt P, Amaducci L, Sorbi S, Piacentini S, Stewart GD, Hobbs WJ, Conneally M, Gusella JF: The genetic defect causing familial Alzheimer's disease maps on chromosome 21. Science 235:885, 1987
121. Tanzi RE, Gusella JF, Watkins PC, Bruns GAP, St George-Hyslop P, Van Keuren ML, Patterson D, Pajan S, Kurnit DM, Nere RL: Amyloid β-protein gene; cDNA, mRNA distributions, and genetic linkage near the Alzheimer locus. Science 235:880, 1987
122. Tanzi RE, St George-Hyslop PH, Haines JL, Polinsky RJ, Nee L, Foncin JF, Nere RL, McClatchey AI, Conneally PM, Gusella JF: The genetic defect in familial Alzheimer's disease is not tightly linked to the amyloid β-protein gene. Nature 329:156, 1987
123. Tawara S, Nakazato M, Kangawa K, Matsuo H, Araki S: Identification of amyloid prealbumin variant in familial amyloidotic polyneuropathy (Japanese type). Biochem Biophys Res Commun 116:880, 1983
124. Terry RD, Gonatas NK, Weiss M: Ultrastructural studies in Alzheimer's presenile dementia. Am J Pathol 44:269, 1964
125. Van Broeckhoven C, Genthe AM, Vandenberghe A, Horsthemke B, Backhoreus H, Raeymaekers P, Van Hul W, Wehnert A,

Ghenens J, Cras P, Bruyland M, Martin JJ, Salbaum M, Multhaup G, Masters CL, Beyreuther K, Gurling HMD, Mullan MJ, Holland A, Barton A, Irving N, Williamson R, Richards SJ, Hardy JA: Failure of familial Alzheimer's disease to segregate with the A4 amyloid gene in several European families. Nature 329:153, 1987

126. van Duinen SG, Castaño EM, Prelli F, Bots GThAB, Luyendijk W, Frangione B: Hereditary cerebral hemorrhage with amyloidosis in patients of Dutch origin is related to Alzheimer disease. Proc Natl Acad Sci USA 84:5991, 1987
127. Vinters HV: Cerebral amyloid angiopathy: a critical review. Stroke 18:311, 1987
128. Wallace MR, Dwulet FE, Conneally PM, Benson MD: Biochemical and molecular genetic characterization of a new variant prealbumin associated with hereditary amyloidosis. J Clin Invest 78:6, 1986
129. Wattendorff AR, Bots GThAM, Went LN, Endtz LJ: Familial cerebral amyloid angiopathy presenting as recurrent cerebral haemorrhage. J Neurol Sci 55:121, 1982
130. Weingarten MD, Lockwood AH, Huo SY, Kirschner MW: A protein factor essential for microtubule assembly. Proc Natl Acad Sci USA 72:1858, 1975
131. Westermark P, Shirahama T, Skinner M, Brun A, Cameron R, Cohen AS: Immunohistochemical evidence for the lack of amyloid P component in some intracerebral amyloids. Lab Invest 46:457, 1982
132. Westermark P, Wernstedt C, O'Brien TD, Hayden DW, Johnson KH: Islet amyloid in type 2 human diabetes mellitus and adult diabetic cats contains a novel putative polypeptide hormone. Am J Pathol 127:414, 1987
133. Wischik CM, Crowther RA, Stewart M, Roth M: Subunit structure of paired helical filaments in Alzheimer's disease. J Cell Biol 100:1905, 1985
134. Wisniewski K, Jervis GA, Moretz RC, Wisniewski HM: Alzheimer neurofibrillary tangles in diseases other than senile or presenile dementia. Ann Neurol 5:288, 1979
135. Wisniewski HM, Narang HK, Terry RD: Neurofibrillary tangles of paired helical filaments. J Neurol Sci 27:173, 1976
136. Wisniewski HM, Wen GY: Substructures of paired helical filaments from Alzheimer's disease neurofibrillary tangles. Acta Neuropathol (Berl) 66:173, 1985
137. Wong CW, Quaranta V, Glenner GG: Neuritic plaques and cerebrovascular amyloid in Alzheimer's disease are antigenically related. Proc Natl Acad Sci USA 82:8729, 1985
138. Wood JG, Mirra SS, Pollock NJ, Binder LI: Neurofibrillary tangles of Alzheimer disease share antigenic determinants with the axonal microtubule-associated protein tau (τ). Proc Natl Acad Sci USA 83:4040, 1986
139. Yen SH, Dickson DW, Crowe A, Butler M, Shelanski ML: Alzheimer's neurofibrillary tangles contain unique epitopes and epitopes in common with the heat-stable microtubule associated proteins tau and MAP_2. Am J Pathol 126:81, 1987
140. Zemer D, Pras M, Sohar E, Modan M, Cabili S, Gafni J: Colchicine in the prevention and treatment of the amyloidosis of familial mediterranean fever. N Engl J Med 314:1001, 1986

Biology of Disease

Receptor-Mediated Endocytosis and Intracellular Processing of Insulin: Ultrastructural and Biochemical Evidence for Cell-Specific Heterogeneity and Distinction from Nonhormonal Ligands

ROBERT M. SMITH AND LEONARD JARETT

Department of Pathology and Laboratory Medicine, University of Pennsylvania School of Medicine, Philadelphia, Pennsylvania

INTRODUCTION

The purpose of this review is to present biochemical and ultrastructural evidence which demonstrate that differences exist between the binding, internalization and intracellular processing of insulin and other types of ligands such as LDL and alpha-2-macroglobulin. In addition, other data will show that there is substantial cell-specific heterogeneity among different cell types in the processing of the insulin-receptor complex.

Binding of macromolecules to receptors on cell surfaces and receptor-mediated endocytosis of the ligand-receptor complex are ubiquitous processes shared by different types of ligands and cell-types with diverse functions. It has been suggested that receptor-mediated endocytosis[1] of all ligands on all cell types could be achieved using the same mechanism (3, 74, 113). Results from many biochemical studies demonstrated that certain common features of endocytosis and processing did exist for a variety of ligands. Studies showed receptor internalization was temperature and, generally, energy dependent. The effects of various inhibitors on ligand and receptor processing have provided substantial information about mechanisms controlling the endocytosis and recycling of receptors. In several of these studies the intracellular accumulation of different ligands was affected in the same way by various inhibitors (11, 16), again supporting the concept of a universal mechanism of endocytosis. The theory of receptor recycling was proposed since it was a frequent finding that the intra-

[1] The terms "receptor-mediated endocytosis", "internalization", and "uptake" will be used synonymously throughout this article.

cellular accumulation of ligand exceeded the number of available receptors (19, 45, 72) and that receptor endocytosis rarely resulted in substantially decreased numbers of membrane receptors except in the case of EGF receptors (18).

Our understanding of the mechanisms of receptor-mediated internalization and intracellular ligand processing was greatly advanced by ultrastructural studies of LDL uptake in fibroblasts by Anderson, Brown, Goldstein and colleagues (reviewed in Ref. 40). Based on their findings a universal model was developed which included three essential features: (a) the concentrative endocytosis of ligands in coated pits on the cell membrane; (b) lysosomal processing of the ligand; and (c) recycling of receptors to the cell membrane for reutilization in the endocytotic process. This model has been discussed in several reviews (86, 112, 113, 114). Subsequent studies provided evidence that several ligands including asialoglycoprotein (29, 118), EGF (18, 19, 74), and α-2-macroglobulin (74, 113), were internalized and processed in a similar manner.

While these biochemical and ultrastructural studies supported the concept of a universal mechanism of receptor-mediated endocytosis, several laboratories, including our own, investigated the cellular processing of hormonal and other nonhormonal ligands and found significant differences from the LDL model. These differences were demonstrated both biochemically and morphologically and suggested that receptors for functionally different types of ligands may have different mechanisms controlling ligand and/or receptor internalization and intracellular processing. Some of these differences include internalization of the ligand receptor complex predominantly in non-coated pinocytotic invaginations[2] (2, 6, 77, 93, 96, 99, 100, 103), recycling of both the ligand and receptor (9, 28, 50, 105), absence of significant lysosomal degradation of the ligand (15, 61), and differing effects of inhibitors on ligand or receptor internalization or processing (30, 43, 87). In addition, studies of insulin processing in different cell types utilizing several inhibitors suggested that functionally different cells or tissues may have cell-specific internalization mechanisms and different routes of intracellular processing (23, 94). These findings make a universal mechanism of receptor-mediated endocytosis and intracellular ligand processing as proposed in the LDL model highly unlikely.

INITIAL CELL MEMBRANE LIGAND-RECEPTOR INTERACTION

The first step analyzed in a study of receptor-mediated endocytosis is the binding of ligands to receptors on the cell surface and the events that immediately follow. Along with chemical and structural characteristics which convey ligand recognition specificity to receptors there may exist factors responsible for differences in their endocytotic properties. Recent studies using modified insulin receptors suggest that a portion of the receptor may be necessary for internalization (89). The existence of such factors can be deduced from differences in the sites of action of different ligands and the role the receptor plays in the cell's response to the ligand.

Receptors for hormones serve multiple roles. The first, shared by all types of receptors, is to recognize and bind the ligand. Secondly, as a result of ligand occupancy, hormone receptors undergo a chemical or structural modification which results in the generation of "second messengers." Lastly, a relatively small percentage of the bound hormone may be internalized. In contrast to hormones, a large number of nonhormonal[3] ligands including LDL, asialoglycoprotein, viruses, and protease-complexes have few if any documented effects on cellular metabolism directly resulting from binding to their respective receptor. These ligands are invariably internalized and translocated to an appropriate intracellular site where they are processed, utilized or exert their biologic action. This major functional difference in the ligand-receptor interaction is characteristic of different classes of ligands which, in this review, will be called hormonal or nonhormonal ligands, respectively. Some of the differences between these types of receptors may result from the major structural differences of the cytoplasmic portion of receptors such as LDL and α-2-macroglobulin or insulin, IGF I and EGF (20, 40, 108, 109, 110, reviewed in Ref. 35). Viewed in this context, it would not be surprising if significant differences existed between the mechanisms or pathways of endocytosis and intracellular processing of hormone receptors and nonhormonal substances.

Sites of Insulin Action

The binding of insulin to its receptor on the cell surface is generally considered to be sufficient to trigger the pleiotropic effects of the hormone (reviewed in Ref. 35). Some direct effects of insulin, however, on intracellular organelles, particularly "growth factor effects" in the nucleus, have been demonstrated (reviewed in Ref. 86). Some of insulin's effects are detected within seconds after the hormone binds to the receptor, whereas other effects occur minutes or hours later. The initial event following insulin binding to the receptor α-subunit is the activation of the tyrosine kinase and the phosphorylation of tyrosine residues on the β-subunit (65). Several lines of evidence suggest that insulin stimulated tyrosine kinase activity may be a prerequisite for all subsequent insulin action (88) and perhaps receptor internalization (89). Other studies have shown that some of the intracellular effects of insulin controlling carbohydrate, lipid and protein metabolism were mimicked by, and may result from, the generation of a mediator substance now known to be a phosphooligosaccharide derived from a PI-glycan (66) which was rapidly released from the cell membrane after the binding of the hormone to its recep-

[2] The terms "noncoated pinocytotic invagination" and "pinocytotic invagination" will be used synonymously throughout this manuscript.

[3] The term "non-hormonal ligands" as used in this article refers to a general class of endogenous substances such as LDL, asialoglycoprotein, α-2-macroglobulin, mannose-6-phosphate and transferrin. "Hormonal ligands" refers to insulin, glucagon, ACTH, epinephrine, prolactin, and others specifically named in context. "Growth factors" refers to epidermal, insulin-like, nerve and platelet-derived growth factors (EGF, IGF's, NGF, and PDGF, respectively). Steroid receptors are specifically excluded from this discussion.

tor (reviewed in Ref. 42). It has also been suggested that the internalization of insulin and its receptor, and their translocation to nuclei or other intracellular sites, may be responsible for some of the long-term effects of the hormone (4, 34, 85, 101). Despite decades of investigation into insulin action, there is much that remains unclear concerning the complex mechanisms which cause the diverse metabolic effects of the hormone.

Biochemical Characterization of the Insulin Receptor

Since the first step in insulin's action is its binding to a cell membrane receptor, a great deal of investigation has centered on determining the characteristics of insulin binding. Biochemical investigations using ^{125}I-insulin have shown that the insulin-receptor interaction appeared to be similar in many different cell types. Virtually all studies revealed a curvilinear Scatchard plot of binding data which was interpreted in several ways: evidence of negative cooperativity (13), multiple binding sites with different affinities and capacities and other phenomena (17, 51).

Subsequently, the structure of the insulin receptor was determined using several different techniques (64, 84, 117) including gene cloning (20, 108). The insulin receptor has been shown to be composed of two α-subunits (molecular weight = 135,000) and two β-subunits (molecular weight = 95,000) linked by disulfide bonds to give the heterotetrameric structure of the membrane receptor (reviewed in Refs. 35, 53). With but one possible exception (46, 116) the insulin receptor isolated from a variety of sources has been virtually identical.

Ultrastructural Characterization of the Organization of Insulin Receptors

In the mid 1970s, while this and other laboratories were biochemically characterizing the insulin receptor, others were using electron-dense ligands and electron microscopy to assess the distribution of lectin, toxin, and immunoglobulin receptors on cell surfaces (7, 14, 80). In order to carry out correlative biochemical and ultrastructural investigations of the insulin receptor, this laboratory prepared a covalently linked ferritin-insulin complex which retained the biologic and immunologic activity of native insulin (55). The method of preparing the ferritin-insulin complex has been improved (97), including the eliminating ferritin oligomers which resulted in monomeric ferritin-insulin (Fm-I) (58). Recently, a novel colloidal-gold insulin complex was developed (95). The complex differs from previously described gold-insulin ligands (1, 76) in that the number of insulin molecules attached to each gold particle has been significantly reduced. The reduction in the number of insulin molecules resulted in a ligand with receptor binding and biologic activities virtually identical with native insulin. Furthermore, with fewer insulin molecules on each gold particle potential artifacts that might result from a highly multivalent ligand were avoided (81, 83).

The numerous similarities found in the biochemical characterization of the insulin receptor from various sources suggested that the ultrastructural observations of insulin receptors should be identical on all cells, particularly if the organization of receptors in the cell membrane had any relationship to receptor affinity and characteristics such as the curvilinear Scatchard plot. Rat adipocytes were being utilized to study insulin action by several laboratories because the cells are relatively easy to isolate in large numbers and insulin affects many of their metabolic processes. Our studies began by documenting the organization[4] of insulin receptors on the surface of adipocyte plasma membranes (55, 58) and intact adipocytes (56).

The number of insulin receptors/cell are significantly less than those of lectins or immunoglobulins. Therefore, the number of Fm-I receptors observed was less than in ultrastructural studies of lectin (7, 80) or immunoglobulin (14) receptors. Quantitative analysis of the number of insulin receptors observed morphologically was virtually identical with the number calculated from biochemical ^{125}I-insulin binding studies (57).

Figure 1 is a composite electron micrograph demonstrating the steady-state organization of insulin receptors on rat adipocytes. The Fm-I particles were found in the glycocalyx overlying the cell membrane. Some of the receptors were found as single molecules but the majority were in groups of two or more receptor sites. Grouped receptors were defined by computer assisted analysis (27) as receptors located within 400 Å of another occupied receptor. The groups of insulin receptors may have resulted from microaggregation of single receptors after receptor occupancy similarly to the microaggregation of immunoglobulin receptors (14). Studies were performed on both isolated plasma membranes and intact adipocytes to investigate the formation of the receptor groups and similar results were obtained (58). Figure 2 shows the results of a quantitative analysis of receptor organization on intact rat adipocytes incubated for various times with Fm-I. Since receptors remain mobile at 4° C (93, 113), one set of the cells was chemically fixed (prefixed) prior to the addition of Fm-I to preserve the native distribution of the unoccupied receptors. Prefixation was performed on these and other cells under conditions that did not affect specific ^{125}I-insulin binding (58, 93), but was sufficient to prevent the ligand-induced aggregation of ferritin-concanavalin A (58). Approximately 65% of the insulin receptors were grouped on the prefixed adipocytes and at all time points between 2 and 60 minutes on unfixed cells. Unlike receptors for lectins and immunoglobulins, there was no evidence of time-dependent or occupancy-induced microaggregation of the insulin receptor. The percentage of insulin receptors in groups was independent of insulin concentration in the range of 20 to 400 ng/ml which suggested that the groups were not

[4] The term "organization" of receptors as used in this manuscript refers to the location of occupied insulin receptors relative to other occupied receptors. "Distribution" of receptors refers to the location of receptors with respect to specific cellular structures, *i.e.*, microvilli, pinocytotic invaginations, endosomes, etc. Since Fm-I has been shown to have the same receptor specificity as native insulin (97), insulin receptors and Fm-I receptors are used synonymously. As with ^{125}I-insulin, Fm-I identifies only occupied insulin receptors and it is to be understood that this entire discussion refers only to receptors occupied by the Fm-I molecule.

a function of the percent of total receptors occupied (27, 58, 93). The observations from these studies indicated that insulin receptors existed in naturally formed small groups before and independently from the binding of the hormone. This was the first indication, from morphologic studies, that a difference may exist between insulin and other types of receptors.

Ultrastructural studies performed with human placental syncytial trophoblast (78) confirmed the existence of grouped insulin receptors on another insulin responsive tissue. As a result of these two studies it appeared that insulin receptors on insulin-sensitive cells would share a common ultrastructural organization, even though they might be different from lectin and immunoglobulin receptors.

The steady-state organization of Fm-I receptors on liver plasma membranes was analyzed next (54). In contrast to the predominantly grouped insulin receptors on adipocytes, almost 60% of the receptors on the liver membranes were single molecules with the remainder in natural groups. This was the first indication of cell-specific ultrastructural differences in the organization of insulin receptors on different insulin-sensitive cells.

The initial organization and mobility of insulin receptors was investigated on a variety of other cell types including 3T3-L1 adipocytes (93), H4IIEC3 hepatoma cells (102), IM-9 lymphocytes and human fibroblasts (100). Figure 3 compares the initial organization of Fm-I receptors on these four cell types to that found on rat adipocytes. The rat adipocyte (and placenta as discussed above) proved to be unique in having a large percentage of its insulin receptors initially in natural groups. On each of the other cell types 60 to 80% of the insulin receptors were initially single molecules. Contrary to the results seen in Figure 2, when the cells with predominantly single receptors were incubated at 37° C, all

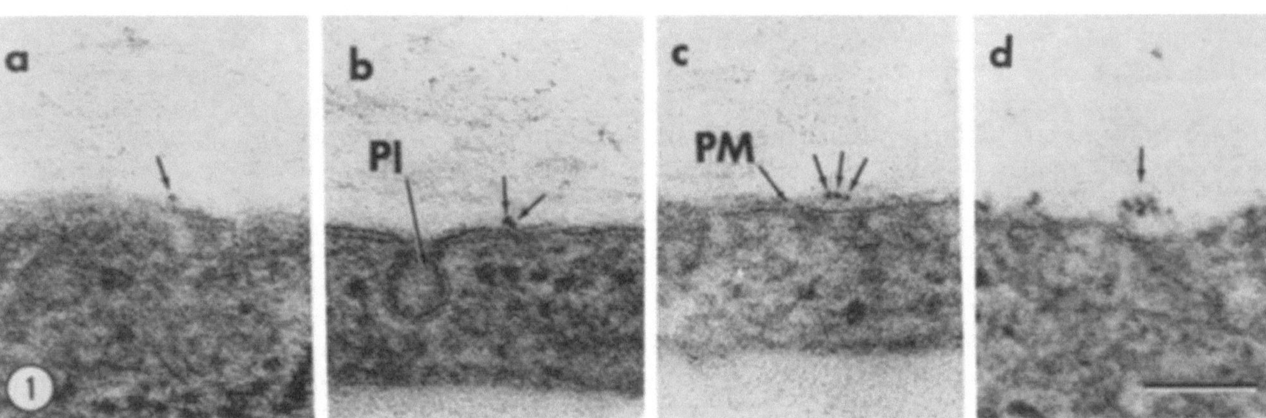

FIG. 1. Electron micrograph demonstrating the organization of ferritin-insulin receptor sites on intact rat adipocytes. Ferritin-insulin molecules (*arrows*) were found in the glycocalyx of the plasma membrane as single molecules (*a*) or, predominantly, in groups of 2 to 6 molecules (*b* to *d*). *PI*, pinocytotic invagination; *PM*, plasma membrane. Bar, 0.1 μm.

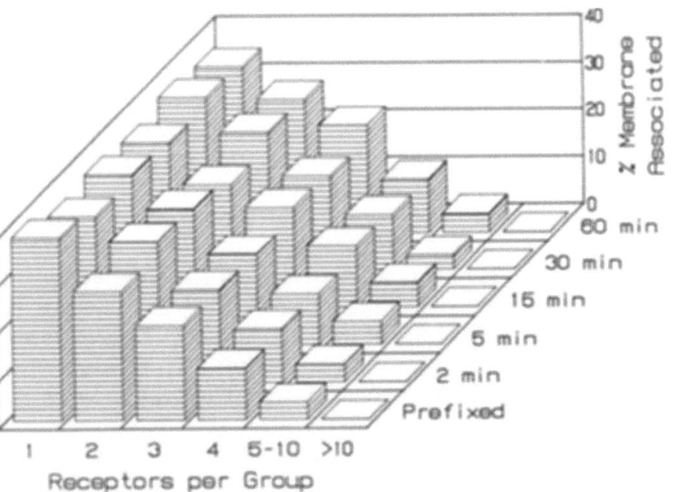

FIG. 2. Organization of ferritin-insulin receptor sites on intact rat adipocytes. Cells were incubated with saturating concentrations of Fm-I for 2 to 60 minutes at 37° C (30 minutes for prefixed cells), washed and prepared for electron microscopy. The prefixed condition provides the organization in the native or unoccupied state. The number of receptor sites/group was analyzed and is expressed as a percentage of the total membrane-associated ferritin particles. No difference in receptor organization was found between prefixed cells or unfixed cells at any time point.

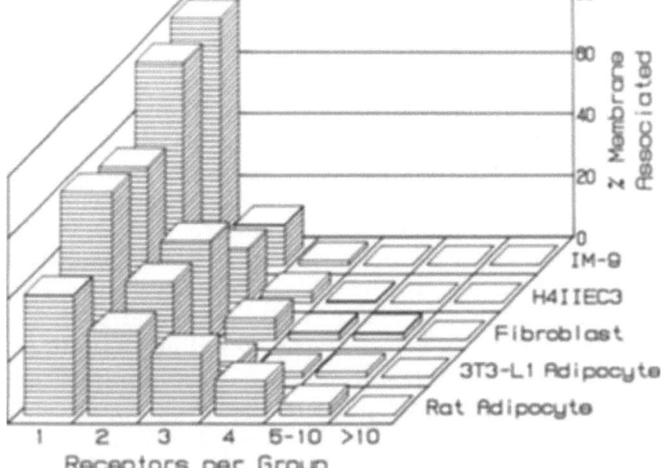

FIG. 3. Difference in the initial organization of ferritin-insulin receptor sites on five cell types. All cells were prefixed and incubated with saturating concentrations of Fm-I for 30 minutes at 37° C, washed and prepared for electron microscopy. The number of receptor sites/group was analyzed and is expressed as a percentage of the total membrane-associated ferritin particles. All cells except the rat adipocyte had a greater percentage of single or nongrouped insulin receptors than grouped receptors in the native or unoccupied state.

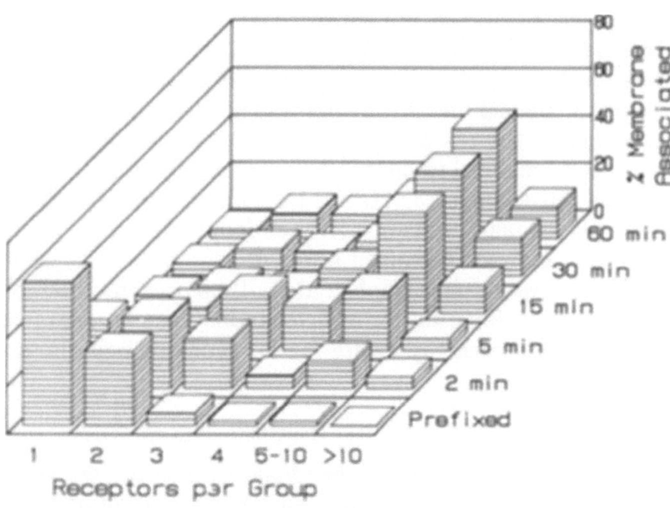

FIG. 4. Organization of ferritin-insulin receptor sites on 3T3-L1 adipocytes. Experimental conditions were the same as in Figure 2. The prefixed cells demonstrate that insulin receptors are not grouped initially. The unfixed cells demonstrate that occupied insulin receptor microaggregate, and within 15 minutes groups of 5 to 10 receptor sites predominated.

showed a marked microaggregation of the occupied receptors. There were only small quantitative differences between these cell types and the reorganization of receptors on the 3T3-L1 adipocyte is representative (Fig. 4). Within 2 minutes, the percentage of single receptors had been reduced by 50%. By 15 minutes, steady-state had been achieved with approximately 90% of the receptors in groups with more than two receptor molecules.

Characteristics of the Naturally Formed Groups of Insulin Receptors

The naturally formed groups of insulin receptors observed on rat adipocytes were investigated to determine the mechanisms controlling the receptor organization. It was reasoned that cytoskeletal proteins, probably microfilaments, might be involved in forming or maintaining the groups as had been implicated in the clustering of lectin and immunoglobulin receptors (106). Cytochalasin B, an agent known to disrupt groups of aggregated receptors (79) possibly through its effect on microfilaments (111), caused a dose-dependent disruption of the groups of Fm-I receptors (59) which suggested that microfilaments did indeed play a role in the organization of the insulin receptor. However, cytochalasin D, a more potent microfilament inhibitor failed to effect receptor organization (75, 111). The most plausible explanation for the differences between the effects of the two cytochalasins was that disulfide bonds and not microfilaments were involved in maintaining the groups. Cytochalasin B has been shown to bind to thiols (70), a property not shared by cytochalasin D.

The disulfide bond hypothesis was tested using dithiothreitol (DTT) and *n*-ethylmaleimide (NEM) treatment of adipocyte plasma membranes (60) before incubating with Fm-I. Both agents caused a significant increase in the number of single insulin receptors, with a corresponding decrease in the number of receptor groups. Disruption of the insulin receptor groups by DTT could be reversed by oxidized glutathione, whereas the effects of NEM were nonreversible. NEM treatment following DTT resulted in a greater decrease in the number of groups than either agent alone. The degree of disruption caused by cytochalasin B, DTT and NEM were comparable. These results suggested that disulfide bonds between adjacent insulin receptors, or between the Fm-I receptors and neighboring protein molecules in the plasma membrane of the rat adipocyte, were responsible for the natural groups of receptors.

Since the ultrastructural studies demonstrated that the organization of the insulin receptors could be altered by disulfide reduction or thiol alkylation, the effects of these treatments on insulin binding was investigated biochemically to determine whether receptor organization was related to binding characteristics (91). Treatment of adipocyte plasma membranes with DTT (0.1 to 1 mM) caused up to a three-fold increase in ^{125}I-insulin binding at low hormone concentrations and the normally curvilinear Scatchard plot was linearized. Both the high and low affinity binding sites were affected resulting in a single site with an intermediate affinity. In contrast, in liver plasma membranes, DTT had no effect on the curvilinear Scatchard plot and increased ^{125}I-insulin binding by only 10 to 20%.

The lack of a significant effect on liver plasma membranes was also observed by Jacobs and Cuatrecasas (52). In addition, they found that DTT treatment of placental membranes resulted in decreased insulin binding and a linearized Scatchard plot. Therefore, three different tissues, with different insulin receptor organizations, showed three different biochemical responses to DTT. These results were the first biochemical evidence that demonstrated a significant cell-specific behavioral difference in insulin receptors.

Shechter *et al.* (92), investigated a possible relationship between the organization of insulin receptors and biochemical characteristics of insulin binding by studying the effects of low concentrations of anti-insulin antibodies on insulin binding to liver and adipocyte plasma membranes. They observed that the bivalent antibody increased insulin binding significantly on liver plasma membranes and linearized the Scatchard plot but that monovalent Fab had no effect. However, when adipocytes were incubated under similar conditions no effects of anti-insulin antibody were observed. Shechter *et al.* (92) concluded that the bivalent antibody externally cross-linked the insulin receptors on liver, changing the overall receptor affinity, and that receptors on the adipocyte were not affected since they were already in microaggregates.

Ultrastructural studies (71) confirmed Shechter's hypothesis. Anti-insulin antibody, over a narrow concentration range, decreased the number of single Fm-I receptors on liver plasma membranes by approximately 50%. The number of receptors in groups of more than two receptor molecules was more than doubled. However, anti-insulin antibody failed to have any effect on the organization of insulin receptors on rat adipocytes.

This last observation raised several questions concerning the mobility of the insulin receptor in adipocytes.

Quite clearly, if the insulin receptors in liver membranes could be microaggregated by anti-insulin antibody, the receptors in liver membranes were mobile. However, if the occupied receptors on adipocytes could not be induced to group, did this demonstrate that they were not mobile? This question has still not been completely resolved. Since the effects of cytochalasin and DTT were reversible, that is, the dispersed receptors reformed groups when cytochalasin B was removed from the incubation media or the cells were incubated with oxidized glutathione after DTT treatment, a certain degree of receptor mobility must be present. The most plausible explanation is that the single insulin receptors are indeed mobile but that they are scattered so widely across the adipocyte cell surface that few single receptors came together to be cross-linked by the anti-insulin antibody. Computer analysis of the distance between receptors demonstrated that the single receptors formed from the disruption of natural groups were significantly closer to other receptors, though not grouped, than the rest of the widely distributed single receptor sites (27), which may explain their ability to reform groups even in the absence of an external cross-linking agent. The large groups of receptors probably have decreased mobility due to their large size and the increased resistance of such groups to diffusion in the lipid bilayer (26).

Summary of Initial Interaction of Insulin with Cell-Membrane Receptors

The data reviewed in the preceding paragraphs demonstrated that, with the exception of the rat adipocyte and the placental syncytial trophoblast, insulin receptors were initially dispersed molecules which rapidly microaggregated after insulin bound to the receptor. Although this might appear to be similar to the observations for α-2-macroglobulin, asialoglycoprotein and other dispersed receptors, as will be shown later the distribution of the microaggregated insulin receptors on most cell types was quite different from that predicted by the LDL model. The studies with disulfide reagents suggested that there was a relationship between the organization of insulin receptors and characteristics of the ligand-receptor interaction, however the importance of receptor organization in insulin action remains unclear. Since receptors were always grouped in intact cells at steady-state, it is tempting to speculate that microaggregation of receptors is necessary for insulin's effects, and such speculations have been made based on other observations (63). The naturally formed groups of insulin receptors on the adipocyte may account for the number of apparent "spare receptors" and the exquisite sensitivity of these cells to insulin if the occupancy of a single receptor in each group could stimulate the neighboring receptor kinases or result in phosphorylation of the remaining receptors in the group.

INSULIN RECEPTOR REDISTRIBUTION AND ENDOCYTOSIS

Several reviews of receptor-mediated endocytosis have been published (4, 40, 86, 112, 114). With few exceptions those articles have reinforced the concept of a universal model based on the uptake of LDL. A common finding in studies of nonhormonal ligands was that the receptor was located in, or, if dispersed, concentrated over, coated areas in the cell membrane prior to endocytosis. In some cases, more than 50% of the membrane associated ligand has been localized in coated pits making up only 2 to 3% of the cell surface (3, 113, 114). This process has been referred to as "concentrative endocytosis" and is an essential component of an efficient endocytosis system. In the following paragraphs data will be presented which should establish that no single endocytotic process or intracellular pathway exists for all types of ligands, especially insulin.

Initial Distribution of Insulin Receptors

In documenting the endocytosis of insulin we compared not only the changes in receptor organization, summarized above, but the initial and time-dependent changes in distribution of insulin receptors on specific cell membrane domains in several cell types. In Figure 5 the initial distribution of insulin receptors on five different cells is compared. All of these cells were prefixed to prevent movement of the occupied insulin receptors. The differences in initial receptor distribution were almost entirely due to structural differences among the cells. Isolated rat adipocytes have no microvilli and are smooth, almost round cells. Pinocytotic invaginations and coated pits account for 15 and 0.3%, respectively, of the adipocyte cell surface (96). On the other cell types, microvilli made up approximately 40% of the cell surface area, pinocytotic invaginations about 5 to 10% and coated pits 1 to 2%.

The Fm-I bound to groups of insulin receptors distributed randomly on the surface of the rat adipocyte. Approximately 13% of the membrane-associated receptors

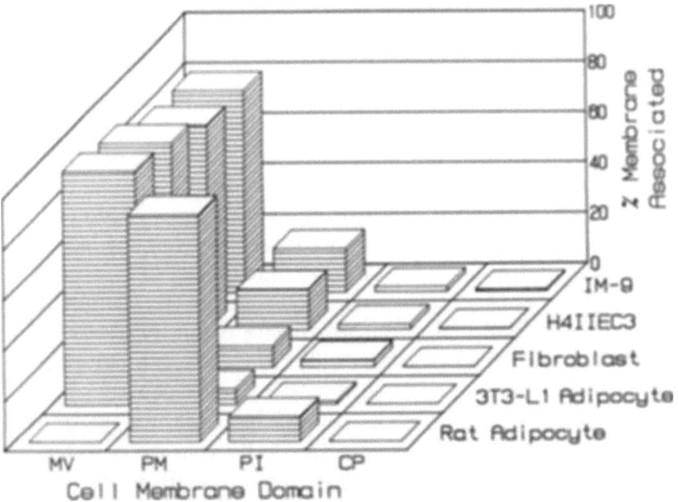

FIG. 5. Difference in the initial distribution of ferritin-insulin receptor sites on five cell types. All cells were prefixed and incubated with saturating concentrations of Fm-I for 30 minutes at 37° C, washed and prepared for electron microscopy. The distribution of receptor sites on microvilli (*MV*), undifferentiated plasma membrane (*PM*), pinocytotic invaginations (*PI*) or coated pits (*CP*) was analyzed and is expressed as a percentage of the total membrane-associated ferritin particles. The vast majority of receptors were initially located on microvilli on those cells with microvilli. Isolated rat adipocytes have no microvilli.

were found in pinocytotic invaginations; none were found in coated pits. On the other four cell types, Fm-I bound preferentially to single insulin receptors located almost exclusively on the microvilli. Preferential binding to microvilli has also been observed in other cell types including human fibroblasts and other hepatoma cell lines (our unpublished observations).

Redistribution of Occupied Insulin Receptors and Localization to Endocytotic Structures

As shown in Figure 6, the time-dependent redistribution of insulin receptors on the rat adipocyte was minimal. There was a small increase in the percentage of Fm-I molecules associated with apparent pinocytotic invaginations (98, 99). The concentration of Fm-I on plasma membrane domains was determined at various time points and the receptor concentration remained stable on the plasma membrane at approximately 25 receptors/μm^2. In pinocytotic invaginations, receptor concentration increased from 13.6 to the same level as on the plasma membrane within 10 minutes. There was no time-dependent increase in the concentration of the ligand in coated pits. Furthermore, the concentration of Fm-I particles in the coated pits on adipocytes was significantly lower than on other areas of the cell surface which suggested that insulin receptors may be excluded from the coated pits. Since the concentration of insulin receptors in the pinocytotic invaginations was no greater than the concentration on the rest of the plasma membrane, it was concluded that receptor-mediated endocytosis of insulin in the rat adipocyte was a random, not concentrative, process.

The redistribution of insulin receptors was assessed on 3T3-L1 adipocytes (93). As shown in Figure 7, within 2 minutes, a substantial percentage of the occupied receptors had migrated from the microvilli to the undifferentiated plasma membrane and a steady-state distribution between the microvilli and plasma membrane was

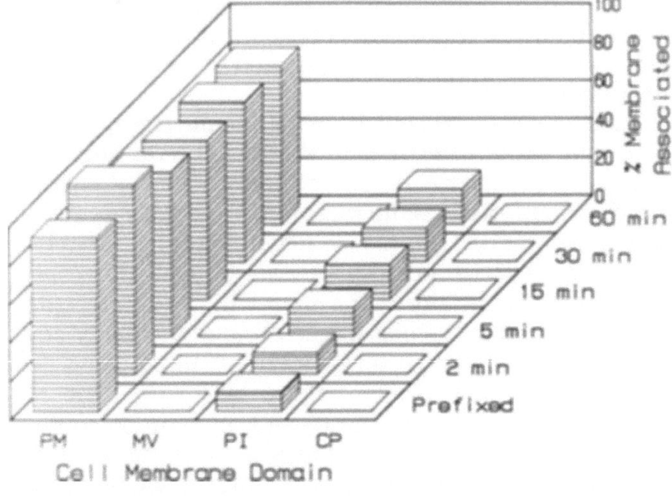

Fig. 6. Redistribution of occupied ferritin-insulin receptors on intact rat adipocytes. Experimental conditions were the same as in Figure 2. A slight decrease was found in the percentage of Fm-I receptors on the plasma membrane (*PM*) along with a corresponding increase in receptors in pinocytotic invaginations (*PI*). No receptors were observed in coated pits (*CP*) at any time point.

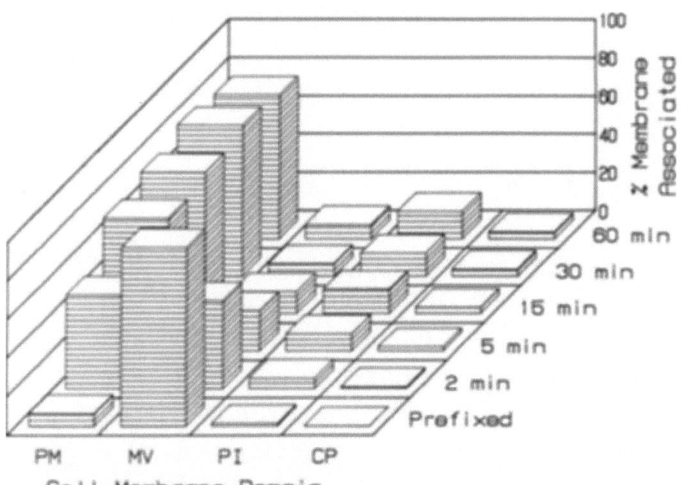

Fig. 7. Redistribution of occupied ferritin-insulin receptors on 3T3-L1 adipocytes. Experimental conditions were the same as in Figure 4. The occupied insulin receptors moved from microvilli (*MV*) to the undifferentiated plasma membrane (*PM*). A steady-state distribution was attained within approximately 5 minutes. Insulin receptors were observed in pinocytotic invaginations (*PI*) and in coated pits (*CP*) in proportion to the amount of surface area each of these domains contribute to the cell surface.

seen between 5 and 10 minutes. There was a time-dependent increase in the percentage of receptors in pinocytotic invaginations and in coated pits. However, the total amount of Fm-I in each of those structures was approximately proportional to the amount of cell surface area contributed by each type of endocytotic structure. The concentration of Fm-I receptors in pinocytotic invaginations and coated pits did not exceed the concentration of receptors on the undifferentiated plasma membrane. These data showed that insulin receptors were randomly redistributed and endocytosed in both pinocytotic invaginations and coated pits, as opposed to being concentratively endocytosed. Although these studies did not address differences in the rates of endocytosis via pinocytotic invaginations or coated pits, the fact that pinocytotic invaginations were at least 10 times more plentiful suggested that endocytosis via coated pits contributed only a small fraction of the intracellular hormone.

Redistribution of insulin receptors on the IM-9 lymphocyte (100) was, in most respects, similar to that found in the 3T3-L1 adipocyte. There was one significant difference. As the Fm-I occupied receptors microaggrated and migrated from the microvilli to the plasma membrane, large numbers of receptors were shed from the cell surface as shown in Figure 8. The Fm-I particles were almost always on the exterior of the electron-dense material, which was believed to be similar to the glycocalyx of the cell membrane. It has been previously reported that insulin receptors on IM-9 cells were water soluble and could be purified from the incubation media (24) and the observed shedding supports this concept. The IM-9 lymphocyte has been used for a large number of biochemical studies characterizing insulin's interaction with its receptor. One of the well-defined characteristics of that interactions is receptor down regulation

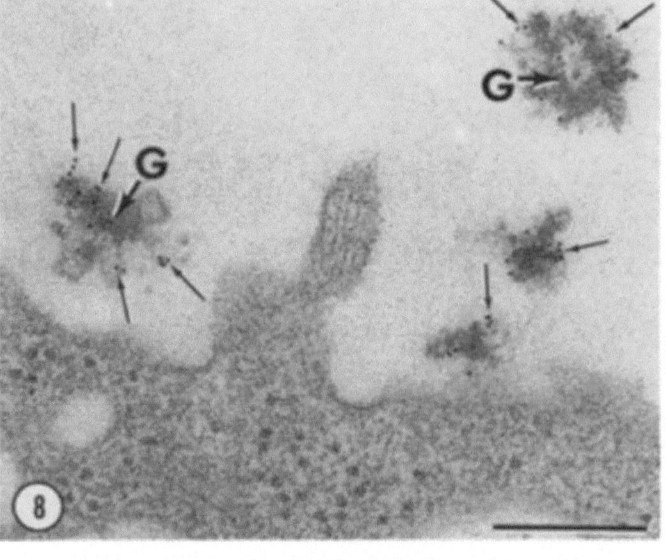

FIG. 8. Electron micrograph demonstrating shedding of occupied ferritin-insulin receptors from IM-9 lymphocytes. Cells were incubated with Fm-I for 30 minutes at 37° C and prepared for electron microscopy. Substantial amounts of glycocalyx-like material (*G*) was observed which was apparently shed from the cell surface. Fm-I particles (*arrows*) were observed primarily on the periphery of this material. Bar, 0.2 μm.

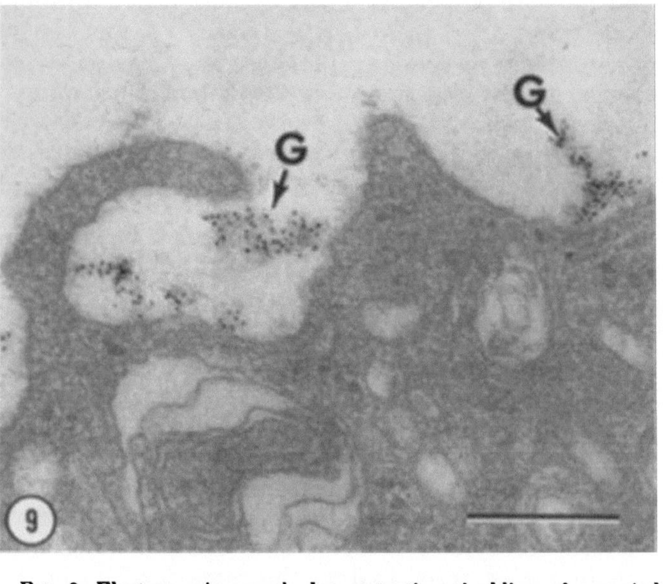

FIG. 9. Electron micrograph demonstrating shedding of occupied ferritin-insulin receptors from H4IIEC3 hepatoma cells. Cells were incubated with Fm-I for 30 minutes at 37° C and prepared for electron microscopy. A small amount of glycocalyx-like material (*G*) was observed which was apparently shed from the cell surface. In contrast to the Fm-I binding in the material shed from the IM-9 lymphocyte, the Fm-I particles were found distributed almost evenly throughout the glycocalyx-like material. Bar, 0.2 μm.

(25). Our observations would suggest that significant numbers of insulin receptors are lost from the cell surface due to shedding of the insulin-receptor complex, not due to internalization of the insulin-receptor complex (see Figure 11).

The redistribution of receptors on the H4IIEC3 hepatoma cell line was also comparable to the 3T3-L1 adipocyte with a rapid decrease in the number of receptors on the microvilli accounted for by an increase in receptors on the plasma membrane (102). The relative distribution of receptors in pinocytotic invaginations and coated pits was proportional to the surface area contributed by these structures. The concentration of Fm-I molecules in each structure indicated that neither the invaginations nor coated pits concentrated the insulin receptor. Once again, insulin receptor-mediated endocytosis was random, not concentrative. There was a small amount of shedding of receptors from the cell surface of hepatoma cells (Fig. 9), however the arrangement of the Fm-I molecules in the electron-dense material was different than that observed in IM-9 lymphocytes. The Fm-I particles were found distributed throughout the glycocalyx clump, rather than on the exterior. A major difference was found in receptor redistribution on the hepatoma cell, unlike any of the previously examined cell types. Insulin receptors on H4IIEC3 hepatoma cells formed relatively large microaggregates on the cell surface. These aggregates appeared to be internalized when the distal tips of microvilli fused with the cell membrane and formed a macrophagosome. This process resulted in large amounts of Fm-I being internalized into large endosomes.

Investigations of other cultured cell lines, including H35 hepatoma cells and human fibroblasts showed patterns similar to that observed with the 3T3-L1 adipocyte. In studies investigating the development of insulin receptors in mouse embryos (47), a significantly different distribution of receptors was observed. At steady-state, insulin receptors on blastocyst stage embryos were found in small groups on the membrane of the trophoblasts, with few single receptors on microvilli projecting into the zona pellucida. There were few pinocytotic invaginations observed, however, coated areas of the membrane were prevalent and contributed 5 to 8% of the cell surface. Unlike the other cells studied, insulin receptors were concentrated over these coated areas. In developing mouse embryos endocytosis of the insulin-receptor complex was concentrative and appeared to mediated almost entirely by coated pits.

In summary, redistribution of insulin receptors fell into four major categories (Table 1). The rat adipocyte, which lacked microvilli, showed only minor changes in the distribution of insulin receptors. Cells with numerous microvilli (H4IIEC3 and H35 hepatoma cells, IM-9 lymphocytes, 3T3-L1 adipocytes and human fibroblasts) bound insulin initially on the microvilli. Insulin receptors rapidly moved to the plasma membrane. At steady-state, the insulin receptors on all cells except the adipocyte and trophoblast of the mouse embryo blastocyst were randomly distributed over the plasma membrane, pinocytotic invaginations and coated pits. The rat adipocyte appeared to exclude insulin receptors from the coated pits while insulin receptors were concentrated in the coated pits on mouse embryo cells. These variations suggested that cell-specific mechanisms controlled the internalization process of insulin receptors.

TABLE 1. INITIAL AND STEADY-STATE DISTRIBUTION OF INSULIN RECEPTORS ON VARIOUS CELL TYPES

Cell type	Distribution	
	Initial	Steady-state
Rat adipocyte	Plasma membrane and invaginations	Plasma membrane and invaginations
3T3-L1 Adipocyte, H35 hepatoma, H4IIEC3 hepatoma and human fibroblasts	Microvilli and plasma membrane	Plasma membrane, invaginations, microvilli and coated pits
IM-9 lymphocytes	Microvilli and plasma membrane	Plasma membrane and microvilli
Mouse embryo trophoblast	Plasma membrane and coated pits	Coated pits, plasma membrane and microvilli

The initial distribution of insulin receptors was determined with cells that were prefixed before the addition of monomeric ferritin-insulin or colloidal-gold-insulin. The prefixed cells were incubated for 30 to 45 minutes with ligand. Steady-state distribution was determined after normal (unfixed) cells were incubated with ligand for 30 to 45 minutes at 37° C. The electron-dense particles were analyzed on the basis of their association with four discrete morphologic areas of the cell membrane: microvilli, pinocytotic invaginations, coated pits, and (the remaining unspecialized surface) plasma membrane.

ULTRASTRUCTURAL COMPARISON OF INSULIN AND α-2-MACROGLOBULIN INTERNALIZATION ON RAT ADIPOCYTES

The lack of Fm-I particles in coated pits on rat adipocytes was contrary to the model proposed for receptor-mediated endocytosis (3, 40, 112, 113) and raised several possibilities. The comparatively low number of coated pits on the adipocyte may have been non-functional and the cell may have adapted the relatively high number of pinocytotic invaginations to overcome this deficiency. Another alternative suggested was that the coated pits may turn over so rapidly that our chance of observing Fm-I in those structures was unlikely. If that were true, very few coated pits could never the less internalize substantial amounts of insulin. Lastly, insulin receptors could be different from other receptors and utilize pinocytotic invaginations rather than coated pits as their primary endocytotic structure. The last question had been addressed by documenting the random endocytosis of insulin in coated pits in different cell types (100) which had higher concentrations of coated pits. Therefore, we needed to establish whether the apparent exclusion of insulin from coated pits on adipocytes was in fact an exclusion or whether coated pits were nonfunctional. This was accomplished by comparing the endocytosis of insulin and α-2-macroglobulin since α-2-macroglobulin is internalized exclusively by coated pits on fibroblasts (113).

A colloidal-gold α-2-macroglobulin-methylamine complex (Au-a2M) was prepared and its distribution compared to that of Fm-I on the cell surface (32). When adipocytes were incubated at 4° C to prevent ligand internalization, but permit maximal accumulation of ligand in endocytotic structures, over 17% of the Au-a2M was localized over coated pits and only 0.1% was found in pinocytotic invaginations (Table 2). At the same time approximately 9% of the Fm-I was in pinocytotic invaginations and only 0.6% was in coated pits. Given the relative amount of surface area of these structures, these data indicate that at 4° C, α-2-macroglobulin receptors were concentrated over 50-fold in the adipocyte coated pits and were greater than 99% excluded from pinocytotic invaginations. On the other hand insulin was randomly distributed between both coated pits and pinocytotic invaginations. When the cells were incubated for 30 minutes at 37° C, the percentage of total cell-associated ligand in the coated pits decreased for both α-2-macroglobulin and insulin as shown in the lower half of Table 2. This decrease was most probably due to the rapid internalization of the coated pit at 37° C which prevented the accumulation of ligand seen in the cells incubated at 4° C. In spite of the decrease, α-2-macroglobulin receptors were still concentrated (6.5×) in coated pits, whereas insulin receptors were excluded or simply not detected. Calculations performed on the basis of these observations indicated that greater than 99% of the internalized α-2-macroglobulin was internalized via coated pits and 99% of the insulin entered via pinocytotic invaginations. These comparative ultrastructural data provided conclusive evidence that coated pits were functional on rat adipocytes and that receptors for different ligands can

TABLE 2. COMPARISON OF THE DISTRIBUTION OF α-2-MACROGLOBULIN AND INSULIN RECEPTORS IN RAT ADIPOCYTE INVAGINATIONS AND COATED PITS

	α-2-Macroglobulin	Insulin
Cells incubated at 4° C		
Percentage of ligand associated with:		
Pinocytotic invaginations	0.1	8.7
Coated pits	17.7	0.6
Relative concentration in:		
Pinocytotic invaginations	0.007	0.83
Coated pits	52.2	1.06
Cells incubated at 37° C		
Percentage of ligand associated with:		
Pinocytotic invaginations	0.9	2.6
Coated pits	2.6	0.0
Relative concentration in:		
Pinocytotic invaginations	0.06	1.36
Coated pits	6.6	0.0

Rat adipocytes were incubated with colloidal gold α-2-macroglobulin-methylamine or monomeric ferritin-insulin for 90 minutes at 4° C or 30 minutes at 37° C. Receptor distribution was determined and expressed as a percentage of the total membrane-associated ligand. "Relative Concentration" in pinocytotic invaginations and coated pits compares the amount of ligand associated with those areas of the plasma membrane in relationship to the amount that each of those domains contributes to the total cell surface. A random distribution would result in a value of approximately 1.0; values greater than 1.0 suggest ligand concentration in a domain, whereas values less than 1.0 imply an exclusion.

have entirely different endocytotic pathways on the same cell type.

Biochemical Evidence of Differences in Insulin Binding or Endocytosis and Intracellular Processing

Several laboratories have used agents which inhibit extracellular and lysosomal proteases (30, 38, 43, 44, 50, 61, 104), formation of coated vesicles (11, 30, 43, 87), acidification of endosomes (30, 43, 50, 87, 107) and energy production or utilization (82, 107) in order to block steps in the processing of insulin and other ligands. While this should be an excellent method of determining the sequential route of receptor-mediated endocytosis, when inhibitors affect more than one process, or affect undocumented processes, the interpretation of the data becomes difficult. Despite this problem, and with some reservations, we investigated the effects of a number of these agents on insulin uptake in different cell types (23, 94).

Bacitracin is a cyclic polypeptide antibiotic which has been used at a concentration of about 1 mM to inhibit the proteolytic degradation of insulin (38, 44, 104). The effects of bacitracin on insulin binding and degradation were determined in several different cell types (23). Bacitracin was shown to inhibit both cell associated and media degradation of insulin in different cell types, although concentrations yielding half-maximal inhibition varied from 25 to 250 μM. When insulin binding was measured at concentrations of bacitracin greater than 250 μM, bactracin increased insulin binding to rat adipocytes, but decreased cell associated insulin in 3T3-L1 preadipocytes and adipocytes, human fibroblasts and H4IIEC3 hepatoma cells. This effect was temperature dependent and seen only when cells were incubated at 24 to 37° C. As shown in Figure 10, when cells were incubated with concentrations of bacitracin causing half-maximal inhibition of insulin degradation, intracellular accumulation of insulin was slightly increased in rat adipocytes and decreased by 40 to 70% in H4IIEC3 hepatoma cells, and 3T3-L1 preadipocytes and adipocytes. Intracellular accumulation was only slightly decreased in human fibroblasts and unaffected in IM-9 lymphocytes. These data suggested that cell-specific differences exist either in the processes or proteases that bacitracin affects or in the processing of insulin by these cells.

Chloroquine has been used by numerous investigators to prevent the "lysosomal" processing of ligands. Current evidence suggests that one of the effects of chloroquine may be at an earlier intracellular step, perhaps in acidic organelles (12). When treated with chloroquine all cells, except H4IIEC3 hepatoma cells and IM-9 lymphocytes, showed a significant increase in both total cell associated insulin and intracellular insulin (Fig. 11) (94).

Methylamine and dansylcadaverine which reportedly affect endocytosis of ligands via coated pits by inhibiting transglutaminase activity (11) had no effects on intracellular accumulation of insulin in rat adipocytes or 3T3-L1 preadipocytes (94). Intracellular accumulation of insulin in 3T3-L1 adipocytes was increased by methylamine and decreased by dansylcadaverine. Both agents decreased insulin accumulation slightly in fibroblasts. Methylamine decreased, while dansylcadaverine increased, insulin accumulation in H4IIEC3 hepatoma

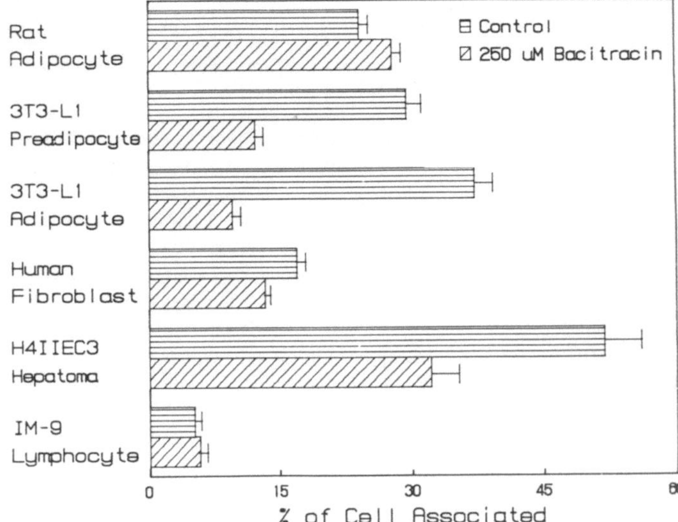

FIG. 10. Effect of 250 μM bacitracin on intracellular accumulation of ^{125}I-insulin in various cell types. Cells were preincubated for 15 minutes at 37° C with 250 μM bacitracin. ^{125}I-insulin (2 ng/ml) was added and the cells incubated an additional 30 minutes. The intracellular accumulation of insulin was determined and expressed as a percentage of total cell associated. Under control conditions intracellular accumulation of insulin ranged from greater than 50% (H4IIEC3 hepatoma cells) to less than 10% (IM-9 lymphocytes) of total cell associated. Bacitracin significantly reduced intracellular accumulation in 3T3-L1 preadipocytes and adipocytes, human fibroblasts and H4IIEC3 hepatoma cells. Intracellular accumulation of ^{125}I-insulin was increased by bacitracin in rat adipocytes and there was no effect on IM-9 lymphocytes.

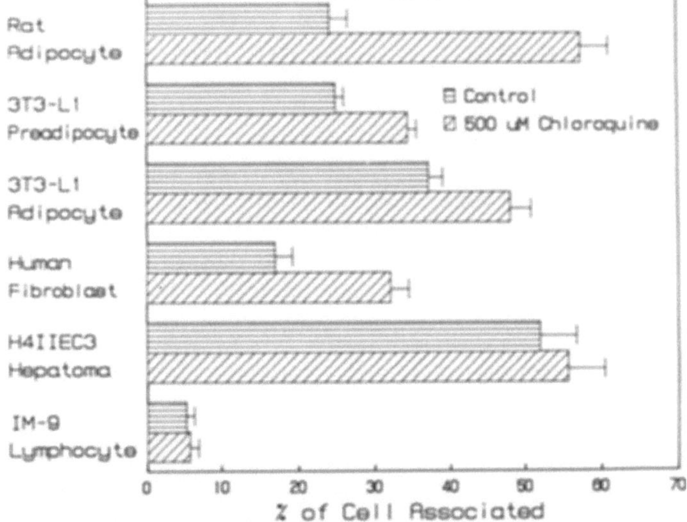

FIG. 11. Effect of 500 μM chloroquine on intracellular accumulation of ^{125}I-insulin in various cell types. Experimental conditions were as described in Figure 10 except the cells were preincubated with 500 μM chloroquine. The magnitude of chloroquine's effect varied greatly between different cell types. Intracellular accumulation was increased greatest in rat adipocytes but significant increases were found in 3T3-L1 preadipocytes and adipocytes, and human fibroblasts. Chloroquine did not affect intracellular accumulation of ^{125}I-insulin in H4IIEC3 hepatoma cells or IM-9 lymphocytes.

cells. IM-9 cells were not affected. The effect of these agents could not be consistently correlated with the amount of Fm-I that would be internalized via coated pits.

Biochemical Comparison of α-2-Macroglobulin and Insulin Internalization in Rat Adipocytes and H35 Hepatoma Cells

Insulin and α-2-macroglobulin processing in rat adipocytes was compared by Gliemann and Sonne (30) using various inhibitors. Their results demonstrated striking differences between the effects of inhibitors on the two ligands. In summary, cell associated insulin was increased by colchicine, vinblastine, monensin, and chloroquine, whereas α-2-macroglobulin was decreased by each of these inhibitors. Leupeptin, a lysosomal protease inhibitor, had no effect on insulin accumulation or degradation but increased α-2-macroglobulin accumulation and decreased its degradation. NH_4Cl, methylamine, dansylcadaverine and dinitrophenol decreased α-2-macroglobulin binding and degradation without having a significant effect on insulin binding or processing. Equal concentrations of cyanide blocked all α-2-macroglobulin binding and degradation, while inhibiting only about 50% of insulin's association and degradation. These data indicate that the mechanisms controlling the association of these two ligands, their internalization and their intracellular processing are substantially different.

We have investigated differences in the processing of α-2-macroglobulin and insulin in H35 hepatoma cells. Many of our findings (Table 3) were similar to those of Gliemann and Sonne (30). We were particularly interested in the differences in the effects of chloroquine and monensin, two agents that should sequester the ligand-receptor complex in intracellular organelles, and increase cellular accumulation of both insulin and α-2-macroglobulin. Cells were incubated for 30 minutes at 37° C with chloroquine or monensin in the absence of ligand, chilled to 4° C, and ^{125}I-insulin or α-2-macroglobulin was added to measure ligand binding to cell surface receptors. As shown in Table 4, chloroquine and monensin resulted in a decrease in the number of α-2-macroglobulin receptors expressed on the cell surface without affecting insulin receptors.

This observation suggested another striking difference between the internalization of the two receptors. α-2-Macroglobulin receptors apparently were internalized constitutively in the absence of bound ligand. Therefore, in the presence of agents which inhibit receptor recycling, the number of receptors available on the cell surface decreased rapidly. On the other hand, no detectable decrease in insulin receptors suggested that those receptors were internalized only after insulin bound. It was possible that the failure to observe a decrease in insulin binding was due to a large number of "spare receptors" and the low concentration of insulin used to measure binding. This was tested by incubating chloroquine or monensin treated cells with saturating concentrations of insulin (1 μg/ml) for 4 hours at 4° C. No decrease in insulin binding was found in the chloroquine or monensin treated cells which suggested that no significant constitutive internalization of the insulin receptor occurred during the incubation at 37° C in the presence or absence of chloroquine or monensin.

Table 3. Effects of Inhibitors on the Intracellular Accumulation of ^{125}I-Insulin or ^{125}I-α-2-Macroglobulin-Methylamine in H35 Hepatoma Cells

Inhibitor	Insulin	α-2-Macroglobulin
	(% of Control)	
500 μM Chloroquine	249.8 ± 25.1	62.5 ± 0.9
25 μM Monensin	353.5 ± 28.1	30.2 ± 9.5
100 μg/ml Leupeptin	99.2 ± 3.8	140.1 ± 9.1
100 μM Cyto. D	103.7 ± 7.6	34.9 ± 9.0
5 mM NaN_3	100.9 ± 6.7	23.7 ± 2.6
20 mM NaN_3	102.1 ± 7.8	9.1 ± 0.8
5 mM DNP	100.2 ± 7.2	10.3 ± 1.2
20 mM DNP	94.6 ± 6.6	4.1 ± 1.3
5 mM KCN	98.7 ± 4.5	9.6 ± 4.5
20 mM KCN	64.1 ± 8.2	1.5 ± 1.1

H35 hepatoma cells were incubated with the indicated agent for 30 minutes before the addition of either ^{125}I-insulin or ^{125}I-α-2-macroglobulin methylamine. The cells were incubated for an additional 30 minutes at 37° C. Intracellular accumulation of insulin was assessed by removing surface bound hormone with an acidic buffer wash; surface bound α-2-macroglobulin methylamine was removed by a 1 mM EDTA wash.

Table 4. Effect of Chloroquine or Monensin Pretreatment on ^{125}I-Insulin or ^{125}I-α-2-Macroglobulin-Methylamine Binding to Cell Surface Receptors on H35 Hepatoma Cells

Ligand	Addition	Preincubation temperature (° C) 4	37
		(% of Control)	
^{125}I-Insulin			
	500 μM Chloroquine	114.5 ± 4.5	112.5 ± 5.4
	25 μM Monensin	117.6 ± 5.8	109.4 ± 4.5
^{125}I-α-2-Macroglobulin-methylamine			
	500 μM Chloroquine	99.8 ± 5.3	72.6 ± 4.5
	25 μM Monensin	92.9 ± 7.5	50.9 ± 5.6

H35 hepatoma cells were preincubated for 30 minutes at the indicated temperature with the agent shown. The cells were chilled to 4° C and saturating concentrations of ^{125}I-insulin or ^{125}I-α-2-macroglobulin were added and the cells were incubated for 90 minutes. Since internalization of the ligand-receptor complex was negligible at 4° C (data not shown), cell-associated ligand represents binding to available receptors on the cell surface.

Intracellular Pathways of Ligand and Receptor Processing

At one time it was widely believed that insulin was not internalized (10) because insulin's effects were caused by binding to a cell membrane receptor. This concept gradually changed as a result of several observations. Biochemical subcellular fractionation studies by Bergeron, Posner, and colleagues (5), Goldfine and colleagues (36) and others (31, 49) demonstrated that insulin could bind to various isolated intracellular organelles including nuclei, nuclear membranes, and Golgi (reviewed in Ref. 34).

Some of these studies were not generally accepted because of the difficulty in assessing potential plasma membrane contamination of the subcellular fractions. Furthermore, the existence of intracellular proteins capable of binding insulin did not prove that insulin, located on or outside the cell membrane, could enter the cell. This latter question was resolved when cell fractionations performed after cells were incubated with ^{125}I-insulin found insulin in vesicles, and in Golgi and Golgi-like fractions although little or no insulin was found in lysosomes or nuclei (reviewed in Refs. 4, 37, 48). The internalization of insulin into hepatocytes, IM-9 lymphocytes, and adipocytes was documented morphologically using autoradiography (86) and monomeric ferritin-insulin (100). A number of laboratories have now used biochemical and ultrastructural techniques to demonstrate insulin internalization in a variety of cell types.

Determining Intracellular Pathways of Insulin-Receptor Complexes

Several laboratories have studied the internalization of insulin using biochemical methods and have published sometimes conflicting data concerning the intracellular localization of insulin. Differences in intracellular location of insulin have also been found in morphologic studies. These reports have been reviewed (4, 35, 37, 48, 86). Insulin in a variety of cell types has been localized in vesicles of various sizes, densities and enzymatic characteristics, in "lysosomes" and similar organelles, in Golgi and related vesicles and in nuclei. Demonstrating the intracellular pathway using either biochemical or ultrastructural techniques is a difficult task due to a number of problems.

When subcellular fractionation is used to localize either receptors or insulin, actual or perceived cross contamination between subcellular fractions inevitably complicates the analysis. When morphological analyses are used several problems arise. A large number of terms almost synonymous with "endosomes" have been introduced. Some of these terms are attempts to define a specific vesicular structure by size, appearance (multivesicular body) or shape (tubular vesicle). Other investigators describe structures on the basis of histochemical characteristics (acidic organelles, phosphatase-positive lysosomes, etc.). This leads to some difficulty in comparing the localization of ligands in one study to another study using different terminology for, perhaps, the same structures. The precision in localizing the ligand by light or electron microscopy is necessarily limited to the resolution of the technique involved. Although autoradiography may be less precise (because the grain may be 1000 Å from the hormone (90)) than electron-dense ligands (ferritin or gold conjugates), autoradiography has been used successfully by many laboratories. Finally, the accuracy of any determination made by ultrastructural techniques can be severely handicapped by the size of the sample analyzed. To illustrate this point, a single datum point in a biochemical binding assay may be derived from the average of as many as 10^9 to 10^{12} receptors. That large a sample size is not practical, nor is it necessary, in morphologic studies. The limits of detection in ultrastructural studies are several orders of magnitude more sensitive than in biochemical analyses. We have generally analyzed 1200 to 3000 receptor sites/experiments condition while others have used less (21) coupled with computer analysis.

In almost all studies, labeled insulin has been used to analyze the distribution of both hormone and its receptor. However, dissociation of insulin from the receptor, whether in response to decreased pH in acidic organelles or in the same manner as at the cell surface, may make speculations on the location of the receptor suspect. The use of photoaffinity labeled ^{125}I-insulin (8, 22, 45) can eliminate the dissociation of insulin from its receptor as long as the 95% or more of the bound insulin which does not become crosslinked to the receptor (116) is thoroughly removed from the cell membrane before endocytosis begins. If the noncross-linked insulin is not removed there is little advantage in using the photoaffinity ligand.

Ultrastructural Analysis of the Intracellular Processing of Insulin in Rat Adipocytes

The time-dependent uptake of Fm-I was found to occur exclusively in pinocytotic invaginations which became small endosomes (98, 99). At later times Fm-I was found in larger endosomes, multivesicular bodies and lysosome-like structures. The time course of Fm-I accumulation is shown in Figure 12. Fm-I accumulation in pinocytotic invaginations and endosomes reached a steady state between 10 and 15 minutes. Steady-state in multivesicular bodies and lysosome-like structures did not occur for another five minutes. The amount of Fm-I was greatest in pinocytotic invaginations and the least in a multivesicular bodies and lysosomes. The differences in the amount of insulin in the successive intracellular compartments, in addition to the differences in time to steady-state, suggested that the Fm-I was being recycled through an endosome compartment to the plasma mem-

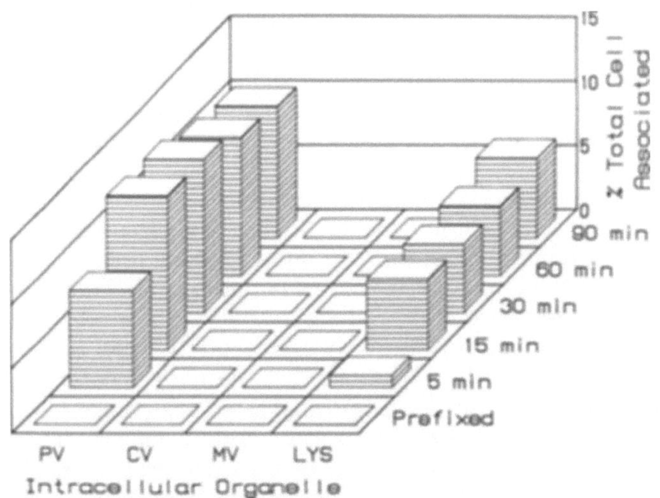

FIG. 12. Intracellular distribution of ferritin-insulin particles in rat adipocytes. Experimental conditions were the same as in Figure 2 except cells were incubated 5 to 90 minutes at 37° C. The majority of intracellular Fm-I particles were found in small pinocytotic vesicles (*PV*). No Fm-I particles were observed in coated vesicles (*CV*). Approximately 7% of the total cell associated Fm-I particle were found in multivesicular bodies and lysosomes (*LYS*).

branes in structures which appeared to be pinocytotic invaginations. Less than 10% of the cell associated Fm-I was found in lysosomes at steady state.

The addition of chloroquine resulted in several changes. As many investigators have reported, chloroquine increased the intracellular accumulation of insulin in adipocytes (see Fig. 11). A morphologic comparison of normal cells and cells treated with chloroquine show significant differences in the appearance of cytoplasmic organelles (115). In rat adipocytes, the number of multivesicular bodies and lysosome-like structures were increased. Various cytoplasmic structures (endosomes, endoplasmic reticulum, and Golgi) were enlarged with swollen cisternae. Morphometric analysis showed that chloroquine had no effect on the amount of Fm-I in small or large endosomes but increased the amount of Fm-I in the multivesicular bodies and lysosomes from approximately 7% in the control to 23% of the cell associated Fm-I (98). These studies suggested that chloroquine increased intracellular insulin by inhibiting the turnover or normal sequential development of multivesicular bodies and lysosomes, resulting in an increased number of these structures containing Fm-I, as well as preventing degradation of the insulin within the lysosome.

Ultrastructural Comparison of Intracellular Processing of Insulin in Other Cell Types

Given the differences in insulin receptor redistribution between adipocytes and other cell types such as H4IIEC3 hepatoma cells, 3T3-L1 adipocytes and IM-9 lymphocytes, one might expect to see differences in the intracellular pathways. Insulin internalization in IM-9 lymphocytes was difficult to quantify in the manner described for adipocytes due to the low amount of insulin internalized by this cell (see Fig. 11). However, insulin was found in small and large endosomes and in multivesicular bodies (100). Lysosome-like structures were rarely seen and less than 5% had any Fm-I (as compared with 24% of adipocyte lysosomes containing Fm-I molecules).

Over 30% of Fm-I receptors on H4IIEC3 hepatoma cells were internalized into large macrovesicles or phagosomes (Fig. 13). Less than 10% and 5% of the receptors were in endosomes and lysosomes, respectively. Only 3% of the Fm-I particles were seen in apparent coated vesicles. Chloroquine treatment caused the same type of morphologic changes in the number and structure of intracellular organelles as was seen in adipocytes but failed to increase the amount of Fm-I in the phagosomes and had no significant effect on the number of particles in lysosomes (102).

Insulin internalization into 3T3-L1 adipocytes (Fig. 14) was similar qualitatively to that seen in rat adipocytes. The major differences were that about 2% of the cell associated ligand was found in apparent coated vesicles and approximately 15% was found in multivesicular bodies and lysosomes. The amount of Fm-I in multivesicular bodies and lysosomes was considerably higher in 3T3-L1 adipocytes than in the other cells studied, and was even higher than the amount found in the endosomes. This suggested that more of the insulin may be translocated to the multivesicular bodies and lysosomes and less recycled to the cell surface.

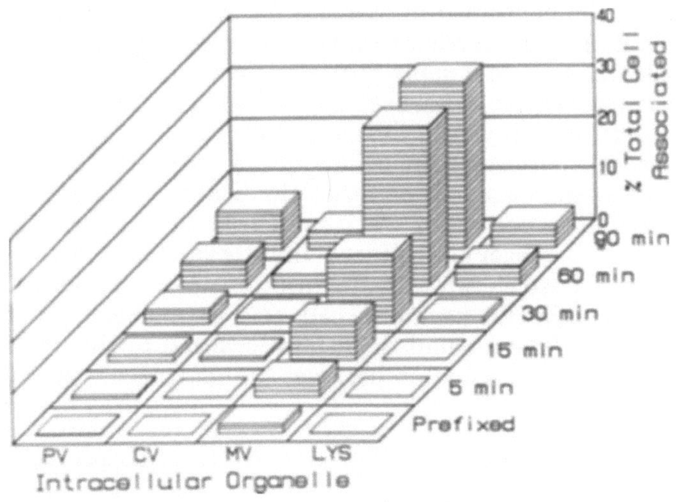

Fig. 13. Intracellular distribution of ferritin-insulin particles in H4IIEC3 hepatoma cells. Experimental conditions were the same as in Figure 12. The vast majority of the internalized Fm-I particles was found in unique structures identified as macrovesicles (*MV*) which apparently originated from the internalization of Fm-I aggregates by macropinocytosis. Fm-I was also found in pinocytotic vesicles (*PV*), coated vesicles (*CV*), and multivesicular bodies and lysosomes (*LYS*).

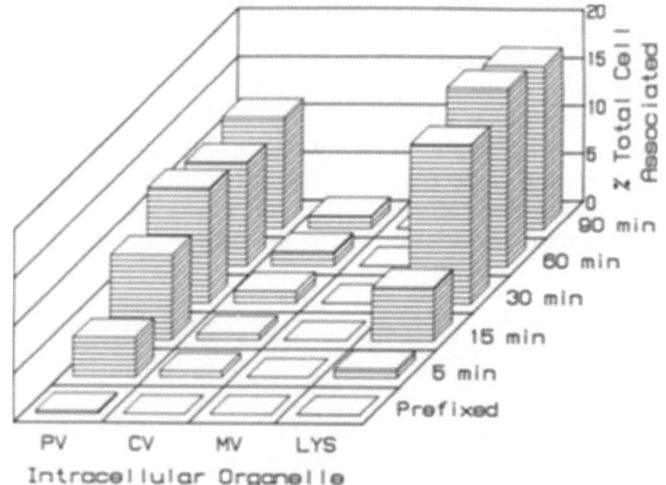

Fig. 14. Intracellular distribution of ferritin-insulin particles in 3T3-L1 adipocytes. Experimental conditions were the same as in Figure 12. The 3T3-L1 adipocyte differed from the rat adipocyte (Figure 12) by having some Fm-I particles in coated vesicles (*CV*) and by accumulating more Fm-I in multivesicular bodies and lysosomes (LYS) than in the vesicular structures.

Translocation of Insulin and Insulin-Receptor Complexes to Nuclei

While analyzing the intracellular distribution of insulin in the 3T3-L1 adipocyte, Fm-I particles were detected in the nucleus. This led to a detailed biochemical and ultrastructural study of nuclear accumulation in 3T3-L1 adipocyte nuclei (101). Nuclear accumulation was shown to be time- and temperature-dependent. Whereas steady-state levels of Fm-I were reached in all other intracellular organelles within 15 to 20 minutes, Fm-I accumulation in nuclei continued to increase for at least 90 minutes. Multiple Fm-I particles were generally found in the same general area, invariably near a nuclear pore and in or at the edge of the condensed chromatin (Fig. 15). Autoradiographic studies utilizing photoaffinity labeled ^{125}I-insulin, performed in collaboration with Olefsky and colleagues, demonstrated that the ligand, along with at least some portion of the insulin receptor, was translocated to nuclei of cultured hepatocytes (85). Recent studies have shown that ^{125}I-insulin is also translocated to nuclei in H35 hepatoma cells (our unpublished observations). The amount of insulin localized to the nuclei has been estimated at between 3 and 10% of the cell associated.

BIOLOGIC FUNCTIONS OF INTERNALIZATION

Nonhormonal Ligands

The primary, and perhaps sole, purpose of receptor-mediated internalization of nonhormonal ligands is to deliver specific macromolecules to intracellular sites where they are utilized or degraded.

Insulin and Other Hormonal Ligands

It has been suggested that the purpose for the internalization of insulin and other hormones was primarily for hormone degradation or in some cases for regulating the number of hormone receptors (41). In both instances, those functions would protect the cell from high concentrations of hormone either by decreasing the amount of the hormone or decreasing the number of receptors, and thus the hormone effects, on the cell. However, the extent of lysosomal degradation of insulin differs in various cell types and often has been far less efficient than the degradation of other ligands. In endothelial cells there is no detectable intracellular degradation of insulin (15, 61, 103). Several studies have demonstrated that substantial insulin degradative activity is found associated with the cell membrane (44) or in the cytosol (39) rather than in the lysosomes. Down regulation of insulin receptors may be related to other processes, such as receptor shedding in IM-9 lymphocytes or effects of experimental agents on receptor recycling (73).

Several different types of studies have attempted to demonstrate that internalization of insulin was unrelated to the metabolic effects of the hormone. These studies included linking insulin to large impermeable molecules (10), using anti-receptor antibodies which mimic insulin action (62) and the use of inhibitors of receptor internalization (69). These studies, either singularly or collectively, have not conclusively proved that internalization of the hormone-receptor complex was totally unrelated to some metabolic effect.

In contrast, several studies have demonstrated that insulin can directly affect enzyme activities and nuclear functions in isolated subcellular fractions (33). Recently, Khan *et al.* (67) and Klein *et al.* (68) reported that insulin receptor kinase is in an activated state in intracellular endosomes. These observations raise some intriguing possibilities concerning potential intracellular effects of insulin as illustrated in Figure 16. If the intracellular pathway were able to deliver insulin or the insulin-receptor complex to an intracellular site of action, as we and others have demonstrated, might not the hormone,

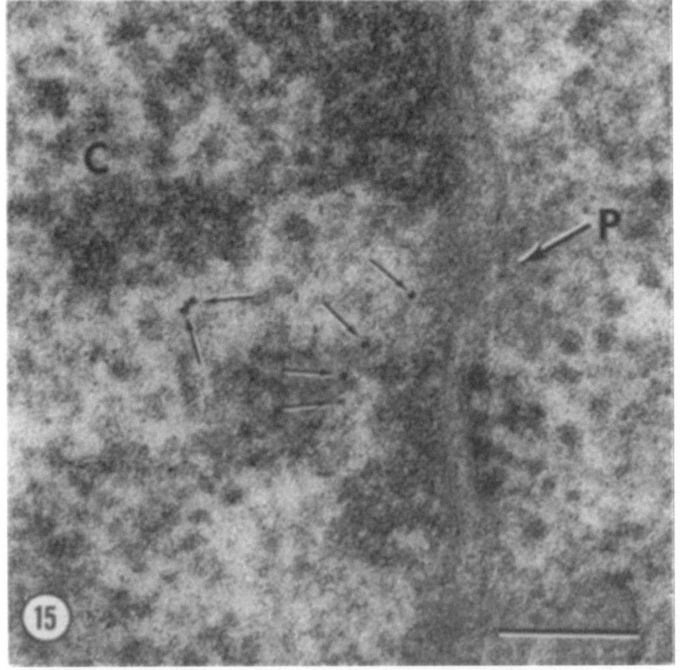

FIG. 15. Electron micrograph demonstrating nuclear accumulation of ferritin-insulin. 3T3-L1 adipocytes were incubated for 90 minutes at 37° C with 200 ng/ml of Fm-I prepared for electron microscopy. Fm-I particles (*arrows*) observed in the nucleus were located near a nuclear pore (*P*) and were most frequently associated with the condensed chromatin (*C*). Bar, 0.1 μm.

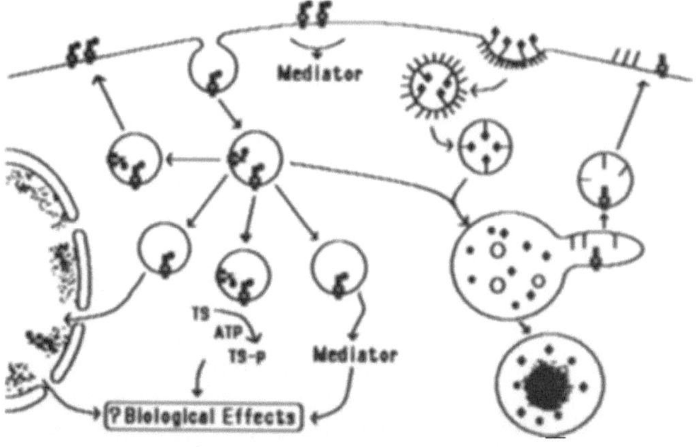

FIG. 16. Schematic model demonstrating nonhormonal and hormonal receptor-mediated internalization and intracellular processing. Illustrated on the right of the model is the concentrative, coated-pit route of internalization of ligands such as LDL and alpha-2-macroglobulin. The left side depicts the interaction of insulin with its receptor on the cell surface and the generation of mediators, including (but not shown) the phosphorylation of the receptor's beta subunit. Occupied insulin receptors are internalized in a non-concentrative manner in pinocytotic invaginations and, based on the cell type, in coated pits (not shown). Internalized occupied insulin receptors apparently follow multiple intracellular pathways which include lysosomal processing, nuclear accumulation and rapid recycling. The pathways, or the proportion of ligand in the pathways, varies in different types of cells and therefore may be cell-specific. It is proposed that the movement throughout the cytoplasm of small vesicles containing occupied insulin receptors provides a mechanism for bringing the activated tyrosine kinase of the beta subunit, or generated mediators, to cytoplasmic sites of insulin action eliciting biological effects.

the activated tyrosine kinase or "second messenger" have an effect on the intracellular systems? In particular, given the evidence that kinase activation and substrate phosphorylation may play an important role in insulin's action, the intracellular distribution of several hundred endosomes each containing a few insulin receptors with activated tyrosine kinases, may bring these kinases into contact with numerous potential intracellular substrates. If metabolic effects are regulated by the generation of low molecular weight mediators at the plasma membrane, could not the endosome also generate the same mediators and regulate metabolic events? Finally, the endosome can carry insulin and its receptor to the nucleus where they may be involved in gene regulation. These speculations need to be resolved in order to more fully understand the possible roles on insulin internalization.

SUMMARY

This review has presented some of the data which indicate that there are substantial differences in the mechanisms of receptor-mediated uptake and intracellular processing of ligands. Data from various laboratories indicate that receptor-mediated endocytosis is not necessarily synonymous with the concentrative, coated-pit-mediated internalization of ligand-receptor complexes. That differences exist both between the internalization of different types of ligands on the same cell type and between different types of cells for same ligand has clearly been documented. The differences in mechanisms or structures involved in receptor-mediated endocytosis have been demonstrated both biochemically and ultrastructurally. The reasons for these two diverse internalization pathways utilizing coated and non-coated membrane domains are not known and require further investigation to substantiate or disprove hypotheses presented here and elsewhere. Similarly, while differences in intracellular routing of hormonal and non-hormonal ligands and their receptors certainly exist, the factors controlling the itinerary of the ligand or its receptor need to be identified. The differences in ligand-receptor processing already demonstrated should indicate that interpretation of the results of future studies must be made with a great deal of caution and conservatism particularly when attempting to apply knowledge of one ligand and cell system to pharmacologically, ultrastructurally, or physiologically dissimilar systems.

Address reprint requests to: Leonard Jarett, M.D., Simon Flexner Professor and Chairman, Department of Pathology and Laboratory Medicine, Hospital University of Pennsylvania, 3400 Spruce Street, Philadelphia, PA 19104.

REFERENCES

1. Ackerman GA, Wolken KW: Histochemical evidence for the differential surface labeling, uptake and intracellular transport of a colloidal gold-labeled insulin complex by normal human blood cells. J Histochem Cytochem 29:1137, 1981
2. Ackerman GA, Yang J, Wolken KW: Differential surface labeling and internalization of glucagon by peripheral leukocytes. J Histochem Cytochem 31:433, 1983
3. Anderson RGW, Brown MS, Goldstein JL: Role of the coated endocytic vesicle in the uptake of receptor-bound low density lipoprotein in human fibroblasts. Cell 10:351, 1977
4. Bergeron JJM, Cruz J, Khan MN, Posner BI: Uptake of insulin and other ligands into receptor-rich endocytic components of target cells: the endosomal apparatus. Ann Rev Physiol 47:383, 1985
5. Bergeron JJM, Evans WH, Geschwind II: Insulin binding to rat liver Golgi fractions. J Cell Biol 59:771, 1973
6. Bergmann JS, Carney DH: Receptor-bound thrombin is not internalized through coated pits in mouse embryo cells. J Cellular Biochem 20:247, 1982
7. Bretton R, Wicker R, Bernhard W: Ultrastructural localization of concanavalin A receptors in normal and SV40-transformed hamster and rat cells. Int J Cancer 10:397, 1972
8. Carpentier JL, Gazzono H, Van Obberghen E, Fehlmann M, Freychet P, Orci L: Intracellular pathway followed by the insulin receptor covalently coupled to ^{125}I-photoreactive insulin during internalization and recycling. J Cell Biol 102:989, 1986
9. Chvatchko Y, Van Obberghen E, Fehlmann M: Internalization and recycling of insulin receptors in hepatoma cells; absence of regulation by receptor occupancy. Biochem J 222:111, 1984
10. Cuatrecasas P: Interaction of insulin with the cell membrane: the primary action of insulin. Proc Natl Acad Sci USA 63:450, 1969
11. Davies PJA, Davies DR, Levitzki A, Maxfield FR, Milhaud P, Willingham MC, Pastan IH: Transglutaminase is essential in receptor mediated endocytosis of alpha-2-macroglobulin and polypeptide hormones. Nature 283:162, 1980
12. de Duve C: Lysosomes revisited. Eur J Biochem 137:391, 1983
13. De Meyts P, Roth J, Neville DM, Jr, Gavin JR, III, Lesniak MA: Insulin interaction with its receptor: experimental evidence for negative cooperativity. Biochem Biophys Res Commun 55:154, 1973
14. de Petris S, Raff MC: Distribution of immunoglobulin on the surface of mouse lymphoid cells as determined by immunoferritin electron microscopy. Antibody-induced, temperature dependent redistribution and its implications for membrane structure. Eur J Immunol 2:523, 1972
15. Dernovsek KD, Bar RS, Ginsberg BH, Lioubin MN: Rapid transport of biologically intact insulin through cultured endothelial cells. J Clin Endocrinol Metab 58:761, 1984
16. Dickson RB, Schlegel R, Willingham MC, Pastan I: Binding and internalization of alpha-2-macroglobulin by cultured fibroblasts; effects of monovalent ionophores. Exp Cell Res 142:127, 1982
17. Donner DB: Regulation of insulin binding to isolated hepatocytes: correction for bound hormone fragments linearizes Scatchard plots. Proc Natl Acad Sci USA 77:3176, 1980
18. Dunn WA, Connolly TP, Hubbard AL: Receptor-mediated endocytosis of epidermal growth factor by rat hepatocytes: receptor pathway. J Cell Biol 102:24, 1986
19. Dunn WA, Hubbard AL: Receptor-mediated endocytosis of epidermal growth factor by hepatocytes in the perfused rat liver: ligand and receptor dynamics. J Cell Biol 98:2148, 1984
20. Ebina Y, Ellis L, Jarnagin K, Ederly M, Graf L, Clauser E, Ou J-H, Masiarz F, Kan YW, Goldfine ID, Roth RA, Rutter WJ: The human insulin receptor cDNA: the structural basis for hormone-activated transmembrane signalling. Cell 40:747, 1985
21. Fan JY, Carpentier JL, Van Obberghen E, Blackett NM, Grunfeld C, Gorden P, Orci L: The interaction of ^{125}I-insulin with cultured 3T3-L1 adipocytes: quantitative analysis of by the hypothetical grain method. J Histochem Cytochem 31:859, 1983
22. Fehlmann M, Carpentier JL, LeCam A, Thamm P, Saunders D, Brandenburg D, Orci L, Freychet P: Biochemical and morphological evidence that insulin receptor is internalized with insulin in hepatocytes. J Cell Biol 93:82, 1982
23. Gansler TS, Smith RM, Jarett L: Cell type-specific variability of bacitracin's effects on insulin binding and intracellular accumulation. Diabetes 35:392, 1986
24. Gavin JR III, Buell DN, Roth J: Water-soluble insulin receptors from human lymphocytes. Science 178:168, 1972
25. Gavin JR III, Roth J, Neville DM, Jr., De Meyts P, Buell DN: Insulin-dependent regulation of insulin receptor concentrations: a direct demonstration in cell culture. Proc Natl Acad Sci USA 71:84, 1974
26. Gershon ND: Model for capping of membrane receptors based on boundary surface effects. Proc Natl Acad Sci USA 75:1357, 1978
27. Gershon ND, Smith RM, Jarett L: Computer assisted analysis of ferritin-insulin receptor sites on adipocytes and the effects of cytochalasin B on groups of insulin receptor sites. J Membr Biol 58:155, 1981
28. Gueze HJ, Slot JW, Strous GJAM, Peppard J, von Figura K, Hasilik A, Schwartz AL: Intracellular receptor sorting during endocytosis: comparative immunoelectron microscopy of multiple receptors in rat liver. Cell 37:195, 1984

28. Gueze HJ, Slot JW, Strous GJAM, Peppard J, von Figura K, Hasilik A, Schwartz AL: Intracellular receptor sorting during endocytosis: comparative immunoelectron microscopy of multiple receptors in rat liver. Cell 37:195, 1984
29. Geuze HJ, Slot JW, Strous GJAM, Schwartz AL: The pathway of the asialoglycoprotein-ligand during receptor-mediated endocytosis: a morphological study with colloidal gold/ligand in the human hepatoma cell line, Hep G2. Eur J Cell Biol 32:38, 1983
30. Gliemann J, Sonne O: Uptake and degradation of insulin and alpha-2-macroglobulin-trypsin complex in rat adipocytes. Evidence for different pathways. Biochim Biophys Acta 845:124, 1985
31. Goidl JA: Insulin binding to isolated liver nuclei from obese and lean mice. Biochem 18:3674, 1979
32. Goldberg RI, Smith RM, Jarett L: Insulin and alpha-2-macroglobulin-methylamine undergo endocytosis by different mechanisms in rat adipocytes: I. Comparison of cell surface events. J Cell Physiol 133:203, 1987
33. Goldfine ID: Effects of insulin on intracellular functions. In Biochemical Actions of Hormones, Vol VIII, edited by Litwack G, p 273. New York, Academic Press, Inc, 1981
34. Goldfine ID: Interaction of insulin, polypeptide hormones, and growth factors with intracellular membranes. Biochim Biophys Acta 650:53, 1981
35. Goldfine ID: The insulin receptor: molecular biology and transmembrane signalling. Endocrin Rev 8:235, 1987
36. Goldfine ID, Smith GJ: Binding of insulin to isolated nuclei. Proc Natl Acad Sci USA 73:1427, 1976
37. Goldfine ID, Jones AL, Hradek G, Kriz BM, Wong KY: Entry of insulin into target cells. In Hormones in Normal and Abnormal Human Tissues, edited by Fotherby K, Pal SB, p 503. New York, Walter de Gruyter, 1981
38. Goldfine ID, Williams J, Bailey A, Wong KY, Iwamoto Y, Yokono K, Baba S, Roth RA. Degradation of insulin by isolated pancreatic acini: evidence for cell surface protease activity. Diabetes 33:64, 1984
39. Goldstein BJ, Livingston JN: An evaluation of the importance of lysosomal and neutral cytosol proteases in insulin degradation by adipocytes. Endocrinology 109:963, 1981
40. Goldstein JL, Brown MS, Anderson RGW, Russell DW, Schneider WJ: Receptor-mediated endocytosis: concepts emerging from the LDL receptor system. In Annual Review of Cell Biolology, Vol 1, edited by Palade GE, p 1. Palo Alto, CA, Annual Reviews, Inc., 1985
41. Gordon P, Carpentier J-L, Freychet P, Orci L: Internalization of polypeptide hormones: mechanism, intracellular localization and significance. Diabetologia 18:263, 1980
42. Gottschalk WK, Jarett L: Intracellular mediators of insulin action. Diabetes Metab Rev 1:229, 1985
43. Haigler HT, Willingham MC, Pastan I: Inhibitors of ^{125}I-epidermal growth factor internalization. Biochem Biophys Res Commun 94:630, 1980
44. Hammons GT, Smith RM, Jarett L: Inhibition by bacitracin of rat adipocyte plasma membrane degradation of ^{125}I-insulin is associated with an increase in plasma membrane bound insulin and a potentiation of glucose oxidation by adipocytes. J Biol Chem 257:11563, 1982
45. Heidenreich KA, Brandenburg D, Berhanu P, Olefsky JM: Metabolism of photoaffinity-labeled insulin receptors by adipocytes; role of internalization, degradation, and recycling. J Biol Chem 259:6511, 1981
46. Heindenreich KA, Zahniser NR, Berhanu P, Brandenburg D, Olefsky JM: Structural differences between insulin receptors in the brain and peripheral target tissues. J Biol Chem 258:8527, 1983
47. Heyner S, Rosenblum IY, Wikarczuk ML, Smith RM: Receptor-mediated uptake of gold-labeled insulin by early mouse embryos (abstr). J Biol Chem 105:256, 1987
48. Horuk R, Olefsky JM: Post-binding events in insulin action. Mol Cell Endocrinol 42:1, 1985
49. Horvat A, Li E, Katsoyannis PG: Cellular binding sites for insulin in rat liver. Biochem Biophys Acta 382:609, 1975
50. Huecksteadt T, Olefsky JM, Brandenburg D, Heidenreich KA: Recycling of photoaffinity-labeled insulin receptors in rat adipocytes; dissociation of insulin-receptor complexes is not required for receptor recycling. J Biol Chem 261:8655, 1986
51. Jacobs S, Cuatrecasas P: The mobile receptor hypothesis and "cooperativity" of hormone binding; application to insulin. Biochim Biophys Acta 433:482, 1976
52. Jacobs S, Cuatrecasas P: Disulfide reduction converts the insulin receptor of human placenta to a low affinity form. J Clin Invest 66:1424, 1980
53. Jacobs S, Cuatrecasas P: Insulin receptor: structure and function. Endocr Rev 2:251, 1981
54. Jarett L, Schweitzer JB, Smith RM: Insulin receptors: differences in structural organization on adipocyte and liver plasma membranes. Science 210:1127, 1980
55. Jarett L, Smith RM: Electron microscopic demonstration of insulin receptors on adipocyte plasma membranes utilizing a ferritin-insulin conjugate. J Biol Chem 249:7024, 1974
56. Jarett L, Smith RM: Ultrastructural localization of insulin receptors on adipocytes. Proc Natl Acad Sci USA 72:3256, 1975
57. Jarett L, Smith RM: Ultrastructural approaches to the study of hormone receptors: the use of ferritin-insulin in the localization of biologically relevant insulin receptors. In Cell Membrane Receptors for Viruses, Antigens and Antibodies. Polypeptide Hormones and Small Molecules, edited by Beers RF Jr, Bassett EG, p 91. New York, Raven Press, 1976
58. Jarett L, Smith RM: The natural occurrence of insulin receptors in groups on adipocyte plasma membranes as demonstrated with monomeric ferritin-insulin. J Supramol Struct 6:45, 1977
59. Jarett L, Smith RM: Effect of cytochalasin B and D on groups of insulin receptors and on insulin action in rat adipocytes. J Clin Invest 63:571, 1979
60. Jarett L, Smith RM: Partial disruption of naturally occurring groups of insulin receptors on adipocyte plasma membranes by dithiothreitol and n-ethylmaleimide: the role of disulfide bonds. Proc Natl Acad Sci USA 80:1023, 1983
61. Jialal I, King GL, Buchwald S, Kahn CR, Crettaz M: Processing of insulin by bovine endothelial cells in culture; internalization with degradation. Diabetes 33:794, 1984
62. Kahn CR: The role of insulin receptors and receptor antibodies in states of altered insulin action. Proc Soc Exp Biol Med 162:13, 1979
63. Kahn CR, Baird KL, Jarrett DB, Flier JS: Direct demonstration that receptor crosslinking or aggregation is important in insulin action. Proc Natl Acad Sci USA 75:4209, 1978
64. Kasuga M, Hedo JA, Yamada KM, and Kahn CR: The structure of insulin receptor and its subunits; evidence for multiple nonreduced forms and a 210,000 possible proreceptor. J Biol Chem 257:10392, 1982
65. Kasuga M, Karlsson FA, Kahn CR: Insulin stimulates the phosphorylation of the 95,000-dalton subunit of its own receptor. Science 215:185, 1982
66. Kelly KL, Mato JM, Merida I, Jarett L: Glucose transport and anti-lipolysis are differentially regulated by the polar head group of an insulin sensitive glycophospholipid. Proc Natl Acad Sci USA 84:5793, 1987
67. Khan MN, Savole S, Bergeron JJ, Posner BI: Characterization of rat liver endosomal fractions. *In vivo* activation of insulin-stimulable receptor kinase in these structures. J Biol Chem 261:8462, 1986
68. Klein HH, Freidenberg GR, Matthaei S, Olefsky JM: Insulin receptor kinase following internalization in isolated rat adipocytes. J Biol Chem 262:10557, 1987
69. LeCam A, Maxfield F, Willingham M, Pastan I: Insulin stimulation of amino acid transport in isolated rat hepatocytes is independent of hormone internalization. Biochem Biophys Res Commun 88:873, 1979
70. Lienhard GE, Wardzala LJ: Cytochalasin B reacts with thiols. FEBS Lett 64:69, 1976
71. Lyen KR, Smith RM, Jarett L: Differences in the ability of anti-insulin antibody to aggregate monomeric ferritin-insulin occupied receptor sites on liver and adipocyte plasma membranes. Diabetes 32:648, 1983
72. Marshall S, Green A, Olefsky JM: Evidence for recycling of insulin receptors in isolated rat adipocytes. J Biol Chem 256:11464, 1981
73. Marshall S, Olefsky JM: Tris (hydroxymethyl) aminomethane permits the expression of insulin-induced receptor loss in isolated rat adipocytes. Biochem Biophys Res Commun 102:646, 1981
74. Maxfield FR, Schlessinger J, Shechter Y, Pastan I, Willingham MC: Collection of insulin, EGF and alpha-2-macroglobulin in the same patches on the surface of cultured fibroblasts and common internalization. Cell 14:805, 1978
75. Mimura N, Asano A: Actin-related gelation of Ehrlick tumour

cell extracts is reversibly inhibited by low concentrations of Ca^{2+}. Nature (Lond) 272:273, 1978
76. Moll UM, Thun CH, Pfeiffer EF: Colloidal gold-labeled insulin complex, characterization and binding to adipocytes. Histochemistry 86:83, 1986
77. Montesano R, Roth J, Robert A, Orci L: Non-coated membrane invaginations are involved in binding and internalization of cholera and tetanus toxins. Nature 296:651, 1982
78. Nelson DM, Smith RM, Jarett L: Nonuniform distribution and grouping of insulin receptors on the surface of human placental syncytial trophoblast. Diabetes 27:530, 1978
79. Nicolson G: Transmembrane control of the receptors on normal and tumor cells. I. Cytoplasmic influence over cell surface components. Biochim Biophys Acta 457:57, 1976
80. Nicolson GL, Smith JR, Hyman R: Dynamics of toxin and lectin receptors on a lymphoma cell line and its toxin-resistant variant using ferritin-conjugated, ^{125}I-labeled ligand. J Cell Biol 78:565, 1978
81. Oda Y, Kasi K-I, Ishii S-I: Studies on the specific interaction of concanavalin A and saccharides by affinity chromatography: application of quantitative affinity chromatography to a multivalent system. J Biochem 89:285, 1981
82. Olefsky JM, Kao M: Surface binding and rates of internalization of ^{125}I-insulin in adipocytes and IM-9 lymphocytes. J Biol Chem 257:8667, 1982
83. Perelson AS, DeLisi C: Receptor clustering on a cell surface. I. Theory of receptor cross-linking by ligands bearing two chemically identical functional groups. Math Biosci 48:71, 1980
84. Pilch PF, Czech MP: The subunit structure of the high-affinity insulin receptor. Evidence of disulfide linked receptor complex in fat cell and liver plasma membranes. J Biol Chem 255:1722, 1980
85. Podlecki DA, Smith RM, Kao M, Tsai P, Huecksteadt T, Brandenburg D, Lasher RS, Jarett L, Olefsky JM: Nuclear translocation of the insulin receptor; a possible mediator of insulin's long term effects. J Biol Chem 262:3362, 1987
86. Posner BI, Khan MN, Bergeron JM: Endocytosis of peptide hormones and other ligands. Endocr Rev 3:280, 1982
87. Potau N, Bailey AC, Roach E, Williams JA, Goldfine ID: Methylamine and monensin do not block insulin internalization but do influence the intracellular distribution and action of insulin in pancreatic acini from diabetic mice. Endocrinology 115:205, 1984
88. Rosen OM: After insulin binds. Science 237:1452, 1987
89. Russell DS, Gherzi R, Johnson EL, Chou C-K, Rosen OM: The protein-tyrosine kinase activity of the insulin receptor is necessary for insulin-mediated receptor down regulation. J Biol Chem 262:11833, 1987
90. Salpeter MM, Fertuck HC, and Salpeter EE: Resolution in electron microscope autoradiography. III. Iodine^{125}I, the effect of heavy metal staining, a reassessment of critical parameters. J Cell Biol 72:161, 1977
91. Schweitzer JB, Smith RM, and Jarett L: Differences in organizational structure of insulin receptor on rat adipocyte and liver plasma membranes: role of disulfide bonds. Proc Natl Acad Sci USA 77:4692, 1980
92. Shechter Y, Chang K, Jacobs S, Cuatrecasas P: Modulation of binding and bioactivity of insulin by anti-insulin antibody: relation to possible role of receptor self-aggregation in hormone action. Proc Natl Acad Sci USA 76:2720, 1979
93. Smith RM, Cobb MH, Rosen OM, Jarett L: Ultrastructural analysis of the organization and distribution of insulin receptors on the surface of 3T3-L1 adipocytes: rapid microaggregation and migration of occupied receptors. J Cell Physiol 123:167, 1985
94. Smith RM, Gansler TS, Laudenslager NH, Shah N, Jarett L: Heterogeneous effects of inhibitors of receptor processing on insulin binding and intracellular accumulation in various cell types. Lab Invest 55:593, 1986
95. Smith RM, Goldberg RI, Jarett L: Preparation and characterization of a colloidal gold-insulin complex with binding and biological activities identical to native insulin. J Histochem Cytochem, 36:359, 1988
96. Smith RM, Jarett L: Morphological characterization of insulin receptor distribution by ferritin-insulin and the route of uptake of ferritin-insulin into adipocytes. In Current Views on Insulin Receptors, edited by Andreani D, De Pirro R, Lauro R, Olefsky J, Roth J, p 197. New York, Academic Press, 1981
97. Smith RM, Jarett L: A simplified method of producing biologically active monomeric ferritin-insulin for use as a high resolution ultrastructural marker for occupied insulin receptors. J Histochem Cytochem 30:650, 1982
98. Smith RM, Jarett L: Ultrastructural basis for chloroquine-induced increase in intracellular insulin in adipocytes: alteration of lysosomal function. Proc Natl Acad Sci USA 79:7302, 1982
99. Smith RM, Jarett L: Quantitative ultrastructural analysis of receptor-mediated insulin uptake into adipocytes. J Cell Physiol 115:199, 1983
100. Smith RM, Jarett L: Tissue-specific variation in insulin receptor dynamics. In Insulin, Its Receptor and Diabetes, edited by Hollenberg MD, p 105. New York, Marcel Dekker, Inc., 1985
101. Smith RM, Jarett L: Ultrastructural evidence for the accumulation of insulin in nuclei of intact 3T3-L1 adipocytes by an insulin-receptor mediated process. Proc Natl Acad Sci USA 84:459, 1987
102. Smith RM, Laudenslager NH, Shah N and Jarett L: Insulin binding and processing by H4IIEC3 hepatoma cells: ultrastructural evidence for a unique route of internalization and processing. J Cellular Physiol 130:428, 1987
103. Solenski NJ, Williams SK: Insulin binding and vesicular ingestion in capillary endothelium. J Cell Physiol 124:87, 1985
104. Sonne O, Gliemann J: The mechanism of receptor-mediated degradation of insulin in isolated adipocytes: indirect evidence for a non-lysosomal pathway. Mol Cell Endocrinol 31:315, 1983
105. Suzuki K, Kono T: Internalization and degradation of fat cell-bound insulin. Separation and partial characterization of subcellular vesicles associated with iodoinsulin. J Biol Chem 254:9786, 1979
106. Taylor RB, Duffus WPH, Raff MC, dePetris S: Redistribution and pinocytosis of lymphocyte surface immunoglobulin molecules induced by anti-immunoglobulin antibody. Nature (London) New Biol 233:225, 1971
107. Ueda M, Robinson FW, Smith MH, Kono T: Effects of monensin on insulin processing in adipocytes; evidence that the internalized insulin-receptor complex has some physiological activities. J Biol Chem 260:3941, 1985
108. Ullrich A, Bell JR, Chen EY, Herrera A, Petruzzelli LM, Dull TJ, Gray A, Coussens L, Liao Y-C, Tsubokawa M, Mason A, Seeburg PH, Grunfeld C, Rosen OM, Ramachandran J: Human insulin receptor and its relationship to the tyrosine kinase family of oncogenes. Nature 313:756, 1985
109. Ullrich A, Coussens L, Hayflick JS, Dull TJ, Gray A, Tam AW, Lee J, Yarden Y: Human epidermal growth factor receptor cDNA sequence and aberrant expression of the amplified gene in A431 epidermoid carcinoma cells. Nature 309:418, 1984
110. Ullrich A, Gray A, Tam AW, Yang-Feng T, Tsubokawa M, Collins C, Henzel W, LeBon T, Kathuria S, Chen E, Jacobs S, Franke U, Ramachandran J, Fujita-Yamaguchi Y: Insulin-like growth factor I receptor primary structure: comparison with insulin receptor suggests structural determinants that define functional specificity. EMBO J 5:2503, 1986
111. Weihing RR: Cytochalasin B inhibits actin-related gelation of HeLa cell extracts. J Cell Biol 71:303, 1976
112. Wileman T, Harding C, and Stahl, P: Receptor-mediated endocytosis. Biochem J 232:1, 1985
113. Willingham MC, Maxfield FR, Pastan IH: alpha-2-Macroglobulin binding to the plasma membrane of cultured fibroblasts; diffuse binding followed by clustering in coated regions. J Cell Biol 82:614, 1979
114. Willingham MC, Pastan IH: Receptor-mediated endocytosis of hormones in cultured fibroblasts. In Receptor-Mediated Binding and Internalization of Toxins and Hormones, edited by Middlebrook JL, Kohn LD, p 135. New York, Academic Press, 1981
115. Wisner-Gebhart AM, Brabec RK, Gray RH: Morphometric studies of chloroquine-induced changes in hepatocytic organelles in the rat. Exp Mol Pathol 33:144, 1980
116. Yip CC, Moule ML, Yeung CWT: Characterization of insulin receptor subunits in brain and other tissues by photoaffinity labeling. Biochem Biophys Res Commun 96:1671, 1980
117. Yip CC, Moule ML, Yeung CWT: Subunit structure of insulin receptor of rat adipocytes as demonstrated by photoaffinity labeling. Biochem 21:2940, 1982
118. Zeitlin PL, Hubbard AL: Cell surface distribution and intracellular fate of asialoglycoproteins: a morphological and biochemical study of isolated rat hepatocytes and monolayer cultures. J Cell Biol 92:634, 1982

Biology of Disease

Gastrin-Releasing Peptide (Mammalian Bombesin) Gene Expression in Health and Disease

Mary E. Sunday, Lee M. Kaplan, Etsuro Motoyama, William W. Chin, and Eliot R. Spindel

Departments of Pathology and Medicine, Brigham & Women's Hospital, Massachusetts General Hospital, and Harvard Medical School; Departments of Anesthesiology and Pediatrics, Children's Hospital of Pittsburgh

INTRODUCTION

In recent years much attention has been focused on gastrin-releasing peptide (GRP), the mammalian homologue of bombesin, both as a neuroregulatory hormone and as a tissue-specific growth factor in normal and neoplastic tissues. This paper will analyze the distribution and role of GRP in normal mammalian tissues and examine the potential involvement of GRP in diverse pathologic processes.

ISOLATION AND CHARACTERIZATION OF BOMBESIN AND GASTRIN-RELEASING PEPTIDE

GRP is the 27-amino acid mammalian homologue of the 14-amino acid amphibian peptide bombesin (Fig. 1). Bombesin was originally isolated from the skin of the frog *Bombina bombina* in 1971 by Erspamer and coworkers (3). In amphibians, three families of bombesin-like peptides have been characterized: the bombesins, the ranatensins, and the phyllolitorins, all of which have closely related amino acid sequences at their carboxy (C) termini (3, 32, 33, 142). Within frog skin, these peptides are present in myoepithelial "poison" glands under positive noradrenergic control where they have been postulated to play a role in defense against predators (142). Thus far, a mammalian equivalent of bombesin (GRP) and a mammalian equivalent of ranatensin (neuromedin B) have been identified. Little is yet known about the physiology or pathology of neuromedin B. This discussion will accordingly be limited to GRP.

Using anti-bombesin antisera, radioimmunoassays were developed and bombesin-like immunoreactivity (BLI) was identified in the brain, lung and gut of several mammalian species (142). In 1979, the 27-amino acid mammalian homologue of bombesin was isolated from porcine stomach using the release of gastrin as a bioassay (93). This gave rise to the name "gastrin-releasing peptide" or GRP, although this peptide possesses numerous other physiologic effects (detailed below). Both bombesin and GRP include a conserved C-terminal heptapeptide (Fig. 1) which is required for immunogenicity as well as for high affinity receptor binding and biologic activity (171). In addition, the C-terminal methionine must be amidated in order to be recognized by antibodies and cellular receptors (70).

27-amino acid GRPs have now been isolated from avian proventriculus (92), canine small intestine (127), and human pulmonary tumors (112). The structure of human GRP has been established by amino acid sequencing (127) and by molecular cloning (143). The sequence of rat GRP has been determined by molecular cloning (80) and differs from human GRP by the addition of two amino acids within the amino terminus of the molecule, giving rise to a 29-amino acid peptide. The 4 mammalian GRPs thus far identified contain 15 identical amino acids at the C-terminus; avian GRP differs from them by only 2 amino acids in this region (142). A 10-amino acid peptide corresponding to the C-terminal decapeptide of GRP has been isolated from porcine spinal cord (95), canine small intestine (127), and a human pulmonary carcinoid tumor (143). It is thought to be a tryptic cleavage product of GRP and is now termed GRP-10 (the earlier designation, "neuromedin C," has been discontinued). Both GRP and GRP-10 share all of the bioactivity of bombesin, as determined by structure-activity analyses (129) which map the bioactive region to the highly conserved C-terminal 7 to 10 amino acids.

Most researchers now refer to mammalian bombesin as GRP and the term bombesin is reserved strictly for the amphibian peptide (142). Antibodies to amphibian bombesin do not distinguish between GRP-27 and GRP-10 in radioimmunoassays or immunohistochemical analyses. No additional mammalian peptides have been identified which react with anti-bombesin antisera. Hence bombesin-like immunoreactivity in mammalian species appears to be comprised only of these two forms of GRP.

STRUCTURE OF THE GRP GENE AND mRNAs

mRNAs encoding human GRP were originally isolated by Spindel *et al.* (143, 144, 147) from a pulmonary carcinoid rich in bombesin-like immunoreactivity and subsequently confirmed by Battey and co-workers in four of seven small cell lung carcinoma (SCCL) cell lines and one of two metastatic SCCL tumors (136). cDNA sequencing and S_1 nuclease analysis have revealed three distinct GRP mRNA species (Fig. 2), each of which encodes human GRP (detailed below). Thus, human GRP (hGRP) is encoded as part of a larger precursor peptide (preproGRP) which includes a signal peptide, GRP, and a C-terminal extension peptide (CTEP). The three mRNA species differ only in the region encoding the CTEP, giving rise to three putative CTEP species (see Fig. 2).

A single human GRP-encoding gene has been identified (143) and localized to chromosome 18 (107). Sequence analysis demonstrates that the gene is comprised of three exons (146). The three distinct mRNA species are generated from the primary transcript of this gene by use of alternative splicing patterns (see Fig. 2). Hu-

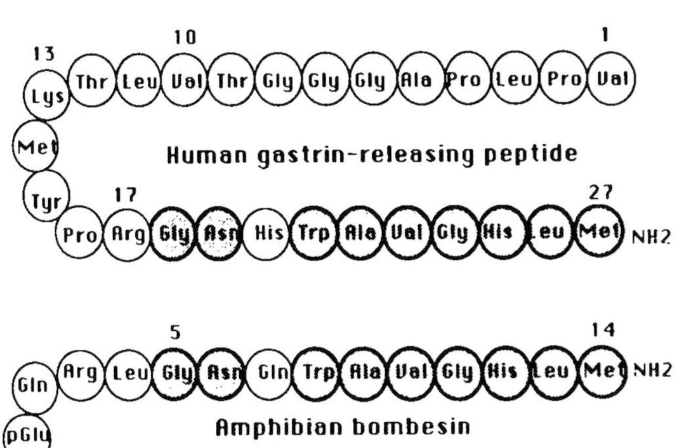

FIG. 1. The amino acid sequences of human GRP and amphibian bombesin. Conserved amino acids are shaded in gray and amidation of the conserved carboxy-terminal methionine residue is indicated.

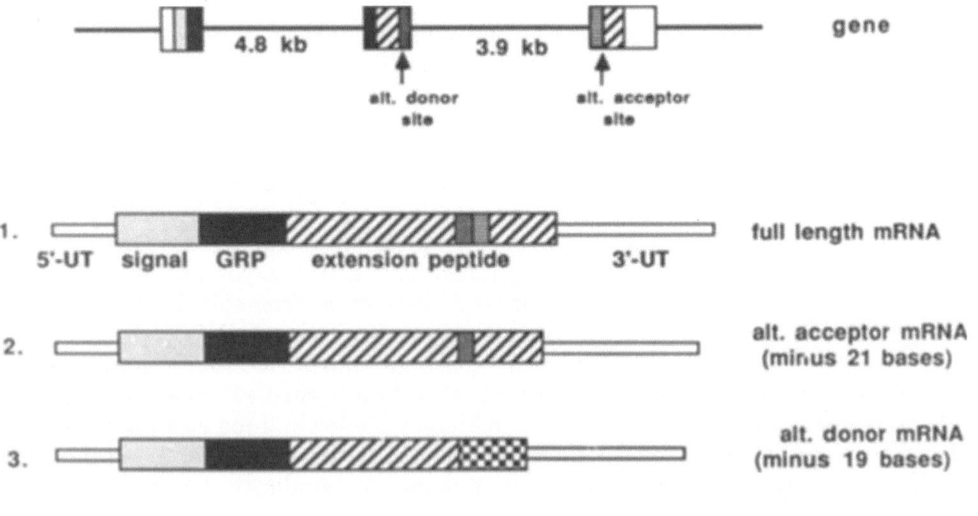

FIG. 2. Diagram of the human GRP gene and mRNAs. The human GRP gene is 10 kb with 2 introns of 4.8 and 3.9 kb as shown. The first intron interrupts the coding sequence for GRP. The two *stippled boxes* flanking intron 2 depict the 19 and 21 base pair sequences which can be alternately spliced out of the gene transcript to yield the 3 mRNAs shown. If neither box is removed the full-length mRNA (form 1) results; if the right-hand box is deleted, then the minus 21 base mRNA (form 2) results; and if the left hand box is deleted, then the minus 19 base mRNA (form 3) results. The *checkered box* at the *right hand* terminal of the mRNA form 3 indicates the new terminal 17 amino acid sequence resulting from the changed reading frame after the 19 base deletion (because a deletion of 19 bases is not evenly divisible by 3).

man GRP mRNA species forms 1, 2 and 3 appear to be present in the same relative ratio of about 60:5:35 in all tissues examined, including benign and malignant pulmonary tumors, fetal and adult lung, stomach and brain (146).

In contrast, only one mRNA species encoding rat GRP has been identified. This mRNA is most similar to mRNA form 3 of human GRP (Fig. 2) (80). There is strong amino acid conservation between the rat and human GRP genes in both the GRP-encoding and the carboxy-terminal extension peptide of GRP (CTEP)-encoding portions, suggesting a possible physiologic role for one or more of the CTEPs (80).

Antibodies directed against the hGRP CTEPs also detect the precursor hormone(s), proGRP, whereas antibodies to bombesin or GRP only detect the mature cleaved and amidated peptide. Detection of the GRP prohormone may be of considerable usefulness both in understanding the biology of these peptides and in diagnostic surgical pathology.

TISSUE DISTRIBUTION AND PHYSIOLOGY OF GRP IN NORMAL MAMMALS

Using antisera against amphibian bombesin which cross-react equally well with GRP, GRP has been demonstrated to be widely distributed in mammalian tissues. Highest concentrations are found in pulmonary neuroendocrine cells of human fetal lung (20, 97, 121, 145, 151, 161, 179), neurons of the central nervous system (CNS) (131), and gut myenteric plexuses (29, 171).

Lung

The highest levels of GRP are present in human fetal and neonatal lung, as demonstrated by both RIA and immunohistochemistry (20, 97, 121, 145, 151, 161, 179). The concentration of the immunoreactive peptides is higher in fetal than in neonatal lungs (161), such that levels decline in parallel with the observed decrease in the number of pulmonary neuroendocrine cells. This time course suggests a possible role for bombesin-like peptides in control of lung development. Moreover, recent studies have suggested that GRP may be a growth factor for both normal and neoplastic pulmonary cells (19, 173, 182).

In situ hybridization and immunohistochemical analyses of fetal and neonatal lung identified GRP mRNAs and peptide as early as 8 weeks gestation in pulmonary neuroendocrine (NE) cells and neuroepithelial bodies. GRP is located predominantly at branch points of bronchioles, but not in primitive air saccules or mature alveoli in neonates (145). As shown in Fig. 3*A*, *in situ* hybridization of fetal lung at 9.5 weeks of gestation with a ^{35}S-labeled GRP cRNA probe revealed GRP mRNA exclusively in NE cells within larger proximal airways. Analysis of serial sections revealed GRP peptide in 20 to 80% of these cells (Fig. 3*B*), which at this developmental stage represent single Kulchitsky-type NE cells. In slightly older fetuses (10.5 to 15 weeks) there was similar hybridization in proximal airways with additional less intense foci in distal (smaller) airways. By 15 weeks, most of the proximal foci also contained GRP peptide, whereas only 25% of distal foci contained detectable GRP peptide. Polak and colleagues (118) and our laboratory have recently demonstrated immunoreactive proGRP colocalizing in many of the same cells as GRP mRNA even in the earliest fetuses, suggesting that part of the lag in the appearance of GRP may be due to a delay in posttranslational processing (*i.e.*, cleavage and amidation) of the prohormone (79), as well as a a delay in mRNA translation.

In midgestation fetal lung (18 to 23 weeks gestation), there are numerous pulmonary NE cells containing GRP peptide as well as mRNA, with *in situ* hybridization signals strong both proximally and distally (Figs. 3*C* and *D*). The vast majority of pulmonary NE cells contained both GRP mRNA and peptide (153).

Although neonatal lung contains multiple GRP-immunoreactive NE cells until at least 3 to 6 months of age (145, 151, 179), similar to midgestation fetuses, the number of foci hybridizing to GRP mRNA probes is considerably less than in fetal lung; most of these foci in neonates were located in the distal respiratory tree. The number of cells containing GRP mRNA and peptide is shown as a function of developmental time in Figure 4. Thus, both peptide and mRNA positive cells reach peak levels by 16 to 30 weeks gestation. The number of peptide-positive cells remains elevated for about 6 months after birth. This is consistent with radioimmunoassay (RIA) determinations of total GRP levels in fetal and neonatal lung (20, 121, 161). In contrast, the number of cells containing detectable mRNA declines considerably by birth. Similar results have been obtained using blot hybridization analysis (145), suggesting that lower GRP mRNA levels in neonates is due in part to fewer cells synthesizing GRP mRNA and in part to decreased mRNA synthesis by individual cells.

In order to confirm the apparent time-dependent shift in GRP mRNA hybridization from predominantly proximal to distal locations within the airways, the intensity of the hybridizing signal was determined by grain density analysis. In early gestation (8 to 15 weeks), hybridization was most intense in the proximal lung, whereas in the neonate, when relatively fewer foci of hybridization were apparent, hybridization was more intense distally than proximally (Fig. 5). These data suggest that in the developing lung, activation of the GRP gene follows a proximal to distal progression, paralleling the growth of the airways. Whether GRP gene products (GRP or CTEP) play a role in the continued growth of airway epithelium during extension of peripheral airways is currently under investigation (118, 148).

GRP and calcitonin (CT) have been demonstrated to be colocalized in many of the same pulmonary NE cells (150, 151, 163) and are generally present in the same neurosecretory granules (150). However, there are different developmental kinetics for the appearance of the two hormones in human fetal lung, with GRP detectable by 8 to 10 weeks gestation (145, 151), whereas CT is not demonstrated until 24 to 28 weeks (151). The significance of this association is not presently known.

GRP immunoreactivity has also been observed in human and guinea pig alveolar macrophages (181; M. E. Sunday, unpublished data). However, we have been un-

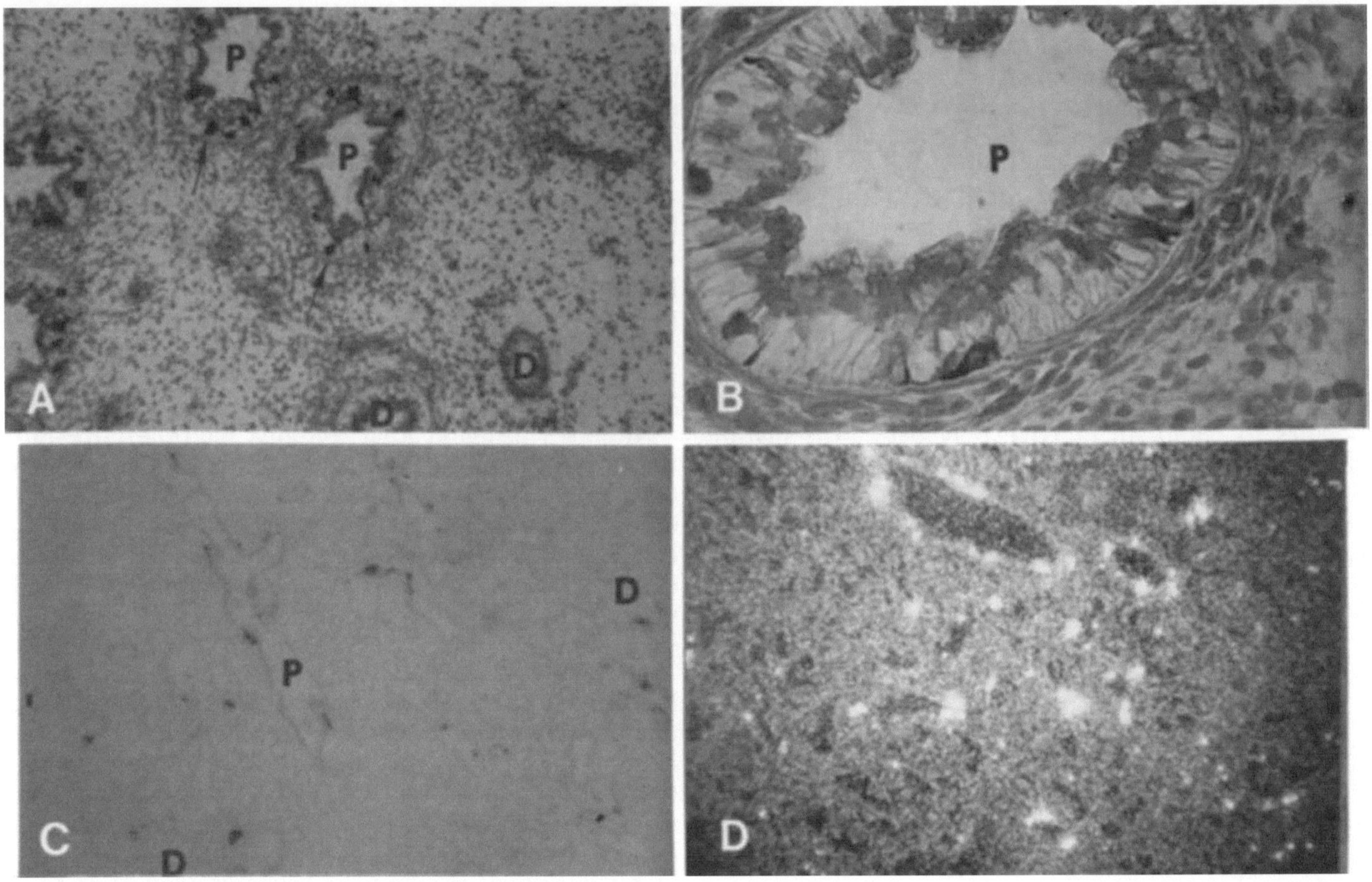

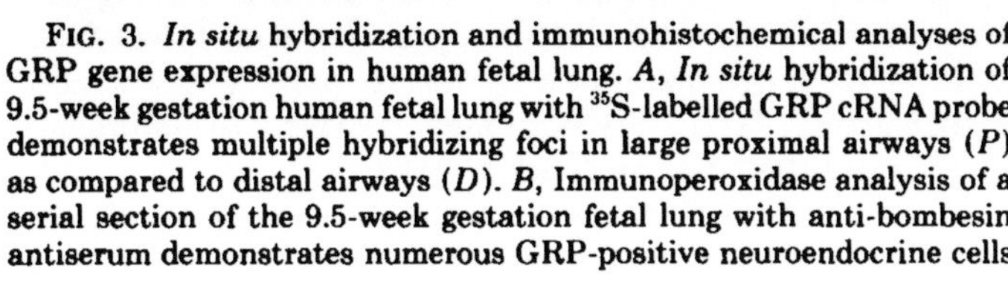

FIG. 3. *In situ* hybridization and immunohistochemical analyses of GRP gene expression in human fetal lung. *A*, *In situ* hybridization of 9.5-week gestation human fetal lung with ^{35}S-labelled GRP cRNA probe demonstrates multiple hybridizing foci in large proximal airways (*P*) as compared to distal airways (*D*). *B*, Immunoperoxidase analysis of a serial section of the 9.5-week gestation fetal lung with anti-bombesin antiserum demonstrates numerous GRP-positive neuroendocrine cells of the Kulchitsky type, which were also present only in large proximal airways. *C*, *In situ* hybridization of 23-week gestation lung demonstrates numerous GRP-positive neuroendocrine cells in both large proximal and smaller distal bronchioles. *D*, Darkfield view of same slide shown in Figure 3*C* shows positive cells as white signals on a dark background Figure 3*A*, ×100; *B*, ×400; *C*, ×63; *D*, ×100.

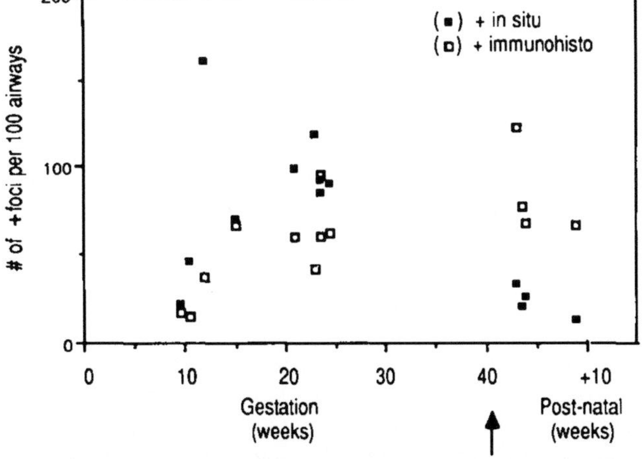

FIG. 4. Time-course of GRP *in situ* hybridizing and immunostaining foci normalized to airway number. GRP mRNA or peptide containing foci were quantitated as described previously (25). Age is shown on lower axis. An *arrow* indicates pre- *versus* postnatal periods. (Reprinted with permission from the Journal of Clinical Investigation 80:1172–1179, 1987).

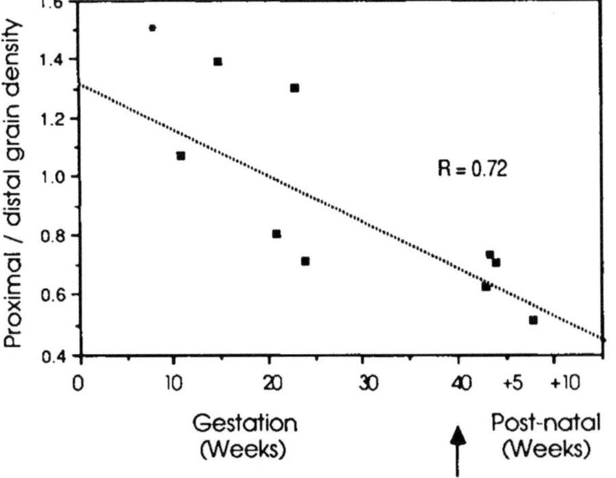

FIG. 5. Time-course of relative intensity of proximal versus distal *in situ* hybridization in developing lung. Grain density of hybridizing foci and identification of airways as proximal or distal was determined as described previously (25). *, point for which hybridization was observed only in proximal airways. The correlation coefficient for a least-squares regression analysis was 0.72 with $p < 0.05$. (Reprinted with permission from the Journal of Clinical Investigation 80:1172–1179, 1987).

able to identify GRP mRNAs by either blot or *in situ* hybridization analyses of human bronchoalveolar lavage (BAL) macrophages even after adherence to plastic. It is possible that GRP immunoreactivity detected in human peripheral blood monocytes only after 1 hour of adherence to plastic (181) may represent conversion of ingested proGRP to mature GRP during culture. Of note, low to moderate levels of GRP immunoreactivity have been measured in BAL fluid from normal adult lung compared with high levels from the lungs of cigarette smokers; these levels in BAL fluid are not correlated with the numbers of BAL macrophages present (1). Although these studies are preliminary, the lack of GRP-specific mRNA suggests that it is more likely that BAL macrophages contain GRP ingested from sloughed pulmonary neuroendocrine cells and/or from bronchial secretions.

Several studies suggest that GRP is involved in control of growth in normal lung. Willey, Lechner, and Harris (182) demonstrated that GRP stimulates the clonal growth of normal adult bronchial epithelial cells *in vitro*. Weber *et al.* (173) and Cuttitta *et al.* (19) have observed GRP-stimulated growth of SCCL cells *in vivo* and in cell culture. Further, this growth could be inhibited by a monoclonal antibody to the bioactive C-terminus of GRP (19). Since many of these SCCL cell lines also secrete GRP, these data suggest the possibility of a positive autocrine effect on the proliferation of certain SCCL cell lines and tumors.

GRP is also a potent mitogen for Swiss 3T3 mouse fibroblasts (133) and for *N-ras*-transfected NIH 3T3 cells (169). The role of GRP in the proliferation of pulmonary fibroblasts is not known.

Bombesin has also been demonstrated to cause bronchoconstriction within the guinea pig lung which cannot be inhibited by antagonists of acetylcholine, histamine, or serotonin (56). High tissue levels of GRP during the perinatal period suggest that there may be a role for GRP in neonatal circulatory adaptation. Given intracerebrally to cats, bombesin increases minute volume due to an increased tidal volume without a change in respiratory rate (47). In a rat model, central administration of bombesin causes apneusis-like alterations in breathing pattern (109). Thus, there are probably several physiologic roles of GRP in fetal and neonatal lung, both related to growth processes and also to circulatory and ventilatory adaptations.

THYROID

GRP immunoreactivity has been detected in several tumors of thyroidal C cells (medullary carcinomas of the thyroid, MCTs) (43, 55, 66, 68, 90, 120, 140, 186). In order to determine whether the GRP gene is expressed in normal neuroendocrine cells of the thyroid, we analyzed fetal and pediatric thyroids (154) for both GRP mRNA and peptide (Fig. 6). Mean levels of total thyroidal GRP immunoreactivity, which were low in mid-gestation fetuses (19 to 22 weeks gestation) and early neonates (<0.5 pg/mg), were nearly 10-fold higher in specimens taken between 3 weeks and 5 months of age (3.3 ± 1.3 pg/mg). Peak levels occurred at about 2 months of age. Levels of GRP immunoreactivity in the thyroid decreased by 8 months of age and were consistently low thereafter (<1 pg/mg). Calcitonin levels determined on the same thyroids were about 100-fold greater than GRP levels at all ages, with a linear correlation between GRP and CT levels (R = 0.98).

In situ hybridization and immunohistochemical analyses reveal that thyroidal C cells contain GRP mRNA and peptide (Figs. 7 and 8). Immunoperoxidase examination of serial tissue sections (Fig. 7*A* and *B*) revealed colocalization of GRP and CT immunoreactivity in many individual C-cells of fetal and neonatal thyroid (Fig. 7). Although 70% of fetal and neonatal CT-positive C cells also contain GRP peptide and mRNA (Figs. 8*A* and 9),

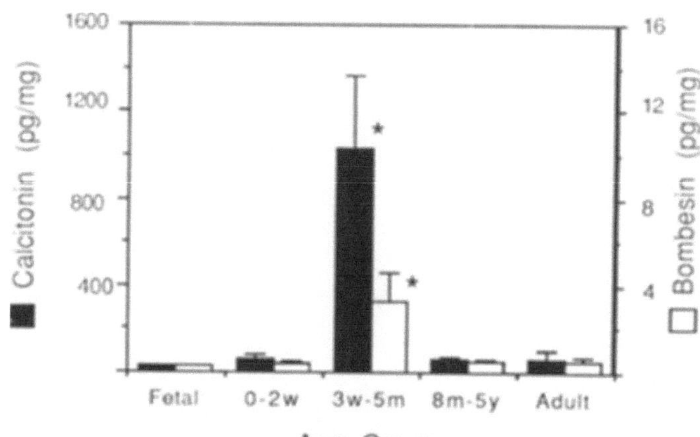

FIG. 6. Quantitative radioimmunoassay of calcitonin (CT) and GRP (bombesin-like immunoreactivity) in developing human thyroid. The peptide fraction was purified from acid extracts of one fresh thyroid lobe from each case, and assayed for total CT and GRP by the double antibody method (53). The age groups represent: 3 fetuses (19 to 21.5 weeks); 5 newborns (8 hours to 2 weeks old); 7 infants (3 weeks to 5 months old); 3 older pediatric cases (8 months, 4 years, and 5 years old); and 4 adults (29 to 95 years old). *Bars* depict mean values as pg/mg wet weight of tissue ± SEM, *, $p < 0.01$. (Reprinted with permission from Endocrinology, 1988 (Ref. 154)).

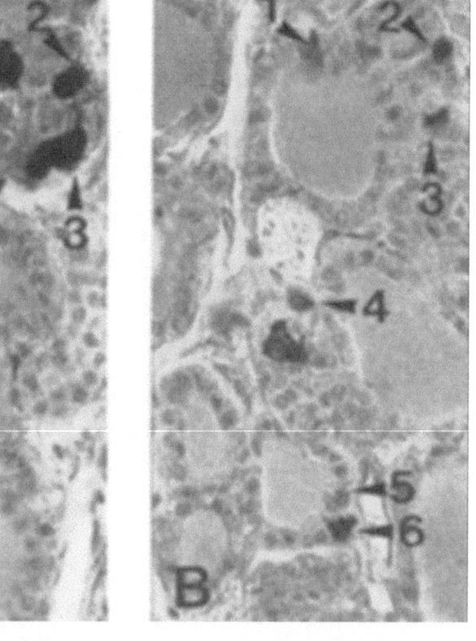

FIG. 7. Immunostaining for calcitonin and GRP in neonatal thyroid. Neonatal thyroid (1 day old) in which serial 3-μm sections were immunostained for calcitonin (*A*) and GRP (*B*) are shown. *Numbers* with *arrows* indicate the same cell in corresponding sections. (Reprinted with permission from Endocrinology, 1988 (Ref. 154)). ×500.

<20% of C cells in adult thyroid contain detectable GRP peptide and mRNA (Figs. 8*B* and 9). It is interesting that the earliest fetus examined by histochemistry, which was 12 weeks gestation, had five times more cells containing GRP than CT. This observation suggests that GRP may precede CT in the thyroid as well as in the lung (151). More early fetuses will have to be analyzed to confirm this point.

In summary, during development, peak GRP levels occur in neonatal thyroid. The increase in GRP and CT levels in neonatal thyroid is apparently due to both increased numbers of C cells and elevated concentrations of GRP and CT/cell. The 10-fold decline in CT and GRP in thyroids of older children and adults appears to be due primarily to the dilutional effect of growth of colloid-containing thyroid follicles (about a 10-fold increase in size), since the concentration of C cells is 10-fold greater in human neonatal thyroid than in adult thyroid and the absolute number of C cells is similar in both neonates and adults (183). Paradoxically, the decreased proportion of C cells containing detectable GRP in adult thyroid suggests that there is about a 3-fold higher concentration of GRP/GRP-positive C cell in adults as compared with neonates. This implies that adult C cells store GRP peptide, which is analogous to GRP peptide storage in pulmonary neuroendocrine cells in neonates (145).

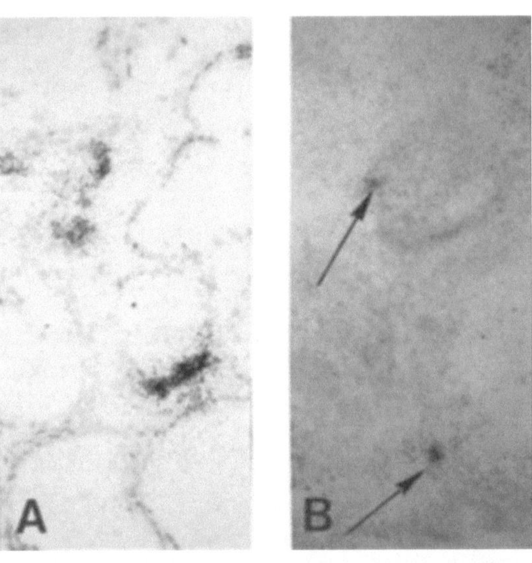

FIG. 8. *In situ* hybridization of human thyroid with GRP anti-sense cRNA probe. *A*, Thyroid from 5-month-old infant demonstrates strong autoradiographic signals throughout the parafollicular and follicular regions, corresponding to abundant GRP mRNAs in C-cells (×400). *B*, Thyroid from 49-year-old patient demonstrates weak *in situ* signals in relatively few foci (arrows), corresponding to scant GRP mRNA (×250). (Reprinted with permission from Endocrinology, 1988 (Ref. 154). Figure 8*A*, ×400; 8*B*, ×250.

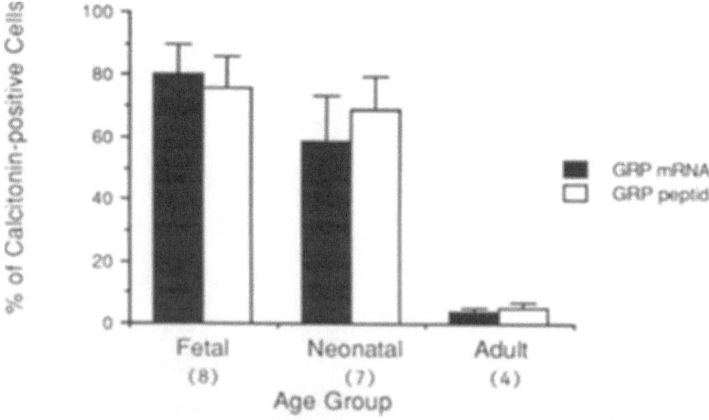

FIG. 9. Percentages of GRP-positive C cells in thyroid from different age groups. Histograms summarize the numbers of GRP-positive C cells as a percentage of CT-positive C cells in serial sections according to age groups: 8 fetuses (19.5 to 23.5 weeks gestation); 7 neonates (1 day to 5 months old); and 5 histologically normal adults without thyroid tumors (24 to 95 years old). *, $P < 0.01$. (Reprinted with permission from Endocrinology, 1988 (Ref. 154).

Despite these observations, the function of GRP in normal thyroidal development is not known. It is possible that GRP plays a role as a thyroid growth factor analogous to its effects in the lung (19, 173, 182). In preliminary experiments, a human medullary carcinoma cell line was found to form larger tumor colonies *in vitro* in the presence of bombesin, but this effect was observed only with early cell passages (54). In mouse thyroid development, mitoses of C cells were only observed in the first 4 weeks of neonatal life (174), suggesting that the neonatal period may be associated with thyroidal cell proliferation. This may be correlated with maximal GRP gene activation in the developing thyroid during the neonatal period.

Central Nervous System

GRP is found in several groups of neurons in mammalian brain and spinal cord (10, 46, 94, 100, 101, 104, 113, 114, 131, 168). Highest concentrations of GRP immunoreactivity are detected in the hypothalamus (10, 168, 171), with lower levels in the midbrain and brainstem. GRP immunoreactivity is barely detectable in the cerebellum. GRP immunostaining in the hypothalamus is localized in neuronal cell bodies of the suprachiasmatic nucleus and the parvocellular region of the paraventricular nucleus; it is also localized in the lateral aspect of the nucleus tractus solitarius and in several pontine and medullary regions (113, 114, 131). Moody and co-workers (10, 113) have also described high levels of GRP in the rat hypothalamus, but found even higher concentrations in the substantia gelatinosa trigemini and nucleus tractus solitarius. They observed intermediate levels in the arcuate nucleus and the interpeduncular nucleus, and lower concentrations in other hypothalamic regions, central grey, amygdala and substantia nigra.

During fetal rat brain development, GRP is virtually undetectable until birth (94). The concentration increases rapidly after birth, first in the caudal and later in rostral brain regions, with GRP immunostaining reaching adult levels by the second to third postnatal week (46, 104). Interestingly, GRP receptors apparently precede GRP, with receptors being detectable in fetal rat brain (104). The presence of specific receptors suggests that these peptides function as neurotransmitters or neuroregulatory hormones in the brain. Supporting this contention, subcellular fractionation studies have shown GRP to be associated with synaptosomes; release of GRP from rat brain hypothalamic slices is triggered by K^+-mediated depolarization and pharmacologic agents in a Ca^{++}-dependent manner (104).

Administration of GRP or bombesin to whole animals elicits a wide range of central homeostatic and behavioral responses including: hypothermia (158); regulation of adrenal epinephrine secretion, blood sugar, and cardiac function (35); alterations in gastric acidity (125, 170); anorexia (44); and grooming behavior (17). These functions are consistent with the high levels of GRP found in hypothalamic and brainstem nuclei (10, 113, 114, 168) and support a significant neuroregulatory role for this peptide.

In rat spinal cord, RIA analyses have revealed that GRP is present at 8-fold higher concentrations in the dorsal horn than the ventral horn (105). These data correlate with the detection of high densities of immunoreactive fibers in the posterior horn in both rat (114) and cat (34). Nearly all of these fibers disappear after rhizotomy (114), providing evidence for their sensory origin. A few GRP-positive nerve terminals persist in the anterior horn and around the central canal after rhizotomy; these fibers may originate from intrinsic spinal cord neurons or from higher levels of the CNS (113). The highest concentration of GRP in the cord is in the dorsal horn of the lower lumbar and sacral regions. This may correlate with the presence of GRP-positive cell bodies in preverterbral sympathetic ganglia (38, 138), the gastrointestinal (GI) and genitourinary tracts (26, 41, 152), and prevertebral ganglia, as well as GRP-positive nerve terminals in the adrenal medulla (35). Some GRP-positive fibers in prevertebral sympathetic ganglia have been shown to be projections from enteric GRP-positive neurons (21), suggesting a possible GRP-mediated communication loop among the gut, prevertebral ganglia and the spinal cord (21, 138, 139).

GRP immunoreactivity has been demonstrated in human and guinea pig pituitary extracts (88) with the highest concentrations in the stalk, moderate amounts in the anterior lobe and lowest levels in the neural lobe. In adult rat pituitary, we have found GRP only in nerve fibers, mainly in the anterior lobe, but not in cell bodies. Human pituitary does not appear to contain GRP mRNA on our Northern blot analyses.

GRP and bombesin have been demonstrated to decrease basal and stimulated secretion of growth hormone (GH), thyrotropin (TSH) and prolactin (PRL) when given intracerebrally to rats (69, 113). Mitsuma, Nogimori, and Chaya (96) found that peripheral administration of bombesin increased hypothalamic thyrotropin-releasing hormone and decreased plasma TSH levels, with no change in plasma thyroid hormone levels. However, Rivier, Rivier, and Vale (128) demonstrated that intravenous administration of bombesin stimulates GH and PRL release in rats. This effect may be mediated via CNS pathways, since they observed no effect of bombesin on GH or PRL release in cultures of normal rat pituitaries (128). Relevant data on this subject are conflicting. A pituitary tumor cell line was demonstrated to release GH and PRL *in vitro* after bombesin stimulation (177) and normal bovine pituitary cells release GH but not PRL when treated with bombesin in culture (6). Similarly, GRP releases GH from cultured rat pituitary cells (122). Further studies are required to clarify the exact role of GRP in regulating pituitary hormone secretion.

Gastrointestinal Tract

GRP is widely distributed in intrinsic neurons throughout the mammalian GI tract (21, 29, 40, 122, 139, 171, 187). Price *et al.* (122) reported high levels of GRP immunoreactivity in human fundus, antrum, pylorus, and pancreas with lower levels in the duodenum, jejunum, terminal ileum, and colon. Similarly, Walsh, Wong, and Dockray (171) found the highest GRP levels in rat fundus and antrum, with lower levels in small bowel and colon. Although bombesin-like immunoreactivity is present in endocrine cells in avian proventriculus and stomach of several species of frog (171), GRP in the mammalian gut appears to be limited to neurons.

Immunocytochemical analyses have localized GRP to cell bodies within the submucosal and myenteric plexuses as well as nerve terminals in smooth muscle of the small intestine and colon (21, 29, 40, 122, 139, 171, 187). In the gastric fundus and antrum, however, GRP is found predominantly in the mucosal plexus (29, 171, 187). In the pancreas, GRP is largely present in intra-pancreatic ganglia, particularly in the periacinar regions (40, 187). On northern blots of human fetal and adult GI tissues, we have found highest levels of GRP mRNA in colon, with moderate levels in stomach and lower levels in duodenum, jejunum, ileum, and pancreas; the levels in adult tissues are lower than in the corresponding fetal tissues, but the relative abundance of GRP mRNA in different GI tissues is the same for fetuses and adults (data not shown). This is in contrast to the highest levels of GRP immunoreactivity reported in stomach, with lower levels in small bowel and colon (122, 171). We have used immunohistochemical and *in situ* hybridization analyses to localize GRP, GRP CTEPs and GRP-specific mRNAs to the submucosal and myenteric plexuses in the colon (Fig. 10*A* to *C*) and in the small intestine, and the mucosal plexus of the stomach (Fig. 10*D*). It will be important to quantitate tissue levels of proGRP by RIA throughout the GI tract, as levels of the GRP-associated CTEPs may correlate more closely with GRP mRNA levels.

The three major effects of GRP on the GI tract are regulation of gut motility, modulation of GI enteropancreatic hormone release, and stimulation of intestinal and pancreatic epithelial growth *in vivo*:

(a) GRP stimulates increased frequency of contractions of gut smooth muscle with resulting slower propulsive forces through the small intestine and colon (119). Administration of monoclonal anti-bombesin antibodies to dogs leads to increased gastric retention (72). This effect is not mediated by gastrin, suggesting that GRP may stimulate gastric emptying directly.

(b) GRP was named in recognition of its effect on promoting gastrin release *in vivo* (5, 93, 142). In addition, intravenous administration of GRP stimulates release of insulin, glucagon, pancreatic polypeptide, somatostatin, and gastric inhibitory peptide (91, 166) in dogs and humans, as well as pancreatic enzyme secretion in humans (4). GRP stimulates gastrin release from isolated gastrin cells (167), enzyme secretion in isolated, perfused pancreas (24), and insulin release from a pancreatic islet cell line (156).

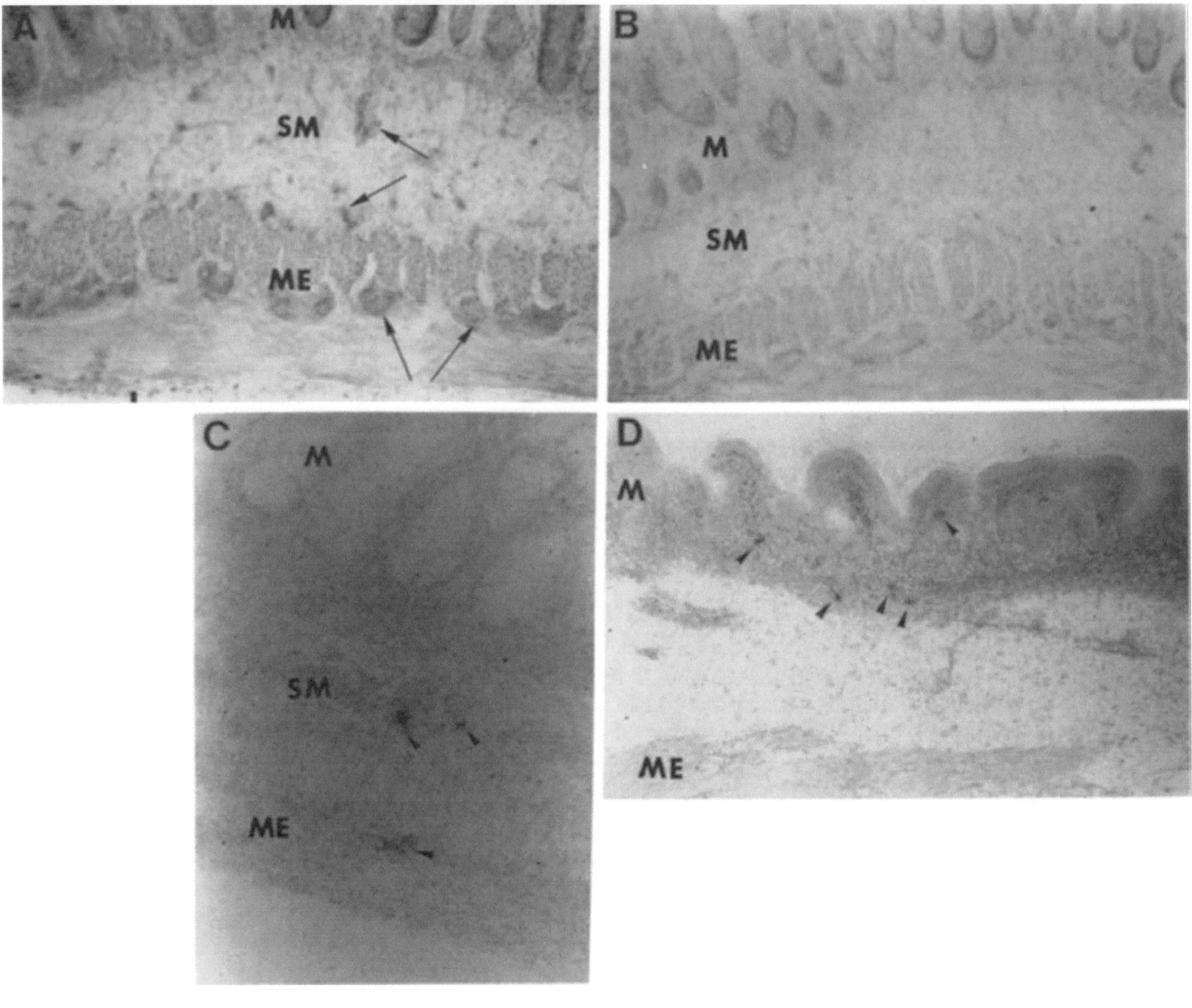

FIG. 10. Immunohistochemistry and *in situ* hybridization for GRP peptide and mRNAs in fetal colon and stomach. *A*, Immunoperoxidase analysis of 18-week gestation human fetal colon with anti-bombesin antiserum and the avidin-biotin technique (Vector Laboratories, Inc.) demonstrates GRP localized to ganglia in the submucosal and myenteric plexuses as indicated by *arrows*. *M*, mucosa; *SM*, submucosa; *ME*, muscularis externa. *B*, Negative control serial section corresponding to Figure 11*A*, run in parallel with the same anti-bombesin antiserum that had been preabsorbed with amphibian bombesin antigen (10 μg/ml). *C*, *In situ* hybridization of the same fetal colon with ^{35}S-labeled GRP cRNA probe shows prominent GRP mRNA-positive cells present in the regions of the submucosal and myenteric plexuses. *D*, *In situ* hybridization of stomach from the same fetus demonstrates GRP-positive cells in the gastric mucosal plexus (*arrows*). Figure 10*A* and *B*, ×250; *C*, ×300; *D*, ×250.

(c) Bombesin administered intravenously (82) or orally (81) to neonatal rats induces hyperplasia of gastrin-containing cells in the antrum as well as hyperplasia of duodenal and pancreatic acinar glands. These effects may be due to GRP acting directly on target cells, as gastrin has been shown to have no effect on growth of gastric mucosa or small intestine in rabbits before weanling (189). The involvement of enteroglucagon or gastrin released after GRP treatment in an *in vivo* model of GRP-induced growth has not yet been evaluated (64). The precise role of GRP in GI growth and development remains to be determined.

BREAST MILK

Significant levels of GRP immunoreactivity have been reported in both human and bovine milk (30, 59, 77, 78). Due to the difficulty in obtaining human lactating breast tissue, we examined bovine udder. Weak to moderate GRP immunoreactivity was demonstrated in cow udder in the apical cytoplasm of cells lining the lactiferous glands (153). Numerous other growth factors have been identified in maternal milk (15, 39, 74, 110, 176, 191) (Table 1). Since orally administered bombesin has been demonstrated to lead to significant GI growth in neonatal

TABLE 1. GROWTH FACTORS IDENTIFIED IN MILK

GRP
Epidermal growth factor
Growth hormone
Growth hormone-releasing hormone
Insulin
Insulin-like growth factors
Nerve growth factor
Thyroid-stimulating hormone
Thyrotropin-releasing hormone
Transforming growth factor, type α

rats (81), these data raise the possibility that milk is an important source of GRP for developing animals.

Genitourinary Tract and Adrenal

GRP has been identified in nerve fibers throughout the female reproductive tract of the rat (41, 152), with highest levels in the vagina and uterus. It is present in nerve cell bodies of the paracervical ganglion formation (138), as well as throughout the bladder (41). We have similarly observed GRP-positive nerve fibers in human uterine smooth muscle by immunocytochemistry. Pharmacologic experiments on isolated uterine and cervical smooth muscle demonstrated concentration-dependent clonic contractions in uterus and cervix elicited by GRP or bombesin, most pronounced in estrogen-treated rats (152). Thus, GRP may have a role in female reproductive functions. Bombesin is also known to induce marked, long-lasting contraction of the rat urinary bladder and ureter (3)

Rare GRP-positive neuroendocrine cells have been demonstrated in human prostate, where they represent fewer than 5% of the neuron-specific enolase-positive cell population (26). Although the function of GRP in prostate is unknown, the detection of GRP immunoreactivity in human seminal fluid suggests a possible role in male reproductive function (164). It is of interest that the number of neuroendocrine cells in the guinea pig prostate increases with increasing age (27).

Although GRP immunoreactivity has been demonstrated in chromaffin cells of bovine adrenal medulla (83), we have been unable to demonstrate GRP mRNA or peptide in human fetal or adult adrenal tissue. However, it is well recognized that GRP acts through sympathetic nerve endings to stimulate epinephrine secretion from the rat adrenal medulla (35).

GRP RECEPTORS

Tissue Distribution

The cellular receptors for bombesin/GRP have been extensively mapped *in vivo* and characterized *in vitro* using both receptor autoradiography (46, 89, 111, 175, 190) and radioreceptor assays (67, 73, 84, 99, 132, 137, 157, 178, 188). These receptors, which we will term "GRP receptors," recognize the conserved C-terminus of bombesin and GRP (142) and are present throughout the CNS, GI tract, and other target organs. The highest concentration of receptors is present on gastrin cells in the antral mucosa (89, 167, 167a), with over 200,000 receptors/antral gastrin cell (167). By autoradiography, GRP receptors are also abundant in the circular muscle and myenteric plexus of the antrum, with lower levels in the circular muscle from the esophagus to the pylorus, longitudinal muscle in ileum and colon, and myenteric plexus in both small and large bowel. Receptors are detected on smooth muscle of bladder, uterus, and seminal vesicles (89). In the rat CNS, GRP binding sites are distributed in discrete regions of gray but not white matter. Highest levels are found in the olfactory bulb and tubercle, nucleus accumbens, hypothalamic nuclei (suprachiasmatic and periventricular), hippocampus, dentate gyrus, nucleus tractus solitarius, and substantia gelatinosa (190). GRP receptors are also present in the dorsal horn of the spinal cord (111), where their distribution corresponds to the location of GRP-positive nerve terminals.

GRP receptors have been most extensively characterized by cross-linking and/or radioreceptor assays using pituitary cells (178), pancreatic islet cell lines (157), normal pancreas (137), small cell carcinoma cell lines (67, 99), and 3T3 fibroblast cell lines (73, 84, 132, 169, 188). Receptors may also be present on monocytes or macrophages, as these cells have been reported to exhibit a chemotactic response to GRP (134). However, no direct demonstration of GRP receptors on these cells has been made.

Biochemistry of GRP Receptors and Second Messenger Pathways

A GRP-binding protein has been isolated from a rat PRL-secreting pituitary cell line (GH_4C_1) (36, 178); it has been shown to be a glycoprotein of about 100 kilodaltons (kd). There are about 3,600 binding sites/cell. In contrast, in insulin-secreting HIT hamster pancreatic cells (36, 157) a smaller GRP-binding protein of about 68 kD has been identified. These cells contain approximately 85,000 binding sites each. Various investigators have reported widely different molecular weights for putative GRP receptors, which are reported to be 78 kd on human SCCL cell lines with about 2,000 sites/cell (99), 65 to 85 kd on 3T3 cells with ~10,000 to 100,000 sites/cell (73, 84, 132, 188), and 75 kd on human glioma cell line GM-340 with ~55,000 sites/cell (73). The significance of these different molecular weights is unknown; in part, they may indicate differential glycosylation, as treatment with *N*-glycanase reduced the apparent molecular weight on 3T3 cells and glioma cells to 45 kd (73). The antral gastrin cells, which have 200,000 binding sites each, have the highest affinity GRP receptor known, with a K_d ~0.01 nM (167). This compares with a GRP receptor K_d ~0.5 nM in human SCCLs (99), ~1.2 nM in rat pituitary cells (178), and ~1.9 nM in NIH 3T3 cells (73).

Whereas most cell surface receptors for peptide or polypeptide ligands act through guanine nucleotide-binding proteins or through tyrosine phosphorylation (188), the GRP receptor has been associated with both of these properties (13, 84, 132, 169). The intracellular transduction mechanism which appears to mediate the effects of GRP in proliferative responses involves activation of the inositol trisphosphate/protein kinase C second messenger pathway (52). Inositol triphosphate and diacylglycerol formation is also a major component of the GRP-induced transduction mechanism leading to insulin secretion from a pancreatic islet cell line (157). Two transduction mechanisms have been implicated in the generation of these intracellular messengers: (a) a guanine nucleotide regulatory protein (G-protein) with GTPase activity (84, 132, 157, 169); and (b) a distinct 115 kd cell surface protein identified in Swiss 3T3 cells and human SCCL cells which becomes tyrosine-phosphorylated in response to bombesin stimulation (13). It is thought that this 115 kd protein may represent a distinct subunit of the GRP receptor and may be especially important in the induction of the mitogenic response to GRP, analogous to activation of tyrosine phosphorylation in response to insulin, epidermal growth factor, platelet-derived growth factor, and other mitogens (132). It is not known whether phosphotyrosine is associated with secretory responses induced by GRP or bombesin on pituitary cells, gastrin cells, or anterior pituitary cells (14). However, tyrosine phosphorylation is not universally associated with the mitogenic response to GRP (57). The explanation for these discrepancies is not known.

Several bombesin/GRP receptor antagonists have been identified which are useful tools in exploring receptor structure and function, as well as potential therapeutic agents (16, 18, 51, 60, 185). While most of these are substance P analogs with high toxicity and low affinity for the GRP receptor ($K_d \sim 10^{-6}$ M) (16, 60, 185), a new series of specific bombesin analogs with either agonist or antagonist properties has recently been generated by reducing peptide bonds in synthetic bombesin (18). The affinities of these new antagonists for the GRP receptor are high, with K_d values as low as 10^{-8} M. These compounds will be useful for further analysis of receptor structure and function.

Potential Role of Oncogene-Encoded Proteins in GRP Receptor Function

In NIH 3T3 fibroblasts, the proliferative effects of bombesin appear to be mediated through the protein product of the cellular *N-ras* oncogene (169). The *ras* gene codes for a plasma membrane protein, p21, whose only known biochemical function is a high-affinity GTPase activity. Although Swiss 3T3 cells proliferate in direct response to bombesin or GRP (133, 169), NIH 3T3 cells, which have far fewer surface receptors for GRP, do not. However, the expression of normal $p21^{N\text{-}ras}$ in these NIH 3T3 cells leads to functional coupling of GRP receptors to stimulated inositol phosphate production and cellular proliferation (169). Thus, *N-ras* p21 may be related to the putative G-protein mediating the cellular effects of GRP after binding to its receptor.

GRP also causes activation of the c-*myc* and c-*fos* oncogenes in 3T3 cells (84, 132). Cumulatively, these data suggest the operation of a cellular pathway triggered by GRP or bombesin, initially involving protein products of the cellular *N-ras* oncogene at the plasma membrane and leading to the expression of at least two additional classes of oncogenes (132).

GRP IN PATHOLOGIC PROCESSES

Lung Diseases

Increased GRP immunoreactivity in neonatal or adult lung is associated with a variety of pathologic conditions (Table 2). These will be discussed according to age groups; most of the pediatric diseases involve regeneration of injured lung and the adult diseases reflect either hyperplasia in response to injury or frank neoplasia.

Pediatric Lung Diseases. Markedly increased numbers of GRP-positive pulmonary neuroendocrine cells are present in children with bronchopulmonary dysplasia as compared with control infants of a similar age (62). This situation stands in contrast to hyaline membrane disease, where low levels of GRP immunoreactivity and low numbers of GRP-containing cells are seen in the lungs of affected infants (42, 62, 151). In acute hyaline membrane disease, airway hypoxia may lead to degranulation of pulmonary neuroendocrine cells containing GRP as well as serotonin and other vasoactive amines (97) with resulting alterations in vasomotor and/or bronchomotor tone (151). Similar changes have been demonstrated in response to airway hypoxia (but not arterial hypoxia) in sheep (76). It is also possible that necrosis and sloughing of airway epithelium contribute to lower GRP levels in hyaline membrane disease (23). Subsequently, airway epithelial regeneration associated with the transition to chronic bronchopulmonary dysplasia is associated with increased numbers of GRP-positive cells (62). Although GRP may be elevated secondary to regeneration of pulmonary neuroendocrine cells, it is postulated that GRP may be a critical growth factor involved in airway epithelial regeneration, since normal bronchial epithelial cells in culture demonstrate a proliferative response to GRP (182).

An increased frequency of GRP-positive pulmonary NE cells was also observed in 16 full-term newborn infants with brainstem damage due to birth asphyxia but without persistent fetal circulation, as compared with 6 control infants with meconium aspiration and persistent fetal circulation (45). It was suggested that intact brainstem function may be essential for the release of GRP from pulmonary neuroendocrine cells as well as for pulmonary vasoconstriction leading to persistent fetal cir-

Table 2. Pulmonary Diseases Associated with Elevated GRP Levels

Infants and Children
Bronchopulmonary dysplasia
Anencephaly
Cystic fibrosis
Bronchiectasis
Adults
(High altitude adaptation)
Cigarette smoking
Chronic obstructive pulmonary disease
Bronchiectasis
Asbestosis
Perineoplastic neuroendocrine cell hyperplasia
Tumorlets (carcinoid type)
Carcinoids
Atypical carcinoids
Small cell undifferentiated carcinomas

culation. These observations also serve to reemphasize that these clinical results are difficult to interpret conclusively; the physiology in perinatal adaptive responses is quite complex.

In an attempt to clarify the kinetics and potential role of GRP gene activation in newborn respiratory distress syndromes, we carried out *in situ* hybridization and immunoperoxidase analyses and quantitated the numbers of positive foci in postmortem lung specimens (Table 3). Chromogranin A immunoreactivity was included as a positive control for pulmonary neuroendocrine cells. Although there are too few cases for conclusive statistical analyses, several trends are notable. First, in the hyaline membrane disease cases, there are generally lower numbers of GRP-positive NE cells present as compared with control infants (see Table 3, Figs. 4 and 11); these data are consistent with previously reported observations (42, 62). Similarly, GRP mRNA was barely detectable or absent in three of four infants with hyaline membrane disease (Fig. 11*A*), two of whom had coexistent pulmonary hypoplasia; in the fourth case, abundant GRP mRNA-containing cells were detected although only a few cells contained GRP peptide. In contrast, 2 infants with bronchopulmonary dysplasia had normal to high levels of both GRP mRNA (Fig. 11*B*) and GRP peptide. These preliminary data suggest that in acute hyaline membrane disease, pulmonary NE cell degranulation and/or necrosis may be accompanied by low GRP mRNA, and that in the transition to chronic bronchopulmonary dysplasia, both GRP mRNA and peptide may be elevated. Interpretation of these cases is often complicated by coexistent pulmonary hypoplasia, which alone may be associated with low GRP mRNA and peptide, perhaps due to a primary lack of pulmonary NE cells (see below). It is possible that elevated levels of GRP mRNA may develop early in airway epithelial regeneration. Carefully controlled animal studies will be required to clarify the time course of GRP gene activation in relation to airway regeneration.

Two infants with idiopathic pulmonary hypoplasia had undetectable GRP mRNA and low to absent GRP peptide (Table 3). Cells containing chromogranin A were also rare or undetectable, indicating a lack of pulmonary NE cells generally. This relative lack of GRP and chromogranin A associated with idiopathic pulmonary hypoplasia suggests that PNECs, and potentially GRP, may be required for normal growth and maturation of the lungs. However, one infant with pulmonary hypoplasia associated with anencephaly (126) had markedly elevated numbers of GRP mRNA- and peptide-positive pulmonary NE cells (Fig. 11*C*). Overall, it appears that pulmonary NE cells and possibly GRP may be necessary but not sufficient for normal growth and development of the lungs. Ongoing investigations in our laboratory will attempt to clarify these initial observations.

In view of the vasoconstrictor action of bombesin, we considered it important to determine whether GRP gene expression is associated with secondary pulmonary hypertensive arteriopathy. GRP *in situ* hybridization and immunohistochemical analyses were carried out on open lung biopsy specimens from infants with congenital heart disease. The results are given in Table 3. There was no correlation between the number of GRP mRNA or peptide-positive cells and relative pulmonary flow (Q_p/Q_s) or resistance (R_p/R_s), pulmonary arterial pressure (P_p), or the Rabinovitch-Reid classification of arterial wall thickness (11, 123, 124). However, all of the cases except one were Heath-Edwards grade I, so we cannot make any assessment of the relationship of GRP gene expression to the grade of pulmonary arteriopathy. There was a trend toward lower numbers of GRP mRNA and peptide-

TABLE 3. GRP GENE EXPRESSION IN RESPIRATORY DISTRESS SYNDROMES

Case group	Gestational age[b] (wk)	Age at Death[c]	PMI[d] (hr)	No. of (+) cells/100 AWs[e] GRP ISH	GRP ICC	ChrA ICC
HMD[a]						
1	24	1 da	7	2	0	0
2	32	1 da	14	53	2	6
3	34*	2 da	16	0	39	40
4	42*	1.5 da	18	0	68	98
BPD						
5	24	2 mo	48	71	56	116
6	28	1 mo	32	35	116	70
Hypo						
7	32	SB	4	0	11	0
8	34	15 min	2	0	0	0
Anenc						
9	30	SB	3	7	115	34
10	34*	SB	24	292	210	54
Contr						
11	FT	SB	32	49	96	32
12	FT	23 da	6	33	122	ND[f]
13	FT	6 wk	6	26	68	ND
14	FT	7 wk	21	20	77	ND
15	FT	2.5 mo	24	9	67	ND

[a] Major clinicopathologic diagnosis are: HMD, hyaline membrane disease; BPD, bronchopulmonary dysplasia; Hypo = pulmonary hypoplasia (defined as lung weight low for age): case 7 with multiple congenital anomalies including laryngeal atresia and renal agenesis, combined lung weight 12 gm (normal 27.1 gm); case 8 with polyhydramnios, combined lung weight 30 gm (normal 38 gm); Anenc = anencephaly; Contr = controls: case 11 with meconium aspiration; case 13 with congenital heart disease; other controls with sudden infant death syndrome. (*) Also had coexistent pulmonary hypoplasia: case 3 with congenital heart disease and relative right lung hypoplasia (right 20 gm, left 75 gm), but sections of left lung only were examined here; case 4 with idiopathic pulmonary hypoplasia, combined lung weight 22 gm (normal 44 gm).

[b] Gestational age is given in weeks. FT = full-term.

[c] Age at death is given in minutes, days (da), weeks (wk), or months (mo); SB = stillborn.

[d] PMI, postmortem interval given in hours.

[e] Tissues were processed by routine fixation in 10% buffered formalin and embedding in paraffin. *In situ* hybridization (ISH) was performed with a ^{35}S-labeled cRNA probe for human GRP to detect cells containing GRP mRNAs as detailed previously (145). Immunocytochemistry for GRP was performed by the avidin-biotin complex immunoperoxidase technique using rabbit antisera to amphibian bombesin (145) and a monoclonal antibody for human chromogranin A (Hybritech, San Diego, California). Controls were as described previously (145).

[f] ND, not determined.

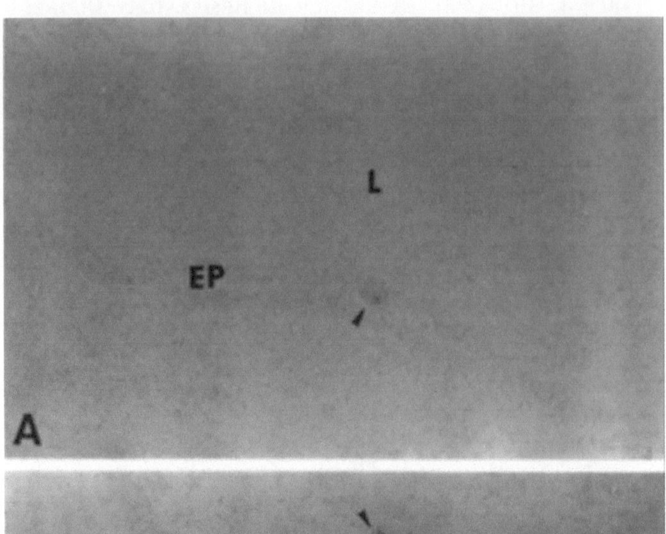

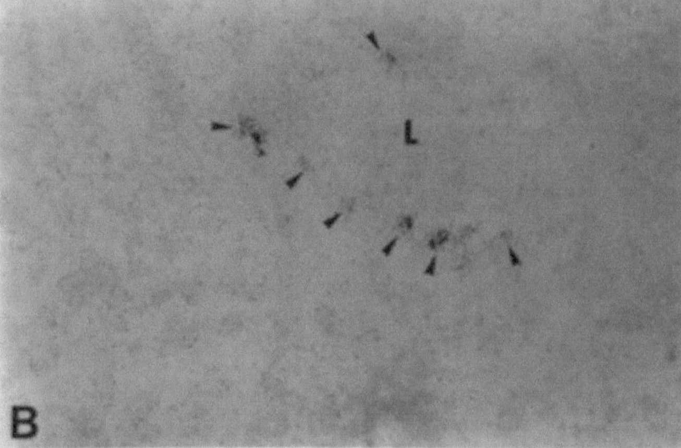

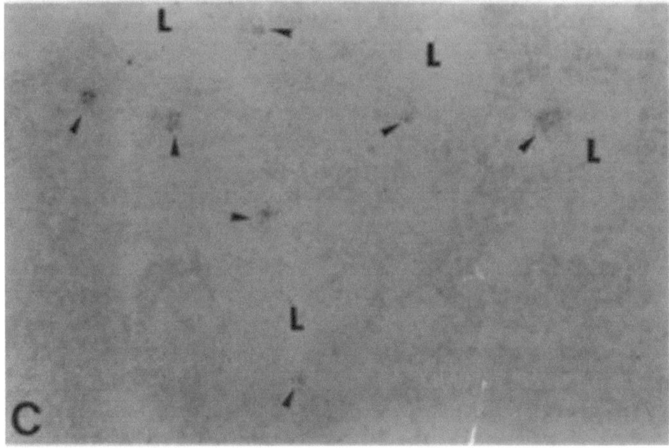

FIG. 11. *In situ* hybridization of pathologic newborn lung specimens for GRP mRNAs. *A*, One-day-old neonate with hyaline membrane disease (case 1 from Table 3) has only rare GRP mRNA-positive neuroendocrine cells (*arrowhead*) present in airway epithelium (*EP*, epithelium; *L*, airway lumen; faintly counterstained with methyl green to better visualize autoradiographic grains). *B*, 2-month-old infant with bronchopulmonary dysplasia (case 5 from Table 3) has multiple GRP mRNA-positive neuroendocrine cells (*arrowheads*) lining bronchiolar epithelium. *C*, Stillborn infant with anencephaly and pulmonary hypoplasia (case 10 from Table 3) has numerous GRP mRNA-positive cells present throughout the lung (*arrowheads*). Figure 11*A*, and *B*, ×300; *C*, ×250.

positive cells in infants with thicker bronchiolar and pulmonary arterial smooth muscle (Table 3); however, this trend was not statistically significant. Heath *et al.* 50a) have recently demonstrated a progressive increase in the number of bombesin-immunoreactive bronchiolar endocrine cells in a case of primary pulmonary hypertension followed over 5 years up to the stage of plexiform arteriopathy. At this time, we can only conclude that the relationship between GRP levels and pulmonary hypertension remains to be clarified.

Elevated pulmonary GRP immunoreactivity may also be found in children with cystic fibrosis or those subjected to prolonged assisted ventilation (63). This finding may result from neuroendocrine cell hyperplasia in response to airway injury, regeneration, and/or hypoxia.

Adult Lung Diseases, Including Neoplasia. Elevated levels of GRP immunoreactivity may be associated with high altitude adaptation in adults (48) and with hypoxia-induced neuroendocrine cell hyperplasia (76). Elevated GRP levels have also been demonstrated in bronchial lavage fluid from cigarette smokers (1), and in lungs from patients with asbestosis, bronchiectasis, and chronic obstructive pulmonary disease (48, 162, 172). In an animal model of asbestosis, elevated GRP immunoreactivity was observed in rat lung extracts only late in the clinical course, suggesting that GRP probably does not play a primary role in the pathologic progression of this disease (22). In many of these chronic diseases, pulmonary NE cell hyperplasia or pulmonary carcinoid-like tumorlets may be present later in the disease course, possibly triggered by hypoxia and/or pulmonary epithelial injury and regeneration. Prominent GRP immunoreactivity (48) and GRP gene expression (153) have also been demonstrated in NE cell hyperplasias adjacent to both neuroendocrine and non-neuroendocrine lung tumors (Fig. 12*A*). It is not known whether this NE cell hyperplasia precedes or follows the induction of the adjacent tumor. In hamsters, pulmonary NE cell hyperplasia may precede development of squamous cell and adenocarcinomas (86). We have also observed prominent GRP gene expression in a majority of tumorlets in lungs from patients with bronchiectasis (153).

GRP mRNAs and peptide are frequently detected at high levels in human pulmonary carcinoids and SCCLs (9, 12, 31, 49, 50, 102, 103, 117, 130, 135, 136, 141, 143, 160, 184). Although GRP may be detected in sera from patients with SCCL (103), elevated serum GRP levels only rarely give rise to clinical symptoms. There is one case report of a patient with a neuroendocrine tumor producing GRP which gave rise to Cushings syndrome via increased ACTH release (55). However, there is evidence for the involvement of GRP in the biologic behavior of these tumors. In particular, GRP stimulates the clonal proliferation of several SCCL cell lines in culture and in nude mice (19, 173). This proliferation is inhibited by monoclonal antibodies to the bioactive C-terminus of GRP (19), suggesting that an autocrine mechanism may contribute to unregulated cell growth in SCCL.

In most series, about 50 to 70% of pulmonary carcinoids (Fig. 12*B*) (9, 12, 48, 130, 135, 160), but <20% of SCCLs (12, 31, 49, 50, 102, 103, 117, 141, 184), contain GRP immunoreactivity. However, about 70% of some SCCLs contain detectable levels of proGRP, as determined by immunoreactivity for the GRP CTEPs (49, 184). It should be noted that the sensitivity of detection of GRP immunoreactivity varies somewhat, perhaps de-

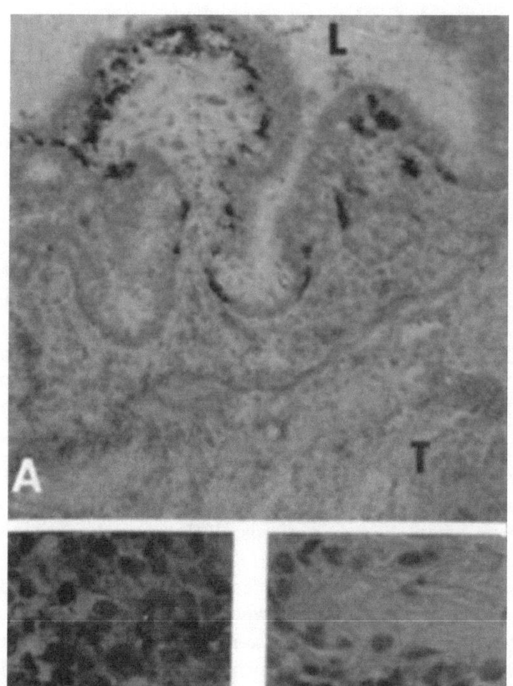

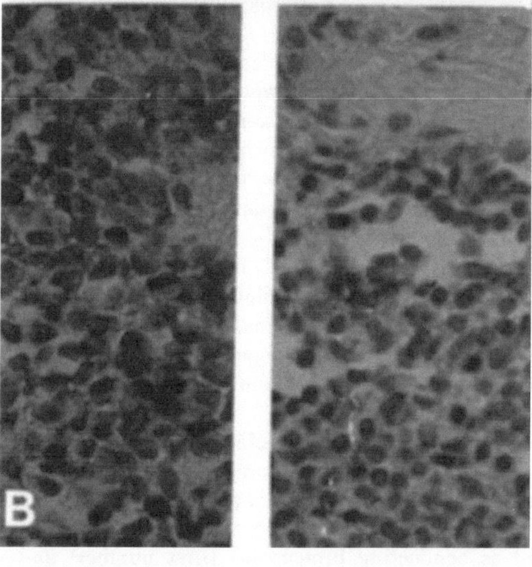

FIG. 12. GRP immunohistochemistry and *in situ* hybridization analyses of pathologic adult lung specimens. *A*, Immunoperoxidase analysis of histologically normal bronchiolar epithelium adjacent to a GRP-negative poorly differentiated adenocarcinoma (labeled *T*, tumor) demonstrates numerous darkly stained GRP-positive neuroendocrine cells and neuroepithelial bodies just below the mucosa (*L*, airway lumen). *B*, Immunoperoxidase analysis of the original pulmonary carcinoid tumor from which GRP mRNAs were isolated (11), stained with anti-bombesin antiserum (*left*) and with the same antiserum preabsorbed with bombesin antigen (10 μg/ml). Figure 12*A*, ×100; *B*, ×400.

pending on the antisera employed, with one group reporting concordant immunostaining for GRP and the CTEPs in about half of SCCLs, both primary and metastatic (61, 148). Using the more sensitive technique of *in situ* hybridization virtually all SCCLs have been found to contain GRP mRNA, reflecting GRP gene activation in these tumors (50). These observations are of diagnostic importance, in that CTEP antisera would augment histochemical diagnosis of a majority of pulmonary SCCLs, as well as extra-pulmonary SCCs (see "GI" section below) (149).

Taken together, these data indicate that GRP gene activation is associated with a majority of SCCLs but that processing of proGRP to GRP may be variable. Present studies aim to determine whether these cells exhibit abnormal post-translational processing and whether GRP CTEPs have a role in tumor growth.

THYROID HYPERPLASIA AND NEOPLASIA

The GRP gene is expressed at high levels not only in normal developing thyroidal cells (154), but also in C cell hyperplasia (Fig. 13*A*) and in MCT (Fig. 13*B*) (43, 55, 66, 90, 120, 140, 186). Suzuki *et al.* (155) have also reported high levels of GRP mRNA in three MCTs, where levels of mRNA correlated closely with levels of GRP peptide measured by RIA.

In 7 of 11 specimens of normal thyroid adjacent to GRP-negative follicular adenomas and papillary carcinomas, the proportion of GRP-positive C cells was increased from less than 20% of the CT-positive C cells to about 60% (154). In one of these 7 specimens, overt nodular and diffuse C cell hyperplasia was also observed (Fig. 13*A*). This finding appears to be analogous to GRP-positive perineoplastic pulmonary NE cell hyperplasia and pulmonary tumorlets in chronically injured lungs (48). It appears to represent perineoplastic activation of the GRP gene in pathologic adult thyroid, and may signify a host response to a neoplastic stimulus, analogous to pulmonary NE cell hyperplasia in diethylnitrosamine-treated hamsters (86). Alternatively, the perineoplastic phenomenon may represent a host response to the tumor, or to diffusible factors elaborated by the tumor itself.

Of note, the highest levels of GRP or CT immunoreactivity seen in adult thyroids without tumors were in patients with hypercalcemia (154). Cell hyperplasia has been reported in hypercalcemic humans (87) and in dogs with induced hypercalcemia (65). As GRP and CT levels are strikingly correlated in thyroid at all ages examined (154), it is possible that GRP and CT synthesis are regulated by similar factors. For instance, elevated calcium levels, which are known to increase CT synthesis and secretion, may also trigger the GRP gene. Studies are planned to determine whether GRP is a marker of generalized C-cells proliferation in response to calcium levels.

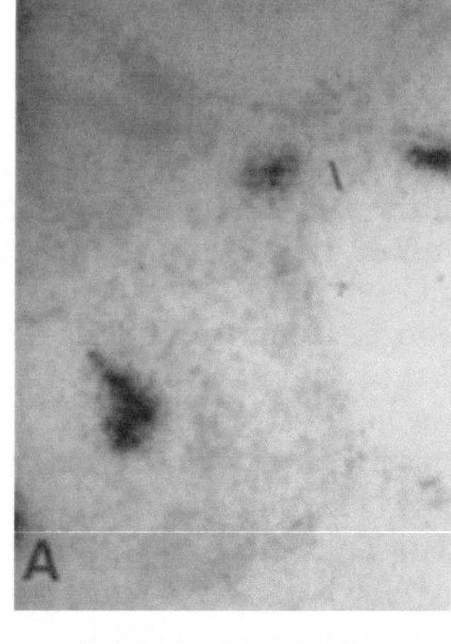

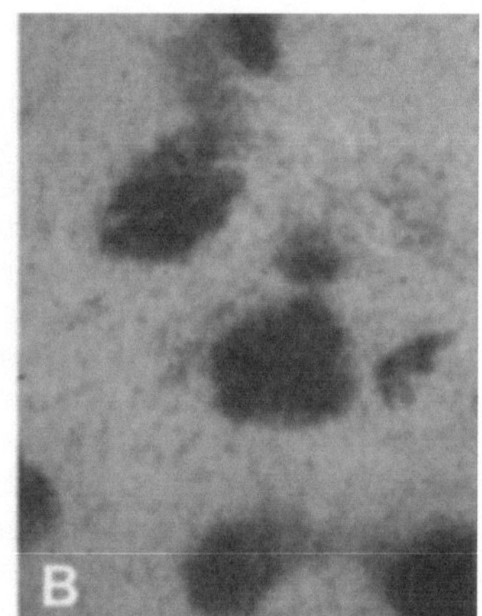

FIG. 13. *In situ* hybridization for GRP mRNAs in hyperplastic and neoplastic thyroidal C cells. *A*, Incidental C cell hyperplasia identified in grossly normal thyroid adjacent to a resected GRP-negative follicular adenoma, demonstrating diffusely scattered clusters of C cell hyperplasia with abundant GRP mRNA. *B*, Medullary carcinoma of the thyroid, with strong [^{35}S]-GRP autoradiographic signals overlying invasive nests of tumor cells, but negative over adjacent connective tissue. (Reprinted with permission from Endocrinology, 1988 (Ref. 154). Figure 13*A*, ×160; *B*, ×200.

Central Nervous System

GRP is present at high levels in most SCCLs metastatic to brain (2). Cerebrospinal fluid (CSF) GRP levels are often significantly elevated in these patients, being detectable in CSF from 21% of patients with parenchymal CNS metastases and 78% of those with meningeal carcinomatosis (116). GRP was undetectable in 52 intrinsic neurological tumors and 7 meningiomas tested (2). However, there is 1 case report of a patient with von Hippel-Lindau syndrome having GRP-positive cells comprising the intervascular cells of hemangioblastomas in cerebellum, retina and spinal cord (58). It is suggested that the histogenesis of these tumors may be neural, particularly since all of the spinal hemangioblastomas in this case occurred in the dorsal root ganglia (58). More cases of this rare syndrome need to be studied to clarify whether this is a general phenomenon.

The concentration of GRP has also been demonstrated to be significantly decreased by RIA of postmortem brain tissue from 25 patients with Parkinson's disease as compared with 25 patients who died without neurologic disease (7). The brain regions affected were the caudate nucleus and globus pallidus, the 2 regions which include the major dopamine terminal fields arising from cell bodies in the substantia nigra. There was no change in GRP levels in substantia nigra or ventral tegmental area of patients with Parkinson's disease, in contrast to the decrease in other neurotransmitters in these regions. The decreases in GRP in the caudate nucleus and globus pallidus may be due to the destruction of GRP-containing nerve terminals in these regions, the destruction of GRP-positive cell bodies in other brain regions that project to the striatum, or to the loss of positive regulation by other neurotransmitters (*e.g.*, dopamine) (7). These alterations in local peptide concentrations may be understood when neuroanatomical pathways of GRP projections in human brain are clarified.

Table 4. GRP Gene Expression in Pulmonary Hypertensive Arteriopathy

Dx[a]	Age (mo)[b]	Number of (+) Cells/100 AWs[c] GRP ISH	GRP ICC	% Av WTh PA[d]	AvThick of BrSmM[e]
					μm
VSD	7	195	752	31.0	1.19, NP
VSD, PDA	6	543	636	41.5	NP, 1.09
VSD, ASD, PDA	2	178	261	50.7	1.94, 2.54
VSD	2	139	269	55.4	1.68, 0.97
VSD, PFO	7	88	207	27.7	0.60, 1.43
VSD	7	273	236	42.5	0.69, NP
VSD	9	11	90	46.1	NP, 3.37
MR	12	88	254	43.2	7.09, NP

[a] Major clinicopathologic diagnoses of open-lung biopsied cases are given abbreviated as: ASD, atrial septal defect; MR, mitral regurgitation; PDA, patent ductus arteriosus; PFO, patent foramen ovale; VSD, ventricular septal defect.

[b] Age is given in months. All cases were Heath-Edwards grade I except the 12-month-old infant, who was grade III.

[c] Open lung biopsy specimens were fixed immediately after removal in 10% buffered formalin and routinely embedded in paraffin. *In situ* hybridization (ISH) and immunocytochemistry (ICC) were performed and the number of positive cells quantitated as described in the legend to Table 3.

[d] Average wall thickness (Av WTh) of pulmonary arteries (PAs) was determined by measuring the medial wall thickness between the internal elastic and external elastic membranes of all 50- to 100-μm arteries in one complete section of each biopsy specimen; the result is expressed as a percentage of the arterial radius from the center of the lumen to the external elastic membrane.

[e] The average thickness of bronchiolar smooth muscle (BrSmM) was determined by measuring (in micrometers) the thickness of bronchiolar smooth muscle in all airways in one complete section of each biopsy specimen; the results are divided according to the type of airway, specified as conducting bronchioles (first number) and respiratory bronchioles (second number). NP, not present in biopsy specimen.

Gastrointestinal Tract

Although normal human gut endocrine cells do not contain detectable GRP, GRP immunoreactivity has been reported in about 60% of intestinal carcinoids (8, 106), occasional islet cell tumors and a single hepatic carcinoid (120). Furthermore, about half of extrapulmonary small cell carcinomas (SCCs) have been demonstrated to have proGRP immunoreactivity, including 11 of 22 of these tumors in esophagus and 1 of 2 in colon; fewer than 10% of these tumors had GRP immunoreactivity (149). These data indicate that one must consider possible extrapulmonary origins for metastatic GRP-positive or proGRP-positive tumors. Although growth stimulation of extrapulmonary SCCs by GRP has not yet been demonstrated, GRP may act as a growth factor for extrapulmonary SCCs analogous to SCCLs. These undifferentiated tumors exhibit similar biologic behavior regardless of location.

Bombesin has been demonstrated to stimulate the growth of preneoplastic acinar cell lesions in early stages of pancreatic carcinogenesis induced by azaserine in rats (85). The role of bombesin-like peptides in GI carcinogenesis remains to be determined for both neuroendocrine and nonneuroendocrine tumors.

There is little evidence that GRP plays a role in the genesis of peptic ulcer disease. Given intravenously, GRP leads to increased acid secretion via gastrin release in all species (70, 75, 97, 166). In contrast, intracerebral administration of GRP decreases acid secretion in rat and dog via central mechanisms (48a, 159, 170, 171). Gastrin, which is the main factor believed to be responsible for the pathologic hypersecretion of the Zollinger-Ellison syndrome, has not been implicated in the pathogenesis of classical peptic ulcer disease (53). In one clinical study, bombesin-stimulated serum gastrin levels were significantly greater in 9 duodenal ulcer patients as compared with 10 similarly treated controls, which suggests that exaggerated release of gastrin after local GRP stimulation could contribute to the hyperactive secretory response in peptic ulcer disease (53). Although no increases in serum GRP levels have been detected in postprandial human subjects (75, 171), GRP could control gastrin release in a paracrine fashion with release from enteric nerve endings directly into blood vessels of the lamina propria (37); such an effect need not lead to elevated serum levels.

Recent preliminary data suggest that bombesin-stimulated exocrine pancreatic secretion may be useful in the diagnosis of chronic pancreatitis (71). Seven patients with chronic pancreatitis had half the volume and bicarbonate output of six healthy controls in response to bombesin infusion. More patients need to be analyzed to determine whether this test would be of clinical utility.

GRP immunoreactivity appears to be normal in patients with inflammatory bowel disease (98). GRP immunoreactivity has been reported to be decreased in the aganglionic segment of colon of neonatal mice with congenital aganglionic colon, suggesting a possible role in this mouse model of Hirschsprung's disease (165).

Breast, Genitourinary Tract, Adrenal, and Skin

Although GRP is present in lactating breast, we have not detected GRP mRNA or peptide by *in situ* hybridization or immunohistochemistry in 5 cases of fibrocystic disease with intraductal hyperplasia and 1 case of lobular hyperplasia. We have also been unable to demonstrate GRP mRNA or peptide in 5 cases of breast carcinoma, including both ductal and lobular subtypes (153). One study has described GRP immunoreactivity in only 1 of 41 breast carcinomas (108).

Despite the presence of rare GRP-positive neuroendocrine cells in normal adult prostate (26), we have not observed any increases in GRP in 5 cases of benign prostatic hyperplasia (BPH), in 6 prostatic adenocarcinomas, or in normal prostate tissue adjacent to 6 prostatic carcinomas (Table 5). One study has demonstrated GRP immunoreactivity in only 1 of 50 prostatic adenocarcinomas, although one-third of these 50 tumors had other neuroendocrine features (28). If anything, there is a decline in the number of neuroendocrine cells in benign prostatic hyperplasia and adjacent to carcinomas, which may represent atrophy of these cells in populations with increasing age. In contrast, an increase in prostatic NECs has been observed in aging guinea pigs (27).

Table 5. GRP and Chromogranin A Immunoreactivity in Normal, Hyperplastic, and Perineoplastic Prostate

Prostate case group[a]	Number of (+) cells/10^3 glands[b]		% of NECs
	GRP	*chrA*	*(+) GRP*[c]
Normal	30 ± 7 (3)	883 ± 97 (3)	3.4 ± 0.8
Benign hyperplasia	4 ± 2 (5)[d]	249 ± 105 (5)[d]	3.0 ± 1.0
Perineoplastic	7 ± 5 (6)[d]	736 ± 301 (6)	1.0 ± 1.0

[a] Normal cases were selected as men (35 to 39 years old) who died with no evidence of prostate pathology. Benign prostatic hyperplasia cases were randomly selected surgical cases undergoing transurethal resection of the prostate (49 to 72 years old). Perineoplastic cases were randomly selected surgical cases undergoing prostatic resections for previously diagnosed prostatic carcinoma (51 to 68 years old).

[b] All tissues were processed by routine fixation in 10% buffered formalin and embedding in paraffin. Immunoperoxidase analysis for GRP and chromogranin A were performed as described in the legend to Table 3. The number of positive cells was counted in an entire section and normalized/10^3 glands, and expressed ± 1 SE.

[c] The percentage of neuroendocrine cells (defined by staining for chromogranin A) which were positive for GRP was calculated.

[d] $p < 0.01$ compared with normal control values, calculated using the paired Student's *t*-test.

Although normal human bladder contains GRP-immunoreactivity only in neurons (41) and normal human adrenal medulla does not appear to contain detectable GRP in either fetuses or adults, GRP immunoreactivity has been reported in a bladder small cell carcinoma (61) and in a small percentage of pheochromocytomas (120, 160). These isolated observations may represent aberrant peptide gene activation in tumors originating from precursor cells of the diffuse neuroendocrine system (115).

Although normal mammalian skin does not contain GRP, one group has reported GRP immunoreactivity in 62% of neuroendocrine carcinomas of the skin (160). In a more detailed analysis (180), 4 of 7 secondary cutaneous neuroendocrine carcinomas (all metastatic from lung) were found to contain GRP immunoreactivity. In contrast, none of 21 primary neuroendocrine carcinomas of the skin ("Merkel cell" carcinomas) was positive for GRP. These observations are of clinical relevance. If a cutaneous tumor contains GRP, one should search for a primary elsewhere, most likely in lung (180) or in the GI tract (8).

CONCLUSIONS

GRP has become recognized as a significant neuroregulatory hormone and growth factor in normal mammals. Its widespread tissue distribution and diverse, potent biologic effects suggest that it plays a major role in modulating homeostatic responses and stimulating cellular proliferation in a developmental and tissue-specific manner. Its role in pathogenesis appears to be related mainly to its properties as a growth factor, especially in lung, where it can induce clonal growth of both normal and neoplastic epithelial cells. One can understand its association with regenerative processes such as bronchopulmonary dysplasia and bronchiectasis, as well as with neoplasia, by hypothesizing that GRP gene activation occurs during fetal lung development and in response to tissue insult or injury (Fig. 14). The resultant pathology represents a spectrum of lesions ranging from neuroen-

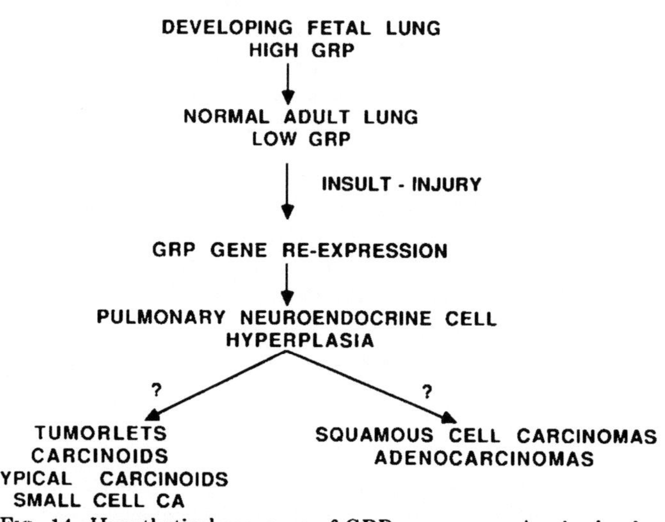

Fig. 14. Hypothetical sequence of GRP gene expression in developing hyperplastic and neoplastic lung. See text for discussion.

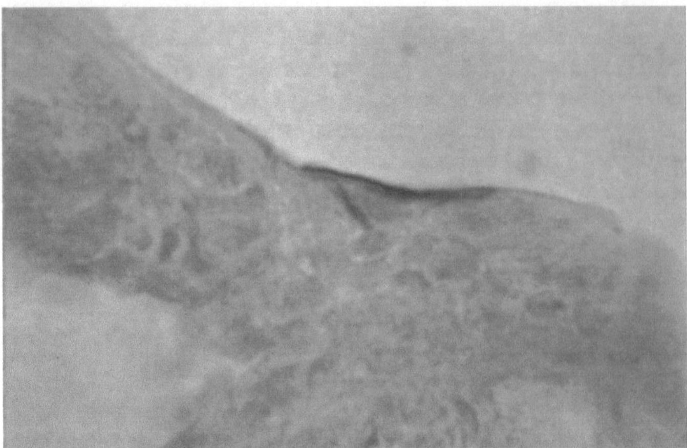

FIG. 15. Immunoperoxidase analysis of neonatal hamster lung. Four-day-old neonatal hamster lung immunostained with anti-bombesin antiserum demonstrates occasional GRP-positive pulmonary neuroendocrine cells. ×1,500.

docrine cell hyperplasia and benign carcinoid tumors to widely metastasizing small cell carcinomas. Although GRP-positive neuroendocrine cells may also be prominent in tissue adjacent to non-neuroendocrine tumors of lung and thyroid, the significance of this association is not known. In order to delineate further the mechanisms involved in these processes, animal models must be explored. In this regard, it is of interest that GRP-positive neuroendocrine cells are easily identified in neonatal hamsters (Fig. 15). Adult hamsters develop pulmonary NE cell hyperplasias as well as neuroendocrine tumors in response to systemic carcinogens. We hope that this model will permit further delineation of the role of GRP in normal development and tumorigenesis.

Other disorders may also be associated with low or absent GRP gene expression, such as idiopathic pulmonary hypoplasia. Defects in GRP receptor number or function may explain observations such as the over-responsiveness to bombesin challenge observed in duodenal ulcer patients. In order to understand the involvement of GRP in such a wide diversity of disease states more clearly, further definition of molecular mechanisms of GRP gene activation and the molecular structure and regulation of the GRP receptor needs to be explored. When we understand the kinetics and mechanisms of GRP activation during normal mammalian embryogenesis and in physiologic states, understanding of the pathophysiology will be close at hand.

Acknowledgments: We are grateful to Dr. Alba Greco for the cases used in Table 2, and to Dr. Hubert Wolfe for helpful discussions. We would also like to thank Drs. Hal Chapman, Eugene Mark, Shirin Nash, Lynne Reid, and Agnes Schonbrunn for reviewing this manuscript.

Address reprint requests to: Mary E. Sunday, M.D., Ph.D., Department of Pathology, Brigham & Women's Hospital, 75 Francis Street, Boston, MA 02115.

REFERENCES

1. Aguayo SM, Kane M, Schwarz MI, King T, Grauer L, Dienhart D, Bunn PA, Miller YE: Bombesin-like immunoreactivity in bronchoalveolar lavage from smokers and interstitial lung disease (abstr). Clin Res 35:530, 1987
2. Allen JM, Hoyle NR, Yeats JC, Ghatei MA, Thomas DGT, Bloom SR: Neuropeptides in neurological tumors. J Neurooncol 3:197, 1985
3. Anastasi A, Erspamer V, Bucci M: Isolation and structure of bombesin and alytesin, two analogous active peptides from the skin of the European amphibians Bombina and Alytes. Experientia 27:166, 1971
4. Basson N, Giri S, Improta G, Lezoche E, Melchiorri P, Percoco M, Speranza V: External pancreatic secretion after bombesin infusion in man. Gut 16:994, 998, 1975
5. Bertaccini G, Erspamer V, Melchiorri P, Sopranzi N: Gastrin release by bombesin in the dog. Br J Pharmacol 52:219, 1974
6. Bicknell R, Chapman C: Bombesin stimulates growth hormone secretion from cultured bovine pituitary cells. Neuroendocrinology 36:33, 1983
7. Bissette G, Nemeroff CB, Decker MW, Kizer JS, Agid Y, Javoy-Agid F: Alterations in regional brain concentrations of neurotensin and bombesin in Parkinson's disease. Ann Neurol 17:324, 1985
8. Bostwick DG, Roth KA, Barchas JD, Bensch KG: Gastrin-releasing peptide immunoreactivity in intestinal carcinoids. Am J Clin Pathol 82:428, 1984
9. Bostwick DG, Roth KA, Evans CJ, Barchas JD, Bensch KG: Gastrin-releasing peptide, a mammalian analog of bombesin, is present in human neuroendocrine lung tumors. Am J Pathol 117:195, 1984
10. Brown M, Allen R, Villarreal J, Rivier J, Vale W: Bombesin-like activity: radioimmunologic assessment in biological tissues. Life Sci 23:2721, 1978
11. Burrows FA, Rabinovitch M: The pulmonary circulation in children with congenital heart disease: morphologic and morphometric considerations. Can Anaesth Soc J 32:364, 1985
12. Chejfec G, Lee I, Warren WH, Gould VE: Bombesin in human neuroendocrine (NE) neoplasms. Peptides 6 (Suppl 3):107, 1985
13. Cirillo DM, Gaudino G, Naldini L, Comoglio PM: Receptor for bombesin with associated tyrosine kinase activity. Mol Cell Biol 6:4641, 1986
14. Comoglio PM: Personal communication.
15. Corps AN, Brown KD: Stimulation of intestinal epithelial cell proliferation in culture by growth factors in human and ruminant mammary secretions. J Endocrinol 113:285, 1987
16. Corps AN, Rees LH, Brown KD: A peptide that inhibits the mitogenic stimulation of Swiss 3T3 cells by bombesin or vasopressin. Biochem J 231:781, 1985
17. Cowan A, Khunawat P, Zhu XZ, Gmerek DE: Effects of bombesin on behavior. Life Sci 37:135, 1985
18. Coy DH, Heinz-Erian P, Jiang N-y, Jensen RT: Progress in the development of competitive bombesin antagonists (abstr). Regul Pept 19:105, 1987
19. Cuttitta F, Carney DN, Mulshine J, Moody TW, Fedorko J, Fischler A, Minna JD: Bombesin-like peptides can function as autocrine growth factors in human small cell lung cancer. Nature 316:823, 1985
20. Cutz E, Chan W, Track NS: Bombesin, calcitonin and leu-enkephalin immunoreactivity in endocrine cells of the human lung. Experientia 37:765, 1981
21. Dalsgaard C-J, Hokfelt T, Schultzberg M, Lundberg JM, Terenius L, Dockray GJ, Goldstein M: Origin of peptide-containing fibers in the inferior mesenteric ganglion of the guinea-pig: immunohistochemical studies with antisera to substance P, enkephalin, vasoactive intestinal polypeptide, cholecystokinin and bombesin. Neuroscience 9:191, 1983
22. Day R, Lemaire I, Masse S, Lemaire S: Pulmonary bombesin in experimentally induced asbestosis in rats. Exp Lung Res 8:1, 1985
23. de la Monte SM, Hutchins GM, Moore GW: Respiratory epithelial cell necrosis is the earliest lesion of hyaline membrane disease of the newborn. Am J Pathol 123:155, 1986
24. Deschodt-Lanckman M, Robberecht P, De Neef P, Lammens M, Christophe J: In vitro action of bombesin and bombesin-like peptides on amylase secretion, calcium efflux, and adenylate cyclase activity in the rat pancreas. J Clin Invest 58:891, 1976
25. Dey RD, Hoffpauir JM: Ultrastructural colocalization of the bioactive mediators 5-hydroxytryptamine and bombesin in endocrine cells of human fetal airways. Cell Tissue Res 246:119, 1986
26. di Sant'Agnese PA: Calcitonin-like immunoreactive and bombesin-like immunoreactive endocrine-paracrine cells of the human prostate. Arch Pathol Lab Med 110:412, 1986

27. di Sant'Agnese PA, Davis NS, Chen M, deMesy Jensen KL: Age-related changes in neuroendocrine (endocrine-paracrine) cell population and the serotonin content of the guinea pig prostate. Lab Invest 57:729, 1987
28. di Sant'Agnese PA, de Mesy Jensen KL, O'Toole K: Neuroendocrine differentiation in prostatic carcinoma (abstr). Lab Invest 54:16, 1986
29. Dockray GJ, Vaillant C, Walsh JH: The neuronal origin of bombesin-like immunoreactivity in the rat gastrointestinal tract. Neuroendocrinol 4:1561, 1979
30. Ekman R, Ivarsson S, Jansson L: Bombesin, neurotensin and pro-opio-melanotropin immunoreactants in human milk. Regul Pept 10:99, 1985
31. Erisman MD, Linno RI, Hernandez O, DiAngustine RP, Lazarus LH: Human lung small cell carcinoma contains bombesin. Proc Natl Acad Sci USA 79:2379, 1982
32. Erspamer V, Falconieri Erspamer G, Massanti G, Endean R: Active peptides in the skins of one hundred amphibian species from Australia and Papua New Guinea. Comp Biochem Physiol 77C:99, 1984
33. Erspamer V, Melchiorri P, Falconieri Erspamer G, Montecucchi PC, de Castiglione R: Phyllomedusa skin: a huge factory and store-house of a variety of active peptides. Peptides 6 (Suppl 3):7, 1985
34. Fiddes JC, Goodman HM: The cDNA for the β-subunit of human chorionic gonadotropin suggests evolution by gene by read-through into the 3'-untranslated region. Nature 286:684, 1980
35. Fisher LA, Cave CR, Brown MR: Central nervous system cardiovascular effects of bombesin in conscious rats. Am Physiol Soc 248:H425, 1985
36. Fischer JB, Schonbrunn A: The bombesin receptor is coupled to a guanine nucleotide binding protein which is insensitive to pertussis and cholera toxins. J Biol Chem 263:2808, 1988
37. Furness JB, Miller AS, Costa M: Bombesin-like peptides in the enteric plexuses (abstr). Regul Pept 19:109, 1987
38. Fuxe K, Agnati LF, McDonald T, Locatelli V, Hokfelt T, Dalsgaard C-J, Battistini N, Yanaihara N, Mutt V, Cuello AC: Immunohistochemical indications of gastrin releasing peptide-bombesin-like immunoreactivity in the nervous system of the rat. Codistribution with substance P-like immunoreactive nerve terminal systems and coexistence with substance P-like immunoreactivity in dorsal root ganglion cell bodies. Neurosci Letters 37:17, 1983
39. Gaull GE, Wright CE, Isaacs CE: Significance of growth modulators in human milk. Pediatrics 75:142, 1985
40. Ghatei MA, George SK, Major JH, Carlei F, Polak JM, Bloom SR: Bombesin-like immunoreactivity in the pancreas of man and other mammalian species. Experientia 40:884, 1984
41. Ghatei MA, Gu J, Allen JM, Polak JM, Bloom SR: Bombesin-like immunoreactivity in female rat genito-urinary tract. Neurosci Letters 54:13, 1985
42. Ghatei MA, Sheppard MN, Henzen-Logman S, Blank MA, Polak JM, Bloom SR: Bombesin and vasoactive intestinal polypeptide in the developing lung: marked changes in acute respiratory distress syndrome. J Clin Endocrinol Metab 57:1226, 1983
43. Ghatei MA, Springall DR, Nicholl CG, Polak JM, Bloom SR: Gastrin-releasing peptide-like immunoreactivity in medullary thyroid carcinoma. Am J Clin Pathol 84:581, 1985
44. Gibbs J, Bourne EM: Effect of bombesin on feeding behavior. Life Sci 37:147, 1985
45. Gillan JE, Pape KE, Cutz E: Association of changes in bombesin immunoreactive neuroendocrine cells in lungs of newborn infants with persistent fetal circulation and brainstem damage due to birth asphyxia. Pediatr Res 20:828, 1986
46. Gillati M, Moody T: The development of rat brain bombesin-like peptides and their receptors. Dev Brain Res 15:286, 1984
47. Gillis RA, Jensen RT, Buller A, DaSilva AMT, Hamosh P, Holtman JR: Central respiratory and cardiovascular effects of bombesin (abstr). Fed Proc 42:358, 1983
48. Gould VE, Linnoila RI, Memoli VA, Warren WH: Neuroendocrine components of the bronchopulmonary tract: hyperplasias, dysplasias, and neoplasms. Lab Invest 49:519, 1983
48a. Gunion MW, Tache Y: Bombesin microinfusion into the paraventricular nucleus suppresses gastric acid secretion in the rat. Brain Res 422:118, 1987
49. Hamid QA, Addis BJ, Springall DR, Ibrahim NB, Ghatei MA, Bloom SR, Polak JM: Expression of the C-terminal peptide of human pro-bombesin in 361 lung endocrine tumours, a reliable marker and possible prognostic indicator for small cell carcinoma. Virchows Arch [A] 411:185, 1987
50. Hamid QA, Bishop AE, Springall DR, Adams C, Giaid A, Denny P, Ghatei M, Legon S, Cuttita F, Rode J, Spindel E, Bloom SR, Polak JM: Detection of human pro-bombesin mRNA in small cell carcinoma of the lung: in situ hybridisation with cRNA probe. Cancer in press, 1988
50a. Heath D, Smith P, Gosney J, Mulcahy D, Fox K, Yacoub M, Harris P: The pathology of the early and late stages of primary pulmonary hypertension. Br Heart J 58:204, 1987
51. Heinz-Erian P, Coy DH, Tamura M, Jones SW, Gardner JD, Jensen RT: [D-Phe12]bombesin analogues: a new class of bombesin receptor antagonists. Am J Physiol 252:G439, 1987
52. Heslop JP, Blakeley DM, Brown KD, Irvine RF, Berridge MJ: Effects of bombesin and insulin on inositol (1,4,5) trisphosphate and inositol (1,3,4) trisphosphate formation in Swiss 3T3 cells. Cell 47:703, 1986
53. Hirschowitz BI, Tim LO, Helman CA, Molina E: Bombesin and G-17 dose responses in duodenal ulcer and controls. Dig Dis Sci 30:1092, 1985
54. Hofler H, Klimpfinger M, Ruhri C, Pfragner R, Spindel ER, Putz B, Wirnsberger G: Medullary thyroid carcinoma: characterization of neuroendocrine gene and oncogene expression. Lab Invest 56:31A, 1987
55. Howlett TA, Hale AC, Price J, Doniach I, Rees LH, Wass JAH, Besser GM: Pituitary ACTH-dependent Cushing's syndrome due to ectopic production of a bombesin-like peptide by a medullary carcinoma of the thyroid. Clin Endo 22:91, 1985
56. Impicciatore M, Bertaccini G: The bronchoconstrictor action of the tetradecapeptide bombesin in the guinea-pig. J Pharm Pharmac 25:872, 1973
57. Isacke CM, Meisenhelder J, Brown KD, Gould KL, Gould SJ, Hunter T: Early phosphorylation events following the treatment of Swiss 3T3 cells with bombesin and the mammalian bombesin-related peptide, gastrin-releasing peptide. EMBO J 5:2889, 1986
58. Ismail SM, Jasani B, Cole G: Histogenesis of haemangioblastomas: an immunocytochemical and ultrastructural study in a case of von Hippel-Lindau syndrome. J Clin Pathol 38:417, 1985
59. Jahnke GD, Lazarus LH: A bombesin immunoreactive peptide in milk. Proc Natl Acad Sci USA 81:578, 1984
60. Jensen RT, Jones SW, Folkers K, Gardner JD: A synthetic peptide that is a bombesin receptor antagonist. Nature 309:61, 1984
61. Jensen S, Cuttitta F, Winton T, Patterson GA, Chamberlain D, Ihde D, Linnoila I: Concordant expression of gastrin-releasing peptide (GRP) and GRP gene associated peptides (GGAPs) in primary and metastatic human small cell lung cancers (SCLCs): an immunohistochemical analysis (abstr). Regul Pept 19:116, 1987
62. Johnson DE, Loch JE, Elde RP, Thompson TR: Pulmonary neuroendocrine cells in hyaline membrane disease and bronchopulmonary dysplasia: Pediatr Res 16:446, 1982
63. Johnson DE, Wobken JD, Landrum BG: Changes in bombesin, calcitonin and serotonin immunoreactive pulmonary neuroendcrine cells in cystic fibrosis and after prolonged mechanical ventilation. Am Rev Respir Dis 137:123, 1988
64. Johnson LR: Regulation of gastrointestinal growth. In Physiology of the Gastrointestinal Tract, Ed 2, edited by Johnson LR, pp 301–333. New York, Raven Press, 1987
65. Kameda Y, Hideki O, Horino M: Ontogeny of immunoreactive somatostatin in thyroid C cells from dogs and guinea pigs. Anat Rec 208:89, 1984
66. Kameya T, Bessho T, Tsumuraya M, Yamaguchi K, Abe K, Shimosato Y, Yanaihara N: Production of gastrin-releasing peptide by medullary carcinoma of the thyroid. Virchows Arch [A] 401:99, 1983
67. Kane M: Direct evidence for a membrane-associated receptor for a bombesin-like peptide in human small cell lung carcinoma H345 cells. Chest 91 (Suppl): 14, 1987
68. Kendall CH, Homer CE, Bishop AE, Polak JM: Age-related peptide production by human thyroid C cells: An immunohistochemical study. Virchows Arch [A] 410:97, 1986
69. Kentroti S, McCann SM: The effect of gastrin-releasing peptide on growth hormone secretion in the rat. Endocrinology 117:1363, 1985

70. Knigge U, Holst JJ, Knuhtsen S, Petersen B, Krarup T, Holst-Pedersen J, Christiansen PM: Gastrin-releasing peptide: pharmacokinetics and effects on gastro-entero-pancreatic hormones and gastric secretion in normal men. J Clin Endocrinol Metab 5902:310, 1984
71. Koch TR, Carney JA, Go VL: Distribution and quantitation of gut neuropeptides in normal intestine and inflammatory bowel diseases. Dig Dis Sci 32:369, 1987
72. Kovacs TOG, Mulshine JL, Cuttitta F, Maxwell V, Walsh JH: The effects of long-term immunoneutralization of bombesin on gastric function in dogs (abstr). Regul Pept 19:120, 1987
73. Kris RM, Hazan R, Villines J, Moody TW, Schlessinger J: Identification of the bombesin-receptor on murine and human cell by cross-linking experiments. J Biol Chem 262:11215, 1987
74. Kulski JK, Hartmann PE: Milk insulin, GH and TSH: relationship to changes in milk lactose, glucose and protein during lactogenesis in women. Endocrinol Exp (Bratisl) 17:317, 1983
75. Lambert JR, Hansky J, Soveny C, Hunt P: Comparative effects of bombesin and porcine gastrin-releasing peptide in the dog. Dig Dis Sci 29:1036, 1984
76. Lauweryns JM, Cokelaere M, Lerut T, Theunynck P: Cross-circulation studies on the influence of hypoxia and hypoxaemia on neuro-epithelial bodies in young rabbits. Cell Tissue Res 193:373, 1978
77. Lazarus LH, Gaudino G, Wilson WE: Erspamer V: An immunoreactive peptide in milk contains bombesin-like bioactivity. Experienta 42:822, 1986
78. Lazarus LH, Wilson WE, Gaudino G, Irons BJ, Guglietta A: Evolutionary relationship between nonmammalian and mammalian peptides. Peptides 6 (Suppl 3):295, 1985
79. Lebacq-Verheyden AM, Coelingh K, Coligan J, Battey J: Processing of the human prepro-gastrin releasing peptide hormone (GRP) expressed in Swiss 3T3 mouse embryo fibroblasts and in a baculovirus/insect cell system (abstr). Regul Pept 19:122, 1987
80. Lebacq-Verheyden AM, Krystal G, Markowitz S, Way J, Sausville E, Battey J: Molecular analysis of the expression of mammalian prepro-gastrin releasing peptide genes (abstr). Regul Pept 19:122, 1987
81. Lehy T: Influence of bombesin on GI cell growth (abstr). Regul Pept 19:123, 1987
82. Lehy T, Puccio F, Chariot J, Labeille D: Stimulating effect of bombesin on the growth of gastrointestinal tract and pancreas in suckling rats. Gastroenterology 90:1942, 1986
83. Lemaire S, Chouinard L, Mercier P, Day R: Bombesin-like immunoreactivity in bovine adrenal medulla. Regul Pept 13:133, 1986
84. Letterio JJ, Coughlin SH, Williams LT: Pertussis toxin-sensitive pathway in the stimulation of c-myc expression and DNA synthesis by bombesin. Science 234:1117, 1986
85. Lhoste EF, Longnecker DS: Effect of bombesin and caerulein on early stages of carcinogenesis induced by azaserine in the rat pancreas. Cancer Res 47:3273, 1987
86. Linnoila RI, Becker KL, Silva OL, Snider RH, Moore CF: Calcitonin as a marker for diethylnitrosamine-induced pulmonary endocrine cell hyperplasia in hamsters. Lab Invest 51:39, 1984
87. LiVolsi VA, Feind CR, LoGerfo P, Tashjian AH Jr.: Demonstration by immunoperoxidase staining of hyperplasia of parafollicular cells in the thyroid gland in hyperparathyroidism. Metabolism 37:550, 1973
88. Major J, Ghatei M, Bloom S: Bombesin-like immunoreactivity in the pituitary gland. Experentia 39:1158, 1983
89. Mantyh PW, Mantyh CR, Giraud AS, Soll AH, Walsh JH, Vigna SR: Localization of specific binding sites for bombesin and related peptides in the gastrointestinal tract (abstr). Regul Pept 19:125, 1987
90. Matsubayashi S, Yanaihara C, Ohkubo M, Fukata S, Hayaski Y, Tamai H, Nakagawa T, Miyauchi A: Kuma, K, Abe, K, Suzuki, T, and Yanaihara, N Gastrin-releasing peptide immunoreactivity in medullary thyroid carcinoma. Cancer 53:2471, 1984
91. McDonald TJ, Ghatei MA, Bloom SR, Adrian TE, Mochizuki T, Yanaihara C, Yanaihara N: Dose-response comparisons of canine plasma gastroenteropancreatic hormone responses to bombesin and the porcine gastrin-releasing peptide. Regul Pept 5:125, 1983
92. McDonald TJ, Jornvall H, Ghatei M, Bloom SR, Mutt V: Characterization of an avian gastric (proventricular) peptide having sequence homology with the porcine gastrin-releasing peptide and the amphibian peptides bombesin and alytesin. FEBS Lett 122:45, 1980
93. McDonald TJ, Jornvall H, Nilsson G, Vagne M, Ghatei M, Bloom SR, Mutt V: Characterization of a gastrin releasing peptide from porcine non-antral gastric tissue. Biochem Biophys Res Commun 90:227, 1979
94. McGregor G, Woodhams P, O'Shaughnessy D, Ghatei M, Polak J, Bloom S: Developmental changes in bombesin, substance P, somatostatin and vasoactive intestinal polypeptide in the rat brain. Neurosci Lett 28:21, 1982
95. Minamino N, Kangawa K, Matsuo H: Neuromedin B is a major bombesin-like peptide in rat brain: regional distribution of neuromedin B and neuromedin C in rat brain, pituitary and spinal cord. Biochem Biophys Res Commun 124:925, 1984
96. Mitsuma T, Nogimori T, Chaya M: Bombesin inhibits thyrotropin secretion in rats. Acta Endocrinol 108:79, 1985
97. Modlin IM, Lamers CB, Walsh JH: Stimulation of canine pancreatic polypeptide, gastrin, and gastric acid secretion by ranatensin, litorin, bombesin nonapeptide and substance P. Regul Pept 1:279, 1981
98. Montesani C, D'Amato A, Chiappalone S, Narilli P, Procacciante F: Bombesin as exocrine pancreatic stimulator in healthy and chronic pancreatitis subjects (abstr). Regul Pept 19:127, 1987
99. Moody TW, Carney DN, Cuttitta F, Quattrocchi K, Minna JD: High affinity receptors for bombesin/GRP-like peptides on human small cell lung cancer. Life Sciences 37:105, 1985
100. Moody TW, O'Donohue TL, Jacobwitz DM: Biochemical localization and characterization of bombesin-like peptides in discrete regions of rat brain. Peptides 2:75, 1981
101. Moody TW, Pert CB: Bombesin-like peptides in rat brain: quantitation and biochemical characterization. Biochem Biophys Res Commun 90:7, 1979
102. Moody TW, Pert CB, Gazdar AF, Carney DN, Minna JD: High levels of intracellular bombesin characterize human small-cell lung carcinoma. Science 214:1246, 1981
103. Moody TW, Russell EK, O'Donohue TL, Linden CD, Gazdar AF: Bombesin-like peptides in small cell cancer: biochemical characterisation and secretion from a cell line. Life Sci 32:487, 1983
104. Moody T, Thoa N, O'Donohue T, Pert C: Bombesin-like peptides in rat brain: Localization in synaptosomes and release from hypothalamic slices. Life Sci 26:1707, 1980
105. Moody TW, Thoa NB, O'Donohue TL, Jacobowitz DM: Bombesin-like peptides in rat spinal cord: biochemical characterization, localization and mechanism of release. Life Sci 29:2273, 1981
106. Nash SV, Said JW: Gastroenteropancreatic neuroendocrine tumors. J Clin Pathol 86:415, 1986
107. Naylor SL, Sakaguchi AY, Spindel ER, Chin WW: Human gastrin-releasing peptide gene is located on chromosome 18. Somat Cell Molec Genet 13:87, 1987
108. Nesland JH, Holm R, Johannessen JV, Gould VE: Neurone specific enolase immunostaining in the diagnosis of breast carcinomas with neuroendocrine differentiation. Its usefulness and limitations. J Pathol 148:35, 1986
109. Niewoehner DE, Levine AS, Morley JE: Central effects of neuropeptides on ventilation in the rat. Peptides 4:277, 1983
110. Noda K, Umeda M, Ono T: Transforming growth factor activity in human colostrum. Jpn J Cancer Res 75:109, 1984
111. O'Donohue TL, Massari JV, Pazoles CJ, Chronwall BM, Shults CW, Quirion R, Chase TN, Moody TW: A role for bombesin in sensory processing in the spinal cord. J Neurosci 12:2956, 1984
112. Orloff MS, Reeve JR Jr, Ben-Avram CM, Shively JE, Walsh JH: Isolation and sequence analysis of humán bombesin-like peptides. Peptides 5:865, 1984
113. Panula P: Histochemistry and function of bombesin-like peptides. Med Biol 64:177, 1986
114. Panula P, Yang H-YT, Costa E: Neuronal location of the bombesin-like immunoreactivity in the central nervous system of the rat. Regul Pept 4:275, 1982
115. Pearse AGE: The cytochemistry and ultrastructure of polypeptide hormone producing cells of the APUD series, and the embryologic, physiologic and pathologic implications of the concept. J Histochem Cytochem 17:303, 1969
116. Pedersen AG, Becker KL, Bach F, Snider RH, Gazdar AF, Sorensen PS, Bunn PA, Hansen HH: Cerebrospinal fluid bombesin and

calcitonin in patients with central nervous system metastases from small-cell lung cancer. J Clin Oncol 4:1620, 1986
117. Pert CB, Schumacher UK: Plasma bombesin concentrations in patients with extensive small cell carcinoma of the lung. Lancet 1:509, 1982
118. Polak JM: Personal communication.
119. Porreca F: Centrally-initiated gastrointestinal motor effects of bombesin (abstr). Regul Pept 19:133, 1987
120. Price J, Kruseman AC, Doniach I, Howlett TA, Besser GM, Rees LH: Bombesin-like peptides in human endocrine tumors: quantitation, biochemical characterisation and secretion. J Clin Endocrinol Metab 60:1097, 1985
121. Price J, Penman E, Bourne GL, Rees LH: Characterisation of bombesin-like immunoreactivity in human fetal lung. Regul Pept 7:315, 1983
122. Price J, Penman E, Wass JAH, Rees LH: Bombesin-like immunoreactivity in human gastrointestinal tract. Regul Pept 9:1, 1984
123. Rabinovitch M, Haworth SG, Castaneda AR, Nadas AS, Reid LM: Lung biopsy in congenital heart disease: a morphometric approach to pulmonary vascular disease. Circulation 58:1107, 1978
124. Rabinovitch M, Haworth SG, Vance Z, Vawter G, Castaneda AR, Nadas AS, Reid LM: Early pulmonary vascular changes in congenital heart disease studied in biopsy tissue. Hum Pathol 11 (Suppl):499, 1980
125. Ravetch JV, Kirsh IR, Leder P: Evolutionary approach to the question of immunoglobulin heavy chain switching: Evidence from cloned human and mouse genes. Proc Natl Acad Sci USA 77:6734, 1980
126. Reale FR, Esterly JR: Pulmonary hypoplasia: a morphometric study of the lungs of infants with diaphragmatic hernia, anencephaly, and renal malformations. Pediatrics 51:91, 1973
127. Reeve JR Jr, Walsh JH, Chew P, Clark B, Hawke D, Shively JE: Amino acid sequences of three bombesin-like peptides from canine intestine extracts. J Biol Chem 258:5582, 1983
128. Rivier C, Rivier J, Vale W: The effect of bombesin and related peptides on prolactin and growth hormone in the rat. Endocrinology 102:519, 1978
129. Rivier JE, Brown MR: Bombesin, bombesin analogues and related peptides: effects on thermoregulation. Biochemistry 17:1766, 1978
130. Roth KA, Evans CJ, Weber E, Barchas JD, Bostwick DG, Bensch KG: Gastrin-releasing peptide-related peptides in a human malignant lung carcinoid tumor. Cancer Res 43:5411, 1983
131. Roth KA, Weber E, Barchas JD: Distribution of gastrin releasing peptide-bombesin-like immunostaining in rat brain. Brain Res 251:277, 1982
132. Rozengurt E: Early signals in the mitogenic response. Science 234:161, 1986
133. Rozengurt E, Sinnett-Smith J: Bombesin stimulation of DNA synthesis and cell division in cultures of Swiss 3T3 cells. Proc Natl Acad Sci USA 80:2936, 1983
134. Ruff M, Schiffmann E, Terranova V, Pert CB: Neuropeptides are chemoattractants for human tumor cells and monocytes: a possible mechanism for metastasis. Clin Immunol Immunopathol 37:387, 1985
135. Said JW, Vimadalal S, Nash G, Shintaku IP, Heusser RC, Sassoon AF, Lloyd RV: Immunoreactive neuron-specific enolase, bombesin, and chromogranin as markers for neuroendocrine lung tumors. Hum Pathol 16:236, 1985
136. Sausville EA, Lebacq-Verheyden AM, Spindel ER, Cuttita F, Gazdar AF, Battey JF: Expression of the gastrin-releasing peptide gene in human small cell lung cancer. J Biol Chem 261:2451, 1986
137. Scemama JL, Zahidi A, Fourmy D, Fagot-Revurat P, Vaysse N, Pradayrol L, Ribet A: Interaction of [125I]-Tyr-4-bombesin with specific receptors on normal human pancreatic membranes. Regul Pept 13:125, 1986
138. Schultzberg M: Bombesin-like immunoreactivity in sympathetic ganglia. Neuroendocrinology 2:363, 1983
139. Schultzberg M, Dalsgaard C-J: Enteric origin of bombesin immunoreactive fibres in the rat coeliac-superior mesenteric ganglion. Brain Res 269:190, 1983
140. Sikri KL, Varndell IM, Hamid QA, Wilson BS, Kameya T, Ponder BA, Lloyd RV, Bloom SR, Polak JM: Medullary carcinoma of the thyroid. An immunocytochemical and histochemical study of 25 cases using 8 separate markers. Cancer 56:2481, 1985
141. Sorensen GD, Bloom SR, Ghatei MA, Del Prete SA, Cate CC, Pettingill OS: Bombesin production by small cell carcinoma of the lung. Regul Pept 4:59, 1982
142. Spindel ER: Mammalian bombesin-like peptides. Trends Neurosci 9:130, 1986
143. Spindel ER, Chin WW, Price J, Rees LH, Besser GM, Habener JF: Cloning and characterization of cDNAs encoding gastrin-releasing peptide. Proc Natl Acad Sci USA 81:5699, 1984
144. Spindel ER, Krane IM: Molecular biology of bombesin-like peptides: Comparison of cDNAs encoding human gastrin-releasing peptide, human neuromedin B and amphibian ranatensin. Ann NY Acad Sci, in press 1988
145. Spindel ER, Sunday ME, Hofler H, Wolfe HJ, Habener JF, Chin WW: Transient elevation of mRNAs encoding gastrin-releasing peptide (GRP), a putative pulmonary growth factor, in human fetal lung. J Clin Invest 80:1172, 1987
146. Spindel ER, Zilberberg MD, Chin WW: Analysis of the gene and multiple mRNAs encoding human gastrin-releasing peptide (GRP): alternate RNA splicing occurs in neural and endocrine tissue. Molec Endo 1:224, 1986
147. Spindel ER, Zilberberg MD, Habener JF, Chin WW: Two prohormones for gastrin-releasing peptide are encoded by two mRNAs differing by 19 bases. Proc Natl Acad Sci USA 83:19, 1986
148. Springall DR, Hamid Q, Ghatei MA, Bhatnagar M, Ibrahim NBN, Cuttitta F, Bloom SR, Polak JM: Expression of C-flanking peptide of human pro-bombesin in pulmonary endocrine cells and their tumors (abstr). Regul Pept 19:139, 1987
149. Springall DR, Ibrahim NBN, Rode J, Sharpe MS, Bloom SR, Polak JM: Endocrine differentiation of extra-pulmonary small cell carcinoma demonstrated by immunohistochemistry using antibodies to PGP 9.5, neuron-specific enolase and the C-flanking peptide of human pro-bombesin. J Pathol 150:151, 1986
150. Stahlman MT, Jones M, Gray ME, Kasselberg AG, Vaughn WK: Ontogeny of neuroendocrine cells in human fetal lung. III. An electron microscopic immunohistochemical study. Lab Invest 56:629, 1987
151. Stahlman MT, Kasselberg AG, Orth DN, Gray ME: Ontogeny of neuroendocrine cells in human fetal lung: II. An immunohistochemical study. Lab Invest 52:52, 1985
152. Stjernquist M, Ekblad E, Owman C, Sundler F: Neuronal localization and motor effects of gastrin-releasing peptide (GRP) in rat uterus. Regul Pept 13:197, 1986
153. Sunday ME: Tissue-specific distribution of the mammalian bombesin gene. Ann NY Acad Sci, in press 1988
154. Sunday ME, Wolfe HJ, Roos BA, Chin WW, Spindel ER: Gastrin-releasing peptide (GRP) gene expression in developing, hyperplastic, and neoplastic human thyroidal C-cells. Endocrinology 122:1551, 1988
155. Suzuki M, Yamaguchi K, Abe K, Adachi N, Nagasaki K, Asanuma F, Adachi I, Kimura S, Terada M, Taya Y, Matsuzaki J, Keizaburo M: Detection of gastrin-releasing peptide mRNA in small cell lung carcinomas and medullary thyroid carcinomas using synthetic oligodeoxyribonucleotide probes. Jpn J Clin Oncol 17:157, 1987
156. Swope SL, Schonbrunn A: Bombesin stimulates insulin secretion by a pancreatic islet cell line. Proc Natl Acad Sci USA 81:1822, 1984
157. Swope SL, Schonbrunn A: Characterization of ligand binding and processing by bombesin receptors in an insulin-secreting cell line. Biochem J 247:731, 1987
158. Tache Y, Brown M: On the role of bombesin in homeostasis. Trends Neurosci 5:431, 1982
159. Tache Y, Ishikawa T, Gunion M, Reybould E: Bombesin: central nervous system action to inhibit gastric secretion (abstr). Regul Pept 19:140, 1987
160. Tamai S, Kameya T, Yamaguchi K, Yanai N, Abe K, Yanaihara N, Yamazaki H, Kageyama K; Peripheral lung carcinoid tumor producing predominantly gastrin-releasing peptide (GRP). Cancer 52:273, 1983
161. Track NS, Cutz E: Bombesin-like immunoreactivity in developing human lung. Life Sci 30:1553, 1982
162. Tsutsumi Y, Osamura RY, Watanabe K, Yanaihara N: Immunohistochemical studies on gastrin-releasing peptide- and adrenocorticotropic hormone-containing cells in the human lung. Lab Invest 48:623, 1983

163. Tsutsumi Y, Osamura RY, Watanabe K, Yanaihara N: Simultaneous immunohistochemical localization of gastrin releasing peptide (GRP) and calcitonin (CT) in human bronchial endocrine-type cells. Virchows Arch [A] 400:163, 1983
164. Ulisse S, Gnessi L, Fabbri A, Jannini EA, Moretti C, Bonifacio V, Di Luca Sidizzi A, Fraioli F, Isidori, A: Bombesin-like immunoreactivity in human seminal fluid (abstr). Regul Pept 19:143, 1987
165. Vaillant C, Bu'Lock A, Dimaline R, Dockray GJ: Distribution and development of peptidergic nerves and gut endocrine cells in mice with congenital aganglionic colon, and their normal littermates. Gastroenterol 82:291, 1982
166. Varner AA, Modlin IM, Walsh JH: High Potency of bombesin for stimulation of human gastrin release and gastric acid secretion. Regul Pept 1:289, 1981
167. Vigna SR, Giraud A, Soll AH, Walsh JH, Mantyh PW: Characterization of bombesin receptors on canine antral gastrin cells (abstr). Regul Pept 19:144, 1987
167a. Vigna SR, Mantyh CR, Giraud AS, Soll AH, Walsh JH, Mantyh PW: Localization of specific binding sites for bombesin in the canine gastrointestinal tract. Gastroenterology 93: 1287, 1987
168. Villarreal JA, Brown MR: Bombesin-like peptide in hypothalamus: chemical and immunological characterization. Life Sci 23:2729, 1978
169. Wakelam MJO, Davies SA, Houslay MD, McKay I, Marshall CJ, Hall A: Normal p21N-ras couples bombesin and other growth factor receptors to inositol phosphate production. Nature 323:173, 1986
170. Walsh JH: Role of gastric bombesin-like peptides and related gene products in gastric secretory function (abstr). Regul Pept 19:143, 1987
171. Walsh JH, Wong HC, Dockray GJ: Bombesin-like peptides in mammals. Fed Proc 38:2315, 1979
172. Watanabe H, Kobayashi H, Honma K, Ohnishi Y, Iwafuchi M: Diffuse panbronchiolitis with multiple tumorlets. A quantitative study of the Kultschitzky cells and the clusters. Acta Pathol Jpn 35:1221, 1985
173. Weber S, Zuckerman JE, Bostwick DG, Bensch KG, Sikic BI, Raffin TA: Gastrin-releasing peptide in a selective mitogen for small cell lung carcinoma in vitro. J Clin Invest 75:306, 1985
174. Wechbanjong N, McMillan PJ, Dalgleish AE: Influence of development on the number of calcitonin-containing cells in the mouse thyroid. Am J Anat 154:477, 1979
175. Welton ML, Mantyh CR, Gates TS, Popper P, Vigna SR, Maggio JE, Passaro E, Mantyh PW: Localization of bombesin receptors in human gastrointestinal tract using quantitative receptor autoradiography (abstr). Regul Pept 19:144, 1987
176. Werner H, Amarant T, Fridkin M, Koch Y: Growth hormone releasing factor-like immunoreactivity in human milk. Biochem Biophys Res Commun 135:1084, 1986
177. Westendorf JM, Schonbrunn A: Bombesin stimulates prolactin and growth hormone release by pituitary cells in culture. Endocrinology 110:352, 1982
178. Westendorf JM, Schonbrunn A: Characterization of bombesin receptors in a rat pituitary cell line. J Biol Chem 258:7527, 1983
179. Wharton J, Polak JM, Bloom SR, Ghatei MA, Solcia E, Brown MR, Pearse AGE: Bombesin-like immunoreactivity in the lung. Nature 273:769, 1978
180. Wick MR, Millns JL, Sibley RK, Pittelkow MR, Winkelmann RK: Secondary neuroendocrine carcinomas of the skin. An immunohistochemical comparison with primary neuroendocrine carcinoma of the skin ("Merkel cell" carcinoma). J Am Acad Dermatol 13:134, 1985
181. Wiedermann CJ, Goldman ME, Plutchok JJ, Sertl K, Kaliner MA, Johnston-Early A, Cohen MA: Bombesin in human and guinea pig alveolar macrophages. J Immunol 137:3928, 1986
182. Willey JC, Lechner JF, Harris CC: Bombesin and the C-terminal tetradecapeptide of gastrin-releasing peptide are growth factors for normal human bronchial epithelial cells. Exp Cell Res 153:245, 1984
183. Wolfe HJ, DeLellis RA, Voelkel EF, Tashjian AH Jr.: Distribution of calcitonin-containing cells in the normal neonatal human thyroid gland: a correlation of morphology with peptide content. J Clin Endocrinol Metab 41:1076, 1975
184. Wood SM, Wood JR, Ghatei MA, Sorenson GD, Bloom SR: Is bombesin a tumour marker for small-cell carcinoma? Lancet 1:690, 1982
185. Yachnis AT, Crawley JN, Robert JT, McGrane MM, Moody TW: The antagonism of bombesin in the CNS by substance P analogues. Life Sci 35:1963, 1984
186. Yamaguchi K, Abe K, Adachi I, Suzuki M, Kimura S, Kameya T, Yanaihara N: Concomitant production of immunoreactive gastrin-releasing peptide and calcitonin in medullary carcinoma of the thyroid. Metabolism 33:724, 1984
187. Yanaihara N, Yanaihara C, Mochizuki T, Iwahara K, Fujita T, Iwanaga T: Immunoreactive GRP. Peptides 2:185, 1981
188. Zachery I, Rozengurt E: Identification of a receptor for peptides of the bombesin family in Swiss 3T3 cells by affinity cross-linking. J Biol Chem 262:3947, 1987
189. Zahavi I, Kelly J, Gall DG: Role of gastrin and cholecystokinin in the ontogenic development of the gastrointestinal tract. Biol Neonate 45:97, 1984
190. Zarbin MA, Kuhar MJ, O'Donohue TL, Wolf SS, Moody TW: Autoradiographic localization of (125-I-Tyr4)bombesin-binding sites in rat brain. J Neurosci 5:429, 1985
191. Zwiebel JA, Bano M, Nexo E, Salomon DS, Kidwell WR: Partial purification of transforming growth factors from human milk. Cancer Res 46:933, 1986

Biology of Disease

Morphology and Biochemistry of Bone Remodeling: Possible Control by Vitamin D, Parathyroid Hormone, and Other Substances

William E. Huffer

Department of Pathology, University of Colorado Health Sciences Center, Denver, Colorado

INTRODUCTION

Abnormal levels of parathyroid hormone and vitamin D and its metabolites play important roles in the pathogenesis of a morphologically diversified spectrum of clinically important metabolic bone diseases. Deficiency of 1,25$(OH)_2$ vitamin D_3 has been associated with osteomalacia (95, 197, 309, 310), types I and II osteoporosis (265), and osteitis fibrosa with osteopenia (166) or osteosclerosis (2, 129, 145). Experimentally, high levels of parathyroid (PTH) cause osteitis fibrosis in association with either osteopenia (304) or osteosclerosis (294, 304) depending on how the PTH is administered (304). Chronic exposure to 1,25$(OH)_2$ vitamin D_3 can also cause osteosclerosis (337) or osteopenia and, paradoxically, osteomalacia (136, 337). Thus, perturbations of calcitropic hormones in the same direction can produce diverse morphologic responses, and conversely, similar morphologic responses can occur in response to perturbations of calcitropic hormones in the opposite direction.

These apparently paradoxical results are presumably explained by complex direct and indirect effects of the calcitropic hormones on bone remodeling, the focal coordinated activity of osteoclasts and osteoblasts that maintains the structural integrity of the skeleton. In recent years, there have been significant advances in our understanding of this process and its controls. Much of the control is local and involves substances other than the calcitropic hormones (217). The general nature of these local controls has been defined in part by cell cultures with relatively pure lines of osteoclasts and osteoblasts which have expanded our concepts of the osteoblastic phenotype and better defined the functional capacities and controls of the osteoclast. Such studies have shown that in addition to their traditional role in synthesizing and secreting macromolecular components of bone matrix, osteoblasts elaborate short range message(s) that mediate osteoclastic responses to bone resorbing agents including PTH. They also synthesize, release, and incorporate into bone matrix, substances capable of exerting immediate or delayed autocrine and paracrine control of bone formation and resorption. They participate directly in matrix resorption via synthesis, secretion, and incorporation into the matrix of neutral collagenase and other metalloproteinases, and influence the activity of these enzymes by synthesizing and releasing activators and inhibitors.

Osteoclasts resorb mineral and matrix of bone, utilizing lysosomal enzymes in an acidic environment. Their resorptive activity is inhibited by calcitonin and prostaglandins, stimulated by osteoblast messages, and not affected directly by PTH or vitamin D metabolites.

This review summarizes the studies forming the basis of the conclusions above and attempts to put them in the perspective of the histologic organization and growth kinetics of bone remodeling units. Possible points of interaction of PTH and vitamin D metabolites in this hypothetical model, and the model's relevance to a few examples of metabolic bone diseases with abnormal PTH and vitamin D metabolism are discussed briefly.

THEORETICAL BASIS OF BONE REMODELING

Bone remodeling occurs at anatomic foci called bone remodeling units (BRUs) (261). Anatomically they are replacement osteons forming new Haversian systems in cortical bone (173) and Howship's lacunae forming new bone packets in trabecular bone (83, 84).

Bone remodeling at a previously quiescent bone surface includes an activation phase, occurring between the application of remodeling stimuli and the onset of osteoclastic resorption, a resorptive phase including the time osteoclasts are actively resorbing the bone surface, a reversal phase during which mononuclear cells occupy the resorptive surface, and bone forming, and mineralizing phases during which the resorption space is refilled with new bone matrix and mineral (12, 83, 84, 160).

The processes described above are controlled by long, intermediate, and short range messages influencing proliferation, differentiation, migration, attachment, and subsequently rates and duration of work by cells of osteoclastic and osteoblastic lineage. The term coupling refers to the usually obligatory temporal and spatial relationship between bone formation and prior bone resorption. Parfitt (238) stressed the biology of the BRU as the basis of coupling. Coupling agents were restricted to those influencing osteoblast recruitment (238). Others use the term to describe messages generated by osteoclastic activity that influence osteoblastic proliferation, migration, differentiation, matrix synthesis, and cessation of synthesis (217). Coupling has also been used to describe the balance between depth of resorption and the amount of bone refilling the resorption space (149). Since the magnitude of those parameters depend on recruitment, life span and work efficiency of both osteoclasts and osteoblasts, this usage encompasses all short or intermediate range messages that explain why osteoclasts and osteoblasts generally perform their functions sequentially in the same site. This latter usage is consistent with recent data indicating that many messages to osteoclasts are transmitted via osteoblasts or related cells.

HISTOLOGIC ORGANIZATION OF OSTEONS AND ENDOSTEAL BRUs

Osteons are cylindrical tunnels formed by a moving tuft of osteoclast-rich fibrovascular tissue known as the cutting cone. The bone removed by the cutting cone is subsequently replaced by osteoblast-rich tissue known as the closing cone (157). These terms are apt because the resorbing and bone-forming surfaces of each of these functional subunits of an osteon approximate the walls of two cones with a common base a short distance from the resorptive end of the osteon (Figs. 1 and 2).

Osteons sectioned longitudinally after labeling with multiple timed doses of tetracycline show that the length of the cutting cone is constant as is the short segment of uncalcified bone (osteoid) between the base of the cutting cone and calcified bone (152, 153, 172, 301) (Fig. 1). The diameter of the osteon at the base of the cutting cone is the same as the diameter of the completed refilled osteon, a fact that can be appreciated because of the presence of a distinctive cement line that is deposited at the end of the resorptive phase of osteonal remodeling (172, 173).

These observations have been combined with measurements of the radial and longitudinal separation of bands of tetracycline to show that the mean longitudinal rates of resorption, formation, and mineralization are equal and constant at 30 to 50 μm/day. The radial resorption rate is approximately 10 μm/day and the radial formation and mineralization rates equal at approximately 1 μm/day with a delay of approximately 10 days between formation and mineralization (152, 153, 301). Because of this delay in mineralization an osteoid seam 10 μm wide extends from the base of the cutting cone to the point along the longitudinal axis of the closing cone where bone formation and mineralization are complete (Fig. 2).

These data can be used to calculate durations of bone formation and resorption. If the average radius of completed osteons (mean wall thickness (MWT)) is known, the length of time it takes for osteoblasts to refill any site along the axis of the osteon with new bone is the duration of bone formation, σ_f (105) and is calculated from the formula σ_f = MWT/MR where MR is the average radial (appositional) mineralization rate, the distance between two tetracycline labels divided by the number of days between labels. In a perfectly oriented osteon, σ_f could also be determined by measuring the longitudinal bone formation rate and the distance from the base of the cutting cone to the point at which bone replacement has been completed. If the longitudinal resorption and formation rates are equal, the amount of time required for the cutting cone to complete the work of radial resorption, σ_r can be determined by the formula

$$\sigma_r = \sigma_f \times \frac{\text{length of cutting cone}}{\text{length of closing cone}}$$

or as a good approximation,

$$\sigma_r = \sigma_f \times \frac{\text{resorption surface}}{\text{formation surface}} \quad (106)$$

As pointed out by Jaworski and Hooper (151) σ_f and

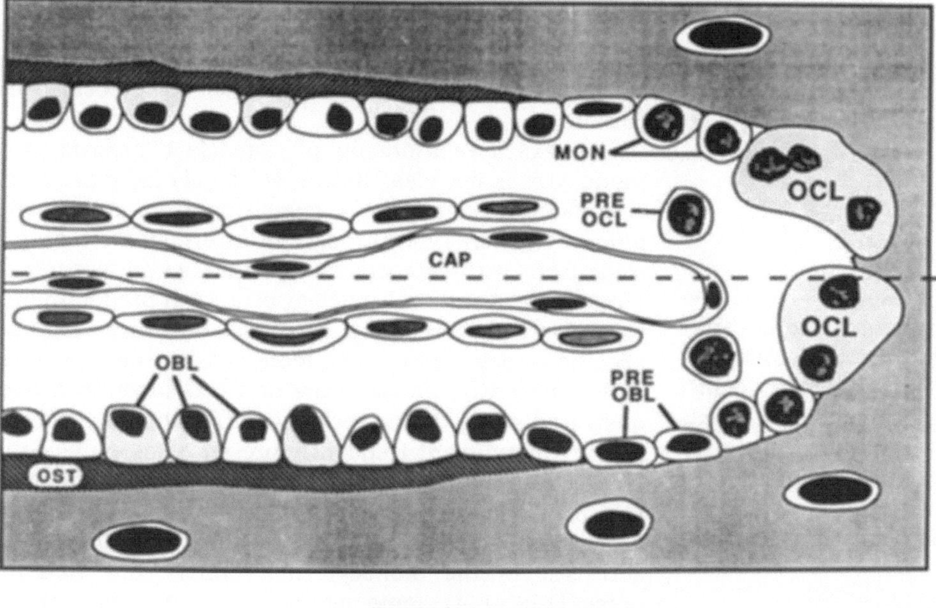

FIG. 1. Diagram of the histology of bone remodeling. The figure is a camera lucida drawing of an osteon. An endosteal BRU is basically an osteon bisected along its longitudinal axis (– – –) with marrow and/or a layer of bone lining cells forming the bisection surface. Two osteoclasts (*OCL*) form the apex of the resorptive or cutting cone. The reversal zone is occupied by spindle-shaped preosteoblasts (*PREOBL*), large mononuclear preosteoclasts (*PREOCL*) and smaller reversal phase monocytes (*MON*). The bone forming or closing cone contains osteoblasts (*OBL*) on an osteoid surface (*OST*). Loose vascular connective tissue with capillaries (*CAP*) is the source or transmitter of precursors of these cells.

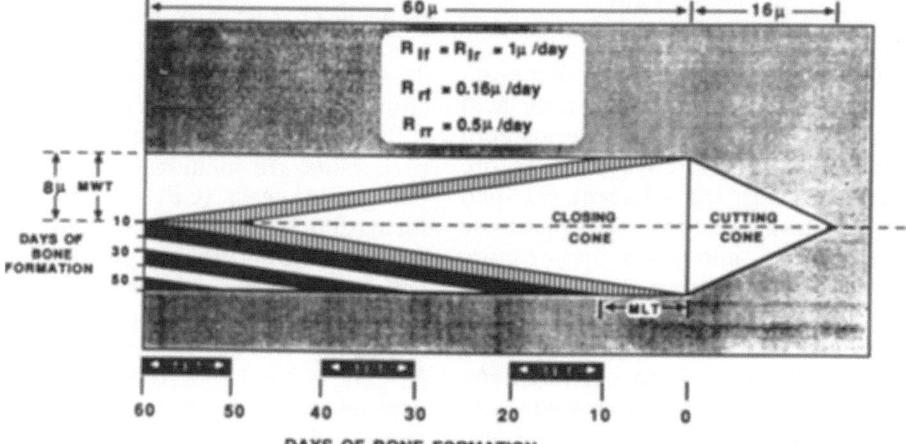

FIG. 2. Diagram of remodeling kinetics. An osteon (*whole figure*) or an endosteal BRU (*bottom half* of figure) is moving from left to right according to principles demonstrated experimentally in tetracycline-labeled canine osteons (152, 153, 301). The length of the cutting cone, the length of unmineralized osteoid (*vertical stripes*) between the base of the cutting cone and mineralized bone, and the width of the osteoid (bone forming) surface are constant with time and the radius of the base of the cutting cone equals the radius (*MWT*) of completely refilled and remineralized osteons (*MWT*). These observations are the basis of calculating longitudinal and radial bone formation and resorption rates and durations from measurements of the dimensions of osteons and lengths and radial separation of bands of tetracycline (black) deposited in mineralized bone during timed labeling periods. Tetracycline deposition is depicted only in the *lower half* of the figure which corresponds to an endosteal BRU. In this figure, the longitudinal rates of formation and resorption (R_{lf}, and R_{lr}, respectively are 1 μm/day and the corresponding radial rates (R_{rf}, and R_{rr}, respectively) 0.16 and 0.5 μm/day. In real osteons or endosteal BRUs longitudinal rates of formation and resorption are equal at 40 to 50 μm/day, and radial rates approximately 1 and 10 μm/day for forming and resorbing surfaces, respectively. As a consequence, osteons and endosteal bone remodeling units are much longer than they are deep, and bone forming surfaces much more extensive than bone resorbing surfaces. The mineralization lag time (*MLT*) is the time between deposition and mineralization of the matrix.

σ_r determined by these methods are not estimates of the life span of a remodeling unit. The life span of a remodeling unit is the length of time that bone remodeling continues in a longitudinal direction and may reflect the life span of osteoclasts in the cutting cone (151). Theoretically, it could be determined from measurements of the longitudinal bone formation rate and the total length of a completed osteon.

These concepts are also applicable to the histomorphometry of endosteal surfaces where BRUs are randomly oriented in space and longitudinal rates of work are generally not evaluated by direct measurements (106). The exact 3-dimensional anatomy of endosteal BRUs has not been studied extensively (147) but is thought to be essentially the same as that of osteons (148). An endosteal BRU can be represented as an osteon bisected along its longitudinal axis. One surface is formed by the layer of cells that normally separate bone surfaces from marrow, the bone lining cells (211). This conceptual view of endosteal BRUs as units in which resorption progresses linearly across bone surfaces and bone formation of progressively greater duration occurs at progressively greater distances from the resorption front is clearly expressed in diagrams of their function (12, 84, 160).

Figure 2 shows that the extent of resorptive or forming surfaces are dependent on both longitudinal and radial work rates and durations. If longitudinal rates always increase or decrease together and to the same extent, then the ratio of resorbing to forming surfaces is determined by radial work and durations rates. It is therefore important to determine what biological events determine radial and longitudinal work rates and durations.

ORIGIN AND DISTRIBUTION OF OSTEOCLASTS AND OSTEOBLASTS AND THEIR PRECURSORS

The last section of this paper presents several hypotheses about the functional organization and controls of BRUs. One is that longitudinal resorption is controlled by proliferation, emigration, and fusion of osteoclast precursors, and subsequent work by osteoclasts, whereas radial resorption is controlled by similar processes involving so-called reversal phase monocytes and preosteoblasts. In order to understand the basis of these hypotheses it is necessary to consider the origin of osteoclasts and monocytes.

Origin and Distribution of Osteoclast Precursors

The immediate osteoclast precursor in mice is a postmitotic mononuclear cell with tartrate-resistant acid phosphatase activity that is first seen in the periosteum of fetal mouse metatarsal bones at 17 days, 1 day before the appearance of osteoclasts in the adjacent calcified cartilage (281). DNA synthesizing osteoclast precursors appear earlier, at days 15 to 16, and divide one or more times before giving rise to the postmitotic precursor (280, 281). Osteoclast precursors first appear in mouse embryos at 8 to 9 days in the yolk sac, are present along with other hematopoietic precursors in the 11-day liver, and by 17 days are present in all fetal tissues tested (312). They persist in some connective tissues in young animals, but in adults appear to be confined to hematopoietic lymphoid tissues (312). In young animals, including humans, demonstration of nuclear and cytoplasmic markers in host osteoclasts after blood borne transplants of bone marrow (57, 200), spleen (199, 201), liver (200), and thymus (201) further demonstrate that osteoclast precursors are present in hematopoietic and lymphoid tissues and can be carried via the blood stream.

Ficoll-Hypaque isolated peripheral blood monocytes from normal 6-week-old mice do not contain osteoclast precursors demonstrable by co-culture with 17 day mouse metatarsals (25). Since the latter technique is capable of demonstrating osteoclast formation from DNA synthesizing or postmitotic precursors, these studies indicate that the young mouse blood does not normally contain circulating early precursors, and that mature monocytes are not late postmitotic preosteoclasts. In addition, hatchling chick blood does not contain cells capable of giving rise to osteoclasts under culture conditions which maintain an osteoclast phenotype in cells derived from the endosteum of 19-day chick tibae (233). On the other hand, mice whose bone resorption has been stimulated with 1α-OH vitamin D_3 can incorporate peripheral blood monocytes into marrow osteoclasts *in vivo* (315) and monocytes isolated from the blood of laying hens can fuse with osteoclasts from the same hens *in vitro* (347). Thus, osteoclast precursors are not normally present in the peripheral blood of mature animals, but under circumstances of increased remodeling, some of the cells isolated with blood monocytes can act as osteoclast precursors.

The exact relationship of osteoclast precursors to monocytes is not clear. Baron *et al.* (11) have presented convincing evidence for a transition from cells with a monocyte phenotype through an intermediate mononuclear form with osteoclastic and monocytic features, to mononuclear and multinuclear cells with predominantly osteoclastic features (11). They also demonstrated nonspecific esterase activity (a monocyte marker) in osteoclasts. Recently, Fc receptors and IgG have been demonstrated along the osteoclastic ruffled border (247) refuting an argument frequently presented as evidence for lack of relationship between osteoclasts and monocytes (139). In addition, although there is generally poor reactivity of osteoclasts with monoclonal antibodies characteristic of the monocyte/macrophage line and *vice versa* (143, 144) some monoclonal antibodies against osteoclasts react with monocytes and their polykaryons but not other cell types (143, 236) and *vice versa* (3). These observations thus favor a developmental relationship between osteoclasts and monocytes.

There is good evidence that early murine osteoclast precursors are included among pluripotential hematopoietic stem cells (CFU-S) (26, 283). *In vitro* osteoclast formation from the most highly purified marrow stem cell populations requires pre-incubation with a stem cell-activating fraction, interleukin-3 (Il-3) (283). In long-term baboon marrow cultures supported by low dose $1{,}25(OH)_2$ vitamin D_3, pretreatment with GM-CSF and M-CSF (CSF-1) increased proliferation of osteoclasts precursors (189). These factors are thought to support growth of granulocyte/monocyte and monocyte colony-forming units, respectively. These results suggested that the point of divergence between osteoclasts and monocytes might be the premonocyte stage (217). However, in shorter cultures of fetal mouse long bones, pretreatment with GM-CSF or Il-3 decreased the number of recently replicated osteoclast precursors incorporated into osteoclasts by subsequent PTH stimulation (182). The total number and percentage of recently replicated granulocytes and monocytes was increased. Scheven, Visser, and Nijweide (282) have shown that Il-3 stimulates osteoclast formation from purified stem cells only if present early in culture (282). Prolonged exposure results in lower osteoclast production. These latter two studies favor an earlier point of divergence between osteoclasts and monocytes as suggested by others (144, 312).

Origin and Distribution of Cells of the Osteoblastic Phenotype

The osteoblast phenotype has been defined by study of osteoblast-like cells in culture (5, 184, 191, 267). Osteoblasts have receptors for PTH (7, 288, 311), $1{,}25(OH)_2$ vitamin D_3 (51, 194, 239, 328), glucocorticoids (92), epidermal growth factor (EGF) (225), prostaglandins (PG) (75), and estrogen, progesterone, and androgens (81, 82). Important functional characteristics include increased synthesis of cyclic AMP (184, 191), decreased type I collagen synthesis (168, 335) and decreased alkaline phosphatase (191) synthesis in response to PTH. Osteoblast-like cells also show increased bone glutamic acid containing protein (BGP) synthesis in response to 1,25$(OH)_2$ vitamin D_3 (248) and make and mineralize bone matrix *in vitro* (77) and *in vivo* in diffusion chambers (6, 24).

The precursors of these cells in adult animals are part of the marrow stromal stem cell system (237) which also includes several other cell lines including fibroblastic cells synthesizing type I collagen, reticular cells synthesizing type III collagen, and poorly classified cells synthesizing both types (15). Stem cells generating bone tissue are present throughout the marrow but are more prevalent near bone surfaces (76).

The properties of cloned populations from osteosarcomas (191, 267) suggest origin from a spectrum of stem cells giving rise to cell lines ranging from a mixture of reticular and fibroblastic cells through varying proportions of fibroblastic and osteoblastic-like cells to cells closely approximating the osteoblastic phenotype (237). The clonal MC3T3-E1 line from normal newborn mouse calvarium, however, has a mixture of cells and tissues which may represent the precursors and maturing cells which make up the cell population of the osteogenic subline of CFU-F (237).

Cells released early in the sequential digestion or mechanical separation of embryonic and neonatal skeletal tissues were originally designated osteoclast-like on the basis of sensitivity to calcitonin and other biochemical characteristics (184, 335). They are, however, not osteoclast-like as shown by histology and assay for osteoclast precursors (25). They may include osteogenic stem cells since they are derived from the periosteum and have biochemical and receptor characteristics distinguishing them from fibroblasts and relating them with preosteoblasts and osteoblasts (G. C. Wong, submitted for publication). Recently another cell line derived from long term murine marrow has been suggested as an osteoblastic stem cell line (221). It fulfills many of the functional and biochemical criteria for osteoblasts but lacks PTH receptors.

Variations in cAMP or alkaline phosphatase synthesis in response to agents known to interact with osteoblastic cells via receptors have been demonstrated among clones from primary outgrowths of rat calvariae (339) or from various established normal or neoplastic osteoblastic cell lines (22, 269). It is not known whether such clones represent subpopulations of different osteoblast-like lineages, different stages of differentiation of a single lineage (22), or artifacts of culture (333).

ORIGIN, DISTRIBUTION, IDENTITY AND FUNCTION OF CELLS OF BRUs

One hour after pulse-labeling with tritiated thymidine, labeled nuclei are present in elongated cells identified as preosteoblasts at the base of the cutting cone of canine osteons (151) (Fig. 1). Most of these labeled cells remain on the osteoid surface for at least 13 days as a discrete band of mature osteoblasts seen at progressively greater distances from the cutting cone. Label first appears in osteocytes beneath this band at 9 days.

Labeled cells identified as mononuclear osteoclast precursors also appear at the base of the cone in 1 hour but there is a delay of 12 to 24 hours before labeled osteoclast nuclei are seen (151). Peak osteoclast labeling occurs at 96 hours and then falls off to low levels by 13 days. These and other studies indicate that the osteoclast population of cutting cones consists of a stable population of cells with a nuclear turnover rate of 8%/day (150).

The putative osteoclast precursors at the base of the cone are located at a site corresponding to the reversal zone of endosteal BRUs. The cells in this region of endosteal BRUs have been termed reversal phase monocytes (8, 12, 84). They are thought to be the same as mononuclear phagocytes replacing osteoclasts at the resorption surface in a model of synchronized remodeling induced on the periosteal surface of rat maxillae by pulling the opposing mandibles (11, 12, 316, 317). In this system a surface previously covered by osteoblasts continuously laying down new bone becomes completely mineralized while the osteoblasts atrophy and are subsequently replaced sequentially by preosteoclasts, osteoclasts, reversal phase monocytes and new osteoblasts. It is a model in which new populations of cells change over a broad surface as a function of time and does not involve movement in space as is the case with osteons and endosteal BRUs. Because the appearance of reversal phase cells on the surface coincides with the appearance of a cement line (317), it has been suggested they initiate coupling by elaboration of the cement line (12, 317). The developmental origin of reversal phase monocytes is not clear. They have tartrate-resistant acid phosphatase activity similar to the osteoclasts preceding them on the resorption surface so it has been suggested that they are osteoclast fission products (12). However, in the same model system, the putative mononuclear osteoclast precursors also have tartrate-resistant acid phosphatase activity (11), an observation substantiated in other model systems developed to demonstrate osteoclast precursors (281). These data thus indicate that reversal phase monocytes have similarities to osteoclast precursors.

It is also possible, however, that mononuclear cells in the reversal zone of endosteal BRUs are members of the monocyte/macrophage lineage. Such cells respond to chemotactic stimuli generated by PTH-induced bone resorption (216, 218) adhere to bone surfaces by clear zones and resorb the bone (13, 161) and have acid phosphatase activity (144, 161). However, mature monocytes don't develop ruffled borders (42, 161), don't form resorption bays typical of osteoclasts *in vitro* (42) are not inhibited by calcitonin (43, 45), and lack most of the surface antigens of osteoclasts as discussed above.

It is thus unclear whether reversal phase monocytes are osteoclast precursors, osteoclast fission products, monocytes, or a mixture of these different functional cells. Whatever their origin, there is good morphological evidence that bone resorption continues when reversal phase monocytes are on the resorbing surface. On trabecular surfaces of normal human iliac bone the mean depth of resorption under osteoclasts is approximately

20 μm, under reversal phase monocytes, 50 μm, and under preosteoblasts, 63 μm (84). Those findings and the additional demonstration that the mean depth of resorption of completed osteons is also approximately 63 μm indicates that resorption continues while the reversal phase monocytes are on the surface, but not after the preosteoblasts reach the surface (84).

These data indicate that BRUs contain mature osteoblasts and osteoclasts which form and resorb bone, respectively, a population of mononuclear cells which probably include post-mitotic osteoclast precursors, a related or separate population of mononuclear phagocytes which resorb bone radially, and preosteoblasts which give rise to osteoblasts. The latter may also be involved in radial bone resorption as detailed further below.

CELLULAR BIOCHEMISTRY OF BONE REMODELING

Traditionally bone resorption has been assigned to osteoclasts, and bone formation to osteoblasts. Recent studies have shown that osteoclasts are capable of resorbing all components of bone but cells of the osteoblastic lineage also participate in matrix resorption. In addition, osteoblastic cells also produce short range messages that may exert important controls on the functions of both osteoclasts and osteoblasts. These studies are summarized below.

Bone Resorption by Osteoclasts

Heersche (132) postulated that osteoclasts resorb noncollagenous proteins and mineral components of bone leaving collagen to be removed by some other cell type. This hypothesis is supported by some of the observations cited in previous sections. However, there is now clear evidence that osteoclasts can resorb all the components of bone matrix as well as its mineral (20).

Scanning electron microscopy has demonstrated osteoclastic resorption tracks passing through mineralized and nonmineralized surfaces (158, 159) and isolated osteoclasts deep within resorption lacunae in the midst of disrupted collagen fibers (47, 158). Studies of bone prelabeled with radioactive proline and calcium have demonstrated that isolated osteoclasts resorb both components of bone, releasing mineral earlier than organic matrix (20). Approximately 40% of the labeled proline was recovered as [^{3}H]-trans-4-hydroxyproline, indicating that nearly 90% of osteoclast-solubilized [^{3}H] was from collagenolysis. The products were too small to represent neutral mammalian collagenase activity and no immunoreactive collagenase was detectable in media or osteoclasts. Equally important, collagenolytic activity by osteoclast lysates showed maximal activity at pH 4.0 and none above pH 5.0.

These data are consistent with earlier work by Vaes and co-workers who concluded that resorption of the organic matrix of bone explants may be due to enzyme systems other than collagenase (101). At that time, bone resorption did not correlate with accumulation of collagenase in the media (101) and they showed inhibition of bone resorption with inhibitors of thiolproteinases without affecting collagenase activity (61).

Resorption by isolated osteoclasts takes place beneath the ruffled border and within the confines of the clear zone. The ruffled border is a complex area of finger-like projection interdigitating with disrupted collagen fibers and mineral crystals of the bone surface (140). This is a zone of active secretion of lysosomal enzymes including ATPase (118) and acid phosphatase (116, 209). During PTH-induced activation of osteoclasts, the appearance of acid phosphatase activity extracellularly and in the matrix coincides with the development of the ruffled border and is seldom seen outside of the resorptive zone delineated by the clear zone (209). The ruffled border is also a site of endocytosis of exogenous markers (117), bone hydroxyapatite (206), and in humans with pyknodysostosis, collagen fibers (87).

The formation of a ruffled border by activated osteoclasts is associated with development of an organelle-free clear zone adjacent to the plasma membrane and completely encircling the ruffled border (140). This zone contains actin-like filaments oriented perpendicular to the bone surface (165). The plasma membrane of the clear zone is in contact with and follows the contours of the nonresorbed bone adjacent to that in contact with the ruffled border, and is thought to function as a seal around the ruffled border (37, 140). A complete clear zone is absent from inactive osteoclasts in rats (140) but regions of ectoplasm similar to the clear zone maintain contact with bone in inactive avian osteoclasts (206).

Scanning electron microscopic studies show sharply demarcated resorption pits somewhat smaller in diameter than the osteoclasts (47, 159). Resorption can be intermittent or continuous as the osteoclasts move across the bone surface, and the depth of resorption minimal or deep (47). The rate of movement of resorbing osteoclasts has been estimated at less than 10 μm/hour (159), the same order of magnitude as the 40 to 50 μm/day measured in 2° osteons by tetracycline labeling.

Scanning electron microscopy supports the concept that the seal provided by the clear zone effectively prevents diffusion of acid away from the resorption site, since the margins of resorption bays are very sharp (159). Specific adherence of the clear zone to bone surfaces has been demonstrated in PTH-stimulated rat long bone resorption by exposing the cultures to hypertonic solution (271). *In vitro* studies with isolated chicken osteoclasts have shown that cell-substratum (glass) adherence utilizes proteins similar to those present in other cell types (vimentin, F-actin, fibrin, α-actin, viniculin), but the exact arrangement of these proteins is, so-far, unique to osteoclasts (196).

Direct measurements by micropuncture and indirect immunofluorescent techniques have shown that the osteoclast resorption bay has an acidic pH (9, 88). Antigens cross-reacting with H^+-ATPases have been demonstrated on the extracellular surface of the osteoclast ruffled border (9, 112) and in lysosomal membranes of osteoclasts and other bone cells (9) but not at other sites on the osteoclast cell membrane (9). Antigens cross-reacting with Na^+K^+-ATPase occur on all parts of the osteoclast membrane including the ruffled border and clear zone (10). These results suggest that osteoclasts utilize an ATPase driven proton pump, perhaps in conjunction with Na^+/K^+ or Ca^{2+} pumps, to deliver hydrogen ions to the resorption bay and facilitate the action of lysosomal enzymes which are also released there (10). Hydrogen ions could be provided by carbonic anhydrase activity which is high in osteoclasts (109, 300). Inhibitors of carbonic anhydrase also inhibit PTH-stimulated bone resorption (212). Carbonic anhydrase is also localized in the ruffled border of normal and PTH-treated chick osteoclasts and diminishes in that location after calcitonin treatment (33). PTH treatment of osteoclasts increases their activity in a dose-dependent manner, an effect blocked by carbonic anhydrase inhibitors (1).

Thus, there is good evidence that osteoclasts remove both the organic and inorganic components of bone at an acid pH, and that this activity is carried out in a highly directed fashion under the ruffled border by lysosomal enzymes and hydrogen ions synthesized and secreted by the osteoclasts. These findings do not rule out Heersche's hypothesis that helper cells might play a role in bone resorption. There is in fact strong evidence that matrix synthesizing cells (fibroblast-like cells in Heersche's original hypothesis) may play a role in bone resorption.

Bone Resorption by Osteoblasts

Many studies have demonstrated synthesis and secretion of neutral collagenase by bone organ cultures (59, 278, 321). Immunohistochemical studies of bone cultures (273, 274) and isolated osteoblast-like cells (275) and isolation of collagenase from cultures of calvarial osteoblast-like cells (130, 234, 235, 275) cloned osteogenic cells (275) and osteogenic sarcoma cells (234, 235) have established that osteoblasts are the major source of collagenase.

Collagenase occurs in minute amounts, in cell or organ culture supernatants, usually in a latent, but sometimes in an active form, depending on culture conditions and isolation procedures (277). A new isolation procedure has yielded sufficient collagenase from fetal mouse calvariae to digest all the collagen in the explant within a few days (78). Synthesis of collagenase as an inactive proenzyme has been demonstrated in a cell free system using rabbit synovial cell mRNA (222), with osteoblast-like cells from mouse calvariae (276). Another latent enzyme, procollagenase activator (321) can be activated by cathepsin B, plasmin and kallikrein but not by carboxy-peptidase B, cathepsin C or D, or thrombin (79). A similar proactivator in rabbit synovial medium is activated by trypsin, 4-amino-phenylmercuric acetate, or by sequential removal and replacement of Ca^{2+} or other bivalent cations (323).

Neutral collagenase is one of a group of metalloproteinases synthesized, secreted and activated by mechanisms similar to those described above (108, 285). They are stimulated by agents which modify cellular cyclic AMP levels (94). Other members include proteoglycanase with activity against chondroitin sulfate-binding sites of proteoglycan aggregate, and other substrates (108), and gelatinase with activity against denatured collagen and other substrates (220).

The active forms of these enzymes are all bound and irreversibly inhibited by a widely distributed enzyme known as tissue inhibitor of metalloproteinases (TIMP) which usually is synthesized by the same organ (34) and cell cultures (235) that synthesize the metalloproteinases. However, a human osteoblastic cell line producing TIMP but not collagenase has been described (264). One control of connective tissue degradation may be based on the balance between TIMP and metalloproteinase production (263).

There has been controversy about the role of metalloproteinases in bone resorption. Sakamoto and Sakomoto (277) suggested that bone resorption is the result of sequential matrix (phase I) and mineral (phase II) resorption, carried out by neutral proteases (exemplified by collagenase) from osteoblasts and related cells, and acid and lysosomal enzyme production by osteoclasts, respectively. Depth of resorption according to this theory would depend on the number of cycles of each phase. In support of this theory are studies showing that collagenase is synthesized and released by osteoblast-like cells in response to PTH stimulation (130) and other substances stimulating bone resorption (63, 155, 156, 234, 235). Mi/mi osteopetrotic mice have unreactive osteoclasts but have a collagenolytic response to PTH restricted to the noncalcified collagen pool (155). Normal mouse bones degrade collagen and release calcium and thiolproteinases in response to PTH, lipopolysaccharide and interleukin-1 (Il-1). These responses are absent from mi/mi bone and so are probably mediated by osteoclasts. Degradation of non-mineralized collagen occurring only in response to PTH in both normal and mi/mi bone thus seems to represent a second nonosteoclast-mediated mechanism of collagenolysis (156).

Sakomoto and Sakamoto (277) have maintained that there is a correlation between bone resorption and release of collagenase by bone explants (reviewed in reference 277). Recently others have shown that dichloromethylenebisphosphonate inhibits PTH-stimulated development of resorption lacunae, loss of calcium, and lysosomal enzyme release more than it inhibits collagen (hydroxyproline) release (62). Bisphosphonates do not decrease heparin-induced collagenase release. This suggests that bisphosphonates inhibit osteoclastic secretion of lysosomal enzymes and degradation of mineralized matrix but not osteoblastic collagenase production and degradation of unmineralized matrix (62). Conversely, a new synthetic inhibitor of collagenase and related metalloproteinases, CI-1, inhibits PTH-induced collagen matrix resorption in mouse embryo calvarial explants without affecting lysosomal enzyme secretion, adding additional evidence that collagenase plays a separate role in a bone resorption (60). With an improved extraction technique a 3-fold increase in calvarial procollagenase content and increased bone resorption was demonstrable after PTH stimulation. These effects were blocked by cyclohexamide but not indomethacin. Calcitonin inhibited resorption without affecting PTH-induced procollagenase synthesis (60). Further studies have shown that the PTH response is duplicated by culturing calvariae with $1,25(OH)_2$ vitamin D_3, prostaglandin (PG) E_2, interleukin-1α, tumor necrosis factor, catabolin, retinoic acid, or endotoxin (63).

How and when collagenase acts is not clear. As noted above, metalloproteinases are activated by proteinases including plasmin. Since osteoblasts product plasminogen activator in response to PTH (126) collagenase could be activated during hormonally induced resorption (138). Latent collagenase is extracted from non-stimulated calvariae subsequent to extraction of mineral and is not extracted from adult human and bovine bone without demineralization (78) indicating that latent collagenase is present in mineralized bone. In PTH-stimulated calvariae increased latent collagenase is recovered in the first tissue extract (the noncalcified matrix pool) and is not demonstrable in the culture media (63, 78). These findings imply that the increased collagenase is incorporated in latent form into nonmineralized bone matrix (63). TIMP is demonstrable in the culture media but not the matrix of PTH-stimulated calvaria (78) suggesting either that it is not incorporated into the bone or that the extraction procedure alters its properties so that it no longer inhibits collagenase activity.

These findings suggest that some of the collagenase synthesized in response to PTH stimulation may not contribute to the current wave of resorptive activity but instead be deposited in bone for release and activation during a subsequent cycle of remodeling as suggested by Mechanic (204). It is possible that inhibitor synthesis and release prevents degradation of newly synthesized bone matrix by combining with collagenase activated during PTH stimulation.

On the other hand, as suggested in the final section of this review, secretion and activation of collagenase by proliferating osteoblasts might contribute to radial resorption of BRUs.

It is also possible that the layer of osteoid normally separating quiescent bone lining cells from calcified bone surfaces (211) is a target for collagenase as a mechanism of osteoclastic activation as suggested by Chambers and others (37, 40, 41, 48, 60, 277). Osteoid could be removed by bone lining cells, either by secreting procollagenase, proactivator and plasminogen activator, or by secreting plasminogen activator which could act on latent procollagenase and proactivator stored in the osteoid during a previous remodeling cycle.

This hypothesis is based on *in vitro* studies showing that isolated osteoclasts fail to resorb osteoid-covered surfaces but actively resorb the mineralized surfaces exposed by collagenase digestion (40, 41). Also, osteoclasts resorb mineralized but not demineralized bone explants *in vivo* (113, 114). This osteoid barrier hypothesis suggests that exposure to calcified surfaces activates osteoclasts, and that osteoblasts are the cells that remove the collagen to expose calcified surfaces. Evidence was provided *in vitro* where co-cultures of rat calvarial mononuclear cells 70 to 85% positive for alkaline phosphatase stimulated bone resorption by isolated osteoclasts (41). Parathyroid treatment of the calvarial cells enhanced osteoclastic resorption whereas demineralization of the osteoid-free bone had the opposite effect.

Other observations, however, indicate that these mechanisms may not be crucial osteoclastic controls. Osteoclasts have been shown to resorb bone of all phases of mineralized bone, ranging from osteoid to heavily mineralized matrix (159). In young adult rabbits, virtually all osteoclasts on the femoral endosteal surface are in contact with fully mineralized bone and show none of the morphologic features of activated osteoclasts. They resemble osteoclasts exposed to calcitonin (185). Similar observations have also been described in laying hens (206, 208). In addition, scanning electron microscopic studies *in vitro* (159) and *in vivo* (158) fail to show disruption of osteoid in the vicinity of osteoblasts during bone resorption. More recent *in vitro* studies of bone resorption by mixed populations of osteoclasts and osteoblast-like cells have provided no evidence of bone resorption by osteoblasts or of modification of the bone substrate by osteoblasts to account for subsequent increased resorption by osteoclasts (203). Although calcified bone is probably the preferred substrate of osteoclasts, resorption of osteoid is not the only mechanism to provide such a surface. In the study of synchronized remodeling discussed above, tetracycline labeling showed that the osteoid surface was transformed to a mineralized surface by continued mineralization rather than by digestion (316).

BONE FORMATION

Bone matrix synthesis is carried out by cells of the osteoblastic lineage. The matrix proteins synthesized by osteoblasts are inferred in part by identification of components extracted and purified from bone, and in part by demonstrating synthesis by osteoblast-like cells *in vitro* and *in vivo*. These include type I collagen (284, 326, 330) a vitamin K-dependent γ-carboxyglutamic acid containing protein known as BGP or osteocalcin (128, 229, 249, 250), a phosphoprotein-binding hydroxylapatite and collagen, osteonectin (97), proteoglycans (97, 98, 102, 133), and sialoproteins (98, 99) including osteopontin which contains amino acid sequences identical with the binding site for fibronectin (232).

These proteins have been shown to be synthesized by bone tissue or osteoblast-like cells, or have been demonstrated in osteoblasts by immunohistochemical techniques. Since the gene for type I collagen is the same throughout the body it has been suggested that the genetic specificity of bone is based on the noncollagenous proteins (319). To date BGP and bone sialoprotein appear to be specific for bone and dentin, but bone proteoglycans, and osteonectin have been demonstrated in other tissues, or their mRNA has been demonstrated in cell types other than those of osteoblastic phenotype (reviewed in reference 319).

The functions of most of these proteins is uncertain. Osteopontin induces binding and spreading of rat osteosarcoma cells which is inhibited by synthetic peptides with the fibronectin binding sequence, suggesting a role in attachment (251, 290). Osteonectin (319) and sialoproteins (134) might play a role in mineralization of bone. BGP has been shown to have a functional domain determined by the gla-helix producing calcium binding, and a chemoattractant activity for mononuclear leukocytes determined by the carboxy-terminal β-sheet (128,

192, 216) and as described below may be related to bone mineralization via vitamin D_3 controlled mechanisms.

Ultrastructural studies have shown that type I collagen synthesis and secretion by osteoblasts is similar to that described in other cell types when studied by autoradiography (330) or by immunohistochemistry with antibody specific for the carboxyl propeptides of type I collagen (336). Label appears sequentially in rough endoplasmic reticulum, secretory granules, and finally, prebone (osteoid). *In vivo* type I procollagen secretion by osteoblasts is also similar to that in fibroblasts (195, 318) and odontoblasts (162) in that procollagen fibrils are demonstrable in intracytoplasmic secretory granules (336). Apparently these cytoplasmic fibrillary aggregates are not obligatory for type I collagen secretion since they are not demonstrable in cultured fibroblasts (246). Organization of procollagen into collagen fibrils occurs in osteoid in association with cleavage of procollagen peptides since antibody staining of these fragments is demonstrable in osteoid but not in mineralized bone (336). The subsequent organization of these fibrils into collagen fibers occurs at a distance from the osteoblasts concomitantly with changes in distribution of ground substance and the number and distribution of osteoblast processes (100). These observations do not support the concept that osteoblasts have a strong influence on the assembly and orientation of collagen fibrils and fibers (160). Osteoblasts are unlike fibroblasts in which the organization and growth of collagen fibrils appears to be influenced by the formation of long rows of secretory granules oriented by deep folds in the cell membrane (318) and are more like odontoblasts in secreting single or only a few fused granules without any particular influence of the cell on their orientation (336).

Osteocalcin has been identified by immunohistochemistry in calcified bone of adult and embryonic rat bone (120), and calf bone (19). In calf bone, both osteonectin and osteocalcin are associated particularly with collagen fibers. In newborn rats, osteocalcin is demonstrable in osteoblasts and mineralized bone but not in osteoid at the light microscopic level (23). Ultrastructural studies show immunoreactivity over osteoid and predentin, strong staining of mineralized bone, and variable staining of osteoblastic rough endoplasmic reticulum and Golgi regions (27, 198). Rat bone 44K bone phosphoprotein (bone sialoprotein I, osteopontin) is demonstrable in the Golgi but not the rough endoplasmic reticulum or in secretory granules of rat osteoblasts (198).

CONTROLS OF BONE REMODELING

Osteoblastic Control of Bone Resorption by Osteoclasts

In 1981 Rodan and Martin (266) hypothesized that bone resorbing substances might act indirectly via messages generated by stimulation of osteoblasts. Since then it has been shown that osteoblastic messages generally increase but can potentially decrease bone resorption by osteoclasts.

In intact bones and in bone organ cultures PTH (142, 258), vitamin D_3, and its metabolites (256, 258) and prostaglandins (253, 307) all increase bone resorption and cyclic AMP synthesis, whereas calcitonin decreases bone resorption while increasing cyclic AMP production (103, 219). *In vitro* PTH and 1,25$(OH)_2$ vitamin D_3 have no effects on bone resorption or motility of isolated osteoclasts (39, 44), whereas calcitonin, and PGI_2, PGE_1, and PGE_2 all inhibit bone resorption and motility (38, 39, 43–46).

These findings with isolated osteoclasts are consistent with studies showing that osteoclasts lack receptors for vitamin D_3 (205) and PTH (7, 288) and that mammalian osteoclasts have receptors for calcitonin (228, 329). Chicken osteoclasts don't have calcitonin receptors (227) and chicken osteoclasts do not exhibit the cyclic AMP response seen in mammalian osteoclasts in response to calcitonin (226). In addition, bone resorption by isolated chicken osteoclasts is not inhibited by synthetic chicken calcitonin (64). Although PG receptors have not been directly demonstrated on osteoclasts, a cAMP response to PG provides indirect evidence for their presence (38).

Chambers (44) concluded that calcitonin inhibits mammalian osteoclastic resorption directly whereas PTH and 1,25$(OH)_2$ vitamin D_3 stimulate resorption through a cell type absent from the isolated osteoclast preparations. He also proposed a direct inhibitory effect of prostaglandins on osteoclasts and an indirect stimulatory effect mediated by some other cell (44). Two recent studies of PG-stimulated bone resorption in organ cultures have demonstrated an early transient depression of bone resorption followed by a later enhancement which is consistent with this hypothesis (58, 174). The early decrease was a cyclic AMP-mediated process (174).

In contrast, the motility and spreading and bone resorption by isolated osteoclasts is increased when they are co-cultured with osteoblasts and stimulated with PTH (46, 202, 203) or PGs (46). Stimulation of isolated osteoclasts was caused by a soluble factor (195, 203). Conditioned media from osteoblast-like cell cultures also increased bone resorption in organ cultures (244), an effect augmented 2 to 3 times by PTH.

The nature of the soluble factor(s) is unknown. It has been described as small ($500 <$ molecular weight < 1000), resistant to freeze thawing, but heat inactivated (203). Another study describes heat inactivated protease sensitive molecules of molecular weight $\approx 100,000$ whose release is blocked by pretreatment of osteoblast-like cells with cyclohexamide. This activity could be abolished by dialysis against buffers with chelating agents (243).

Recently evidence for osteoblastic mediation of osteoclast responses to other bone resorbing substances has been demonstrated. Recombinant monocyte derived tumor necrosis factor α and lymphocyte-derived tumor necrosis factor β (lymphotoxin) are potent inhibitors of bone collagen synthesis and stimulators of bone resorption (18, 36, 289). Neither substance has significant effects on isolated osteoclasts but in the presence of osteoblastic cells they enhance resorption 2 to 3 times via osteoblastic release of a soluble factor (313). Interleukin-1 has also been shown to be a potent stimulator of bone resorption (68, 119, 131). Both Il-1-α and β and PGs stimulate bone resorption synergistically with PTH (68). Il-1 also stimulates bone resorption synergistically with growth factors via PG synthesis (181) and with tumor necrosis factors (272). This synergism has been attributed to effects of multiple second messengers (68). Il-1 has no effect on isolated osteoclasts but enhances resorption in osteoblast/osteoclast co-cultures (314). Thus, a large number of local and systemic bone resorbing agents have been shown to activate osteoclasts via messages generated by osteoblasts. If prostaglandins synthesized by osteoblasts (see below) are also considered, osteoblast messages can also inhibit osteoclasts.

Osteoclast (Delayed Paracrine/Autocrine) and Osteoblast (Autocrine) control of Bone Formation

Aside from suggestions that the cement line is formed by osteoclast products and may be involved in osteoblast recruitment (12) there is little evidence that osteoclast secretions directly influence osteoblastic activity. There is evidence, however, that substances synthesized and released by osteoblasts influence their proliferative and synthetic activity and therefore could act as autocrine controls of remodeling. These and other osteoblast mitogens and stimulators of matrix synthesis are also present in bone matrix, and released by bone resorption and could act as delayed autocrine/paracrine controls (90). These coupling substances could influence proliferation and migration of osteoblasts, and their precursors (osteoblast recruitment), matrix synthesis (work efficiency), and duration of work (217).

Baylink and co-workers have purified or partially purified substances designated skeletal growth factors stimulating DNA and matrix synthesis by normal osteoblast-rich or osteoblast-like osteosarcoma cultures from extracts of chick embryo (71, 72), human (89–91, 214), and bovine bone (154). Demonstration that similar mitogenic activity was synthesized by chick embryo calvarial cells and released from organ cultures in proportion to ^{45}Ca release suggested a delayed paracrine (or autocrine) mechanism of control (90).

Ethylenediaminetetraacetic acid (EDTA) extracts of bovine and human bone are now known to contain multiple mitogenic factors with activity for several normal, osteoblastic, differentiated osteosarcoma and other normal mesenchymal cell lines (178). Radioimmunoassay identification and quantitation of these activities in EDTA extracts of human femoral heads showed that the most abundant were skeletal growth factor and transforming growth factor β (TGF-β), with smaller amounts of insulin-like growth factor and platelet-derived growth factor (PDGF), but no EGF (177). Human 11 kilodalton (kd) skeletal growth factor stimulates collagen synthesis but inhibits DNA synthesis in a nontransformed well differentiated osteoblast cell line, suggesting that it has separate mitogenic effects on less differentiated (*i.e.*, chick embryo calvarial cells) and matrix synthesis stimulating effects on mature cells (179).

TGF-β is produced by rat calvarial cultures (35) and by osteoblast-like cells (73). It is released during PTH-stimulated bone resorption and is mitogenic for some cells with the osteoblast phenotype (52). It is released from resorbing cultures bound to one or more proteins which inhibit its proliferative effect on normal rat kidney cells and its ability to bind to its receptors (245). It stimulates proliferation of rat osteoblast-like cells additively to that of basic fibroblast growth factor and EGF (52). Effects on differentiation are variable, depending on cell density and interaction with other factors (52). In normal mouse (MC3T3-E1) osteoblasts it increases levels of EGF receptors (320) and inhibits proliferation, alkaline phosphatase activity, and cAMP production in response to PTH (80). EGF in this latter study also inhibits alkaline phosphatase activity but stimulates proliferation. TGF-β has also been reported to decrease alkaline phosphatase activity in rat and human osteosarcoma cells (230, 231).

From these data it is apparent that the possible effects of TGF-β release on synthesis at sites of bone resorption are complex and difficult to predict. It could effect both osteoblastic proliferation and differentiated function positively or negatively depending on interactions with other growth factors and other local environmental conditions. Finally, it could also effect the resorption process biphasically since it has been shown to inhibit osteoclast formation but stimulate ^{45}Ca release (54).

The other growth factors stored in bone may also have a role as coupling agents. IGF-1 or somatomedin-C is a systemic growth factor synthesized in the liver in response to growth hormone but also produced locally by fibroblasts. It also has been shown to be produced in response to growth hormone and 1,25$(OH)_2$ vitamin D_3 from bone organ cultures (32, 299) and osteoblast cultures (86, 334). It stimulates proliferation and collagen synthesis in organ cultures (28, 32) in normal MC3T3-E1 clonal mouse osteoblasts (171) and freshly isolated mouse calvarial osteoblasts (334). The amount of somatomedin activity released into the culture media of osteoblast cultures was 2 to 3 times higher than that from fibroblastic cells derived from the outer layers of the periosteum (334). Osteoblast (334) and bone organ cultures (32) both secrete low (6 to 8 kd) and high (>25 kd) molecular weight IGF-1 activity into the media. Osteoblast mitogenic activity is associated only with the low molecular weight material (334) indicating that the binding protein is inhibitory as is the case with TGF-β.

PDGF is a 28 to 35 kd dimer initially isolated from platelet α granules (65, 66). One of the chains of PDGF is encoded by the sis proto-oncogene (65). It stimulates proliferation of a variety of mesenchymal cells including osteoblasts (53) and increases DNA and protein synthesis in cultured rat calvarine (29). Recently, multiple PDGF-like molecules produced by primary cultures of human osteoblast-like cells were shown to be mitogenic for normal rat kidney cells and human osteoblasts (322). Cytoplasmic RNA from the osteoblast-like cells hybridized with a 5′-sis DNA probe, suggesting the sis-proto-oncogene was expressed in these cells. PDGF molecules, therefore, are another class of potential autocrine coupling agents.

Several other growth factors have been implicated in control of osteoblastic proliferation and matrix synthesis. Bone derived growth factor is an 11,000 daltons factor present in bone and conditioned media from bone organ cultures which stimulates both DNA and type I collagen synthesis in bone organ cultures (30) and also stimulates fibroblast and chondrocyte mitosis. This substance has recently been shown to be identical with β_2 microglobulin (31). Human recombinant β_2 microglobulin was subsequently shown to increase DNA noncollagenous protein, and collagen synthesis in osteoblast-enriched and bone organ cultures. β_2 microglobulin (murine) mRNA was demonstrated in all calvarial cell fractions and in an osteosarcoma cell line.

Monocyte-Macrophage and Lymphocyte Controls of Bone Remodeling

Cells of the monocyte/macrophage and lymphocyte lineage secrete cytokines and other substances capable of regulating bone resorption and bone formation. The principle substances involved include tumor necrosis factor (TNF)-β (lymphotoxin), TNF-α and Il-1 (217). PDGF, basic fibroblast growth factor, EGF, interferon, HEP II, $1,25(OH)_2$ vitamin D_3, and prostaglandins are also produced by monocytes (53).

The osteoblast-mediated effects of TNFs α and β and Il-1 on bone resorption by preformed osteoclasts has been discussed above. γ-Interferon inhibits bone resorption (119). Il-1 stimulates production of osteoclast precursors in long-term cultures of human marrow (302). In this system $1,25(OH)_2$ vitamin D_3 also increases osteoclast formation by causing fusion of osteoclast precursors (190, 270). Recombinant human γ-interferon inhibits osteoclast formation in such cultures, apparently by interfering with vitamin D-induced fusion (302).

The cytokines also influence osteoblasts. In fetal rat calvariae, Il-1, and TNFs α and β increase DNA synthesis and inhibit collagen and noncollagenous protein synthesis. γ-interferon also inhibits collagen synthesis (289). Il-1 has also been shown to suppress collagen and noncollagen protein synthesis, alkaline phosphatase activity, and cell proliferation in an *in vitro* model of bone nodule formation from fetal rat osteoblasts (293). TNF α stimulates fetal rat osteoblast DNA synthesis and inhibits collagen production despite an increase in type I collagen mRNA, indicating that it inhibits collagen synthesis by specific effects on translation independent of its effects of cell replication and gene transcription (36).

Some of the monocyte growth factors (PDGF, basic fibroblast growth factor) have been discussed above in connection with osteoblast controls of remodeling. PDGF stimulates bone resorption in fetal mouse calvariae via prostaglandin synthesis (305). EGF stimulates bone resorption directly (257). Another macrophage product designated HEP II has been shown to possess mitogenic activity for osteoblasts, chondrocytes, and muscle cells, but not for fibroblasts (53).

Prostaglandins. Prostaglandins are ubiquitous short-lived paracrine or autocrine messages synthesized from cell membrane phospholipids in response to physical, hormonal, immunologic and other types of membrane stimuli. The major prostaglandins synthesized by bone organ cultures are the cyclo-oxygenase derivatives of arachidonic acid, PGE_2, $PGF_{2\alpha}$, and PGI_2 (prostacyclin) and thromboxane A_2 (260, 340). Normal cloned mouse osteoblast-like cells (343) and some human osteosarcoma cell lines (286) synthesize PGE_2 and $PGF_{2\alpha}$ whereas cells of the ROS series produce mainly PGE_2 (268). PG synthesis by osteoclasts has not been described but monocytes synthesize and release PGE_2 (70).

A variety of stimuli result in PG synthesis and release in bone or osteoblast cultures. In organ cultures, this includes EGF (296, 306), TGFs α and β (296, 308), and synthetic bovine and human PTH (187, 340). In osteoblast-like cells it includes mechanical stimulation (291, 342), EGF (286, 343) and PTH (187). PTH stimulated PG synthesis is inhibited by $1,25(OH)_2$ vitamin D_3 (187).

The biologic effects of PGs on intact bone have been demonstrated by addition of exogenous PGs or stimulators of endogenous PG synthesis (253). In the latter use it is necessary to show inhibition of the biologic response by inhibitors of PG synthesis. In bone organ cultures exogenous PGs and their metabolites generally increase bone resorption (58, 67, 174, 224, 307). In intact bones PGE_2 increases the size of osteoclasts and their clear zones and ruffled borders, and may increase cell number (142). The effects on resorption, therefore, appear to include enhancement of both osteoclast work efficiency and recruitment.

On the other hand, as described above recent studies have shown an early inhibitor effect of PGE_1 (58) and PGE_2 (174) on resorption in bone organ cultures and a direct inhibitory effect of PGs on isolated osteoclasts (40, 44, 46) which is reversed by co-culture of osteoclasts with osteoblast-like cells (46). It thus appears that PG-induced increases in osteoclast-work efficiency are mediated indirectly by other cell types, one of which has osteoblast characteristics. Monocytes also induce bone resorption in organ cultures via synthesis and release of PGE_2 (70). Stimulation of osteoclasts could be the result of PGE_2 stimulation of osteoblasts, or could involve another intermediate cell line such as lymphocytes which release TNF-β in response to monocyte-derived PG (344–346). As already describes, TNF-β and the monocyte products Il-1 and TNF-α all appear to stimulate osteoclasts via an osteoblast-like cell.

Prostaglandins also influence bone formation. They increase cell replication in secondary cultures of osteoblast-like cells (96) and in a cloned osteoblastic line (125). In the latter study the second messenger did not appear to be cAMP, and agents which increased cAMP decreased DNA synthesis. There is evidence that some prostaglandin effects may involve calcium as a second messenger (21, 74, 327). Clonal osteoblast-like cells increase their collagen and noncollagen protein synthesis, alkaline phosphatase activity, and peptidase activity in response to PGs. At higher doses of PG, these stimulatory effects don't occur (55, 123, 124). These effects on osteoblast-like cells are similar to results in bone organ culture where PGs stimulate collagen synthesis and cell proliferation at concentrations of 10^{-7} (56) and inhibit it at higher concentrations (254).

PTH. The effects of PTH on bone resorption by osteoclasts has been discussed in several contexts above. The effects on preformed osteoclasts (work effectiveness) are indirect, mediated by cells with PTH receptors such as osteoblasts (288) or lymphocytes (242). Cytologic activation of pre-existing osteoclasts by PTH is very rapid (141). The effects of single injections of PTH on quiescent osteoclasts on endosteal surfaces of laying hens (207, 209, 210) or thyroparathyroidectomized rats (142) begin within minutes and return to normal within 24 hours. Development of a ruffled border and clear zone occur between 10 and 40 minutes. Secretion of lysosomal enzymes is demonstrable by 20 minutes (209). Cellular hypertrophy occurs by 90 minutes. Ruffled border and clear zones revert to normal within 6 hours but cellular hypertrophy persists up to 24 hours (141).

Increases in osteoclast number following PTH are slower, beginning at 3 to 6 hours and returning to normal in 72 hours in thyroparathyroidectomized rats (142, 324). In organ cultures increased osteoclast numbers are still demonstrable at 96 hours (93). There is an early increase at 24 to 48 hours due to fusion of mononuclear precursors without DNA synthesis and a later increase due to further fusion of labeled precursors evident at 96 hours (93).

These results indicate that PTH enhances proliferation and fusion of osteoclast precursors. These effects have also been demonstrated in a human with primary hyperparathyroidism who had increased numbers of osteoclasts produced in long-term cultures of his marrow (190). It is not known whether these are direct or indirect effects. Increased fusion might be due to PTH induced elevations in 1,25$(OH)_2$ vitamin D_3 production (217) since 1,25$(OH)_2$ vitamin D_3 is thought to enhance fusion of immediate osteoclast precursors (270, 302). It is also possible that PTH-induced elevation of 1,25$(OH)_2$ vitamin D_3 levels could enhance proliferation of osteoclast precursors since 1,25$(OH)_2$ vitamin D_3 is known to effect formation of hematopoietic stem cells (213, 223, 287). The direction of these effects, however, is unclear. Some workers find enhancement (223) and some suppression (213) of myeloid progenitor colony (CFU-C) growth. The former study indicated that 1,25$(OH)_2$ vitamin D_3 selectively promotes macrophage differentiation since it enhanced growth of macrophage colony forming units (CFU-M) while suppressing growth of combined monocyte-macrophage colonies (CFU-GM) and granulocyte colonies (CFU-G) (223). Others have also found 1,25$(OH)_2$ vitamin D_3 stimulation of macrophage colony proliferation and growth (206). These findings may be relevant to Theshingh's suggestion that the osteoclast is derived from a progenitor of resident tissue macrophages, a line thought by some to be distinct from the monocyte lineage (312).

It is possible that such vitamin D effects on proliferation are mediated through stimulation of the synthesis of cytokines. Il-1 and TNFα induce synthesis of a mixture of granulocyte-macrophage colony-stimulating factors *in vivo* (325) and human Il I-α and β stimulate mouse osteoblast MC3T3-E1 cells to produce macrophage colony-stimulating activity (279). 1,25$(OH)_2$ vitamin D_3 stimulates synthesis of Il-1 by murine macrophages (137). Thus, it is possible that *in vivo* elevated PTH levels could elevate 1,25$(OH)_2$ vitamin D_3 levels which could enhance bone resorption directly by increasing fusion of osteoclast precursors, and either directly or indirectly by increasing proliferation of osteoclast precursors. The latter effects, however, are not obligatory since increased bone resorption in response to PTH occurs in organ cultures pretreated with agents that inhibit DNA synthesis (180).

The effect of PTH on osteoblasts is generally inhibitory. In bone organ cultures collagen (167, 170) and osteocalcin (175) synthesis is inhibited. In osteosarcoma and primary and secondary osteoblast cell cultures PTH decreases alkaline phosphatase (184, 191, 335) and collagen (168, 335) synthesis and decreases DNA synthesis by osteosarcoma cells (241).

In contrast to these results, other workers have demonstrated increased alkaline phosphatase activity in neonatal mouse calvarial bone cells (341) and increased proliferation of human osteoblast-like cells (188) in response to PTH.

As already noted, PTH increases synthesis and release of collagenase and its activators and inhibitors (60, 63, 126, 240, 321). PTH also increases creative kinese activity (292).

Two principle cellular/molecular mechanisms to account for the effects of PTH on osteoblasts have been demonstrated. One is receptor activated synthesis of cAMP (see review by Wong (333)) and the other a rapid increase in intracellular calcium (183, 262, 338). PTH-stimulated cAMP synthesis is attenuated by 1,25$(OH)_2$ vitamin D_3 (50, 169) and enhanced by glucocorticoids (50, 110). There is evidence that one of the effects of increased cytoplasmic calcium is increased phosphorylation of proteins via Ca/phosphatidylserine stimulation of protein kinase C (298). It is not known precisely which of the many biologic effects of PTH are mediated by each of these mechanisms, but it has been shown that there is a poor correlation between cAMP production and bone resorption (135) and a good correlation between the activity of PTh and PTH-fragments to increase cytosolic Ca^{2+} in osteoblast-like cells and their ability to induce bone resorption in bone organ cultures (183).

Vitamin D_3 Metabolites. Vitamin D_3 metabolites play a central role in bone remodeling because they have direct or indirect effects on most of the cells in the bone microenvironment. 1,25$(OH)_2$ vitamin D_3, and 19 nor-10-keto,25-hydroxyvitamin D_3 both stimulate both resorption in bone organ cultures (295, 297). These effects on osteoclastic function appear to be mediated by osteoblasts or other types of cells. Osteoblasts, normal human peripheral blood monocytes, malignant B, and T, and undifferentiated lymphocytes, and activated normal lymphocytes have receptors for 1,25$(OH)_2$ vitamin D_3 (252) but receptors have not been demonstrated on osteoclasts. It is possible that osteoclast precursors have receptors since 1,25$(OH)_2$ vitamin D_3 promotes osteoclast formation in long term marrow cultures by increasing fusion of pre-existing precursors and perhaps by stimulating proliferation of osteoclast precursors as discussed above. These questions will not be settled until the lineage of osteoclasts is more clearly defined.

Although 1,25$(OH)_2$ vitamin D_3 in organ cultures increases osteoclastic size and induces cytologic changes similar to those seen with PTH, prostaglandins, and cytokines (142), to date there has been no demonstration as to how those effects are brought about. As already noted 1,25$(OH)_2$ vitamin D_3 has no effect on isolated osteoclasts (44) but experiments showing activation by co-culture with osteoblasts or other cell types have not been reported. It is possible that activation in organ culture is mediated indirectly via cytokines. In addition, it should be noted that at least two studies could find no stimulation of osteoclasts by $1,25(OH)_2$ vitamin D_3 *in vivo* (107, 331). It is difficult to reconcile these reports with *in vitro* studies showing the opposite results (142, 258, 259).

Vitamin D_3 metabolites have multiple, often biphasic effects on osteoblast function. *In vivo* $1,25(OH)_2$ vitamin D_3 increases osteoblast number and cell size (331). DNA synthesis and proliferation are stimulated by this metabolite in osteoblast-like rat osteosarcoma cells (267) which also show differences in pattern of growth, forming clusters rather than sheets (267). In collagen synthesizing human osteoblast-like cells from vertebral marrow $1,25(OH)_2$ vitamin D_3 inhibits proliferation (17).

Effects of this metabolite on alkaline phosphatase (AP) activity apparently depend on the state of differentiation of the cell (90). In low density rat osteosarcoma cell cultures with low AP activity, $1,25(OH)_2$ vitamin D_3 stimulates synthesis, whereas in high density cultures with high AP activity it has the opposite effect (90, 193). AP activity is also inhibited by $1,25(OH)_2$ vitamin D_3 in osteoblast-like cells from mouse calvariae (335). Studies with neonatal rat calvarial osteoblast-like cells indicate that $1,25(OH)_2$ vitamin D_3 is necessary to prevent loss of alkaline phosphatase activity from proliferating and non-proliferating cells (104). In cultured human bone cells $1,25(OH)_2$ vitamin D_3 stimulated alkaline phosphatase while inhibiting proliferation (17).

In organ cultures of bone $1,25(OH)_2$ vitamin D_3 inhibits collagen formation (127,255, 256). It also decreases collagen synthesis in some osteoblastic cell lines (168, 328, 335) in proportion to receptor levels for the hormone (328). However, in human cells it increases collagen synthesis in parallel with alkaline phosphatase activity and reciprocally with proliferative activity (17).

In fetal rat calvariae (175), rat osteosarcoma cell cultures (248), and in human vertebral osteoblast-like cells (16) $1,25(OH)_2$ vitamin D_3 increases synthesis of BGP. $24,25(OH)_2$ vitamin D_3 has no effect (16). Increased synthesis in each system is first noted at 6 hours and is maximum at 96 hours. Increased synthesis of BGP in response to $1,25(OH)_2$ vitamin D_3 occurs concomitantly with decreased collagen synthesis and is suppressed by PTH and EGF but enhanced by insulin in organ culture (175). It is also suppressed by glucocorticoids (16). Insulin alone has no effect on BGP synthesis (175), whereas PTH alone decreases synthesis (16).

As already discussed, $1,25(OH)_2$ vitamin D_3 is one of the substances that stimulates release of collagenase and its activators and inhibitors.

The effects of $1,25(OH)_2$ vitamin D_3 on osteoblastic second messengers also appear to be biphasic. It has no consistent effect on basal cAMP production but it attenuates the effects of agents such as PTH which stimulate cAMP production (50, 169). The effect appears to be exerted beyond the hormone receptor and nucleotide regulatory components of the adenylate cyclase complex (169).

In high density rat osteogenic sarcoma cell cultures, low doses of $1,25(OH)_2$ vitamin D_3 stimulate intracellular calcium accumulation, whereas higher doses have the opposite effect (163). In low density cultures, similar results occur, but the responses require much higher $1,25(OH)_2$ vitamin D_3 concentrations, *i.e.*, sensitivity increases as cell density increases (163). Similar results are obtained after 15 minutes or 48 hours of exposure to $1,25(OH)_2$ vitamin D_3 (164). The inhibitory effects are dependent on protein synthesis, whereas the stimulatory effects are not (164).

Vitamin D_3 metabolites are also thought to play an important role in bone mineralization. Vitamin D deficiency in animals results in a decrease in bone matrix synthesis and mineralization (14). There is an increase in the relative amount of osteoid because the decrease in mineralization rate is greater than the decrease in bone formation rate (146).

There is controversy about which vitamin D_3 metabolite is important in mineralization (115). In rachitic rats, treatment with $24,25(OH)_2$ vitamin D resulted in improvement of the osteomalacia, apparently by enhancing matrix maturation, without changing bone formation, but the effects couldn't be separated from an increase in serum calcium (115). In another study, vitamin D deficiency resulted in a decrease in mineralization rate as $24,25(OH)_2 D_3$ and $25(OH)D_3$ levels fell, while $1,25(OH)_2 D_3$ levels remained constant. Mineralization could be restored with high doses of $24,25(OH)_2D_3$ or $25(OH)D_3$. The former treatment was ineffective in parathyroidectomized animals, but was again effective if given with PTH (303). $24,25(OH)_2$ vitamin D_3 also was more effective in healing the growth plate cartilage in rats with low phosphate vitamin D_3 deficient rickets (4). Direct injection of $24,25(OH)_2$ vitamin D_3 into rachitic chick tibiae heals both cartilage and bone, but physiologic doses of $1,25(OH)_2$ vitamin D_2 have no effect (176). In contrast, in another study, the healing of rickets in rats correlated with increasing serum $1,25(OH)_2$ vitamin D_3 levels, and $24,25(OH)_2$ vitamin D_3 appeared to have no effect (186). Similar results have been reported in chicks (69).

In recent years it has become apparent that high levels of $1,25(OH)_2$ vitamin D_3 can cause an osteomalacic picture (122, 136, 337). This effect is not reversed by PTH or calcitonin (122). In a recent study rachitic rats on a Ca and P adequate diet healed their rickets on doses of $1,25(OH)_2D_3$ of 1 ng/day, whereas higher doses (5 ng/day) resulted in an accumulation of osteoid resembling the original rickets (107). $1,25(OH)_2D_3$ doses healing rickets did not normalize serum calcium and doses that normalized serum calcium, produced a new rachitic lesion. $1,25(OH)_2$ vitamin D_3 did not effect bone resorption in this study.

The conflicting results above might be related to recent data showing that $1,25(OH)_2$ vitamin D_3 and $24,25(OH)_2$ vitamin D_3 have markedly different effects on serum and bone BGP and calcium levels (332). Both serum and bone levels of BGP fall in vitamin D deficient rachitic rats. Treatment with $1,25(OH)_2$ vitamin D_3 raises serum BGP levels but doesn't restore bone levels of BGP. Treatment with $24,25(OH)_2D_3$ does not alter serum BGP levels but increases bone calcium and BGP to levels above normal (332). These findings suggest that 1,25$(OH)_2$ vitamin D_3 promotes mineralization of bone by increasing synthesis of BGP but 24,25$(OH)_2$ vitamin D_3 is necessary to direct BGP into the matrix where its calcium binding domain facilitates mineralization. It is clear, however, that factors other than levels of vitamin D_3 metabolites and the presence of the γ-carboxyglutamic acid containing domain of BGP in bone matrix are important in mineralization, since vitamin K deficiency does not result in osteomalacia (249).

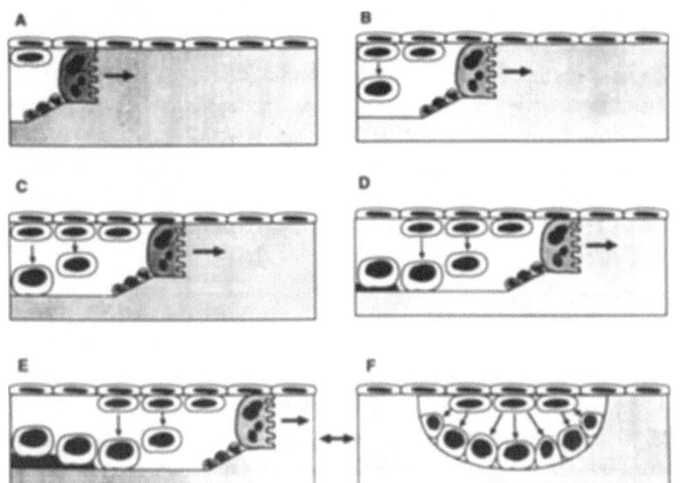

FIG. 4. Recruitment of osteoblasts and the longitudinal rate of bone formation. Longitudinal bone resorption by osteoclasts moves from left to right followed by slower radial resorption to a constant depth by reversal phase monocytes. Osteoblast precursors are thought to be activated near the original bone surface in the vicinity of the osteoclasts and to proliferate and differentiate to reach the resorption surface at a rate normally synchronized with the longitudinal and radial resorption rates so that the length of the reversal phase surface is constant (*C*, *D*, and *E*). Preosteoblasts would then differentiate into matrix synthesizing osteoblasts filling in the resorption space (*D* and *E*). Activation of osteoblasts would be anatomically tied to the longitudinal rate of bone formation but the longitudinal rate of extension of osteoid could be delayed by decreased proliferation or maturation after activation. These changes would increase the length of the reversal phase and/or preosteoblastic surfaces.

A FUNCTIONAL MODEL OF BRUs AND THEIR CONTROL

The studies reviewed above indicate considerable discrepancy and variation *in vivo* and *in vitro* of the effects of vitamin D and PTH on bone. We believe these inconsistencies will ultimately be explained by learning which of the many other substances discussed in this paper are important as local controls of bone remodeling and by showing where and how they act. We also feel that the various osteoblastic cell lines used for *in vitro* studies must ultimately be related to *in vivo* counterparts in BRUs, in the context of the growth characteristics of bone remodeling units. Figures 3, 4, 5, and 6 summarize our concepts about the functional organization of BRUs and possible points of control of bone remodeling by PTH, vitamin D metabolites and other substances discussed in this review.

In order to explain differences in the longitudinal and radial rates and durations of resorption we suggest that osteoclasts are responsible for longitudinal resorption and reversal phase monocytes and preosteoblasts for radial resorption. The rate, duration, and perhaps direction of osteoclastic resorption depend on continuous stimulation of mature osteoclasts and recruitment and fusion of precursors. We place the early osteoclast precursors outside of the BRU under systemic control. They could reach the resorption space via the blood stream or by directed movement from marrow immediately adjacent to the BRU (Fig. 3). Chemoattractants such as the carboxy terminal portion of BGP released by resorptive activity in the BRU might play a role in this process (Fig. 6*A*, arrows 3). The immediate osteoclast precursor are more likely to be in the reversal zone which would likely be a site of strong chemoattractant concentration. As discussed above some of the cells there have histologic and histochemical characteristics of osteoclast precursors. Although on endosteal surfaces osteoclast precursors could be above or in front of osteoclasts, in osteons the only route of access to the osteoclasts is the reversal zone.

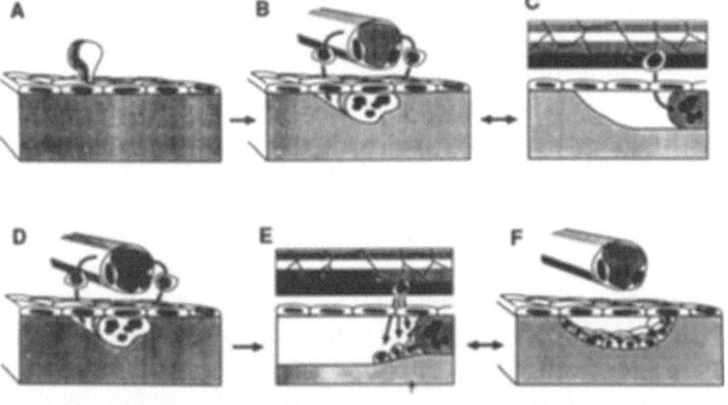

FIG. 3. Possible relationships between osteoclasts and reversal phase monocytes. After activation, a normally quiescent osteoclast (185) (*A*) forms a small cavity beneath the bone lining cells which is progressively enlarged as the osteocyte moves to the right (*C* and *E*) or toward the viewer from the plane of the paper (*B*, *D*, and *F*). Osteoclast precursors in the marrow or blood stream move to a position behind the osteoclast (*B* and *C*) where the immediate postmitotic precursor enters and exits the osteoclast at a rate of 8% of the osteoclast nuclei/day (150) (*C* and *E*). Another population of reversal phase monocytes lines and deepens the resorption surface behind the osteoclast (84), accounting for the slower radial rate of resorption (*E* and *F*). These cells may represent osteoclast fission products (*E*), or a separate population of mononuclear phagocytes entering the resorption bay in a manner similar to preosteoclasts (*D* and *E*). They are probably not osteoclast precursors because their radial resorption would tend to separate them from the longitudinally resorbing osteoclast.

The immediate precursor may be a derivative of a monocytic cell or an independent cell line (Fig. 3) but is unlikely to be a cell independently resorbing bone in a radial direction because that would tend to separate it from the osteoclast if the latter is moving in a longitudinal direction. The mononuclear cells resorbing bone radially could be an independent monocytic cell line replacing osteoclasts at the surface and then leaving the surface as preosteoblasts arrive, or fission products of osteoclasts which continue resorbing independently until they are displaced by preosteoblasts (Fig. 3).

The longitudinal advance of bone forming cells in our view is really a radial centrifugal movement of bone lining cells brought about by their stimulation (activation) in the vicinity of the osteoclast. They proliferate at

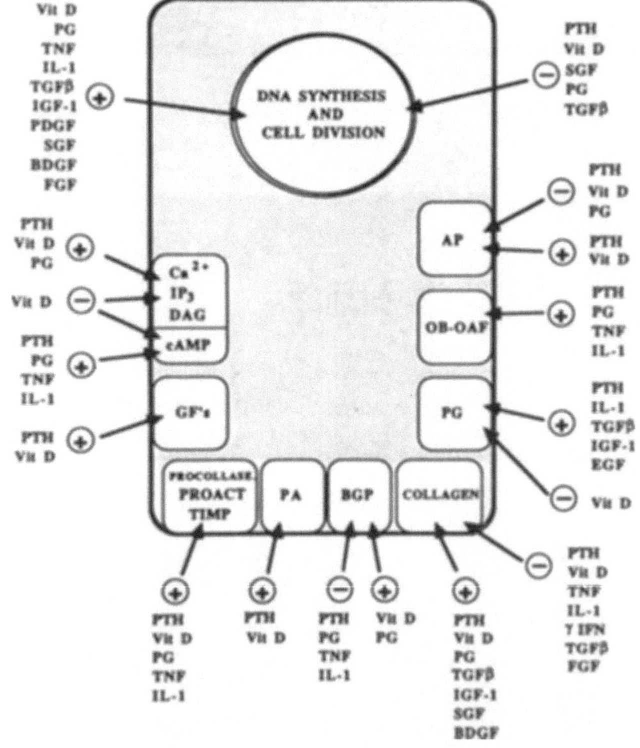

FIG. 5. Osteoblast phenotype and its controls. Cells of the osteogenic lineage are capable of DNA synthesis and cell division and have multiple functional compartments including (a) synthesis of macromolecular matrix components represented by bone glutamic acid containing protein (*BGP*) and type I collagen (b) synthesis of autocrine and paracrine messages represented by undefined factors that activate osteoclasts (*OB-OAF*), prostaglandins (*PG*), and growth factors (GFs) (c) synthesis of metalloproteins, their inhibitors, and their activators, represented by procollagenase (*PROCOLLASE*), and collagenase proactivator (*PROACT*), tissue inhibitor of metalloproteinases (*TIMP*), and plasminogen activator (*PA*) (d) and other substances of poorly defined function such as alkaline phosphatase (*AP*). These activities are controlled internally by receptor mediated synthesis of second messengers including cyclic adenosine 3′:5′-monophosphate (cAMP), intracellular calcium ions (Ca^{2+}), inositol triphosphate (IP_3) and diacylglycerol (*DAG*). They are controlled by a large number of substances whose known effects on DNA synthesis and cell division, synthesis and release of functional molecules, and second messengers are shown. The major controls are the calcitropic hormones parathyroid hormone (*PTH*) and the metabolites of vitamin D (*Vit D*), cytokines including interleukin-1 (*Il-1*), tumor necrosis factors α and β (*TNF*), and γ-interferon (γ*IFN*), prostaglandins (*PG*), and growth factors including skeletal growth factor (*SGF*), transforming growth factor β (TGFβ), insulin-like growth factors (*IGF-1*), epidermal growth factor (*EGF*), acidic and basic fibroblast growth factors (*FGF*), and bone-derived growth factor (*BDGF*), now known to be β_2 microglobulin.

the site they were activated as the osteoclast moves away from them and reversal phase monocytes resorb bone radially in the wake of the advancing osteoclasts (Fig. 4). As their proliferative activity moves them toward the resorption surface, they may contribute to its ultimate depth by elaborating procollagenase, proactivator, and plasminogen activator which could diffuse into bone already demineralized by osteoclasts (Fig. 6*A*, arrows 6).

Once osteoblasts reach the resorptive surface DNA synthesis ceases and synthesis of macromolecular matrix components begins (Fig. 6*B*). The osteoblast would thus begin its matrix synthesizing phase and reverse its own movement in the BRU to a radial centripetal direction (Fig. 4). The osteoblasts subsequent functional life is therefore carried out in approximately the same position at which it is activated relative to the bone as a whole, but at increasingly greater distances from the resorptive portion of its own BRU.

The model proposes that activation of bone remodeling occurs in two stages. The first stage activates all of the bone lining cells, to produce osteoclast activating factors (OB-OAF), throughout the skeleton in the case of hormonal stimulation, or on specific bone surfaces in the cases of changing physical stress or local conditions such as infection or neoplasia. Existing quiescent osteoclasts respond and initiate new BRUs (Figs. 3, and 6*A*, arrows 1) whose activity would continue as long as the lining cells remained activated, or as long as osteoclast precursors were available.

Since osteocytes are generally considered part of the lining cell system (211) they may also produce OB-OAF. This would account for normal osteonal remodeling and tunneling resorption seen in severe pathologic remodeling states such as osteitis fibrosis in renal osteodystrophy (145). Very high levels of PTH which are characteristic of this condition (2) would presumably favor diffusion of hormone into the osteocyte canalicular system. Once a BRU was initiated by surface lining cells releasing OB-OAF, osteoclastic resorption into canalicular systems of activated osteocytes might direct their movement away from the surface.

The second stage in the activation of a bone remodeling cycle would be activation of the bone lining cells to proliferate and differentiate. This is a local phenomenon which could be coupled to movement of the osteoclast by release of matrix growth factors by osteoclastic resorption (Fig. 6*A*, arrows 1).

Possible points of control of this system by PTH, vitamin D, and other substances indicated in Figure 6 and are based on the summary of positive and negative controls of osteoblastic function in Figure 5. Activation of surface lining cells by PTH or other similarly acting substances, particularly the cytokines, would initiate osteoclastic resorption (Fig. 6*A*, arrows 1). As discussed above, the position of $1{,}25(OH)_2$ vitamin D_3 in activating osteoclasts is unclear but it could act on marrow monocytes to induce the synthesis of cytokines which could then activate lining cells to produce OB-OAF. Growth factors stored in the matrix during prior remodeling cycles could initiate proliferation and differentiation to the preosteoblastic level (Fig. 6A, arrows 2). These responses might be enhanced by systemic agents such as $1{,}25(OH)_2$ vitamin D_3 and monocyte products (Fig. 6*A*, arrows 4).

Up to the stage of matrix synthesis it would be appropriate to suppress collagen synthesis with PTH and $1{,}25(OH)_2$ vitamin D_3, BGP synthesis with PTH (Fig. 6*A*, arrows 6) or cytokines (Fig. 6*A*, arrows 5), and stimulate DNA synthesis with $1{,}25(OH)_2$ vitamin D_3 and growth factors (Fig. 6*A*, arrows 2, 4). As already noted synthesis and activation of collagenase would also be appropriate and could be controlled by PTH and $1{,}25(OH)_2$ vitamin D_3 (Fig. 6, arrows 6).

During the matrix synthesizing phase DNA synthesis could be inhibited and collagen synthesis initiated by $1{,}25(OH)_2$ vitamin D_3 and changes in the balance of PTH, autocrine or delayed autocrine/paracrine sub-

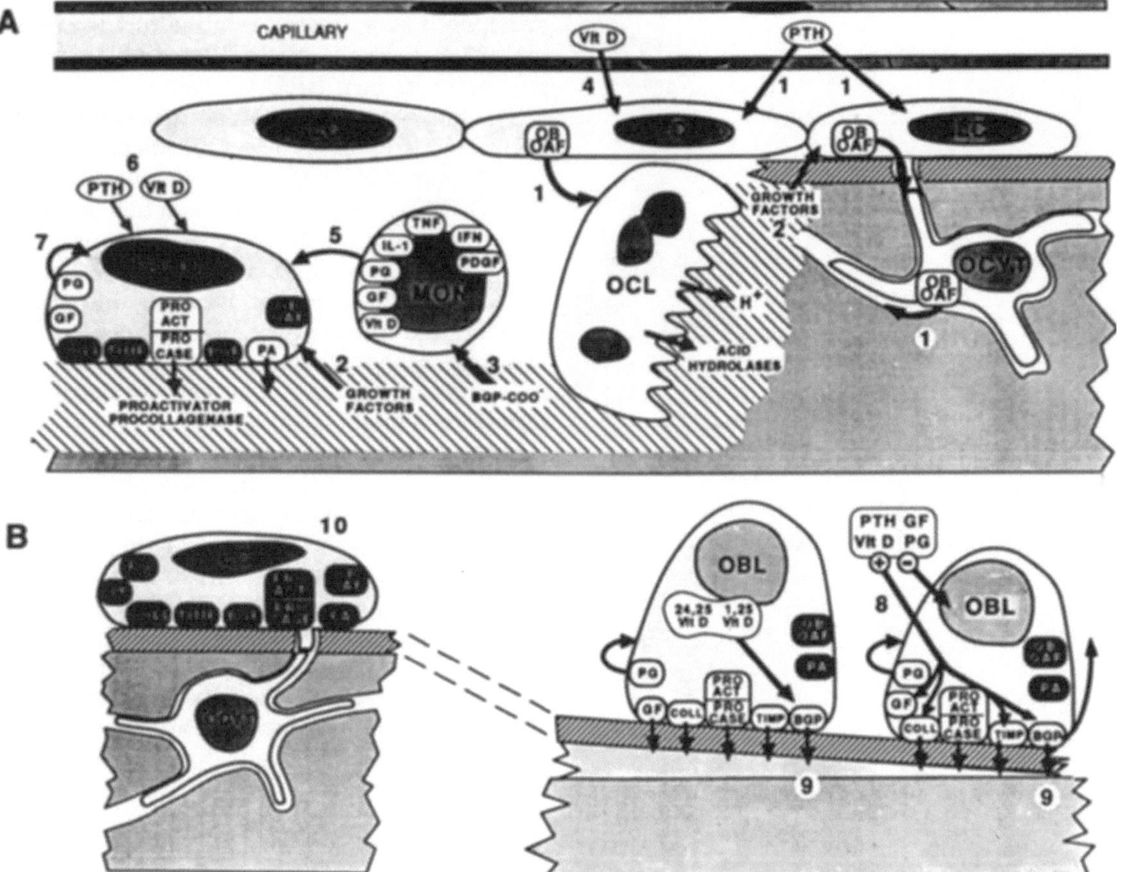

FIG. 6. Hypothetical model of growth and function of bone remodeling units and their controls. *A*, Activation of bone remodeling is viewed as a two-stage process. Widespread activation of bone lining cells and osteocytes by physical forces or hormones (*PTH*) to release osteoclastic activating factors (*OB-OAF*) would stimulate quiescent osteoclasts to longitudinal resorption utilizing hydrogen ions and acid hydrolases (*arrows, 1*). Release of matrix growth factors would further activate bone lining cells locally to proliferate and differentiate (*arrows, 2*). Subsequent steady-state bone remodeling would represent a balance of systemic and local controls. Emigration of preosteoclasts and reversal phase monocytes to the reversal zone might be aided by chemotactic matrix components (*BGP-COO*) released by osteoclastic resorption (*arrows, 3*). Proliferation and differentiation of bone lining cells to preosteoblasts and osteoblasts could be modulated by hormonal stimuli (*arrows, 4*) or cytokines and growth factors from reversal phase monocytes (*arrows, 5*), matrix growth factors (*arrows, 2, 3*), or by release of PGs and growth factors as autocrine controls (*arrows, 7*). These multiple controls could sequentially activate (white) or suppress (black) specific osteoblastic functions. For example, PTH and $1,25(OH)_2$ vitamin D_3 might stimulate collagenase activity and suppress collagen synthesis in preosteoblasts (*arrows, 6*) and stimulate release of prostaglandins or growth factors. *B*, In more mature osteoblasts, prostaglandins, growth factor, $1,25(OH)_2$ vitamin D_3 and PTH acting together might suppress DNA synthesis and initiate matrix synthesis (*arrows, 8*). Changing controls might also modify posttranslational activity. For example, changes in the proportion of vitamin D metabolites might alter BGP secretion so that most of the molecules were incorporated into the matrix rather than appearing in the pericellular space and the blood stream (*arrows, 9*). Both bone resorption and bone formation would cease when the original activating stimulus (PTH) disappeared, allowing bone lining cells and osteocytes to revert to a quiescent state (10). Increases in the number of bone remodeling units would depend on proliferation of osteoclast precursors at a distance from bone surfaces and would result from interactions among hematopoietic stem cells, lymphocytes, and monocytes controlled by hormones, cytokines and growth factors.

stances such as growth factors or prostaglandins (Fig. 6*A*, arrows 7; Fig. 6*B*, arrows 8). Synthesis and deposition within the matrix of BGP could be controlled by $1,25(OH)_2$ vitamin D_3 and $24,25(OH)_2$ vitamin D_3 (Fig. 6*B*, arrows 9). Such controls might be directed primarily at the packaging of secretory products, and determine whether they are directed into the matrix rather than the pericellular space or blood stream. They would also be applicable to growth factors and collagenase which might be anticipated to function directly on cells and matrix during earlier phases of osteoblastic activation and to be deposited in the matrix during later phases.

According to this model, the duration of remodeling in each BRU would depend on the continued presence of the original activating stimulus, PTH for example. Removal of that stimulus would result in cessation of both resorption and formation. Osteogenic cells would cease all of their activity and revert to a quiesent state, either as osteocytes or bone lining cells (Fig. 6*B*, arrows 10). While remodeling was in progress, the duration of bone formation at each site (each plane perpendicular to the direction of movement of the BRU) would be theoretically unlimited on endosteal surfaces but limited by the constraints of the resorption space in osteons.

APPLICABILITY OF THE MODEL TO METABOLIC BONE DISEASES

Determination of the accuracy of this model would require extensive in situ demonstration of specific receptor occupancy, mRNA expression, and translation of osteoblast, osteoclast, and monocyte products in quiescent and activated bone. The overall scheme of the organization of BRUs and some of the predicted effects of $1,25(OH)_2$ vitamin D_3 and PTH seem to be consistent with some histomorphometric studies of bone diseases. For example in primary hyperparathyroidism there is an increased osteoclastic surface, a decreased reversal surface, an increased preosteoblastic surface (85), and an increased bone forming surface with a reduced apposition rate (85, 215). The depth of resorption by osteoclasts is normal but resorption under reversal phase monocytes and preosteoblasts is reduced (85). These results are compatible with an increased longitudinal resorption rate by osteoclasts and either a decreased rate or duration of radial resorption by reversal phase monocytes. The increased preosteoblast surface and reduced apposition rates are consistent with prolonged PTH and $1,25(OH)_2$ vitamin D_3 suppression of matrix synthesis.

While it is not yet possible to specifically explain variable skeletal responses to calcitropic hormones, for example, differences in bone mass in humans (8, 49, 215) or other animals (111, 121, 136, 303, 304) exposed to chronic elevations of PTH or vitamin D_3, it is clear from the studies reviewed in this paper that the explanations must be due to differences in local controls of remodeling. The explanation, therefore, must ultimately include description of the functional anatomy of BRU's.

SUMMARY

The effects of PTH and vitamin D on bone are the result of their direct and indirect effects on the functional cells of bone remodeling units and their precursors. These effects are probably modified or controlled by growth factors, cytokines, and PGs generated locally by the process of bone remodeling.

Bone remodeling includes resorptive and bone forming phases, each with a longitudinal and a radial component of progression in time and space. Longitudinal resorption is rapid, prolonged and is probably carried out by osteoclasts utilizing hydrogen ions and lysosomal enzymes to remove mineral and organic components of bone in a highly localized and directed fashion. Individual osteoclasts are probably long-lived cells with a nuclear and perhaps a cytoplasmic turnover rate of 8%/day, with replenishment coming from preosteoclasts in the reversal zone.

Radial resorption is slower and shorter than longitudinal resorption. It is carried out by reversal phase monocytes whose exact relationship to osteoclasts is not clear. Activated collagenase diffusing from osteogenic cells in the reversal zone could also play a role.

The longitudinal rate of bone formation is probably a measure of the rate of proliferation and differentiation of osteogenic cells at the site at which they were activated. The radial rate of bone formation is a measure of how rapidly osteoblasts synthesize and mineralize bone matrix once they reach the resorption surface.

PTH and vitamin D have no direct effects on mature osteoclasts. They may have direct stimulatory effects on proliferation and differentiation of osteoclast precursors and their fusion with osteoclasts but this is not clear because the ontogeny of osteoclasts *vis a vis* monocytes and other phagocytic cells is still not clear. It is likely that their effects to increase osteoclast precursors involve interactions among lymphocytes, monocytes, and hematopoietic stem cells at a distance from bone remodeling units and are mediated by $1,25(OH)_2$ vitamin D_3 induced synthesis of cytokines and colony-stimulating factors.

Stimulatory effects of PTH, vitamin D, PGs, and cytokines on osteoclasts are mediated by as yet undefined factors produced by osteoblasts. Osteoblasts stimulated by PTH could also inhibit osteoclasts by synthesizing and releasing PGs.

PTH and vitamin D have diverse and often contradictory effects on the functional activity of osteoblast-like cells *in vitro* that are difficult to interpret because the relationship of these cells to osteoblasts *in vivo* is not clear. Most of the PTH and vitamin D effects are duplicated by cytokines, growth factors, and PGs, all of which could be expected to modify osteoblast function in PTH and vitamin D-induced bone remodeling because they are synthesized by cells in remodeling units and these cells have receptors for these substances as well as for PTH and vitamin D. Many of these substances are also present in the matrix and would be expected to be released during the resorptive phase of remodeling.

It is not possible to say how these various factors interact to explain the variable effects of PTH and vitamin D on bone *in vivo*. It is likely that cell/cell and cell/matrix interactions, particularly involving osteoblasts play a major role. This review presents a model to suggest how they might interact. This model could be tested by *in situ* studies trying to show how a cell's position in the BRU correlates with the type and number of receptors that are occupied, which of the osteoblastic synthetic products have been transcribed and are being translated, and where the products are going. This approach might be more productive than trying to prove that an osteoblastic-like cell line with a particular set of phenotypic responses *in vitro* is related to osteoblasts *in vivo*.

Acknowledgments: I wish to thank Nancy Hart and Clairene Mraz for their skillful assistance in manuscript preparation and Phillip Pratt for his technical skill and valuable scientific suggestions in preparing the illustrations.

Address reprint requests to: William E. Huffer, M.D., Dept. of Pathology, B216, University of Colorado Health Sciences Center, 4200 East Ninth Avenue, Denver, CO 80262.

REFERENCES

1. Anderson RE, Jee WSS, Woodbury DM: Stimulation of carbonic anhydrase in osteoclasts by parathyroid hormone. Calcif Tissue Int 37:646, 1985
2. Andress DL, Endres DB, Maloney NA, Kopp JB, Coburn JW, Sherrard DJ: Comparison of parathyroid hormone assays with bone histomorphometry in renal osteodystrophy. J Clin Endocrinol Metab 63:1163, 1986
3. Athanason NA, Bliss E, Gatter KC, Heryet A, Woods GC, McGee JO: An immunohistological study of giant cell tumors of bone: evidence for an osteoclast origin of the giant cells. J Pathol 147:153, 1985
4. Atkin I, Pita JC, Ornoy A, Agundez A, Castiglione G, Howell DS: Effects of vitamin D metabolites on healing of low phosphate vitamin D-deficient induced rickets in rats. Bone 6:113, 1985

5. Auf'mkolk B, Hauschka PV, Schwartz ER: Characteristics of human bone cells in culture. Calcif Tissue Int 37:228, 1985
6. Bab I, Ashton BA, Syftestad GT, Owen ME: Assessment of an *in vivo* diffusion chamber method as a quantitative assay for osteogenesis. Calcif Tissue Int 36:77, 1984
7. Barling PM, Bibby NW: Study of the localization of [^{3}H] bovine parathyroid hormone in bone by light microscopic autoradiography. Calcif Tissue Int 77:441, 1985
8. Baron R, Magee S, Silverglate A, Broadhus A, Lang R: Estimation of trabecular bone resorption by histomorphometry: evidence for a prolonged reversal phase with normal resorption in postmenopausal osteoporosis and coupled increased resorption in primary hyperparathyroidism. In Clinical Disorders of Bone and Mineral Metabolism, edited by Frame B, Petts JT, p 191. Amsterdam Excerpta Medica, 1983
9. Baron R, Neff L, Louvard D, Courtoy P: Acidification and bone resorption: immunocytochemical localization of a lysosomal membrane protein at the ruffled border of osteoclasts. J Cell Biol 101:2210, 1985
10. Baron R, Neff L, Roy C, Boisvert A, Caplan M: Evidence for a high specific concentration of (Na^+,K^+) ATPase in the plasma membrane of the osteoclast. Cell 46:311, 1986
11. Baron R, Neff L, Tran Van P, Nefuss R, Vignerey A: Kinetic and cytochemical identification of osteoclast precursors and their differentiation into multinucleated osteoclasts. Am J Pathol 122:363, 1986
12. Baron R, Vignerey A, Horowitz M: Lymphocytes, macrophages, and the regulation of bone remodeling. In Bone and Mineral Research, edited by Peck WA, p 175. Amsterdam, New York, Oxford, Elsevier, 1984
13. Bar-Shavit Z, Teitelbaum SL, Reitsma P, Hall A, Pegg LE, Trial J, Kahn AJ: Induction of monocyte differentiation and bone resorption by 1,25-dihydroxyvitamin D_3. Proc Natl Acad Sci USA 80:5907, 1983
14. Baylink D, Stauffer M, Wergedal J, Rich C: Formation, mineralization, and resorption of bone in vitamin D deficient rats. J Clin Invest 49:1122, 1970
15. Bentley SA, Alabaster OA, Foidart JM: Collagen heterogeneity in normal human bone marrow. Br J Haematol 48:287, 1981
16. Beresford JN, Gallagher JA, Poser JW, Russell RGG: Production of osteocalcin by human bone cells *in vitro*. Effects of $1,25(OH)_2 D_3$, parathyroid hormone and glucocorticoids. Metab Bone Dis Relat Res 5:229, 1984
17. Beresford JN, Gallagher JA, Russell RG: 1,25-dihydroxy vitamin D_3 and human bone derived cells *in vitro*: effects of alkaline phosphatase, type I collagen and proliferation. Endocrinology 119:1776, 1986
18. Bertolini DR, Nedwin GE, Bringman TS, Smith DD, Mundy GR: Stimulation of bone resorption and inhibition of bone formation *in vitro* by human tumor necrosis factors. Nature 319:516, 1986
19. Bianco P, Hayashi Y, Silvestrini G, Termine JD, Bonucci E: Osteonectin and Gla-protein in calf bone: ultrastructural immunohistochemical localization using the protein A-gold method. Calcif Tissue Int 37:684, 1985
20. Blair HC, Kahn AJ, Crouch IC, Jeffrey JJ, Teitelbaum SL: Isolated osteoclasts resorb the organic and inorganic components of bone. J Cell Biol 102:1164, 1986
21. Boland CJ, Fried RM, Tashjian AH Jr: Measurement of cytosolic free Ca^{2+} concentrations in human and rat osteosarcoma cells: Actions of bone resorption-stimulating hormones. Endocrinology 118:980, 1986
22. Bonewald LF, Gutierrez GE, Mundy GR: Different responses of osteoblastic cell lines to osteotropic factors. J Bone Min Res 2 (Suppl):23, 1987
23. Bronckers ALJJ, Gay S, DiMuzio MT, Butler WT: Immunolocalization of γ-carboxyglutamic acid-containing proteins in developing rat bones. Coll Relat Res 5:273, 1985
24. Budenz RW, Bernard GW: Osteogenesis and leukopoiesis within diffusion chamber implants of isolated bone marrow subpopulations. Am J Anat 159:455, 1980
25. Burger EH, Boonenkamp PM, Nijweide PJ: Osteoblast and osteoclast precursors in primary cultures of calvarial bone. Anat Rec 214:32, 1986
26. Burger EH, Vander Meer JWM, Gevel JS, Gribnau JC, Thesingh CW, van Furth R: *In vitro* formation of osteoclasts from long-term cultures, bone marrow and splenic transplants. J Exp Med 192:651, 1982
27. Camarda AJ, Butler WT, Finkelman RD, Nanci A: Immunocytochemical localization of γ-carboxyglutamatic acid-containing proteins (osteocalcin) in rat bone and dentin. Calcif Tissue Int 40:349, 1987
28. Canalis E: Effects of insulin-like growth factor 1 on DNA and protein synthesis in cultured rat calvaria. J Clin Invest 66:709, 1980
29. Canalis E: Effect of platelet-derived growth factor on DNA and protein synthesis in cultured rat calvaria. Metabolism 30:970, 1981
30. Canalis E, Centrella M: Biological characterization of a bone-derived growth factor. In The Chemistry and Biology of Mineralized Tissues, edited by Butler WT, p 70. Birmingham, AL, Ebsco Media, Inc, 1985
31. Canalis E, McCarthy M, Centrella M: Identity of bone derived growth factor (BDGF) with β_2 microglobulin. J Bone Min Res 2:251, 1987
32. Canalis E, McCarthy M, Centrella M: Characterization of a somatomedin synthesized by rat calvariae. J Bone Min Res 2(Supp 1):248, 1987
33. Cao H, Gay CO: Effects of parathyroid hormone and calcitonin on carbonic anhydrase location in osteoclasts of cultured chick embryonic bone. Experientia 41:1472, 1985
34. Cawston TE, Galloway A, Mercer A, Murphy G, Reynolds JJ: Purification of rabbit bone inhibitor of collagenase. Biochem J 195:155, 1981
35. Centrella M, Canalis E: Isolation of EGF-dependent transforming growth factor (TGβ-like) activity from culture medium conditioned by fetal rat calvariae. J Bone Min Res 2:29, 1987
36. Centrella M, McCarthy T, Canalis E: Tumor necrosis factor (TNFα) inhibits bone collagen synthesis independently of its effects on DNA synthesis and collagen mRNA levels. J Bone Min Res 2(Suppl):35, 1987
37. Chambers TJ: The pathobiology of the osteoclast. J Clin Pathol 38:2417, 1985
38. Chambers TJ, Ali NN: Inhibition of osteoclastic motility by prostaglandins I_2, E_1, E_2 and 6-Oxo-E_1. J Pathol 139:383, 1983
39. Chambers TJ, Athanasou NA, Fuller K: The effect of parathyroid hormone, calcitonin and prostaglandins on osteoclastic spreading and motility. J Endocrinol 102:281, 1984
40. Chambers TJ, Darby JA, Fuller K: Mammalian collagenase predisposes bone surfaces to osteoclastic resorption. Cell Tissue Res 241:671, 1985
41. Chambers TS, Fuller K: Bone cells predispose endosteal surfaces to resorption by exposure of bone mineral to osteoclastic contact. J Cell Sci 76:155, 1985
42. Chambers TJ, Horton MA: Failure of cells of the mononuclear phagocyte series to resorb bone. Calcif Tissue Int 36:556, 1984
43. Chambers TJ, Magnus CJ: Calcitonin alters the behavior of isolated osteoclasts. J Pathol 136:27, 1982
44. Chambers TJ, McSheehy PM, Thomson BM, Fuller K: The effect of calcium regulating hormones and prostaglandins on bone resorption by osteoclasts disaggregated from neonatal rabbit bones. Endocrinology 116:234, 1985
45. Chambers T, Moore A: The sensitivity of isolated osteoclasts to morphological transformation by calcitonin. J Clin Endocrinol Metab 57:819, 1983
46. Chambers TJ, Revell PA, Fuller K, Athanason NA: Prostaglandins act as direct inhibitors and indirect stimulators of osteoclastic motility. Br J Exp Pathol 65:557, 1984
47. Chambers TJ, Revell PA, Fuller K, Athanason NA: Resorption of bone by isolated rabbit osteoclasts. J Cell Sci 66:383, 1984
48. Chambers TJ, Thomson BM, Fuller K: The effect of substrate composition on bone resorption by rabbit osteoclasts. J Cell Sci 70:61, 1984
49. Charhon SA, Delmas PD, Malaval L, Chavassieux PM, Arlot M, Chapuy MC, Meunier PJ: Serum bone Gla-portein in renal osteodystrophy: comparison with bone histomorphometry. J Clin Endocrinol Metab 63:892, 1986
50. Chen TC, Feldman D: Modulation of PTH-stimulated cyclic AMP in cultured rodent bone cells: The effects of $1,25(OH)_2$ vitamin D_3 and its interaction with glucocorticoids. Calcif Tissue Int 36:580, 1984

51. Chen TL, Hirst MA, Feldman D: A receptor-like binding macromolecule for 1α,25-dihydroxycholecalciferol in cultured mouse bone cells. J Biol Chem 254:7491, 1979
52. Chen TL, Mallory JB, Chang SL: Effects of transforming growth factor (TGFβ) and its interactions with bFGF and EGF in rat osteoblast-like (RoB) cells. J Bone Min Res 2 (Suppl):256, 1987
53. Cheng SL, Rifas L, Shen V, Tors B, Pierce G, Duel T, Peck WA: J774A.1 Macrophage cell line produces PDGF-like and non-PDGF-like growth factors for bone cells. J Bone Min Res 2:467, 1987
54. Chenu C, Pfeilschifter S, Mundy GR, Roodman GD: Transforming growth factor-β inhibits formation of osteoclast-like cells in long term human marrow cultures. J Bone Min Res 2:253, 1987
55. Chikuma T, Ishii Y, Kato T, Kodama H, Hakeda Y, Kumegawa M: Effect of prostaglandin E_2 on PZ-peptidase and several other peptidase activities in a clonal osteoblast-like cell line derived from newborn mouse calvaria. J Biochem (Tokyo) 97:1533, 1985
56. Chyun YS, Raisz LG: Stimulation of bone formation by prostaglandin E_2. Prostaglandins 27:97, 1984
57. Coccia PF, Krivit W, Cervenka J, Lawson C, Kersey JH, Kim TH, Nesbit ME, Ramsay NKC, Warketin PI, Teitelbaum SL, Kahn AJ, Brown DM: Successful bone marrow transplantation for infantile malignant osteopetrosis. N Engl J Med 302:701, 1980
58. Conway HH, Diez LF, Raisz LG: Effects of prostacyclin and prostaglandin E_1 (PGE_1) on bone resorption in the presence and absence of parathyroid hormone. Calcif Tissue Int 38:130, 1986
59. Cowen KS, Saromoto M, Sakomoto S: Monensin inhibits both collagenase release and bone resorption in mouse calvaria cultures. Biochem Int 11:273, 1985.
60. Delaisse JM, Eeckhout J, Sear C, Galloway A, McCullagh K, Vaes G: A new synthetic inhibitor of mammalian tissue collagenase inhibits bone resorption in culture. Biochem Biophys Res Commun 133:483, 1985
61. Delaisse JM, Eeckhout Y, Vaes G: Inhibition of bone resorption in culture by inhibitors of thiol proteinases. Science 192:1340, 1980.
62. Delaisse JM, Eeckhout Y, Vaes G: Bisphosphates and bone resorption: effects on collagenase and lysosomal enzyme secretion. Life Sci 37:2291, 1985
63. Delaisse JM, Eeckhout Y, Vaes G: Bone-resorbing agents regulate production of collagenase in bone tissue. J Bone Min Res 2 (Suppl 1):49, 1987
64. Dempster DW, Murrills RJ, Horbert WR, Arnett TR: Biological activity of chicken calcitonin: Effects on neonatal rat and embryonic chick osteoclasts. J Bone Min Res 2:443, 1987
65. Duel TF, Huang JS, Huang SS, Stroobant P, Waterfield MD: Expression of a platelet-derived growth factor-like protein in Simian sarcoma virus transformed cells. Science 221:1348, 1983
66. Deuel TF, Huang JS, Proffitt RT, Baenziger JU, Chang D, Kennedy BB: Human platelet-derived growth factor: purification and resolution into two active protein fractions. J Biol Chem 256:8896, 1981
67. Dewhirst FE: 6-Keto-prostaglandin E_1-stimulated bone resorption in organ culture. Calcif Tissue Int 36:380, 1984
68. Dewhirst FE, Ago JM, Peros WJ, Stashenko P: Synergism between parathyroid hormone and interleukin 1 in stimulating bone resorption in organ culture. J Bone Min Res 2:127, 1987
69. Dickson IR, Hall AK, Jande SS: The influence of dihydroxylated vitamin D metabolites on bone formation in the chick. Calcif Tissue Int 36:114, 1984
70. Dominguez JH, Mundy GR: Monocytes mediate osteoclastic bone resorption by prostaglandin production. Calcif Tissue Int 31:29, 1980
71. Drivdahl RH, Howard GA, Baylink DJ: Extracts of bone contain a potent regulator of bone formation. Biochim Biophys Acta 714:26, 1982
72. Drivdahl RH, Puzas JE, Howard GA, Baylink DJ: Regulation of DNA synthesis in chick calvaria cells by factors from bone organ culture. Proc Soc Exp Biol Med 168:143, 1981
73. D'Souza SM, Ibbotson KJ, Twardzik DR, MacDonald BR, Todaro GJ, Mundy GR: Transforming growth factor β (TGF-β) resorbs bone and is produced by osteoblast-like cells. J Bone Min Res 1:74, 1986
74. Dziak R, Farr D, Zoghby G, Weinfeld N: The effects of calmodulin antagonists on prostaglandin E_2-induced responses in rat calvarial bone cells. Arch Oral Biol 31:391, 1986
75. Dziak RM, Hurd D, Miyasaki Kt, Brown M, Weinfeld N, Hausmann E: Prostaglandin E_2 binding and cyclic AMP production in isolated bone cells. Calcif Tissue Int 35:243, 1983
76. Eaglesom CC, Ashton BA, Allen TD, Owen ME: The osteogenic capacity of bone marrow cells. Cell Biol Int Rep 4:742, 1980
77. Ecarot-Charrier B, Glorieux FH, van der Rest M, Pereira GJ: Osteoblasts isolated from mouse calvaria initiate matrix mineralization in culture. J Cell Biol 96:639, 1983
78. Eeckhout Y, Delaisse JM, Vaes G: Direct extraction and assay of bone tissue collagenase and its relation to parathyroid-hormone-induced bone resorption. Biochem J 233:793, 1986
79. Eeckhout Y, Vaes G: Further studies of procollagenase, the latent precursor of bone collagenase. Biochem J 166:21, 1977
80. Elford PR, Guenther HL, Felix R, Cecchini MG, Fleisch H: Transforming growth factor-β reduces the phenotypic expression of osteoblastic MC3T3-E1 cells in monolayer culture. Bone 8:259, 1987
81. Eriksen EF, Berg NJ, Graham M, Colvard DS, Mann KG, Spelsberg TL, Riggs BL: Multiple sex steroid receptors in cultured human osteoblast-like cells. In International Symposium on Osteoporosis, edited by Jonsen J, Riis B, Christiansen C, p 17. Copenhagen, Glostrup Hospital DK, 1987
82. Eriksen EF, Berg NJ, Graham ML, Mann KG, Spelsberg TC, Riggs BL: Evidence of estrogen receptors in human bone cells. J Bone Min Res 2 (Suppl):238, 1987
83. Eriksen EF, Gundersen HJG, Melsen F, Mosekilde L: Reconstruction of the formation site in iliac trabecular bone in 20 normal individuals employing a kinetic model for matrix and mineral apposition. Metab Bone Dis Relat Res 5:243, 1984
84. Eriksen EF, Melsen F, Mosekilde L: Reconstruction of the resorptive site in iliac trabecular bone: a kinetic model for bone resorption in 20 normal individuals. Metab Bone Dis Relat Res 5:235, 1984
85. Erikson EF, Mosekilde L, Melsen R: Trabecular bone remodeling and balance in primary hyperparathyroidism. Bone 7:213, 1986
86. Ernst IM, Froesch ER: Growth hormone (GH) dependent stimulation of rat osteoblasts in culture is mediated partially by local synthesis of immunoreactive insulin-like growth factor (IGF). J Bone Min Res 2 (Suppl):32, 1987
87. Everts U, Aronson DC, Beersten W: Phagocytosis of bone collagen by osteoclasts in two cases of pycnodysostosis. Calcif Tissue Int 37:25, 1985
88. Fallon MD: Bone resorbing fluid from osteoclasts is acidic—an *in vitro* micropuncture study. In Endocrine Control of Bone and Calcium Metabolism, Vol 8A, edited by Cohn CV, Fujiita JT, Talmage RJ, p 144. Amsterdam, Elsevier, 1984
89. Farley JR, Baylink DJ: Purification of a skeletal growth factor from human bone. Biochemistry 21:3502, 1982
90. Farley JR, Baylink DJ: Evidence that skeletal growth factor may be a paracrine effector of bone volume. In Osteoporosis, Vol 1, edited by Christiansen C, Arnaud CD, Nordin BEC, Parfit AM, Peck WA, Riggs BL, p 423. Amsterdam, Excerpta Medica, 1984
91. Farley JR, Masuda T, Wergedal JE, Baylink DJ: Human skeletal growth factor: characterization of the mitogenic effect on bone cells *in vitro*. Biochemistry 21:3508, 1982
92. Feldman D, Dziak R, Koehler R, Stern P: Cytoplasmic glucocorticoid binding proteins in bone cells. Endocrinology 96:29, 1975
93. Feldman RS, Krieger NS, Tashjian AH: Effects of parathyroid hormone and calcitonin on osteoclast formation *in vitro*. Endocrinology 107:1137, 1980
94. Fell HB, Reynolds JJ, Lawrence LE, Bagga MR, Glauert AM: The promotion and inhibition of collagen-breakdown in organ cultures of pig synovium: the requirement for serum components and the involvement of cyclic adenosine 3′:5′-monophosphate (cAMP). Coll Relatat Res 6:51, 1986
95. Felsenfeld A, Llach F: Vitamin D and metabolic bone disease: a clinicopathologic overview. Pathol Annu 17:383, 1982
96. Feyen JHM, Di Bon A, Van der plas A, Lowik CWGM, Nijweide PJ: Effects of exogenous prostanoids on the proliferation of osteoblasts-like cells *in vitro*. Prostaglandins 30:827, 1985
97. Fisher LW, Tuross N, Termine JD: Purification and characterization of proteoglycans I and II, bone sialoproteins I and II, and osteonectin from human bone. J Bone Min Res 2 (Suppl):181, 1987

98. Fisher LW: The nature of the proteoglycans of bone. In The Chemistry and Biology of Mineralized Tissues, edited by Butler WT, p 188. Birmingham, EBSCO Media, 1985
99. Fisher LW, Whitson SW, Avioli LV, Termine JD: Matrix sialoprotein of developing bone. J Biol Chem 258:12723, 1983
100. Fornasier UL: Transmission electron microscopy studies of osteoid maturation. Metab Bone Dis Relat Res 25:103, 1980
101. Francois-Gillet C, Delaisse JM, Eeckhout Y, Vaes G: Immunoreactive collagenase and bone resorption. Biochim Biophys Acta 673:1, 1981
102. Franzén A, Heinegård D: Proteoglycans and proteins of rat bone: purification and biosynthesis of major noncollagenous macromolecules. In The Chemistry and Biology of Mineralized Tissues, edited by Butler WT, p 132. Birmingham, EBSCO Media
103. Friedman J, Raisz LG: Thyrocalcitonin: inhibitor of bone resorption in tissue culture. Science 150:1465, 1967
104. Fritsch J, Grosse B, Lieberherr M, Balsan S: 1,25-Dihydroxyvitamin D_3 is required for growth-independent expression of alkaline phosphatase in cultured rat osteoblasts. Calcif Tissue Int 37:639, 1985
105. Frost HM: Tetracycline-based histological analysis of bone remodeling. Calcif Tissue Res 3:211, 1969
106. Frost HM: Bone histomorphometry: analysis of trabecular bone dynamics. In Bone Histomorphometry, Techniques and Interpretation, edited by Reicker RR, p 109. Boca Raton, FL, CRC Press, 1983
107. Gallagher JA, Beneton M, Harvey L, Lawson DE: Response of rachitic rat bones to 1,25-dihydroxyvitamin D_3: biphasic effects on mineralization and lack of effect on bone resorption. Endocrinology 119:1603, 1986
108. Galloway WA, Murphy G, Sandy JD, Gaurilovic J, Cawston TE, Reynolds JJ: Purification and characterization of a rabbit bone metalloproteinase that degrades proteoglycan and other connective tissue components. Biochem J 209:741, 1983
109. Gay CV, Ito MB, Schraer H: Carbonic anhydrase activity in isolated osteoclasts. Metab Bone Dis Relatat Res 5:33, 1983
110. Gennari C: Glucocorticoids and bone. In Bone and Mineral Research 13, edited by Peck WA, p 213. Amsterdam, Elsevier, 1985
111. Gera I, Hock JM, Gunness-Hey M, Fonesca J, Raisz LG: Indomethacin does not inhibit the anabolic effect of parathyroid hormone on the long bones of rats. Calcif Tissue Int 40:206, 1987
112. Ghiselli R, Blair H, Teitelbaum SL, Gluck S: Identification of the osteoclast proton pump. J Bone Min Res 2 (Supp 1):275, 1987
113. Glowaki J, Altobelli D, Mulliken JB: Fate of mineralized and demineralized osseous implants in cranial defects. Calcif Tissue Int 33:71, 1981
114. Glowaki J, Cox KA: Osteoclastic features of cells that resorb bone implants in rats. Calcif Tissue Int 35:57, 1986
115. Goodman WG, Baylink DJ, Sherrard DJ: 24,25$(OH)_2D_3$, bone formation, and bone resorption in vitamin D-deficient, azotemic rats. Calcif Tissue Int 36:206, 1984
116. Göthlin G, Ericsson JL: Final structural localization of acid phosphomonesterase in the brush border region of osteoclasts. Histochemie 28:337, 1971
117. Göthlin G, Ericsson JL: Observations on the mode of uptake of thorium dioxide particles by osteoclasts in fracture callus. Calcif Tissue Res 10:216, 1972
118. Göthlin G, Ericsson J: Studies on the ultrastructural localization of adenosine triphosphate activity in fracture callus. Histochemie 35:11, 1973
119. Gowen M, Mundy GR: Actions of recombinant interleukin 1, interleukin 2, and interferon gamma on bone resorption *in vitro*. J Immunol 136:2478, 1986
120. Groot CG, Danes JK, Blok J, Hoogendijk A, Hauschka PV: Light and electron microscopic demonstration of osteocalcin antigen in embryonic and adult rat bone. Bone 7:379, 1986
121. Gunness-Hey M, Hock JM: Increased trabecular bone mass in rats treated with human synthetic parathyroid hormone. Metab Bone Dis Relat Res 5:177, 1984
122. Gunness-Hey M, Hock JM, Gera I, Fonseca J, Poser J, Bevan J, Raisz LG: Human parathyroid hormone (1–34) and salmon calcitonin do not reverse impaired mineralization produced by high doses of 1,25-dihydroxyvitamin D_3. Calcif Tissue Int 38:234, 1986
123. Hakeda Y, Nakatani Y, Hiramatsu M, Kurihara N, Tsunoi M, Ikeda E, Kumegawa M: Inductive effects of prostaglandins on alkaline phosphatase in osteoblastic cells, clone MC3T3-E1. J Biochem 97:97, 1985
124. Hakeda Y, Nakatani Y, Kurinara N, Ikeda E, Maeda N, Kumegawa M: Prostaglandin E_2 stimulates collagen and noncollagen protein synthesis and prolyl hydroxylase activity in osteoblastic clone MC3T3-E1 cells. Biochem Biophys Res Commun 126:340, 1985
125. Hakeda Y, Yoshino T, Natakani Y, Kurihara N, Maeda N, Kumegawa M: Prostaglandin E_2 stimulates DNA synthesis by a cyclic AMP-independent pathway in osteoblastic clone MC3T3-E1 cells. J Cell Physiol 138:155, 1986
126. Hamilton JA, Lingelbach S, Partridge NC, Martin TJ: Regulation of plasminogen activator production by bone resorbing hormones in normal and malignant osteoblasts. Endocrinology 116:2186, 1985
127. Harrison JR, Clark NB: Avian medullary bone in organ culture: Effects of vitamin D metabolites on collagen synthesis. Calcif Tissue Int 35:35, 1986
128. Hauschka PV: Osteocalcin: The vitamin K-dependent Ca^{2+}-binding protein of bone matrix. Hemostasis 16:255, 1986
129. Healy MD, Malluche HH, Goldstein DA, Singer FR, Massry SG: Effects of long-term therapy with calcitriol in patients with moderate renal failure. Arch Intern Med 140:1030, 1980
130. Heath JK, Atkinson SJ, Meikle MC, Reynolds JJ: Mouse osteoblasts synthesize collagenase in response to bone resorbing agents. Biochim Biophys Acta 802:251, 1984
131. Heath JK, Saklatvala J, Meikle MC, Atkinson SJ, Reynolds JJ: Pig interleukin 1 (catabolin) is a potent stimulator of bone resorption *in vitro*. Calcif Tissue Int 37:95, 1985
132. Heersche JNM: Mechanisms of osteoclastic bone resorption: a new hypothesis. Calcif Tissue Res 26:81, 1978
133. Heinegard D, Bjorne-Persson A, Coster L, Franzen A, Gardell S, Malstrom A, Paulsson M, Sandfalk R, Vogel K: The core proteins of large and small interstitial proteoglycans from various connective tissues form distinct subgroups. Biochem J 230:181, 1985
134. Herring GM: The organic matrix of bone. In The Biochemistry and Physiology of Bone, Vol 1, Ed 2, edited by Bourne GH, p 128. London, Academic Press, 1972
135. Herrmann-Erlee MPM, Nijweide JM, van der Meer JM, Ooms MAC: Action of bPTH and bPTH fragments on embryonic bone *in vitro*: dissociation of the cyclic AMP and bone resorbing response. Calcif Tissue Int 35:70, 1983
136. Hock JM, Gunness-Hey M, Poser J, Olson H, Bell NH, Raisz LG: Stimulation of undermineralized matrix formation by 1,25 dihydroxyvitamin D_3 in long bones of rats. Calcif Tissue Int 38:79, 1986
137. Hodler B, Evequoz V, Treschel A, Fleisch H, Stadler B: Influence of vitamin D_3 metabolites on the production of interleukins 1, 2, and 3. Immunobiology 170:256, 1985
138. Hoerman K, Lowik C, van den Ruit M, Verhezen J, Bijuvet OLM: Evidence for induction of bone resorption through osteoblast derived plasminogen activators. J Bone Min Res 2 (Suppl 1):17, 1987
139. Hogg N, Shapiro IM, Jones SJ, Slusarenko M, Boyde A: Lack of Fc receptors on osteoclasts. Cell Tissue Res 212:509, 1980
140. Holtrop ME, King GS: The ultrastructure of osteoclasts and its functional implications. Clin Orthop 123:177, 1977
141. Holtrop ME, King GS, Cox KA, Reit B: Time-related changes in the ultrastructure of osteoclasts after injection of parathyroid hormone in young rats. Calcif Tissue Int 27:129, 1975
142. Holtrop ME, Raisz LG: Comparison of the effects of 1,25 dihydroxycholecalciferol, prostaglandin E_2, and osteoclast activating factor with parathyroid hormone on the ultrastructure of osteoclasts in cultured long bones of rats. Calcif Tissue Int 29:201, 1979
143. Horton MA, Lewis D, McNulty K, Pringle VA, Chambers TJ: Monoclonal antibodies to osteoclastomas (giant cell bone tumors): definition of osteoclast specific cellular antigens. Cancer Res 45:5663, 1985
144. Horton MA, Rimmer EF, Lewis D, Pringle JA, Fuller K, Chambers TJ: Cell surface characterization of the human osteoclast: phenotypic relationship to other bone-marrow derived cell types. J Pathol 144:281, 1984
145. Huffer WE, Kuzela D, Popovtzer MM: Metabolic bone disease in chronic renal failure. I. Dialyzed uremics. Am J Pathol 78:365,

1975
146. Ivey JL, Morey ER, Liu CC, Rader JI, Baylink DJ: Effects of vitamin D and its metabolites on bone. In Vitamin D Biochemical, Chemical and Chemical Aspects Related to Calcium Metabolism, edited by Horman AW, Schaefer H, Coburn JW, DeLuca HF, Fraser D, Grigoleit HD, Herrath DV, p 350. New York, Walter de Gruyter, 1977
147. Jaworski ZFG: Some morphologic and dynamic aspects of remodeling on the endosteal cortical and trabecular surface. Isr J Med Sci 7:491, 1971
148. Jaworski ZFG: Physiology and pathology of bone remodeling. Cellular basis of bone structure in health and in osteoporosis. Orthop Clin North Am 12:485, 1987
149. Jaworski ZFG: Coupling of bone formation to bone resorption: a broader view. Calcif Tissue Int 36:531, 1984
150. Jaworski ZFG, Duck B, Sekaly G: Kinetics of osteoclasts and their nuclei in evolving secondary Haversian systems. J Anat 133:397, 1981
151. Jaworski ZFG, Hooper C: Study of cell kinetics within evolving secondary Haversian systems. J Anat 131:91, 1980
152. Jaworski ZFG, Lok E: The rate of osteoclastic bone erosion in Haversian remodeling sites of adult dog's ribs. Calcif Tissue Res 10:103, 1972
153. Jaworski ZFG, Lok E, Wellington JC: Impaired osteoclastic function and linear bone erosion rate in secondary hyperparathyroidism associated with chronic renal failure. Clin Orthop 107:298, 1975
154. Jennings JC, Mohan S, Baylink DJ: Purification and characterization of a small molecular weight skeletal growth factor (bSGF) from bovine bone matrix proteins. Fed Proc 44:1099, 1985
155. Jilka RL, Cohn DJ: A collagenolytic response to parathormone, 1,25-dihydroxycholecalciferol and prostaglandin E_2 in bone of osteopetrotic (mi/mi) mice. Endocrinology 112:545, 1983
156. Jilka R, Hamilton JW: Evidence for two pathways for stimulation of collagenolysis in bone. Calcif Tissue Int 37:300, 1985
157. Johnson LC: Morphologic analysis in pathology: the kinetics of disease and the general biology of bone. In Bone Biodynamics, edited by Frost HM, p 461. Boston, Little, Brown and Co, 1964
158. Jones SJ, Boyde A: Some morphologic observations on osteoclasts. Cell Tissue Res 185:387, 1977
159. Jones SJ, Boyde A, Ali NN, Machonnachie E: A review of bone cell and substratum interactions. Scanning 7:5, 1985
160. Kahn AJ, Fallon MD, Teitelbaum SL: Structure-function relationships in bone: an examination of events at the cellular level. In Bone and Mineral Research Annual, Vol 2, edited by Peck WA, p 136. Amsterdam, New York, Oxford Elsevier, 1984
161. Kahn AJ, Teitelbaum SL: Endotoxin inhibition of macrophage mediated bone resorption. Calcif Tissue Int 33:269, 1981
162. Karim A, Cournil I, Leblond CP: Immunohistochemical localization of procollagens. II. Electron microscopic distribution of procollagen I antigenicity in the odontoblasts and predentin of rat incisor teeth by a direct method using peroxidase-linked antibodies. J Histochem Cytochem 27:1070, 1979
163. Kim YS, Birge SJ, Avioli LV, Miller R: Cell density-dependent vitamin D effects on calcium accumulation in rat osteogenic sarcoma cells (Ros 17/2). Calcif Tissue Int 41:218, 1987
164. Kim YS, Birge SJ, Avioli LV, Millerr R: Early manifestations of vitamin D effects in rat osteogenic sarcoma cells. Calcif Tissue Int 41:223, 1987
165. King GJ, Holtrop ME: Actin-like filaments in bone cells of cultured mouse calvaria as demonstrated by binding to heavy meromyosin. J Cell Biol 66:445, 1975
166. Kleerekoper M, Villanueva AR, Mathews CHE, Rao DJ, Pumo B, Parfitt AM: PTH mediated bone loss in primary and secondary hyperparathyroidism. In Clinical Disorders of Bone and Mineral Metabolism, edited by Frame B, Potts JT, p 200. Amsterdam, Excerpta Medica, 1983
167. Kream BE, Rowe DW, Gworek SC, Raisz LG: Parathyroid hormone alters collagen synthesis and procollagen mRNA levels in fetal rat calvaria. Proc Natl Acad Sci USA 77:5654, 1980
168. Kream BE, Rowe D, Smith MD, Maher V, Majesk R: Hormonal regulation of collagen synthesis in a cloned rat osteosarcoma cell line. Endocrinology 119:1922, 1986
169. Kubota M, Ng KA, Martin TJ: The effect of 1,25-dihydroxyvitamin D_3 on cyclic AMP responses to hormones in clonal osteogenic sarcoma cells. Biochem J 231:11, 1985
170. Kumegawa M, Ikeda E, Tanaka S, Haneji T, Yora T, Sakagishi Y, Minami N, Niramatsu M: The effects of prostaglandin E_2, parathyroid hormone, 1,25-dihydroxycholecalciferol, and cyclic nucleotide analogs on alkaline phosphatase activity in osteoblastic cells. Calcif Tissue Int 36:72, 1984
171. Kurose H, Seino Y, Yamaoka K, Tanaaka H, Yabuuchi H: Effects of somatomedin C and 1,25-dihydroxyvitamin D_3 on clonal osteoblasts, MC3T3-E1. J Bone Min 2 (Supp 1):22, 1987
172. Lacroix P: The internal remodeling of bones. In The Biochemistry and Physiology of Bone, Vol III, Ed 2, edited by Bourne GH, Ch 3, New York and London, Academic Press, 1971
173. Leblond CP, Weinstock M: Radioautographic studies of bone formation. In The Biochemistry and Physiology of Bone, Vol III, Ed 2, Chapter 5, edited by Bourne GH, New York and London, Academic Press, 1971
174. Lerner UH, Ransjo M, Ljunggren O: Prostaglandin E_2 causes a transient inhibition of mineral mobilization, matrix degradation, and lysosomal enzyme release from mouse calvarial bone *in vitro*. Calcif Tissue Int 40:323, 1987
175. Lian JB, Coutts M, Canalis E: Studies of the hormonal regulation of osteocalcin synthesis in cultured fetal rat calvariae. J Biol Chem 260:8706, 1985
176. Lidor C, Atkin I, Ornoy A, Dekel S, Edelstein S: Healing of rachitic lesions in chicks by 24R,25-dihydroxycholecalciferol administered locally into bone. J Bone Min Res 2:91, 1987
177. Linkhart TA, Jennings JC, Baylink DJ: Identification and quantitation of four distinct growth factors stored in human bone matrix. J Bone Min Res 2:44, 1987
178. Linkhart TA, Jennings JC, Mottan S, Wakley GK, Baylink DJ: Characterization of mitogenic activities extracted from bovine bone matrix. Bone 7:479, 1986
179. Linkhart S, Mohan S, Linkhart TA, Kumegawa M, Baylink DJ: Human skeletal growth factor stimulates collagen synthesis and inhibits proliferation in a clonal osteoblast cell line (MC3T3-E1). J Cell Physiol 128:307, 1986
180. Lorenzo JA, Hock JM, Raisz LG: DNA synthesis is not necessary for osteoclastic responses to parathyroid hormone in cultured fetal rat long bones. J Clin Invest 72:1924, 1983
181. Lorenzo JA, Sousa S: Interleukin-1 synergistically enhances bone resorption stimulated by transforming growth factor β in fetal long bone cultures through prostaglandin synthesis. J Bone Min Res 2 (Suppl 1):376, 1987
182. Lorenzo JA, Sousa S, Forsees JM, Hock JM, Medlock ES: Colony stimulating factors regulate the development of multinucleated osteoclasts from recently replicated cells *in vitro*. J Clin Invest 80:160, 1987
183. Lowik CWGM, van Leeuwen JPTM, van der Meer JM, van Zeeland JK, Scheven BAA, Herrmen-Erlee MPM: A two-receptor model for the activity of parathyroid hormone on osteoclasts. A role for intracellular free calcium and cAMP. Cell Calcium 6:311, 1985
184. Luben RA, Wong G, Cohn DV: Biochemical characterization with parathormone and calcitonin of isolated bone cells. Endocrinology 99:526, 1976
185. Luk SC, Nopajaroonsri C, Simon GT: The ultrastructure of endosteum: a topographic study in young adult rabbits. J Ultrastruct Res 46:165, 1975
186. Lund B, Charles P, Egsmose C, Lund BJ, Melsen F, Mosekilde L, Storn T, Sondergård H, Thode J, Sorensen OH: Changes in vitamin D metabolites and bone histology in rats during recovery from rickets. Calcif Tissue Int 37:478, 1985
187. MacDonald BR, Gallagher JA, Ahnfelt-Ronne I, Beresford VN, Gowen M, Russell RGG: Effects of bovine parathyroid hormone and 1,25-dihydroxyvitamin D_3 on the production of prostaglandins by cells derived from human bone. FEBS Lett 169:49, 1984
188. MacDonald BR, Gallagher JA, Russell RG: Parathyroid hormone stimulates proliferation of cells derived from human bone. Endocrinology 118:2445, 1986
189. MacDonald BR, Mundy GR, Clark S, Wang EA, Kuehl TJ, Stanley ER, Roodman GD: Effects of human recombinant CSF-GM and highly purified CSF-1 on the formation of multinucleated cells with osteoclast characteristics in long-term bone marrow cultures. J Bone Min Res 1:227, 1986
190. MacDonald BR, Takahashi N, McManus CM, Holahan J, Mundy

GR, Roodman GD: Formation of multinucleated cells that respond to osteotropic hormones in long term human bone marrow cultures. Endocrinology 120:2326, 1987

191. Majeska RJ, Rodan SB, Rodan GA: Parathyroid hormone-responsive clonal cell lines from rat osteosarcoma. Endocrinology 107:1494, 1980
192. Malone JD, Teitelbaum SL, Hauschka PV, Kahn AJ: Presumed osteoclast precursors (monocytes) recognize two or more regions of osteocalcin. Calcif Tissue Int 84:511, 1982
193. Manolagas SC, Burton DW, Deftos LJ: 1,25-Dihydroxyvitamin D_3 stimulates the alkaline phosphatase activity of osteoblast-like cells. J Biol Chem 256:7115, 1981
194. Manolagas SC, Taylor CM, Anderson DC: Highly specific binding of 1,25-hydroxycholecalciferol in bone cytosol. J Endocrinol 80:35, 1979
195. Marchi F, Leblond CP: Collagen biogenesis and assembly into fibrils as shown by ultrastructural and ^{3}H-proline radioautographic studies on fibroblasts of the rat foot pad. Am J Anat 168:167, 1983
196. Marchisio PC, Cirillo D, Naldini L, Primavera MV, Teti A, Zamboni-Zallone A: Cell-substratum interaction of cultured avian osteoclasts is mediated by specific adhesion structures. J Cell Biol 99:1696, 1984
197. Marel GM, McKenna MJ, Frame B: Osteomalacia. In Bone and Mineral Research/4, edited by Peck WA, p 335. Amsterdam, Elsevier Science Publishers, 1986
198. Mark MP, Prince LW, Gay S, Austin RL, Bhown M, Finkelman RD, Butler WT: A comparative immunocytochemical study on the subcellular distribution of 44kDa bone phosphoprotein and bone γ-carboxyglutamic acid (Gla)-containing protein in osteoblasts. J Bone Min Res 2:337, 1987
199. Marks SC Jr: Osteopetrosis in the ia rat cured by spleen cells from a normal littermate. Am J Anat 146:331, 1976
200. Marks SC Jr: Studies of the cellular cure for osteopetrosis by transplanted cells. Specificity of the cell type in ia rats. Am J Anat 151:131, 1978
201. Marks SC Jr, Schneider GB: Evidence for a relationship between lymphoid cells and osteoclasts: bone resorption restored in ia (osteopetrotic) rats by lymphocytes, monocytes and macrophages from a normal littermate. Am J Anat 152:331, 1978
202. McSheehy PM, Chambers TJ: Osteoblastic cells mediate osteoclastic responsiveness to parathyroid hormone. Endocrinology 118:824, 1986
203. McSheehy PM, Chambers TJ: Osteoblast-like cells in the presence of parathyroid hormone release soluble factor that stimulates osteoclastic bone resorption. Endocrinology 119:1654, 1986
204. Mechanic GL, Binderman I, Harell A: A novel hypothesis for bone resorption and remodeling. In Current Advances in Skeletogenesis, edited by Silbermann M, Slavkin HC, p 322. Amsterdam, Excerpta Medica, 1982
205. Merke J, Klans G, Hugel U, Waldhem R, Ritz E: No 1,25-dihydroxyvitamin D_3 receptors on osteoclasts of calcium deficient chickens despite demonstrable receptors on circulating monocytes. J Clin Invest 77:312, 1986
206. Miller SC: Osteoclast cell surface changes during the egg-laying cycle in Japanese quail. J Cell Biol 75:104, 1977
207. Miller SC: Rapid activation of the medullary bone osteoclast cell surface by parathyroid hormone. J Cell Biol 76:615, 1978
208. Miller SC: Osteoclast cell surface specializations and nuclear kinetics during egg-laying in Japanese quail. Am J Anat 162:35, 1981
209. Miller SC: The rapid appearance of acid phosphatase activity at the developing ruffled border of parathyroid hormone activated medullary bone osteoclasts. Calcif Tissue Int 37:526, 1985
210. Miller SC, Bowman BM, Myers RL: Morphological and ultrastructural aspects of the activation of avian medullary bone osteoclasts by parathyroid hormone. Anat Rec 208:223, 1984
211. Miller SC, Jee WSS: The bone lining cell: a distinct phenotype? Calcif Tissue Int 41:1, 1987
212. Minkin C, Jennings JM: Carbonic anhydrase and bone remodeling: Sulfonamide inhibition of bone resorption in organ culture. Science 176:1031, 1972
213. Miyaura C, Abe E, Nomura H, Nishii Y, Suda T: 1α,25-Dihydroxivitamin D_3 suppresses proliferation of murine granulocyte-macrophage progenitor cells (CFU-C). Biochem Biophys Res Commun 108:1728, 1982
214. Mohan S, Jennings J, Linkhart T, Taylor A, Baylink D: Purification and characterization of a small molecular weight human skeletal growth factor (hSGF). J Bone Min Res 1:60, 1986
215. Mosekilde L, Melsen F: A tetracycline based histomorphometric evaluation of bone resorption and bone turnover in hyperthyroidism and hyperparathyroidism. Acta Med Scand 244:97, 1978
216. Mundy GR, Poser JW: Chemotactic activity of the gamma-carboxyglutamic acid containing protein in bone. Calcif Tissue Int 35:164, 1983
217. Mundy GR, Roodman GD: Osteoclast ontogeny and function. In Bone and Mineral Research/5, edited by Peck WA, p 246. Amsterdam, New York, Oxford, Elsevier, 1987
218. Mundy GR, Varani J, Orr W, Gondek MD, Ward PA: Resorbing bone is chemotactic for monocytes. Nature (Lond) 275:132, 1978
219. Murad F, Brewer HB, Vaughan M: Effect of thyrocalcitonin on adenosine 3′5′ cyclic monophosphate formation in rat kidney and bone. Proc Natl Acad Sci USA 65:446, 1970
220. Murphy G, McAlpine CG, Poll CT, Reynolds JJ: Purification and characterization of a bone metalloproteinase that degrades gelatin and types IV and V collagen. Biochim Biophys Acta 831:49, 1985
221. Nabell LM, Graz TK: Identification of an osteoprogenitor model, the MS3 cell line. J Bone Min Res 2 (Suppl):19, 1987
222. Magase H, Jackson RC, Brinckerhoff CE, Vater CA, Harris ED Jr: A precursor form of latent collagenase produced in a cell-free system with mRNA from rabbit synovial cells. J Biol Chem 256:11951, 1981
223. Nagler A, Riklis I, Kletter Y, Tatarsky I, Fabian I: Effect of 1,25 dihydroxyvitamin D_3 and retinoic acid on normal human pluripotent (CFU-mix), erythroid (BFU-E), and myeloid (CFU-C) progenitor cell growth and differentiation patterns. Exp Hematol 14:60, 1986
224. Neuman SD, Raisz LG: Effects of the prostacyclin products 6-KETO prostaglandin E_1 and 6-KETO prostaglandin $F_{1}\alpha$, on bone resorption *in vitro*. Prostaglandins Leukotrienes Med 15:103, 1984
225. Ng KW, Partridge NC, Niall M, Martin TJ: Epidermal growth factor receptors in clonal lines of a rat osteogenic sarcoma and in osteoblast-rich rat bone cells. Calcif Tissue Int 35:298, 1983
226. Nicholson GC, Livesey SA, Moseley JM, Martin TJ: Actions of calcitonin, parathyroid hormone and prostaglandin E_2 on cyclic AMP formation in chicken and rat osteoclasts. J Cell Biochem 31:229, 1986
227. Nicholson GC, Moseley JM, Sexton PM, Martin TJ: Chicken osteoclasts do not possess calcitonin receptors. J Bone Min Res 2:53, 1987
228. Nicholson GC, Moseley JM, Sexton PM, Mendelsohn FAO, Martin TJ: Abundant calcitonin receptors in isolated rat osteoclasts; biochemical and autoradiographic characterization. J Clin Invest 78:355, 1986
229. Nishimoto SK, Price PA: Proof that the γ-carboxyglutamic acid-containing bone protein is synthesized in calf bone: comparative synthesis rate and effect of coumadin on synthesis. J Biol Chem 254:437, 1979
230. Noda M, Rodan GA: Type-β transforming growth factor inhibits proliferation and expression of alkaline phosphatase in murine osteoblast-like cells. Biochim Biophys Res Commun 140:56, 1986
231. Noda M, Rodan GA: Transforming growth factor β (TGFβ) regulation of alkaline phosphatase expression in rat and human osteosarcoma cells. J Bone Min Res 2:255, 1987
232. Oldberg A, Franzén A, Heinegård D: Cloning and sequence analysis of rat bone sialoprotein (osteopontin) cDNA reveals an Arg-Gly-Asp cell-binding sequence. Proc Natl Acad Sci USA 33:8819, 1986
233. Osdoby P, Martini MC, Caplan AI: Isolated osteoclasts and their presumed progenitor cell, the monocyte, in culture. J Exp Zool 224:331, 1982
234. Otsuka K, Sodek J, Limeback HF: Synthesis of collagenase and collagenase inhibitors by osteoblast-like cells in culture. Eur J Biochem 145:123, 1984
235. Otsuka K, Sodek J, Limeback HF: Collagenase synthesis by osteoblast-like cells. Calcif Tissue Int 36:722, 1984
236. Oursler MJ, Bell LV, Clevinger B, Osdoby P: Identification of osteoclast specific monoclonal antibodies. J Cell Biol 100:1592, 1985
237. Owen M: Lineage of osteogenic cells and their relationship to the

stromal system. In Bone and Mineral Research/3, edited by Peck WA, p 1. Amsterdam, Elsevier Science Publishers, 1985

238. Parfitt AM: The coupling of bone formation to bone resorption: A critical analysis of the concept and of its relevance to the pathogenesis of osteoporosis. Metab Bone Dis Relat Res 4:1, 1982
239. Partridge NC, Frampton RJ, Eisman JA, Michelangeli VP, Elms E, Bradley TR, Martin TJ: Receptors for 1,25(OH) vitamin D_3 enriched in cloned osteoblast-like rat osteogenic sarcoma cells. FEBS Lett 115:139, 1980
240. Partridge NC, Jeffrey JJ, Erlich LS, Teitelbaum SL, Fliszar C, Welgus HG, Kahn AJ: Hormonal regulation of the production of collagenase and a collagenase inhibitor activity by rat osteogenic sarcoma cells. Endocrinology 120:1956, 1987
241. Partridge NC, Opie AL, Opie RT, Martin TJ: Inhibitor effects of parathyroid hormone on growth of osteogenic sarcoma cells. Calcif Tissue Int 37:519, 1985
242. Perry HM, Chappel JC, Bellorin-Font E, Tamao J, Martin KJ, Teitelbaum SL: Parathyroid hormone receptors in circulating human mononuclear leukocytes. J Biol Chem 259:5531, 1984
243. Perry HM, Hobart NH: Partial characterization of a parathyroid stimulated factor(s) from osteoblast-like cells capable of increasing bone resorption. J Bone Min Res 2 (Suppl):13, 1987
244. Perry HM, Skogen W, Chappel JC, Wilner GD, Kahn AJ, Teitelbaum SL: Conditioned medium from osteoblast-like cells mediate parathyroid hormone induced bone resorption. Calcif Tissue Int 40:298, 1987
245. Pfeilschifter L, Bonewald L, Mundy GR: TGFβ is released from bone with one or more binding proteins which regulate its activity. J Bone Min Res 2 (Suppl):249, 1987
246. Phelps RG, Martinez-Hernandez A, Goldberg B: Ultrastructural immunocytochemical localization of type I procollagen in cultured human fibroblasts. Coll Relat Res 5:405, 1985
247. Pierce AM, Lindskog S: Evidence of capping of Fc receptors on osteoclasts. Calcif Tissue Int 29:109, 1986
248. Price PA, Baukol SA: 1,25-Dihydroxyvitamin D_3 increases serum levels of the vitamin K-dependent bone protein. Biochem Biophys Res Commun 99:928, 1981
249. Price PA, Williamson MK: Effects of Warfarin on bone. Studies on the vitamin K-dependent protein of rat bone. J Biol Chem 256:12754, 1981
250. Price PA, Williamson MK, Otawara Y: Characterization of matrix Gla protein. In The Chemistry and Biology of Mineralized Tissues, edited by Butler WT, p 159. Birmingham, AL, Ebsco Media, Inc, 1985
251. Prince CW, Oosawa T, Butler WT, Tomana M, Bhown AS, Bhown M, Schrohenloher RE: Isolation, characterization and biosynthesis of a phosphorylated protein from rat bone. J Biol Chem 262:2900, 1987
252. Provvedini DM, Tsoukas CD, Deftos LJ, Manolagas SC: 1,25 Dihydroxyvitamin D_3 receptors in human leukocytes. Science 221:1181, 1983
253. Raisz LG, Dietrich JW, Simmons HA, Seyberth HW, Habbard W, Oates JA: Effect of prostaglandin endoperoxides and metabolites on bone resorption *in vitro*. Nature 267:532, 1977
254. Raisz LG, Koolemans-Beynen AR: Inhibition of bone collagen synthesis by prostaglandin E_2 in organ culture. Prostaglandins 8:337, 1974
255. Raisz LG, Kream BE: Regulation of bone formation. N Engl J Med 309:83, 1983
256. Raisz LB, Kream BE, Smith MD, Simmons HA: Comparison of the effects of vitamin D metabolites on collagen synthesis and resorption of fetal rat bone in organ culture. Calcif Tissue Int 32:135, 1980
257. Raisz LG, Simmons HA, Sandberg AL, Canalis E: Direct stimulation of bone resorption by epidermal growth factor. Endocrinology 107:270, 1980
258. Raisz LG, Trummel CL, Holick MF, DeLuca HF: 1,25 Dihydroxycholecalciferol: A potent stimulator of bone resorption in tissue culture. Science 175:768, 1972
259. Raisz LG, Trummel CL, Simmons H: Induction of bone resorption in tissue culture: Prolonged response after brief exposure to parathyroid hormone or 25-hydroxycholecalciferol. Endocrinology 90:744, 1972
260. Raisz LG, Vanderhoek JY, Simmons HA, Kream BE, Nicolaou KC: Prostaglandin synthesis by fetal rat long bone *in vitro*: Evidence for a role of prostacyclin. Prostaglandins 17:905, 1979
261. Rasmussen H, Bordier P: The Physiological and Cellular Basis of Metabolic Bone Disease. p 34. Baltimore, Williams & Wilkins, 1974
262. Reid IA, Civitelli R, Halstead LR, Avioli LV, Hruska K: Parathyroid hormone acutely elevates intracellular calcium in osteoblast-like cells. Am J Physiol 252:E45, 1987
263. Reynolds JJ: Inhibition of production and actions of metalloproteinases. Ann Biol Clin (Paris) 44:188, 1986
264. Rifas L, Halstead LR, Peck WA, Avioli LV, Welgus HG: Human osteoblast-like cells secrete tissue inhibitor of metalloproteinases but not interstitial collagenase. J Bone Min Res 2 (Suppl):147, 1987
265. Riggs BL, Melton LJ, Wahner HW: Heterogeneity of involutional osteoporosis: evidence for two distinct osteoporosis syndromes. In Clinical Disorders of Bone and Mineral Metabolism, edited by Frame B, Potts JT, p 337. Amsterdam, Oxford, Princeton, Excerpta Medica, 1983
266. Rodan GA, Martin TJ: Role of osteoblasts in hormonal control of bone resorption. Calcif Tissue Int 33:349, 1981
267. Rodan GA, Rodan SB: Expression of the osteoblastic phenotype. In Bone and Mineral Research Annual 2, edited by Peck WA, p 244. Amsterdam, Elsevier Science Publishers BV, 1983
268. Rodan SB, Rodan GA, Simons HA, Walenga RW, Feinstin MB, Raisz LG: Bone resorption factor produced by osteosarcoma cells with osteoblastic features is PGE_2. Biochem Biophys Res Commun 102:1358, 1981
269. Roden SB, Wesolowski G, Rodan GA: Phenotypic heterogeneity in two subclones of the human osteosarcoma cell line Sc OS-2. J Bone Min Res 2 (Suppl):20, 1987
270. Roodman GD, Ibbotson KJ, MacDonald BR, Kuehl TJ, Mundy GR: 1,25 Dihydroxyvitamin D_3 causes formation of multinucleated cells with several osteoclast characteristics in cultures of primate marrow. Proc Natl Acad Sci USA 82:8213, 1985
271. Ryder MI, Jenkins SD, Horton JE: The adherence to bone by cytoplasmic elements of osteoclasts. J Dent Res 60:1345, 1981
272. Sabatani M, Garrett IR, Mundy GR: TNF potentiates the effects of interleukin-1 on bone resorption *in vitro*. J Bone Min Res 2 (Suppl):34, 1987
273. Sakamoto M, Sakamoto S: Immunocytochemical localization of collagenase in isolated mouse bone cells. Biomed Res 5:29, 1984
274. Sakamoto S, Sakamoto M: Biochemical and immunohistochemical studies on collagenase in resorbing bone in tissue culture. J Periodont Res 17:523, 1982
275. Sakamoto S, Sakamoto M: Isolation and characterization of collagenase synthesized by mouse bone cells in culture. Biomed Res 5:39, 1984
276. Sakamoto S, Sakamoto M: Osteoblast collagenase: Collagenase synthesis by clonally derived mouse osteogenic (MC3T3-E1) cells. Biochem Int 9:51, 1984
277. Sakamoto S, Sakamoto M: Bone collagenase, osteoblasts, and cell mediated bone resorption. In Bone and Mineral Research 4, Ch 2, edited by Peck WA, Amsterdam, New York, Oxford, Elsevier, 1986
278. Sakamoto S, Sakamoto M, Goldhaber P, Glimcher MJ: Isolation of tissue collagenase from homogenates of embryonic chick bones. Biochem Biophys Res Commun 53:1102, 1973
279. Sato K, Fujii Y, Asano S, Ohtsuki T, Kawakami M, Kasono K, Tsushima T, Shizume K: Recombinant interleukin 1 alpha and beta stimulate mouse osteoblast-like cells (MC3T3-E1) to produce macrophage-colony stimulating activity and prostaglandin E_2. Biochem Biophys Res Commun 141:285, 1986
280. Scheven BAA, Burger EH, Kawilarang-DeHass EWM, Wassenar AM, Nijweide PJ: Effects of ionizing radiation on formation and resorbing activity of osteoclasts *in vitro*. Lab Invest 53:72, 1985
281. Scheven BAA, Kawilarang-DeHass EWM, Wassenar AM, Nijweide PJ: Differentiation kinetic of osteoclasts in the periosteum of embryonic bones *in vivo* and *in vitro*. Anat Rec 214:418, 1986
282. Scheven BAA, Visser JWM, Nijweide PJ: Role of interleukin-3 in regulation of the differentiation of osteoclasts. Bone 7:387, 1986
283. Scheven BAA, Visser JWM, Nijweide PJ. *In vitro* osteoclast generation from different bone marrow fractions, including a highly enriched hematopoietic stem cell population. Nature 321:79, 1986
284. Scott DM, Kent GN, Cohn DV: Collagen synthesis in cultured

osteoblast-like cells. Arch Biochem Biophys 201:384, 1980

285. Sellers A, Reynolds JJ, Meikle MC: Neutral metallo-proteinases of rabbit bone. Separation in latent forms of distinct enzymes that when activated degrade collagen, gelatin, and proteoglycans. Biochem J 171:493, 1978
286. Shupnik MA, Tashjian AH Jr: Epidermal growth factor and phorbol ester actions on human osteosarcoma cells: characterization of responsive and nonresponsive cell lines. J Biol Chem 257:12161, 1982
287. Shezen E, Goldman R: 1 alpha,25-dihydroxyvitamin D_3 augments clonal growth of macrophages from rat bone marrow progenitor cells and modulates their function. Int J Cell Cloning 4:115, 1986
288. Silve CM, Hradek GT, Jones AL, Arnaud CD: Parathyroid hormone receptor in intact embryonic chicken bone: characterization and cellular localization. J Cell Biol 94:379, 1982
289. Smith DP, Gowen M, Mundy GR: Effects of interferon gamma, and other cytokines on collagen synthesis in fetal rat bone cultures. Endocrinology 120:2494, 1987
290. Somerman MJ, Prince CW, Sauk JJ, Foster RA, Butler WT: Mechanism of fibroblast attachment to bone extracellular matrix: role of the 44 kilodalton bone phosphoprotein. J Bone Min Res 2:259, 1987
291. Somjen D, Binderman I, Beyer E, Harell A: Bone remodeling induced by physical stress is prostaglandin E_2 mediated. Biochem Biophys Acta 627:91, 1980
292. Somjen D, Kaye AM, Roden GA, Binderman I: Regulation of creatine kinase activity in rat osteogenic sarcoma cell clones by parathyroid hormone, prostaglandin E_2, and vitamin D metabolites. Calcif Tissue Int 37(6):635, 1986
293. Stashenko P, DesJardins LA, Dewhirst FE: Il-1β is a potent inhibitor of bone formation *in vitro*. J Bone Min Res 2 (Suppl):40, 1987
294. Steen-Hackett L, Gera I, Fonesca J, Raisz LG, Hock JM: Human parathyroid hormone 1-34 increases bone mass in denervated legs of rats. J Bone Min Res 2 (Suppl):57, 1987
295. Stern PH, Horst RL, Gardner R, Napoli JL: 10 Keto or 25-hydroxy substitution confer equivalent *in vitro* bone resorbing activity to vitamin D_3. Arch Biochem Biophys 236:555, 1985
296. Stern PH, Krieger NSA, Nissenson RA, Williams RD, Winkler ME, Derynck R, Strewler GJ: Human transforming growth factor-alpha stimulates bone resorption *in vitro*. J Clin Invest 76:2016, 1985
297. Stewart PJ, Stern PH: Vertebral bone resorption *in vitro*: Effects of parathyroid hormone, calcitonin, 1,25-dihydroxyvitamin D_3, epidermal growth factor, prostaglandin E_2 and estrogen. Calcif Tissue Int 40:21, 1987
298. Stewart PJ, Stern PH: Calcium/phosphatidylserine-stimulated protein phosphorylation in bone: Effect on parathyroid hormone. J Bone Min Res 2:281, 1987
299. Stracke H, Schulz A, Moeller D, Rossol S, Schatz H: Effect of growth hormones on osteoblasts and demonstration of somatomedin C/IGF-I in bone organ culture. Acta Endocrinologica 107:16, 1984
300. Sudquist KT, Leppilamp M, Jarjelin K, Kumpulainfn T, Vaananen HK: Carbonic anhydrase isoenzymes in isolated rat peripheral monocytes, tissue macrophages and osteoclasts. Bone 8:33, 1987
301. Tarahashi H, Norimatsu H: The longitudinal and transverse rate of resorption of the Haversian system in canine bone. In Bone Morphometry, edited by Jaworski JF, p 143. Ottawa, University of Ottawa Press, 1976
302. Takahashi N, Mundy GR, Roodman GI: Recombinant human interferon-gamma inhibits formation of human osteoclast-like cells. J Immunol 137:3544, 1986
303. Tam CS, Heersche JN, Jones G, Murray TM, Rasmussen H: The effect of vitamin D on bone *in vivo*. Endocrinology 118:2217, 1986
304. Tam CS, Heersche JNM, Murray TM, Parsons JA: Parathyroid hormone stimulates the bone apposition rate independently of its resorptive action: differential effect of intermittent and continuous administration. Endocrinology 110:506, 1982
305. Tashjian AH, Hohmann EL, Antoniades HN, Levine L: Platelet derived growth factor stimulates bone resorption via a prostaglandin mediated mechanism. Endocrinology 111:118, 1982
306. Tashjian AH Jr, Levine L: Epidermal growth factor stimulates prostaglandin production and bone resorption in cultured mouse calvaria. Biochem Biophys Res Commun 85:966, 1978
307. Tashjian AH Jr, Tice JE, Sides K: Biological activities of prostaglandin analogues and metabolites on bone in organ culture. Nature 266:645, 1977
308. Tashjian AH, Voelkel EF, Lazzaro M, Singer FR, Roberts AB, Derynck R, Winkler ME, Levine L: α and β human transforming growth factors stimulate prostaglandin production and bone resorption in cultures of mouse calvaria. Proc Natl Acad Sci USA 82:4535, 1985
309. Teitelbaum SL, Bone M, Stein PM, Gilden JJ, Bates M, Boisseau VC, Avioli L: Calcifediol in chronic renal insufficiency. Skeletal Response. JAMA 235:164, 1976
310. Teitelbaum SL, Hruska KA, Shieber W, Debnam JW, Nichols S: Tetracycline fluorescence in uremic and primary hyperparathyroidism. Kidney Int 12:366, 1977
311. Teitelbaum SP, Silve CM, Nyiredy KO, Arnaud CD: Down regulation of parathyroid hormone (PTH) receptors in cultured bone cells is associated with agonist-specific intracellular processing of PTH-receptor complexes. Endocrinology 118:595, 1986
312. Thesingh CW: Formation sites and distribution of osteoclast progenitor cells during the ontogeny of the mouse. Dev Biol 117:127, 1986
313. Thomson BM, Mundy GR, Chambers TJ: Tumor necrosis factors alpha and beta induce osteoblastic cells to stimulate osteoclastic bone resorption. J Immunol 138:775, 1987
314. Thomson BM, Sakalatvala J, Chambers TJ: Osteoblasts mediate interleukin-1 stimulation of bone resorption by rat osteoclasts. J Exp Med 164:104, 1986
315. Tinkler SMB, Linder JE, Williams DM, Johnson NW: Formation of osteoclasts from blood monocytes during 1α-OH-Vit. D stimulated bone resorption in mice. J Anat 133:389, 1981
316. Tran Van P, Vignerry A, Baron R: Cellular kinetic of the bone remodeling sequence in the rat. Anat Rec 202:445, 1982
317. Tran Van P, Vignery A, Baron R: An electron microscopic study of the bone remodeling sequence in the rat. Cell Tissue Res 225:283, 1982
318. Trelstad RL, Hayashi K: Tendon collagen fibrillogenesis: Intracellular subassembly and cell surface changes associated with fibril growth. Dev Biol 71:228, 1979
319. Triffit VT: The special proteins of bone tissue. Clin Science 72:355, 1987
320. Uneno S, Yamamoto I: Transforming growth factor β increases receptor levels for epidermal growth factor in MC3T3-E1 cells (a clonal mouse calvarial osteoblastic cell line). J Bone Min Res 2:30, 1987
321. Vaes G: The release of collagenase as an inactive proenzyme by bone explants in culture. Biochem J 126:275, 1972
322. Valentin-Opran A, Delgado R, Valente T, Mundy GR, Graves DJ: Autocrine production of platelet derived growth factor (PDGF)-like peptides by cultured normal human bone cells. J Bone Min Res 2:254, 1987
323. Vater CA, Nagase H, Harris ED: Pro-activator dependent activation of collagenase induced by treatment with EGTA. Biochem J 237:853, 1986
324. Vignerry A, Baron R: The effects of parathyroid hormone on the osteoclastic pool, bone resorption and formation in rat alveolar bone. Calcif Tissue Res 26:23, 1978
325. Vogel SN, Douches SD, Kaufman EN, Neta R: Induction of colony stimulating factor *in vivo* by recombinant interleukin 1 alpha and recombinant tumor necrosis factor alpha 1. J Immunol 138:2143, 1987
326. von der Mark H, von der Mark K, Gay S: Study of differential collagen synthesis during development of the chick embryo by immunofluorescence. I. Preparation of collagen type I and type II specific antibodies and their application to early stages of the chick embryo. Dev Biol 48:237, 1976
327. Walenga RW, Bergstrom W: Stimulation of calcium uptake in rat calvaria by prostacyclin. Prostaglandin 29:191, 1985
328. Walters MR, Rosen DM, Norman AW, Luben RA: 1,25-Dihydroxyvitamin D receptors in an established bone cell line. J Biol Chem 257:7481, 1982
329. Warshawsky H, Goltzman D, Rouleau MF, Bergeron JM: Direct *in vivo* demonstration by autoradiography of specific binding sites for calcitonin in skeletal and renal tissues of the rat. J Cell Biol 85:682, 1980
330. Weinstock M: Elaboration of precursor collagen by osteoblasts as visualized by radioautography after ^{3}H-proline administration. In Extracellular Matrix Influences on Gene Expression, edited by

Slavkin H, Greulich R, p 119. New York, Academic Press, 1975

331. Weisbrode SE, Capen CC, Norman AW: Light- and electron-microscopic evaluation of the effects of 1,25-dihydroxyvitamin D_3 on bone of thyroparathyroidectomized rats. Am J Pathol 97:247, 1979
332. Wientroub S, Price PA, Reddi AH: The dichotomy in the effects of 1,25-dihydroxyvitamin D_3 and 24,25-dihydroxyvitamin D_3 on bone carboxyglutamic acid-containing protein in serum and bone in vitamin D-deficient rats. Calcif Tissue Int 40:166, 1987
333. Wong GL: Skeletal effects of parathyroid hormone. In Bone and Mineral Research Vol 4, edited by Peck WA, p 103 Amsterdam, Elsevier Science Publishers BV, 1986
334. Wong GL, Kotilar D, Schlaeger D, Vanderpol C: Somatomedin C-like and somatomedin C binding activity are present in and secreted by mouse osteoblasts. J Bone Min Res 2 (Suppl):4, 1987
335. Wong GL, Luben RA, Cohn DV: 1,25-Dihydroxycholecalciferol and parathormone: effects on isolated osteoclast-like and osteoblast-like cells. Science 197:663, 1977
336. Wright GM, Leblond LP: Immunochemical localization of procollagens. J Histochem Cytochem 29:791, 1981
337. Wronski TJ, Halloran BP, Bikle DD, Globus RK, Morey-Holton ER: Chronic administration of 1,25-dihydroxyvitamin D_3: Increased bone but impaired mineralization. Endocrinology 119:2580, 1986
338. Yamada H, Fukase M, Miyanchi A, Tsunenar T, Fujii Y, Tsutsumi M, Fujita T: PTH stimulates cytosolic free calcium in osteoblast-like cell line (MC3T3-E1). J Bone Min Res 25 (Suppl 1):115, 1987
339. Yanaguchi A, Kahn AJ, Clevinger I: Establishment of clonal osteoblastic cell lines showing different phenotypes. J Bone Min Res 2 (Suppl):14, 1987
340. Yang CY, Gonnerman WA, Taylor L, Nimberg RB, Polgar PR: Synthetic human parathyroid hormone fragment stimulates prostaglandin E_2 synthesis by chick calvariae. Endocrinology 120:63, 1987
341. Yee JA: Stimulation of alkaine phosphatase activity in cultured neonatal mouse calvarial bone cells by parathyroid hormone. Calcif Tissue Int 37:530, 1985
342. Yeh CK, Rodan SA: Microtubule disruption enhances prostaglandin E_2 production in osteoblastic cells. Biochim Biophys Acta 927:315, 1987
343. Yokota K, Kusaka M, Ohshima T, Yamamoto S, Kurihara N, Yoshino T, Kumegawa M: Stimulation of prostaglandin E_2 synthesis in clonal osteoblastic cells of mouse (MC3T3-E1) by epidermal growth factor. J Biol Chem 261:15410, 1986
344. Yoneda T, Mundy GR: Prostaglandins are necessary for osteoclast activating factor (OAF) production by activated peripheral blood leukocytes. J Exp Med 149:279, 1979
345. Yoneda T, Mundy GR: Monocytes regulate osteoclast activating factor production by releasing prostaglandins. J Exp Med 150:338, 1979
346. Yoneda T, Mundy GR: Release of the lymphokine osteoclast activating factor requires cyclic AMP accumulation. Calcif Tissue Int 34:204, 1982
347. Zamboni-Zallone A, Teti A, Primarera MV: Monocytes from circulating blood fuse *in vitro* with purified osteoclasts in primary culture. J Cell Sci 66:335, 1984

Section II

Inflammation and Immunity

Biology of Disease

Acute Inflammation and Microthrombosis Induced by Endotoxin, Interleukin-1, and Tumor Necrosis Factor and their Implication in Gram-Negative Infection

MYRON I. CYBULSKY, M. K. WILLIAM CHAN, AND HENRY Z. MOVAT

Departments of Pathology and of Immunology, Medical Sciences Building, University of Toronto, Toronto, Ontario, Canada M5S 1A8

INTRODUCTION

Acute inflammation constitutes the body's principal mode of defense against infection and other harmful agents, and neutrophils are the primary effector cells in this process. When inflammation occurs in response to infection with pathogenic microorganisms, the damage that is often observed locally is a sacrifice aimed to prevent the spread of infectious agents throughout the body. Gram-negative microorganisms elicit a brisk inflammatory reaction which is largely induced by one of their cell wall constituents, endotoxin. The infiltrating neutrophils phagocytose and kill the bacteria. The inflammatory reaction is often associated with severe local microvascular injury and abscess formation. Besides eliciting inflammation, endotoxin can predispose the local microvasculature to thrombosis upon subsequent systemic endotoxemia or complement activation, as demonstrated by the local Shwartzman reaction. Both the inflammatory and the thrombotic phenomena induced by endotoxin are mediated by the local generation of cytokines.

In addition to local effects, endotoxin shed by Gram-negative bacteria can access the circulation resulting in profound systemic effects. Endotoxin has been suggested as the principal causative agent of Gram-negative septic shock and disseminated intravascular coagulation, which are associated with a high mortality. It is also capable of eliciting fever, various components of the acute phase reaction, and a prolonged and profound neutropenia.

In this review, we examine the inflammatory and thrombotic reactions elicited by a Gram-negative bacterium, *Escherichia coli* and by endotoxin, followed by an analysis of the *in vivo* and *in vitro* observations which implicate cytokines as the mediators of these phenomena. We then examine the type and the mechanisms of the resulting microvascular injury and deal briefly with the significance of inflammation in defense against Gram-negative microorganisms.

INFLAMMATION INDUCED BY *E. coli* AND ENDOTOXIN

MORPHOLOGIC OBSERVATIONS

By counting the number of neutrophils in the lymph draining an inflammatory lesion and examining the tissue histologically, injection of *E. coli* was found to elicit a very intense inflammatory reaction, resulting in abscess formation in 24-hour lesions in sheep (64). Similar observations, including the abscess formation, were made subsequently in rabbits, in which ultrastructurally phagocytosed bacteria were demonstrable in neutrophils, often undergoing lysis (69). More recently, the morphology of the inflammatory lesions induced by killed *E. coli* was examined again and the findings correlated with other parameters (for details *vide infra* under "Inflammation and Host Defense in Gram-Negative Infection") (27). When 20 sites were injected simultaneously with *E. coli* (6×10^8/site), a marked neutropenia developed and very few neutrophils were detectable at the injected site, and many extracellular bacteria were detectable histologically. A reinjection of the same large number of bacteria after recovery from the neutropenia (during the neutrophilic phase), resulted in a marked infiltration of the dermis by neutrophils, with very few bacteria, mostly within the phagocytes.

The injection of killed *E. coli* or large doses of endotoxin is followed by severe microvascular injury (*vide infra*, "Endotoxin-Induced Microvascular Injury and Thrombosis"). However, the injection of a large number of live *E. coli* (2×10^{10}/site) or smaller numbers in neutropenic rabbits is associated with necrosis of the dermis at the injection site (18).

Quantitative Studies

Having been able to quantitate increase in vasopermeability (115) and changes in blood flow in inflammation (49), it had become pertinent to quantitate the emigration of neutrophil leukocytes and their accumulation in the lesions (55, 56). The first studies on quantitation and kinetics of the acute inflammatory reaction were done with killed *E. coli*. Neutrophils were isolated from the blood of rabbits, radiolabeled and reinfused intravenously. These studies ascertained that the emigration of neutrophils was transient. The maximal rate of emigration was between 2 to 3 hours and after 6 to 8 hours, the rate of emigration was less than 10% of maximal (Fig. 1*A*). With live *E. coli* (18, 86) and leukocyte chemoattractants (22) neutrophil emigration followed similar kinetics. When blood mononuclear leukocytes were radiolabeled (61), the maximal rate of monocyte accumulation into lesions induced by killed *E. coli* coincided with neutrophils, however monocytes continued to accumulate at approximately 25% of the maximal rate for at least 24 hours (Fig. 1*B*). The absolute number of neutrophils which accumulate in *E. coli* lesions during the first 6 hours greatly exceeds the number of monocytes, as is evident in histologic sections of early lesions. Neutrophils comprise over 30% of the rabbit's circulating leukocytes, whereas monocytes constitute less than 5%. Thus, the delivery of circulating neutrophils to the inflammatory site exceeds monocytes by at least 6-fold. Emigrated neutrophils die relatively early or leave the inflammatory site via lymphatics (64). Monocytes continue to accumulate and undergo transformation into macrophages, thus becoming the predominant cell in the late stages of *E. coli* inflammation.

The skin of rabbits was ideal to quantitate events in an inflammatory reaction because various doses or time points under study could be injected in triplicate or quadruplicate, including positive and negative controls. However, *E. coli* or endotoxin as inflammatory stimuli were suitable also for the study of inflammation in the lung (29, 30) and pleura (53, 54). Moreover, by a further purification of the ^{51}Cr-labeled blood neutrophils, and a comparison of the radiolabeled cells in the blood and in a pleural exudate, the specificity and precision of the quantitative procedure was markedly improved (27). This enabled the expression of the results as the number of infiltrating neutrophils/lesion in relation to the number of circulating neutrophils. The latter was demonstrated to influence the delivery of neutrophils at the inflammatory site. When a large dose of *E. coli* was administered, a profound and prolonged neutropenia developed and neutrophil emigration into the *E. coli*-injected intradermal sites was markedly attenuated (27).

In addition to leukocyte emigration, the injection of *E. coli* induced a transient hyperemia, enhanced vasopermeability, and hemorrhage (69). *E. coli* and endotoxin

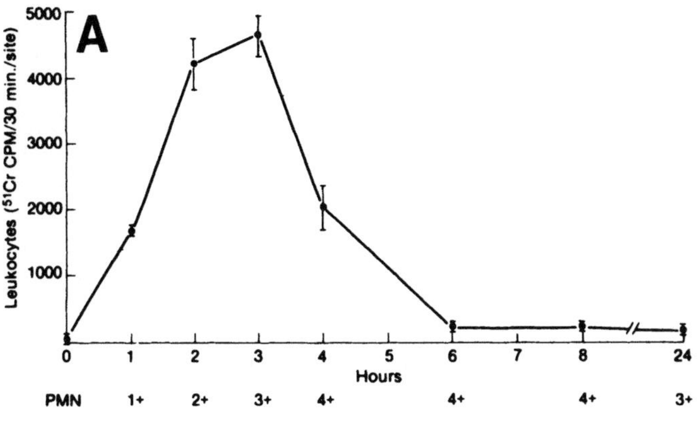

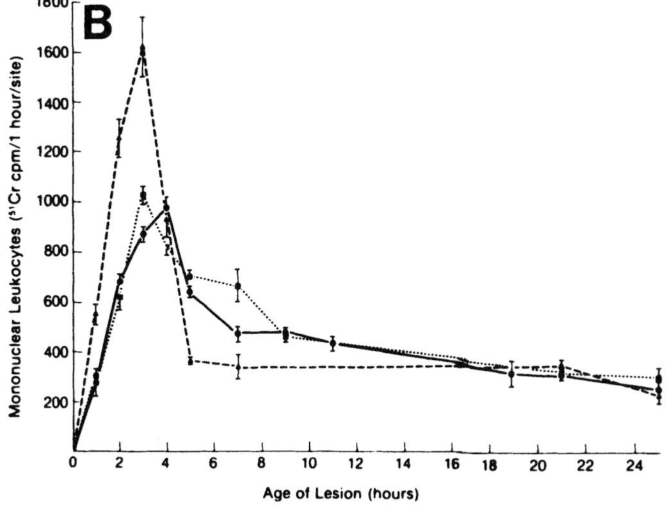

FIG. 1. Kinetics of leukocyte accumulation in rabbit skin. *A*, Rate of neutrophil leukocyte accumulation in inflammatory lesions induced by *E. coli*. Formalin-killed *E. coli* (5×10^8/site) were injected at varying times intradermally and autologous ^{51}Cr-labeled leukocytes were infused 30 minutes before sacrifice. Histologic examination ascertained that during peak emigration, over 90% of the infiltrating cell were neutrophil leukocytes (*PMNs*). Their number in hematoxylin and eosin-stained sections was scored semiquantitatively from 1 to 4+. This is one representative experiment of five. Points are means ± SEM of five replicate sites. Reproduced from Issekutz and Movat, Lab Invest 42:310, 1980. *B*, Mononuclear leukocyte accumulation in inflammatory lesions induced by *E. coli*. Killed *E. coli* (5×10^8/site) were injected intradermally at varying time intervals and ^{51}Cr-labeled mononuclear cells were injected intravenously 1 hour before sacrifice. The results of three experiments are shown. Points are mean ± SEM of triplicate sets. Saline-inoculated sites had 40 cpm, and this was subtracted from each point. By histology, the mononuclear cells were monocytes/macrophages. When ^{51}Cr-labeled lymphocytes were injected intravenously no accumulation was demonstrable. Reproduced from Issekutz *et al.*, Am J Pathol 103:47, 1981, Copyright by the American Association of Pathologists, Inc.

were the most frequent stimuli in inflammation associated with microhemorrhage (68) and microthrombosis (62, 87). Injected *E. coli* or endotoxin readily induce a hemorrhagic inflammatory reaction (69, 87), but this is seldom observed with staphylococcus-induced experimental inflammation (I. J. Cybulsky and H. Z. Movat, unpublished observations). Of all chemotaxins, only activated complement ($C5a_{des\,Arg}$) was capable of eliciting some hemorrhagic response (57, 58, 88). All the procedures mentioned above made use of radiolabeled cells and blood constituents for the quantitation of the inflammatory reaction.

Increase in vascular permeability and hemorrhage in inflammatory reactions induced by killed *E. coli* are neutrophil-dependent components of the reaction, since depletion of circulating neutrophils abrogates the development of vascular injury, quantitated with ^{125}I-albumin and ^{59}Fe-erythrocytes (70). This has been known for some time with respect to immune complex-induced inflammatory reactions associated with vascular injury (reviewed in Refs. 19, 81). The depletion of hemolytic complement and C5 markedly decreases neutrophil emigration, enhanced vasopermeability, and hemorrhage induced by the deposition of immune precipitates (24), however, it only partially inhibits the permeability change induced by *E. coli* and does not influence the neutrophil influx or hemorrhage (70). This suggested a mediating role for complement only in the immune complex-induced inflammatory reaction, and raised the question of a bacterium-derived substance in the mediation of *E. coli*-induced inflammation. Issekutz, Bhimji, and Bertolussi (52) demonstrated that killed *E. coli*-induced inflammation was diminished when the bacteria were treated with polymyxin B (which forms a complex with and inactivates endotoxin) or with anti-endotoxin antibody. Furthermore *E. coli* incubated in heat-inactivated plasma or buffer shed a substance into the supernatant, which induced neutrophil emigration when injected intradermally, but was not chemotactic *in vitro* (51). Polymyxin B or antibody to *O* or core glycolipid antigens diminished the potency of the supernatant (and of endotoxin) to induce neutrophil emigration. Issekutz and Bhimji (51) concluded that the material shed by the *E. coli* was endotoxin. Thus Gram-negative bacteria induce neutrophil emigration by releasing endotoxin which is not directly chemotactic or chemokinetic and at low doses exerts its effect *in vivo* independent of complement. During their growth phase *E. coli* secrete chemotactic formylated peptides (74) and potentially chemotactic lipids. Live *E. coli* induce also a neutrophil-independent tissue injury (18, 59), in which bacterial hemolysins play a role (59).

Attempts were also made to study the relationship between the movement of protein from the vasculature into the extracellular space and the clearance of this protein from the inflammatory site (induced by *E. coli* or other means). This was achieved by quantitating the increase in vascular permeability (^{131}I-albumin) and monitoring simultaneously the disappearance (clearance) of intradermally injected ^{125}I-albumin from inflammatory and control sites (47). It was observed that the removal rates of albumin injected into *E. coli*-induced inflammatory sites (10^2 to 10^6 *E. coli*/site) were not greater than those at sites injected with saline, despite 170 to 700% increases in vasopermeability observed in the inflammatory lesions. In fact, with high doses of *E. coli* (10^8/site) the mobilization of protein from the lesions was significantly reduced. In contrast with other inflammatory stimuli (bradykinin, heat injury) the clearance of extravascular protein from the lesions was enhanced over saline sites, implying a unique mechanism with *E. coli* (and endotoxin)-induced inflammatory edema (47). These observations may have relevance to the development of edema associated with Gram-negative septicemia and have led to studies on the role of lymphatic vessels in inflammatory edema (38, 63).

MEDIATION OF ENDOTOXIN-INDUCED INFLAMMATION

Gram-negative bacteria release (shed) endotoxins, which are lipopolysaccharide-protein complexes (40, 79, 120) and elicit a marked acute inflammatory reaction characterized by intense neutrophil emigration. The hypothesis that endotoxin-induced neutrophil emigration is a mediated process, is based on the knowledge that many of the *in vivo* biologic effects of endotoxin are mediated by host-derived mediators: leukocyte chemoattractants (C5a) and cytokines.

Leukocyte Chemoattractants

To date, substantial evidence has accumulated which suggest that leukocyte chemoattractants do not mediate endotoxin-induced neutrophil emigration. The depletion of complement with cobra venom factor had minimal effects on emigration induced by endotoxin (28) or *E. coli* (70), which indicates that C5a is not a relevant mediator. Picogram quantities of endotoxin are sufficient to elicit detectable neutrophil infiltration into the skin of rabbits and comparisons of molar potencies to leukocyte chemoattractants estimated that endotoxin was at least 1000-fold more potent (22, 26). Moreover, endotoxin did not induce tachyphylaxis to several leukocyte chemoattractants (20, 21, 26). The experiments of McComb, Cybulsky, and Movat (76) demonstrated that endotoxin induces neutrophil emigration by a different mechanism than leukocyte chemoattractants. The onset of neutrophil emigration following the injection of leukocyte chemoattractants was found to be more rapid and unlike endotoxin was not dependent on protein synthesis.

Cytokines: Mediators of the Acute Phase Response

The concept that cytokines are mediators of endotoxin-induced inflammation arose from observations made in conjunction with the acute phase response, which followed various forms of trauma and tissue injury associated with inflammation, but particularly the injection of endotoxin. The acute phase reaction includes fever, leukopenia followed by leukocytosis with neutrophilia, changes in certain heavy metals in the plasma, increase in acute phase proteins (e.g., C-reactive protein, plasma proteinase inhibitors, transport proteins, fibrinogen) in plasma and their secretion in the liver (reviewed in Refs. 67, 81). Kampschmidt and co-workers described in the 60s and 70s a substance, "leukocytic endogenous mediator" which like the earlier described "endogenous pyrogen" and endotoxin, had the capacity to elicit the acute phase response (reviewed in Ref. 65). Both endogenous pyrogen and leukocytic endogenous mediator were shown to be leukocyte-derived, but the cell type was first in question, until monocytes/macrophages were demonstrated as the primary source of interleukin-1 (IL-1), endogenous pyrogen and lymphocyte-activating factor (2, 48, 121). However, more recently good evidence was again presented that neutrophils can synthesize IL-1 (122). Another important source of Il-1 with respect to inflammation is the endothelial cell (71, 92), and the smooth muscle cell (72). Lymphocyte-activating factor (in the thymocyte co-mitogenesis assay) was described in the 70s by immunologists and designated as IL-1 by a group of cellular immunologists (J Immunol 123:2928, 1979). Eventually endogenous pyrogen, leukocytic endogenous mediator and lymphocyte-activating factor were shown to be identical to IL-1, by comparing their biologic and biochemical properties (reviewed in Refs. 33, 34). Recently, tumor necrosis factor (TNF), a cytokine produced by monocytes-macrophages in response to endotoxin was found to possess many of the activities ascribed to IL-1 (6). In view of these observations, the roles of IL-1 and more recently of TNF in mediating neutrophil emigration induced by endotoxin were examined.

Interleukin 1: Mediator of Endotoxin-Induced Neutrophil Emigration

Initial attention was focused on determining whether IL-1 could induce neutrophil emigration *in vivo*. Studies were carried out in which the activities in supernatants of cultured rabbit alevolar macrophages stimulated with opsonized zymosan or lipopolysaccharide, were assayed for neutrophil emigration-inducing activity and activity in the mouse thymocyte comitogenesis assay (25, 28). Fractions from a gel filtration column with low molecular weight showed activity in both assays, with peak activity in 14,000 to 16,000 molecular weight fractions, which corresponded to the MW of IL-1. High molecular weight fractions showed activity only in the neutrophil accumulation assay. Issekutz, Meygeri, and Issekutz (54) have reported similar activity in endotoxin-induced pleural exudates and supernatants of cultured pleural macrophages stimulated with endotoxin. Neutrophil emigration could also be induced with purified murine IL-1 (spirochete-stimulated macrophages, 5, 45), affinity-purified human monocyte-derived IL-1 (25, 26) and recombinant IL-1 preparations (28, 28a, 44, 96a). Observations with recombinant IL-1 are particularly important, since purified monocyte/macrophage-derived preparations may contain trace protein contaminants with biologic activities. Endotoxin contamination of IL-1 preparations has been ruled out by demonstrating stability of endotoxin but not of IL-1 to heating, and inhibition of endotoxin but not IL-1 activity with polymyxin B sulfate. Recently, TNF also has been found to induce neutrophil emigration (3, 28a, 31, 60, 85).

The analysis of the roles of IL-1 and TNF in endotoxin-induced neutrophil emigration is based on (a) comparisons of potencies, (b) kinetic profiles and (c) examination of cross tachyphylaxis. The potencies of both IL-1α and IL-1β approached that of endotoxin (27, 28a) (Fig. 2) and are similar to synthetic lipid A (28a). TNF on the other hand was found to be less potent than the IL-1 species (28, 85) (Fig. 2) and of comparable molar potency to the leukocyte chemoattractants. In earlier studies, leukocyte chemoattractants were found to be at least 1000-fold less potent than endotoxin (21, 26). These experiments suggest that in order to elicit an equivalent magnitude of neutrophil emigration, each molecule of endotoxin would have to generate 1 to 10 molecules of IL-1, 1000 to 10,000 molecules of TNF, or over 1000 molecules of a leukocyte chemoattractant. The latter possibility is not likely at least with regards to $C5a_{des\,Arg}$ or leukotriene B_4 since relatively high concentrations of endotoxin are required for the activation of complement (51) and endotoxin is not a potent stimulator of leukotriene B_4 production (13). The relative amounts of IL-1and TNF production by different cell types remains to be determined, however if both are produced, their effects on neutrophil emigration appear to be synergistic (60, 85) (Fig. 2).

The kinetic profile of neutrophil emigration induced by IL-1, TNF or endotoxin demonstrated a very low rate of emigration in the first 30 minutes (28, 28a). This may represent the time required by the endothelial cells to synthesize proteins adhesive for leukocytes (*vide infra*). After 30 minutes, emigration into sites injected with the cytokines increased dramatically, but remained low for a further 30 minutes into sites injected with endotoxin. These observations suggest that endotoxin may induce the synthesis of a cytokine mediator *in situ*, a process requiring approximately 30 minutes, followed by a further 30 minutes for the synthesis of adhesive proteins by the endothelium. In contrast to the cytokines or endotoxin, leukocyte chemoattractants elicit neutrophil emi-

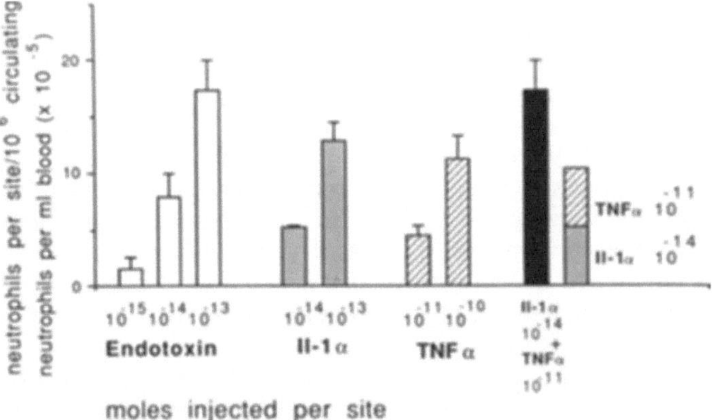

Fig. 2. Neutrophil emigration elicited with endotoxin, IL-1, TNFα or a mixture of the two cytokines, quantitated with ^{51}Cr-labeled neutrophils. The radiolabeled cells circulated for 2 hours after the intradermal injections and entered the inflammatory lesions during that time period. The dose response to two concentrations of IL-1α and TNFα are illustrated. When the lowest concentrations of the two cytokines were injected together, the neutrophil emigration was 69% greater than the additive response induced by each individual cytokine, implying a synergism between IL-1 and TNFα.

gration more rapidly, with significant emigration already detectable within the first 30 minutes after intradermal injections (76).

The term desensitization or tachyphylaxis at the inflammatory site was used in conjunction with reduced responsiveness to an inflammatory agent (20, 21). When dermal sites were reinjected with the same chemotaxin and the neutrophil emigration quantitated with ^{51}Cr-neutrophils after the reinjection (second injection), their number was decreased, compared with sites injected for the first time. Pertinent to this, was the observation that all inflammatory agents tested induced a transient emigration, which had ceased after the 4th hour (22). Thus, inflammatory lesions were initiated 8 hours before sacrifice and restimulated 6 hours later, followed immediately by the quantitation with the intravenously injected radiolabeled neutrophils. The tachyphylaxis was chemotaxin-specific, *i.e.*, sites initiated with *N*-formylmethionylleucylphenylalanine (FMLP) and restimulated with FMLP exhibited a reduced number of accumulated ^{51}Cr-neutrophils. In contrast, when FMLP-initiated sites were restimulated with platelet-activating factor, the same numbers of radiolabeled neutrophils accumulated as at sites injected for the first time with platelet-activating factor. The pathophysiologic role for tachyphylaxis may be to terminate inflammatory responses and to downregulate inflammation to chronically elevated (39) or physiologic (17) levels of cytokines. We utilized tachyphylaxis experiments to establish a potential role for cytokines generated *in situ* by endotoxin. Tachyphylaxis was noted at sites initiated and restimulated with endotoxin (21) and was observed also with natural IL-1 (26) and thereafter with recombinant IL-1 (27, 28a). Tachyphylaxis was dose-dependent; the higher the dose of the first stimulus, the fewer neutrophils accumulated after the reinjection.

Cross-tachyphylaxis was observed between IL-1α and IL-1β and between IL-1 and endotoxin (28a). When dermal sites were first stimulated with endotoxin and reinjected with IL-1, the response to IL-1 was reduced. Diminished neutrophil emigration was also observed when the order of endotoxin and IL-1 injections was reversed. This likely represents the desensitization of tissues to IL-1 generated in response to endotoxin, and implicates IL-1 as a potential mediator of endotoxin-induced neutrophil emigration. Cross-tachyphylaxis was not observed between TNF and endotoxin, suggesting that it is not a relevant mediator of neutrophil emigration.

In all these studies, the leukocytes infiltrating the dermis were almost exclusively neutrophils (Fig. 3).

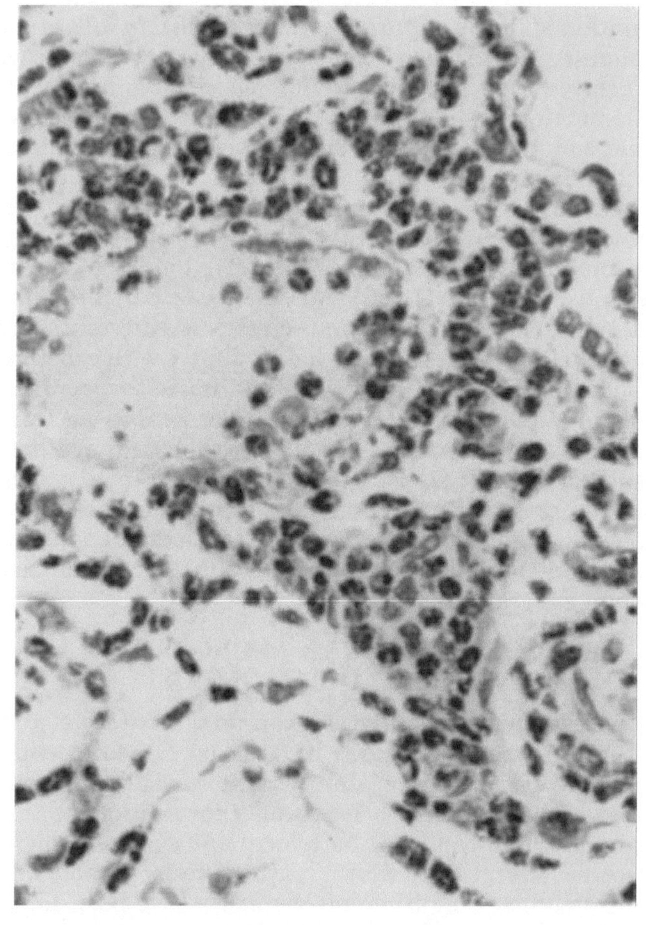

FIG. 3. Dermal inflammatory lesion (18 hours old) induced by the injection of 4 μg IL-1. Almost all the cells infiltrating the perivascular tissue are neutrophils. ×560.

Endotoxin and Cytokine-Induced Endothelial Cell Adhesiveness for Leukocytes

Leukocyte emigration into tissues through the walls of postcapillary venules and small veins can be divided into 3 steps: (a) adhesion of leukocytes to endothelial cells, (b) migration to intercellular junctions and diapedesis, (c) emigration through the endothelial basement membrane and vessel wall into extravascular tissues. An important regulatory step in emigration is the adhesion of leukocytes to endothelial cells, and is dependent both on endothelial and leukocyte mechanisms. Under certain physiologic conditions, leukocytes adhere weakly and transiently to the endothelium, which results in their rolling along venular walls: margination. Under pathologic conditions, particularly inflammation, margination is more pronounced until the leukocytes adhere strongly and eventually emigrate.

The advent of endothelial cell culture has led to *in vitro* studies of leukocyte-endothelial cell adhesion and elucidation of an endothelial cell-dependent adhesive mechanism. Both endotoxin and the cytokines IL-1, TNF and lymphotoxin induce endothelial cells to become adhesive for leukocytes by a mechanism dependent on protein synthesis (11, 37, 41, 103). Similarly, *in vivo* neutrophil emigration induced by endotoxin and IL-1 is dependent on protein synthesis, however this is not the case with leukocyte chemoattractants (76). A specific inducible endothelial cell surface protein designated by Gimbrone, Bevilacqua and colleagues as endothelial-leukocyte adhesion molecule 1 has been identified with two monoclonal antibodies: H4/8 (97) and H18/7 (10). It mediates, in part, neutrophil adherence to stimulated endothelial cells (10, 73). The induction of endothelial-leukocyte adhesion molecule 1 is transient, and endothelial cells become desensitized to restimulation with the same cytokine or endotoxin, when the stimulus has been maintained in the culture medium (97, 98). *In vivo* endothelial-leukocyte adhesion molecule 1 has been identified in delayed type hypersensitivity reactions and in acute inflammatory conditions (23). The functional roles of other endothelial cell activation antigens (43) remain to be determined.

Leukocyte-dependent mechanisms for adhesion are predominantly mediated by a family of cell surface glycoproteins designated "LFA-1/Mac-1/p150,95" by Springer and co-workers (1,106) and CD11/CD18 by the Third International Workshop on Leukocyte Differentiation Antigens. These proteins are heterodimers with a distinct α-subunit (CD11a-c), noncovalently linked to a common β-subunit (CD18). Recurrent life-threatening bacterial infections developed by patients with hereditary deficiency of CD11/CD18 emphasizes its functional importance as reviewed by Anderson and Springer (1). Monoclonal antibodies to CD18 can block neutrophil adhesion to cytokine-stimulated endothelial cells (73, 99) and neutrophil emigration *in vivo* (1a).

ENDOTOXIN-INDUCED MICROVASCULAR INJURY AND THROMBOSIS

As described in the first section on quantitative studies, inflammatory reactions induced by *E. coli* or endotoxin are usually associated with severe injury, manifested by hemorrhage. It has been known for some time that endotoxin can elicit both local and systemic microvascular alterations, whose pathogenesis is not fully understood, and multiple mechanisms have been implicated (reviewed in Refs. 79, 80, 83).

Recent observations indicate that, like the neutrophil emigration, some of the microvascular alterations induced by endotoxin are mediated by IL-1 and TNF, and that neutrophils play a pivotal role in the development of the injury. As described in this review, neutrophil emigration can be induced by subnanogram quantities of endotoxin and both endotoxin and IL-1 are about 1000 times more potent in this respect than chemotaxins. For the elicitation of the classical local Shwartzman reaction, microgram quantities of endotoxin have to be injected locally ("preparative" injection), followed 18 to 24 hours later by an intravenous injection of endotoxin ("challenging" injection). The challenging injection of endotoxin could be substituted by a few procedures, but particularly by the intravascular activation of complement with immune precipitates, zymosan (82), or cobra venom factor (84). Rendering rabbits hypocomplementemic with cobra venom factor prevented the elicitation of a Shwartzman reaction when challenged with immune complexes or zymosan. However, when the intravenous challenge was endotoxin, the decomplementation induced only partial inhibition, implicating mainly complement-independent effects of the infused endotoxin (84). This substitution of endotoxin was more difficult with the preparative injection, until it was observed that with partially purified macrophage-derived IL-1 (presumably containing TNF) a Shwartzman-like reaction could be "prepared" (5, 84). However, when highly purified recombinant IL-1 was injected as a preparative dose, a thrombo-hemorrhagic Shwartzman-like reaction could only be elicited when recombinant TNF was injected simultaneously (84, 85). These lesions were quantitated with ^{59}Fe-erythrocytes (hemorrhage) and ^{111}In-platelets (thrombosis). Interestingly, sites prepared with endotoxin exhibited more thrombosis, and this was corroborated and extended morphologically. In addition to more numerous platelets, considerably more fibrin was seen in the lesions prepared with endotoxin than in those initiated with the cytokines. On the other hand, in the cytokine-induced lesions the hemorrhage was more intense.

These thrombo-hemorrhagic lesions which developed after the intravenous challenge, are superimposed on changes taking place locally after the preparative intradermal injections. In this respect, certain *in vitro* observations are important. These studies indicate that the endothelium plays an active role in coagulation, both in its promotion and inhibition (108). Both IL-1 and TNF can stimulate cultured endothelial cells to produce a tissue factor (thromboplastin)-like activity (8, 9, 93). By inhibiting fibrinolysis, IL-1 may play a role in the fate of a thrombus (12, 91). IL-1 and TNF added together to the endothelial monolayer were found to be additive with respect to induction of procoagulant activity, but *in vivo* with respect to the thrombo-hemorrhagic Shwartzman phenomenon they acted synergistically (84, 85). There is also *in vitro* evidence that endotoxin-stimulated endothelial cells synthesize IL-1 (71, 107). It is thus tempting to speculate that in addition to the inflammatory reaction induced by endotoxin via the cytokines at the injection sites, changes may be taking place at these sites which promote microthrombosis that develops after the intravenous challenge. It has been known for some time that intravenous injection, but particularly reinjection of endotoxin, leads to intravascular coagulation and consumption of clotting factors (80, 90). The reason why the microthrombi and hemorrhage were confined to the "prepared" site was the principal unanswered question, since the studies of Shwartzman (104). One decade ago innumerable intrinsic mediators were believed to be mediating events induced by endotoxin (79). Yet, none of these could fully account for its effects. Today we are still a long way from understanding the molecular events leading to a Shwartzman reaction, but the available evidence strongly suggests that IL-1 and TNF are the principal intrinsic mediators of this endotoxin-induced reaction.

Morphologic observations of the "prepared" sites immediately before intravenous challenge shed some light on the nature of these inflammatory lesions induced by endotoxin or IL-1 plus TNF, and thereby on the events which follow the intravenous challenge. Only when IL-1 and TNF were coinjected was the cellular infiltration comparable to that induced with endotoxin (31, 84, 85). Ultrastructurally, with endotoxin or IL-1 plus TNF, severe injury of venules and small veins was observed in conjunction with varying degrees of degenerative changes in neutrophils, both within and around the vessels. In these neutrophils granules had frequently fused with the cell membrane and were seen free in the lumen or abutting against endothelial cells. The latter exhibited focal or more extensive necrosis and frequently the basement membrane or remnants thereof was devoid of an endo-

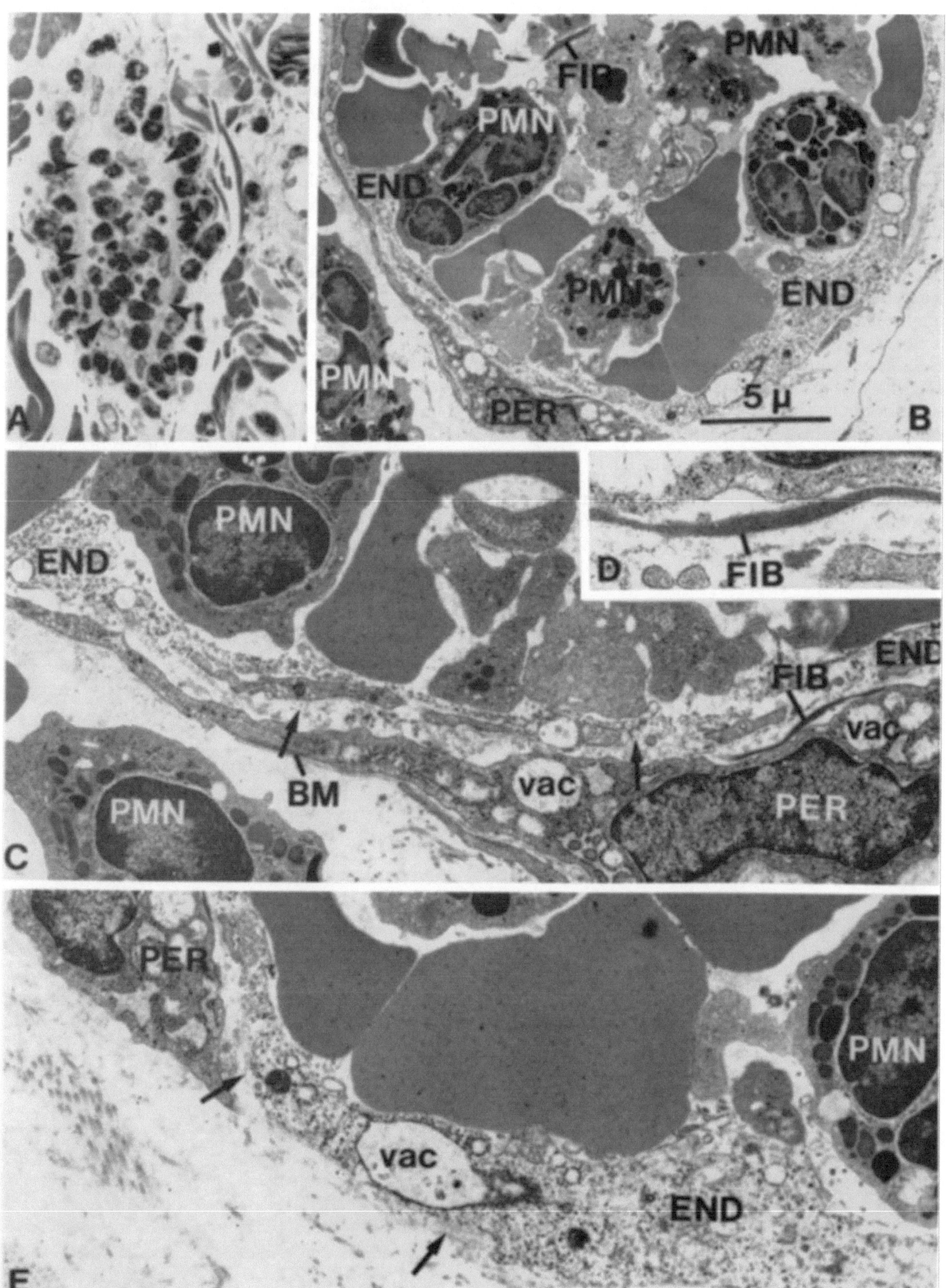

FIG. 4. Example of vessel wall injury. In Figure 4*A* (light microscopy) the endothelium is delineated by *arrowheads*. Neutrophils are present both in the lumen and perivascularly (inside and outside the *arrowheads*). About ½ the vessel is illustrated in the electron micrograph of *B*. Portions of the venular wall are reproduced in *C*, *D*, and *E*. The endothelial cells (*END*) are necrotic and the pericytes (*PER*) intact but vacuolated (*vac*). Some basement membrane (*BM*) surrounds pericytes, but the subendothelial basement membrane is fragmented or absent (*arrows*). Fibrin (*FIB*) is seen in the lumen of *B* and between endothelial cells and pericytes in *C* and *D* (*inset*). Figure 4*A*, ×560; *B*, × 4,125; *C*, ×12,000; *D*, ×33,900; *E*, ×12,000. Reproduced from Movat *et al.*, Am J Pathol 129:463, 1987, Copyright by the American Association of Pathologists, Inc.

thelial lining (Fig. 4). At times, the basement membrane was missing. Erythrocyte extravasation was associated with such changes (Fig. 5). This microvascular injury and the associated inflammatory hemorrhage gradually subsided. However, when a challenging intravenous injection of endotoxin, immune precipitates, zymosan, or cobra venom factor was administered at this time, microthrombi formed and occluded the vessels (Fig. 6). They consisted primarily of aggregated leukocytes, mostly neutrophils, but contained also aggregates of platelets and fibrin and were invariably accompanied by very extensive hemorrhage (85). The neutrophils in these thrombi also exhibited degenerative changes, but these were not seen in the monocytes and occasional lymphocytes. These events could be quantitated with radiolabeled cells and proteins. Early kinetic studies demonstrated that both thrombosis and hemorrhage developed rapidly and subsided 4 to 5 hours after the iv challenge (87).

The mediating role of IL-1 and TNF in the Shwartzman reaction is not fully understood as yet. Our studies on neutrophil emigration indicate that the cytokines, but particularly IL-1, are responsible for the neutrophil infiltration at the prepared site. The neutrophils are instrumental in the development of severe hemorrhage associated with the microvascular injury, because in neutropenic animals, a positive hemorrhagic reaction cannot be elicited (109) and because these cells showed signs of lysis and granule release. The only experimental model in which quantitatively and qualitatively, a similar vessel wall injury could be induced was that in which lysates of neutrophil lysosomes were injected intradermally (89).

There is no evidence in the literature that IL-1 can elicit hemorrhage, but TNF has been described to induce hemorrhagic necrosis of experimental tumors (101) and when massive doses (milligram quantities) were infused in rats, it elicited hemorrhage in several organs (114). Such quantities of TNF induce synthesis of IL-1 *in vitro* and *in vivo* (35), whereas stimulation with IL-1 induces production of IL-1, both *in vivo* and *in vitro* (36, 118). By itself even in very high doses, IL-1 was unable to "prepare" a site for the elicitation of a Shwartzman-like reaction; which was true also of TNF (84, 85). The term TNF is used interchangeably with TNFα and it is identical to cachectin, a substance implicated as the mediator of lethal endotoxin shock (6, 7, 114). By injecting merely microgram quantities, but both cytokines into rabbits, a synergism was demonstrated between IL-1 and TNF in

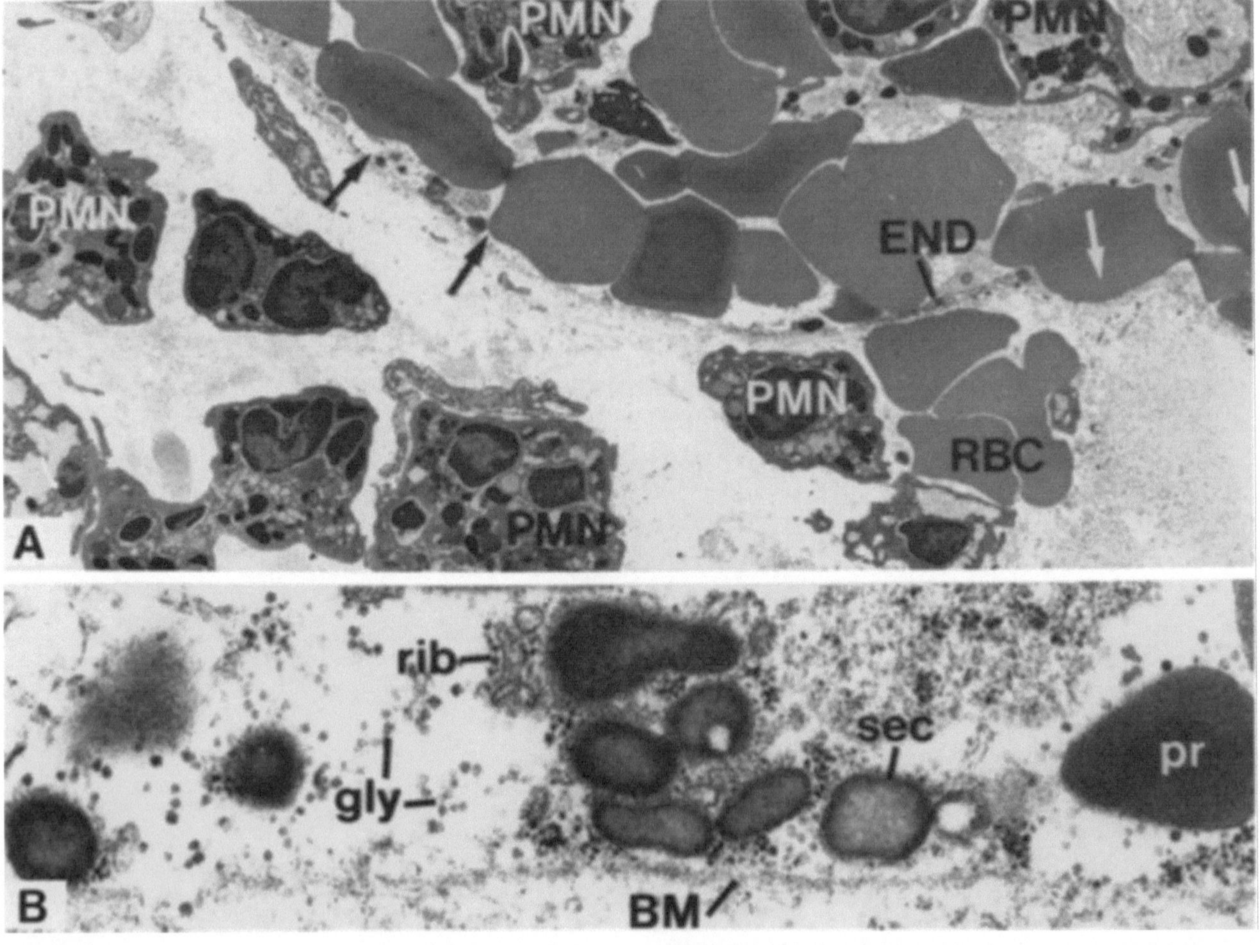

FIG. 5. Example of vessel wall injury. *A*, Most of the lining endothelium is missing. In the *right third* of the illustration, several erythrocytes (*RBC*) are in the perivascular tissue or in the process of crossing the injured vessel wall (*white arrows*). Eight neutrophils (*PMN*) are in the interstitium. *B*, The area between the two *black arrows* in *A*. There are free primary and secondary neutrophil granules (*pr*, *sec*), glycogen (*gly*), and ribosomes (*rib*) in the lumen, above the remnants of the basement membrane (*BM*). *A*, ×3,900; *B*, ×46,000. Reproduced from Movat *et al.*, Am J Pathol 129:463, 1987, Copyright by the American Association of Pathologists, Inc.

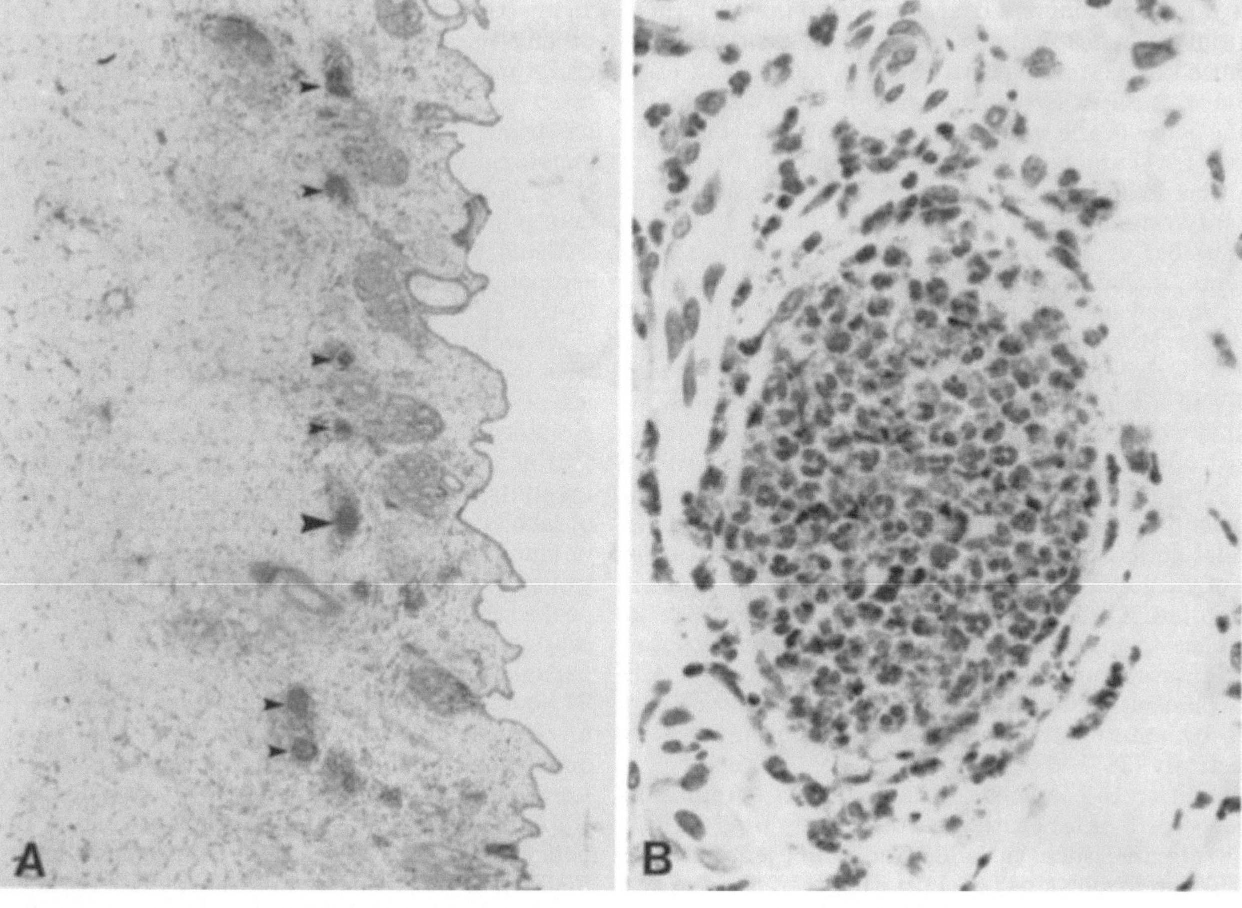

FIG. 6. Shwartzman-like reaction in rabbit skin prepared with intradermal injections of 0.5 μg of IL-1 and 1 μg of TNF. Eighteen hours after the intradermal injections, 10 μg/kg of endotoxin was administered intravenously and the rabbit sacrificed 15 minutes later. *A*, There are numerous venules occluded by microthrombi (small *arrowheads*). *B*, The microthrombi are made up mostly of neutrophils (vessel indicated by large *arrowhead* in *A*). Figure 6*A*, ×35; *B*, ×560.

the induction of a shock-like state with hemorrhagic pulmonary lesions (95). A leukocytopenia and thrombocytopenia were also observed in the last mentioned study and this observation may be important with respect to the intravenous challenging injection in the Shwartzman reaction. The rapid onset and prolonged leukopenia (predominantely neutropenia) observed after endotoxin infusion (29, 109, 110) or injection of *E. coli* (27) may well be mediated by IL-1, or by TNF or by IL-1 acting synergistically with TNF. In keeping with the observations of Okusawa *et al.* (95) on pulmonary changes, when ^{51}Cr-neutrophils were present in the circulation when endotoxin was injected, a large number of these cells were recovered in the lung (29). Furthermore, neutrophils were subsequently mobilized from the bone marrow and many of these ended up in the lungs (30). While the neutropenia after endotoxin or *E. coli* lasted (depending on the dose), from one to several hours, to be able to elicit a protracted shock-like state with leukopenia, Okusawa *et al.* (95) had to follow a bolus (1 μg) by a continuous infusion (5 ng/kg/min each of IL-1 and TNF). Interestingly, when considerably less IL-1 was administered to rats the cytokine was reported to induce only a neutrophilia, whereas TNF induced a neutropenia, followed by two peaks of neutrophilia (the second attributed to intrinsic IL-1 production) (117). There is even a possibility that the intravenous challenge with complement-activating agents may follow a pathway implicating IL-1 and TNF, since *in vitro* C5a and $C5a_{desArg}$ can stimulate blood mononuclear cells to produce IL-1 (94). Potential sources of IL-1 and TNF in the blood are primarily monocytes, and macrophages of the reticular activating system but there is also recent evidence for IL-1 production by neutrophils (111, 122).

INFLAMMATION AND HOST DEFENSE IN GRAM-NEGATIVE INFECTION

With the introduction of antibiotics, Gram-positive infections could be readily controlled, but Gram-negative bacteria became, during the 1950s, problems difficult to deal with, particularly in nosocomial infections (100). Antibiotics have only a limited effect on severe Gram-negative infections such as pneumonia, bacteremia, and septicemia (16, 77). Over a recent 5-year period (1977 to 1981), the mortality in 1,186 episodes of Gram-negative bacteremia was 36.3%, which was no improvement compared with 1924, *i.e.*, the presulfonamide and preantibiotic period (16). Whereas 70% of nosocomial lung infections are attributable to pseudomonas, and 33% to other Gram-negative bacteria, only 5% are caused by

Gram-positive infections (113). Another negative factor is the rapid development of resistance by the bacteria to an antibiotic in hospital-associated infections (102). Sepsis caused by Gram-negative bacteria, alone or in association with other aerobic and anaerobic bacteria, is the leading cause of the syndrome of multiple systems organ failure (4, 14) and is associated with a mortality of 50 to 80%. Should shock occur in association with sepsis, the mortality rate increases to 85 to 90% (105).

A number of bacterial properties contribute to their virulence, including leukocidins, capsules, adhesins, mobility, invasiveness, toxins, iron transport, and serum resistance (15). The diversity of the disease processes due to Gram-negative infection is attributed today mostly to a combination of virulence determinants associated with each bacterial species. For example, only a limited number of *E. coli* strains are usually associated with extraintestinal infections. Urinary tract infections are usually hemolytic (46) and are resistant to the bactericidal action of normal serum (112). One particular class of virulence-associated organelles are known as pili or fimbriae. These hair-like structures foster bacterial adherence to mucosal epithelium via specific receptor-ligand interactions (66). Piliation in *E. coli* permit efficient colonization of the gastrointestinal or genitourinary tracts by enteropathogenic and uropathogenic species respectively (78, 116).

In addition to the above variable factors determining virulence of Gram-negative bacteria, they produce various exotoxins, such as labile and stable enterotoxins (42, 50) and hemolysins (46, 119). However, these microorganisms have one disease-producing factor in common, endotoxin. Whereas the exotoxins are produced and released during bacterial growth, endotoxin is "released" by shedding also from dead bacteria. Release of endotoxin is marked during bacterial lysis (32). Endotoxin or lipopolysaccharide consists of lipid A, a core polysaccharide and the *O*-specific antigen and the biologic activity is known to reside in lipid A. The chemistry of endotoxin was elucidated primarily by Westphal and associates (for reviews see Refs. 40, 120). Endotoxin plays a particularly important role in severe and widespread infections, such as those associated with sepsis and septicemia, in which *E. coli* is the most frequent causative agent (75).

Killed *E. coli* have been shown to shed endotoxin into the medium in which they are suspended (51). Not surprisingly, such bacteria, particularly when deposited in large numbers (20 sites at 6×10^8 bacteria/site) into the dermis, will induce systemic effects attributed to endotoxin, such as fever and neutropenia, followed by neutrophilia (27). Both the magnitude and the duration of the neutropenia were dose-dependent. In these experiments, the number of circulating neutrophils was correlated with the infiltration at the site of *E. coli* injection. Compared with earlier observations where multiple injections of bacteria were administered over a 24-hour period before the quantitation with ^{51}Cr-neutrophils (69), when 20 simultaneous intradermal doses of killed *E. coli* were injected, very few neutrophils emigrated 0 to 4 hours postinjection (during the neutropenic phase). Instead, some influx of neutrophils occurred 6 to 10 hours post-injection (during the neutrophilic phase). When another set of 20 sites was injected 6 hours after the first set of 20 injections (during neutrophilic phase), the rabbits had become refractory to the development of a neutropenia, and a marked accumulation of neutrophils was quantitated in these lesions at 0 to 4 hours (27). The exact roles of various cytokines, and the direct or indirect effects of endotoxin on the levels of circulating neutrophils and their mobilization from the marrow pool remains to be determined.

Using killed *E. coli* has the advantage of fixed and reproducible stimuli. However, within certain dose limits, live *E. coli* elicit essentially similar inflammatory reactions as killed bacteria (86). We extended these studies with live *E. coli*, by comparing the magnitude and kinetics of ^{51}Cr-neutrophil accumulation with the level of circulating neutrophils, the increase in vasopermeability (^{125}I-albumin), and the recovery of bacterial colony-forming units (CFUs) in the dermal lesions of several groups of rabbits: normals, neutropenic (transient or persistent), immunized (active systemic or passive local) (18). Neutrophil emigration and enhanced vasopermeability peaked in 2 to 4-hour-old lesions (2×10^7 or 2×10^8 *E. coli*/site). However, it was essential to elicit at least a partial refractory state to neutropenia by injecting *E. coli* 24 hours before the experiment. This procedure induced a transient mild to moderate neutropenia and a subsequent neutrophilia. With high doses (2×10^{10} *E. coli*/lesion) a protracted neutropenia developed and no neutrophils were delivered to the stimulated sites. Bacterial pour plate colony counts from homogenates of intradermal sites injected with *E. coli*, indicated in normal rabbits early (1 to 2 hours) bacterial multiplication, followed by diminished CFUs at later time points. The decrease in CFUs coincided with the peak emigration of neutrophils into the dermal sites and light and electron microscopy demonstrated phagocytosis of the bacteria by the neutrophils. Animals rendered neutropenic for prolonged periods with nitrogen mustard showed a progressive increase in the numbers of *E. coli* within the intradermal sites, which by 48 hours increased several hundred times over controls. Compared with normals, fewer neutrophils accumulated and there was less plasma exudation. A delayed inflammatory reaction was observed during recovery from neutropenia, as noted already by Issekutz *et al.* (59). As in the lesions with 2×10^{10} *E. coli*/site, in the neutropenic rabbits there was severe dermal necrosis at sites injected with 2×10^7 *E. coli*/site. Animals which were injected with *E. coli* at the time when their circulating neutrophils were recovering from nitrogen mustard treatment, showed only an early (1 to 4 hour) increase in numbers of CFUs, followed by bacterial clearance. Two interesting observations were made in actively immunized animals: no neutropenia developed after the first intradermal injections of *E. coli*, and considerably fewer neutrophils accumulated in the dermis, but interestingly, these were able to cope with bacterial elimination in the same manner as normal controls. Fewer neutrophils accumulated, also with local passive immunization, i.e., when anti-*E. coli* antiserum was deposited at the injection site, but without the capacity to prevent the development of neutropenia.

It was concluded that (a) Neutrophil leukocytes play

a pivotal role in controlling the growth and spread of *E. coli.* (b) In the absence of neutrophils, the bacterial replication is unchecked. (c) In actively immunized rabbits fewer neutrophils can control the infection, (implying that (i) the cellular defense operates more efficiently and (ii) specific antibodies can assist and expedite the clearance of bacteria). (d) Passive transfer of antiserum locally also potentiates the clearance of microorganisms from the site of infection/inflammation. (e) In actively immunized animals no transient neutropenia develops in the circulation.

We propose that cytokines and in particular IL-1 are the principal mediators responsible for mobilizing neutrophils to the inflammatory site where endotoxin is released from Gram-negative bacteria. In immunized animals, fewer neutrophils infiltrated the inflammatory lesions, presumably due to neutralization of endotoxin in the outer wall of the bacteria, leading to less cytokine production, and hence less emigration. Diminished emigration was observed when *E. coli* or endotoxin were treated with antibody or polymyxin B (52). Likewise, when we injected *E. coli* for the first time into actively immunized rabbits, no transient neutropenia developed, probably because the locally liberated endotoxin was bound and this prevented stimulation of IL-1 and TNF synthesis and release. In addition to opsonization, antibody may have another effect in Gram-negative infection, *i.e.*, prevention of a decrease in circulating neutrophils and hence assurance of a constant delivery of neutrophils to the infected site.

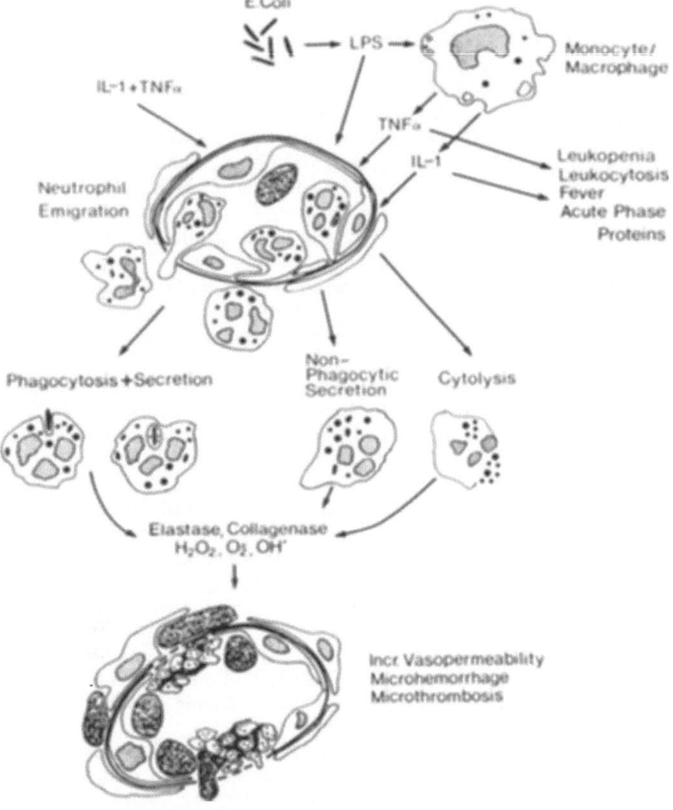

FIG. 7. Diagrammatic representation of events which follow entry of *E. coli* into tissues. The bacteria shed endotoxin (*LPS*) which stimulates monocytes and macrophages (locally and systemically) to synthesize and release IL-1 and TNFα. By acting on the circulating, marginal, and bone marrow pools of neutrophils and their precursors, the cytokines induce neutropenia, followed by neutrophilia (also lymphopenia). These events influence the delivery of neutrophils at the inflammatory site. Other systemic effect of the cytokines are elicitation of fever, acute phase proteins and other components of the acute phase reaction. Through action on the endothelium, IL-1 and TNFα induce neutrophil emigration and accumulation at the site of bacterial multiplication, representing the most important line of defense. IL-1 and TNFα of other sources could also induce neutrophil influx. *In vitro* studies indicate that endotoxin could act directly on the endothelium to induce synthesis and release of IL-1. The emigrated neutrophils release lysosomal enzymes and oxygen radicals by cytolysis, phagocytosis of the bacteria, and secretion and perhaps by nonphagocytic secretion. The severely injured microvessels exhibit increase in vasopermeability, hemorrhage, and thrombosis.

Figure 7 illustrates our concept of the inflammatory events which follows the entry of Gram-negative bacteria into tissues. This diagrammatic presentation disregards exotoxins and emphasizes endotoxin and its effects: generation of host-derived inflammatory mediators and their action locally and systemically.

This work was supported by grants from the Medical Research Council of Canada (MT-1251) and the Heart and Stroke Foundation of Ontario (T082).

Dr. Cybulsky is the recipient of a Medical Research Council of Canada Research Fellowship; present address: Department of Pathology, Vascular Research Division, Brigham and Women's Hospital, Harvard Medical School, 75 Francis Street, Boston, MA 02115.

Dr. Movat is a Career Investigator of the Medical Research Council of Canada.

Address reprint requests to: Henry Z. Movat. M.D., Department of Pathology, University of Toronto, Medical Sciences Building, 1 King's College Circle, Toronto, Ontario M5S 1A8 Canada.

REFERENCES

1. Anderson DC, Springer TA: Leukocyte adhesion deficiency: an inherited defect in the Mac-1 LFA-1, and p150, 95 glycoprotein. Annu Rev Med 38:175, 1987

1a. Arfors K-E, Lundberg C, Lindbom L, Lundberg K, Beatty PG, Harlan JM: A monoclonal antibody to the membrane glycoprotein complex CD18 inhibits polymorphonuclear leukocyte accumulation and plasma leakage *in vivo*. Blood 69:338, 1987

2. Atkins E, Bodel P, Francis L: Release of an endogenous pyrogen *in vitro* from rabbit mononuclear cells. J Exp Med 126:357, 1967

3. Averbrook B, Ulitch T, Jeffes E, Yamato R, Chow G, Masunaka I, Granger G: Human alpha lymphotoxin and TNF induce different types of inflammatory responses in normal tissues (abstr). Fed Proc 46:562, 1987

4. Baue AE, Chaudry IH: Prevention of multiple systems failure. Surg Clin North Am 60:1167, 1980

5. Beck C, Habict GS, Benach JL, Miller F: Interleukin 1: A common endogenous mediator of inflammation and the local Shwartzman reaction. J Immunol 136:3025, 1986

6. Beutler B, Cerami AC: Cachectin. More than a tumor necrosis factor. N Engl J Med 3156:379, 1987

7. Beutler B, Milsark IW, Cerami AC: Passive immunization against cachectin/tumor necrosis factor protects mice from lethal effects of endotoxin. Science 229:869, 1985

8. Bevilacqua MP, Pober JS, Majeau GR, Fiers W, Cotran RS, Gimbrone MA Jr: Recombinant tumor necrosis factor induces procoagulant activity in cultured human vascular endothelium: characterization and comparison with the actions of interleukin. Proc Natl Acad Sci USA 83:4533, 1986

9. Bevilacqua MP, Pober JS, Majeau GR, Cotran RS, Gimbrone, MA Jr: Interleukin 1 (IL-1) induces biosynthesis and cell surface expression of procoagulant activity in human vascular endothelial cell. J Exp Med 160:681, 1984

10. Bevilacqua MP, Pober JS, Mendrick DL, Cotran RS, Gimbrone MA Jr: Identification of an inducible endothelial-leukocyte adhesion molecule. PNAS 84:9238, 1987

11. Bevilacqua MP, Pober JS, Wheeler ME, Cotran RS, Gimbrone

MA Jr: Interleukin-1 acts on cultured human vascular endothelium to increase the adhesion of polymorphonuclear leukocytes, monocytes and related leukocyte cell lines. J Clin Invest 76:2003, 1985
12. Bevilacqua MP, Scheef RR, Gimbrone MA Jr, Loskutoff DJ: Regulation of the fibrinolytic system of cultured vascular endothelium by interleukin 1. J Clin Invest 78:587, 1986
13. Bonny RJ, Humes JL: Physiological and pharmacological regulation of prostaglandin and leukotriene production by macrophages. J Leukocyte Biol 35:1, 1984
14. Borzotta AP, Polk HC Jr: Multiple systems organ failure. Surg Clin North Am 63:315, 1983
15. Brubaker RR: Mechanisms of bacterial virulence. Annu Rev Microbiol 39:21, 1985
16. Bryan CS, Reynolds KL, Brenner ER: Analysis of 1,186 episodes of gram-negative bacteremia in non-university hospitals: the effect of antimicrobial therapy. Rev Infect Dis 5:629, 1983
17. Cannon JG, Dinarello CA: Increased plasma interleukin-1 activity in women after ovulation. Science 227:1247, 1985
18. Chan W, Movat HZ: Microbicidal role of inflammation in Gram negative infection (abstr). Fed Proc, in press 1988
19. Cochrane CG, Janoff A: The Arthus reaction: a model of neutrophil and complement-mediated injury. In The Inflammatory Process, Vol 3, edited by Zweifach BS, Grant L, McCluskey RT, p 85. New York, Academic Press, 1974
20. Colditz IG, Movat HZ: Chemotactic factor-specific desensitization of skin to infiltration by polymorphonuclear leukocytes. Immunol Lett 8:83, 1984
21. Colditz IG, Movat HA: Desensitization of acute inflammatory lesions to chemotaxins and endotoxin. J Immunol 133:2163, 1984
22. Colditz IG, Movat HZ: Kinetics of neutrophil accumulation in acute inflammatory lesions induced by chemotaxins and chemotaxinigens. J Immunol 133:2169, 1984
23. Cotran RS, Gimbrone MA Jr, Bevilacqua MP, Mendrick DL, Pober JS: Induction and detection of a human endothelial activation antigen *in vivo*. J Exp Med 164:661, 1986
24. Crawford JP, Movat HZ, Minta JO, Opas M: Acute inflammation induced by immune complexes in the microcirculation. Exp Mol Pathol 42:175, 1985
25. Cybulsky MI, Colditz IG, Movat HZ: Interleukin 1 activity in the local recruitment of PMNs. Its potential role in endotoxin-induced acute inflammation (abstr). Fed Proc 44:1260, 1985
26. Cybulsky MI, Colditz IG, Movat HZ: The role of interleukin-1 in neutrophil leukocyte emigration induced by endotoxin. Am J Pathol 124:6, 1986
27. Cybulsky MI, Cybulsky IJ, Movat HZ: Neutropenic responses to intradermal injections of *Escherichia coli*. Effects on the kinetics of polymorphonuclear leukocyte emigration. Am J Pathol 124:1, 1986
28. Cybulsky MI, McComb DJ, Dinarello CA, Movat HZ: Mediation by interleukin-1 of neutrophil leukocyte emigration induced by endotoxin. In Leukocyte Emigration and its Sequelae, edited by Movat HZ, p 38. Basel, S Karger AG, 1987
28a. Cybulsky MI, McComb DJ, Movat HZ: Neutrophil leukocyte emigration induced by endotoxin: mediator roles of IL-1 and tumor necrosis factor α. J Immunol, in press 1988
29. Cybulsky MI, Movat HZ: Experimental bacterial pneumonia in rabbits: polymorphonucler leukocyte margination and sequestration in rabbit lungs and quantitation and kinetics of ^{51}Cr-labelled polymorphonuclear leukocytes in *E. coli*-induced lung lesions. Exp Lung Res 4:47, 1982
30. Cybulsky MI, Movat HZ: Application of ^{51}Cr-labelled PMN leukocytes in quantitating PMN kinetics in systemic and local inflammatory mediated processes. Effects of endotoxin, complement and interleukin 1. Surv Synth Pathol Res 1:208, 1983
31. Cybulsky MI, Movat HZ, Dinarello CA: Role of interleukin 1 and tumor necrosis factor α in acute inflammation. Ann Inst Pasteur, (Paris), 138:505, 1987
32. De Voe IW: Egestion of degraded meningococci by polymorphonuclear leukocytes. J Bacteriol 125:258, 1976
33. Dinarello CA: Interleukin-1. Rev Infect Dis 6:51, 1984
34. Dinarello CA: Interleukin-1. Amino acid sequence, multiple biological activities and comparison with tumor necrosis factor (cachectin). Year Immunol 2:68, 1986
35. Dinarello CA, Cannon JC, Wolff SM, Bernheim HA, Beutler B, Cerami A, Figari IS, Palladino MA Jr, O'Connor JV: Tumor necrosis factor (cachectin) is an endogenous pyrogen and induces production of interleukin 1. J Exp Med 163:1433, 1986
36. Dinarello CA, Ikejina T, Warner SJC, Orecole SF, Lonnemann G, Cannon JG, Libby P: Interleukin 1 induces interleukin 1. I. Induction of circulating interleukin 1 in rabbits *in vivo* in human mononuclear cells *in vitro*. J Immunol 139:1902, 1987
37. Dunn CJ, Fleming WE: The role of interleukin-1 in the inflammatory response with particular reference to endothelial cell-leukocyte adhesion. In The Physiologic, Metabolic, and Immunologic Actions of Interleukin-1, edited by Kluger MJ, Oppenheim JJ, Powanda MC, p 45. New York, Alan R Liss, 1985
38. Elias RM, Johnston MG, Hayashi A, Nelson W: Decreased lymphatic pumping after intravenous endotoxin administration in sheep. Am J Physiol 253:183, 1987
39. Gahring L, Baltz M, Pepys MB, Daynes R: Effect of ultraviolet radiation on production of endothelial cell thymocyte-activating factor/interleukin 1 *in vivo* and *in vitro*. Proc Natl Acad Sci USA 81:1198, 1984
40. Galanos CO, Lüderitz O, Rietschel ET, Wesphal O: Newer aspects of the chemistry and biology of bacterial lipopolysaccharides, with special reference to their lipid A component. In Biochemistry of Lipids II, edited by Goodwin TW, p 239. Baltimore MD, University Park Press, 1977
41. Gamble RJ, Harlan JM, Klebanoff SJ, Lopez AF, Vadas MA: Stimulation of the adherence of neutrophils to umbilical vein endothelium by human recombinant tumor necrosis factor. Proc Natl Acad Sci USA 82:8667, 1985
42. Gemmell CG: Comparative studies of the nature and biological activities of bacterial enterotoxins. J Med Microbiol 17:217, 1984
43. Goerd S, Zwadlo G, Schlegel R, Hagemeier H-H, Sorg C: Characterization and expression kinetics of an endothelial cell activation antigen present in vivo only in acute inflammatory tissues. Exp Cell Biol 55:117, 1987
44. Grantstein RD, Margolis R, Mizel SB, Sauder DN: *In vivo* inflammatory activity of epidermal cell-derived thymocyte-activating factor and recombinant interleukin 1 in the mouse. J Clin Invest 77:120, 1986
45. Habicht GS, Beck G: IL-1 is an endogenous mediator of acute inflammation and of the local Shwartzman reaction. In The Physiologic, Metabolic, and Immunologic Actions of Interleukin-1, edited by Kluger MJ, Oppenheim JJ, Powanda MC, p 13. New York, Alan R Liss, 1985
46. Hacker J, Hughes C, Hof H, Goebel W: Cloned hemolysin genes from *Escherichia coli* that cause urinary tract infection determine different levels of toxicity in mice. Infect Immunol 42:57, 1983
47. Hamilton SM, Johnston MG, Fong A, Pepevnak C, Semple JL, Movat HZ: Relationship between increased vascular permeability and extravascular albumin clearance in rabbit inflammatory responses induced with *Escherichia coli*. Lab Invest 55:580, 1986
48. Hanson DF, Murphy PA, Windle BE: Failure of rabbit neutrophils to secrete endogenous pyrogen when stimulated with staphylococci. J Exp Med 151:1360, 1980
49. Hay JB, Johnston MG, Hobbs BB, Movat HZ: The use of radioactive microspheres to quantitate hyperemia in dermal inflammatory sites. Proc Soc Exp Biol Med 150:641, 1975
50. Holmgren J: Toxins affecting intestinal transport processes. In The Virulence of *Escherichia coli*, edited by Sussman M, p 177. London, Academic Press, 1985
51. Issekutz AC, Bhimji S: Role of endotoxin in the leukocyte infiltration accompanying *Escherichia coli* inflammation. Infect Immun 36:558, 1982
52. Issekutz AC, Bhimji S, Bertolussi R: Effect of immune serum or polymyxin B on *Escherichia coli*-induced inflammation and vascular injury. Infect Immun 36:548, 1982
53. Issekutz AC, Megyeri P: Induction of leukocyte infiltration by endotoxin. In Leukocyte Emigration and its Sequelae, edited by Movat HZ, p 24. Basel, S Karger AG, 1987
54. Issekutz AC, Megyeri P, Issekutz TB: Role of macrophage products in endotoxin-induced polymorphonuclear leukocyte accumulation during inflammation. Lab Invest 56:49, 1987
55. Issekutz AC, Movat HZ: Quantitation of neutrophil infiltration *in vivo*. Immunol Lett 1:27, 1979
56. Issekutz AC, Movat HZ: The *in vivo* quantitation and kinetics of rabbit neutrophil leukocyte accumulation in the skin in response

to chemotactic agents and *Escherichia coli*. Lab Invest 42:310, 1980
57. Issekutz AC, Movat HZ: The effect of vasodilatory prostaglandins on polymorphonuclear leukocyte infiltration and vascular injury. Am J Pathol 107:300, 1982
58. Issekutz AC, Movat KW, Movat HZ: Enhancement of vascular permeability and haemorrhage-inducing activity of rabbit $C5a_{des Arg}$: probable role of polymorphonuclear leukocyte lysosomes. Clin Exp Immunol 41:512, 1980
59. Issekutz AC, Ripley M, Rochon Y, Pi-Jimenez E, Wright B: A role for hemolysin in *Escherichia coli*-induced inflammation in granulocytopenic rabbits. J Infect Dis 150:925, 1984
60. Issekutz AC, Wankowicz Z: Synergy between tumor necrosis factor (TNFα) and interleukin 1 (IL-1) in the induction of polymorphonuclear leukocyte emigration (abstr). Fed Proc 46:737, 1987
61. Issekutz TB, Issekutz AC, Movat HZ: The *in vivo* quantitation and kinetics of monocyte migration into acute inflammatory tissue. Am J Pathol 103:74, 1981
62. Jeynes BJ, Issekutz AC, Issekutz TB, Movat HZ: Quantitation of platelets in the microcirculation. Measurement of indium-111 in microthrombi induced in rabbits by inflammatory lesions and related phenomena. Proc Soc Exp Biol Med 165:445, 1980
63. Johnston MG: Interaction of inflammatory mediators with the lymphatic vessel. Pathol Immunopathol Res 6:177, 1987
64. Johnston MG, Hay JB, Movat HZ: Kinetics of prostaglandin production in various inflammatory lesions, measured in draining lymph. Am J Pathol 95:225, 1979
65. Kampschmidt RF: Leukocytic endogenous mediator/endogenous pyrogen. In Infection: The Physiologic and Metabolic Responses of the Host, edited by Powanda MC, Canonico PG, p 403. Amsterdam, Elsevier Science Publisher, 1981
66. Klemm P: Fimbrial adhesions of *Escherichia coli*. Rev Infect Dis 7:321, 1985
67. Koj A: Biologic functions of acute-phase proteins. In The Acute-Phase Response to Injury and Infection, edited by Gordon AH, Koj A, p 145. Amsterdam, Elsevier, 1985
68. Kopaniak MM, Issekutz AC, Burrowes CE, Movat HZ: The quantitation of hemorrhage in the skin: measurement of hemorrhage in the microcirculation in inflammatory lesions and related phenomena. Proc Soc Exp Biol Med 163:126, 1980
69. Kopaniak MM, Issekutz AC, Movat HZ: Kinetics of acute inflammation induced by *E. coli* in rabbits. Quantitation of blood flow, enhanced vascular permeability, hemorrhage and leukocyte accumulation. Am J Pathol 98:485, 1980
70. Kopaniak MM, Movat HZ: Kinetics of acute inflammation induced by *Escherichia coli* in rabbits. II. The effect of hyperimmunization, complement depletion, and depletion of leukocytes. Am J Pathol 110:13, 1983
71. Libby P, Ordovas JM, Auger KR, Robbin HH, Biriny LK, Dinarello CA: Endotoxin and tumor necrosis factor induce interleukin-1 gene expression in adult vascular endothelial cells. Am J Pathol 124:179, 1986
72. Libby P, Ordovas JM, Birinyi LK, Auger KR, Dinarello CA: Inducible interleukin 1 expression in human vascular smooth muscle cells. J Clin Invest 78:1432, 1986
73. Luscinskas FW, Bevilacqua MP, Brock AF, Arnaout MA, Gimbrone MA Jr: Endothelial-leukocyte adhesion: Contributions of endothelial dependent and leukocyte-dependent mechanisms (abstr). Fed Proc, in press 1988
74. Marasco WA, Phan SH, Krutsch H, Showell HJ, Feltner DE, Nairn R, Becker EL, Ward PA: Purification and identification of formyl-methionyl-leucyl-phenylalanine (fMet-Leu-Phe) as the major peptide neutrophil chemotactic factor produced by *Escherichia coli*. J Biol Chem 259:5430, 1984
75. McCabe WR: Gram negative bacteremia. In Infectious Diseases and Medical Microbiology, edited by Braude AI, Davis CE, Fierer J, p 1177. Philadelphia, WB Saunders, 1986
76. McComb DJ, Cybulsky MI, Movat HZ: PMN emigration: protein synthesis dependent and independent mechanisms (abstr). Fed Proc 46:1390, 1987
77. McGowan JE, Barnes MW, Finland M: Bacteremia at Boston City Hospital: occurrence and mortality during 12 selected years (1935–72), with special reference to hospital-acquired cases. J Infect Dis 132:316, 1975
78. Mooi FR, De Graaf FK: Molecular biology of fimbriae of enterotoxigenic *Escherichia coli*. Curr Topics Microbiol Immunol 118:119, 1985
79. Morrison DC, Ulevitch RJ: The effects of bacterial endotoxins on host mediation systems. Am J Pathol 93:526, 1978
80. Movat HZ: Microcirculation in disseminated intravascular coagulation induced by endotoxin. In Handbook of Physiology, Vol IV, The Cardiovascular System, edited by Renkin EN, Michel CC, p 1047. Bethesda MD, American Physiological Society, 1984
81. Movat HZ: The Inflammatory Reaction, Amsterdam, Elsevier, 1985
82. Movat HZ, Burrowes CE: Elicitation of the Shwartzman reaction by a combination of endotoxin and agents which activate the complement system: microvascular events. In Immunopharmacology of Endotoxicosis, edited by Agarwal MK, Yoshida M, p 197. Berlin/New York, Walter de Gruyter and Co, 1984
83. Movat HZ, Burrowes CE: Local Shwartzman reaction: endotoxin-mediated inflammatory and thrombo-hemorrhagic lesions. In Handbook of Endotoxin, Volume 3, Cellular Biology of Endotoxin, edited by Berry LJ, p 260. Amsterdam, Elsevier, 1985
84. Movat HZ, Burrowes CE, Cybulsky MI, Dinarello CA: Role of complement, interleukin-1 and tumor necrosis factor in a local Shwartzman-like reaction. In Leukocyte Emigration and its Sequelae, edited by Movat HZ, p 69. Basel, S Karger AG, 1987
85. Movat HZ, Burrowes CE, Cybulsky MI, Dinarello CA: Acute inflammation and a Shwartzman-like reaction induced by interleukin 1 and tumor necrosis factor. Synergistic action of the cytokines in the induction of inflammatory and microvascular injury. Am J Pathol 129:463, 1987
86. Movat HZ, Cybulsky MI, Colditz IG, Chan MKW, Dinarello CA: Acute inflammation in gram negative infection. Role of endotoxin, interleukin 1, tumor necrosis factor and neutrophils. Fed Proc 46:97, 1987
87. Movat HZ, Jeynes BJ, Wasi S, Movat KW, Kopaniak MM: Quantitation of the development and progression of the local Shwartzman reaction. In Bacterial Endotoxins and Host Response, edited by Agarwal MK, p 179. Amsterdam, Elsevier, 1980
88. Movat HZ, Rettl C, Burrowes CE, Johnston MG: The *in vivo* effect of leukotriene B_4 on polymorphonuclear leukocytes and the microcirculation. Comparison with activated complement ($C5a_{des Arg}$) and enhancement by prostaglandin E_2. Am J Pathol 115:233, 1984
89. Movat HZ, Wasi S: Severe microvascular injury induced by lysosomal releasates of human polymorphonuclear leukocytes. Increase in vasopermeability, hemorrhage, and microthrombosis due to degradation of subendothelial and perivascular matrices. Am J Pathol 121:404, 1985
90. Müller-Berghaus G, Lasch H-G: Microcirculatory disturbances induced by generalized intravascular coagulation. In Handbook of Experimental Pharmacology, Vol 16, Experimental Production of Diseases: Heart and Circulation, edited by Schmier J, Eichler O, p 429. Berlin, Springer-Verlag, 1975
91. Nachman RL, Hajjar KA, Silverstein RL, Dinarello CA: Interleukin 1 induces endothelial cell synthesis of plasminogen activator inhibitor. J Exp Med 163:1260, 1986
92. Nawroth PP, Bank I, Handley D, Cassimeris J, Chess L, Stern D: Tumor necrosis factor/cachectin interacts with endothelial cell receptors to induce release of interleukin 1. J Exp Med 163:1363, 1986
93. Nawroth PP, Stern DM: Modulation of endothelial cell hemostatic properties by tumor necrosis factor. J Exp Med 163:740, 1986
94. Okusawa S, Dinarello CA, Yancey KB, Endres S, Lawley TJ, Frank MM, Burke JF, Gelfand JA: C5a induction of interleukin 1. Synergistic effect with endotoxin or interferon-γ. J Immunol 139:2635, 1987
95. Okusawa S, Gelfand JA, Ikejima T, Connolly RJ, Dinarello CA: Interleukin-1 induces a shock-like state in rabbits: synergism with tumor necrosis factor and the effect of cyclooxygenase inhibition. J Clin Invest, in press 1988
96. Parry SH, Rooke DM: Adhesions and colonization factors of *Escherichia coli*. In The Virulence of *Escherichia coli*, edited by Sussman M, p 79. London, Academic Press, 1985
96a. Pettipher ER, Higgs GA, Henderson B: Interleukin 1 induces leukocyte infiltration and cartilage proteoglycan degradation in

the synovial joint. Proc Natl Acad Sci USA 83:8749, 1986

97. Pober JS, Bevilacqua MP, Mendrick DL, Lapierre LA, Fiers W, Gimbrone MA Jr: Two distinct monokines, interleukin 1 and tumor necrosis factor, each independently induce biosynthesis and transient expression of the same antigen on the surface of cultured human vascular endothelial cells. J Immunol 136:1680, 1986
98. Pober JS, Lapierre LA, Stolpen AH, Brock TA, Springer TA, Fiers W, Bevilacqua MP, Mendrick DL, Gimbrone MA Jr: Activation of cultured human endothelial cells by recombinant lymphotoxin: comparison with tumor necrosis factor and interleukin 1 species. J Immunol 138:3319, 1987
99. Pohlman TH, Stanness KA, Beatty PG, Ochs HD, Harlan JM: An endothelial cell surface factor (s) induced *in vitro* by lipopolysaccharide, interleukin 1 and tumor necrosis factor-increases neutrophil adherence by a CDw18-dependent mechanisms. J Immunol 136:4548, 1986
100. Rogers DE: The changing pattern of life-threatening microbial disease. N Engl J Med 261:677, 1959
101. Ruff MR, Gifford GE: Tumor necrosis factor. Lymphokines 2:235, 1981
102. Sanders CC, Sanders WE Jr: Microbial resistance to newer generation β-lactam antibiotics: clinical and laboratory implications. J Infect Dis 151:399, 1981
103. Schleimer RP, Rutledge BK: Cultured human vascular endothelial cells acquire adhesiveness for neutrophils after stimulation with interleukin 1, endotoxin and tumor-promoting phorbol diesters. J Immunol 136:649, 1986
104. Shwartzman G: Phenomenon of Local Tissue Reactivity and its Immunological, Pathological and Clinical Significance, New York, Paul Hoeber, 1937
105. Sinanan M, Maier RV, Corrico J: Labarotomy for intra-abdominal sepsis in an intensive care unit. Arch Surg 119:652, 1985
106. Springer TA, Dustin ML, Kishimoto TK, Marlin SD: Lymphocyte function-associated LFA-1, CD2, and LFA-3 receptors of the immune system. Annu Rev Immunol 5:223, 1987
107. Stern DM, Bank I, Nawroth PP, Cassimeris J, Kisiel W, Fenton JW II, Dinarello C, Chess L, Jaffe EA: Self-regulation of procoagulant events on the endothelial cell surface. J Exp Med 162:1223, 1985
108. Stern D, Nawroth P, Handley D, Kisiel W: An endothelial cell-dependent pathway of coagulation. Proc Natl Acad Sci USA 82:2523, 1985
109. Stetson CA Jr: Similarities in the mechanisms determining the Arthus and Shwartzman phenomenon. J Exp Med 94:347, 1951
110. Stetson CA Jr, Good RA: Studies on the mechanisms of the Shwartzman phenomenon: Evidence for the participation of polymorphonuclear leukocytes in the phenomenon. J Exp Med 93:49, 1951
111. Tiku K, Tiku ML, Skosey JL: Interleukin 1 production by human polymorphonuclear leukocytes. J Immunol 136:3677, 1986
112. Timmis KN, Boulnois GJ, Bitter-Sauermann D, Cabello FC: Surface components of *Escherichia coli* that mediate resistance to the bactericidal activities of serum and phagocytes. Curr Top Microbiol Immunol 118:197, 1985
113. Tobin MK, Grenvik A: Nosocomial lung infection and its diagnosis. Crit Care Med 12:191, 1984
114. Tracey KJ, Beutler B, Lowry SF, Merryweather J, Wolpe S, Milsark JW, Hariri RJ, Fahey III TJ, Zentella A, Albert JD, Shires GT, Cerami A: Shock and tissue injury induced by recombinant human cachectin. Science 234:470, 1986
115. Udaka K, Takeuchi Y, Movat HZ: Simple method for quantitation of enhanced vascular permeability. Proc Soc Exp Biol Med 133:1384, 1970
116. Uhlin BE, Baga M, Goranson M, Lindberg FP, Lund B, Normark S: Genes determining adhesin formation in uropathogenic *Escherichia coli.* Curr Top Microbiol Immunol 118:163, 1985
117. Ulich TR, del Castillo J, Keys M, Granger GA, Ni R-X: Kinetics and mechanisms of recombinant human interleukin 1 and tumor necrosis factor-α-induced changes in circulating numbers of neutrophils and lymphocytes. J Immunol 139:3406, 1987
118. Warner SJC, Auger KR, Libby P: Interleukin 1 induces interleukin 1. II. Recombinant human interleukin 1 induces interleukin 1 production by adult human vascular endothelial cells. J Immunol 139:1911, 1987
119. Welch RA, Falkow S: Characterization of *Escherichia coli* hemolysins conferring quantitative differences in virulence. Infect Immun 43:156, 1984
120. Westphal O, Jann K, Himmelspach K: Chemistry and immunochemistry of bacterial lipopolysaccharides as cell wall antigens and endotoxins. Prog Allergy 33:9, 1983
121. Windle BE, Murphy PA, Cooperman S: Rabbit polymorphonuclear leukocytes do not secrete endogenous pyrogen or interleukin 1 when stimulated by endotoxin, polyinosine; polycytosine, or muramyl dipeptide. Infect Immunol 39:1142, 1983
122. Yoshinaga M, Goto F, Goto K, Ohkawara S, Kitamura M, Mori S: Triggering of polymorphonuclear leukocytes to produce interleukin-1 at the inflammatory site. In Leukocyte Emigration and its Sequelae, edited by Movat HZ, p 169. Basel, S Karger AG, 1987

Biology of Disease

Role of T Helper Lymphocytes in Autoimmune Diseases

GÉRALD J. PRUD'HOMME AND NOLLAIG A. PARFREY

Department of Pathology, McGill University, Montreal, Canada, H3A 2B4

INTRODUCTION

A large amount of experimental work on autoimmune diseases has been concentrated on the study of autoantibodies, cytotoxic T lymphocytes (CTL), or on deficiencies of T suppressor cells. The purpose of this review is to present evidence that in many autoimmune diseases, either organ-specific or systemic, T helper (Th) lymphocytes play a predominant role. The importance of the Th cell in autoimmune diseases should come as no surprise, in view of the central role that these cells play in almost all immune responses.

The mechanisms by which Th cells contribute to autoimmunity and tissue injury are diverse, and are markedly different in the systemic *versus* the organ-specific autoimmune diseases. For this reason, this review is divided into a section dealing with a number of organ-specific autoimmune diseases, and another section dealing with systemic lupus erythematosus (SLE). Before specifically discussing autoimmune diseases, however, we will briefly review current concepts of Th cell function in the immune system.

THE IMMUNOBIOLOGY OF THE T HELPER LYMPHOCYTE

T Cell Ontogeny

As is well known, T cell precursors (or pro-T cells) are of bone marrow origin. In the thymus, T cell precursors, through a complex process of proliferation and differentiation, give rise to mature T cells which express a T cell receptor (TCR) for antigen (reviewed in reference 2).

Mature peripheral T cells are either CD4 (T4) or CD8 (T8) positive. The most immature thymocytes are negative for both of these antigens. These double negative cells comprise about 3% of thymocytes and are present in the thymic cortex. Double negative cells are able to generate all other thymocytic phenotypes in a sequential manner (2, 52, 79, 155). Of these thymocytes 80% are $CD4^+$, $CD8^+$ (*i.e.*, double positive), and they are located in the cortex. Most of these cells are destined to die within the thymus. Single positive cells expressing the mature CD4 or CD8 phenotype account for about 10 to 15% of thymocytes and are found in the medulla. These probably arise from double positive cells (52, 155), although some favor the suggestion that they arise directly from double negative cells and that all double positive cells form an end pathway destined for death (161).

TCR gene rearrangement and mRNA and protein expression occurs sequentially during thymocyte maturation both within the adult thymus and during fetal development (15, 152, 155). These gene rearrangements resemble those which occur in immunoglobulin genes, and give rise to the mature two-chain (α and β, or γ and δ) TCR.

Whereas the details of the thymocyte maturation are becoming clearer, the development of major histocompatibility complex (MHC) restriction and of self tolerance are areas where hypotheses continue to outnumber established facts. As we will discuss below, the process of antigen recognition by T lymphocytes is complex, and involves simultaneous recognition of self MHC molecules and an antigen. T cells appear to learn to recognize self MHC molecules in the thymus. The injection of antibodies to class II MHC molecules, for example, inhibits the development of Th lymphocytes (88). Although there is conflicting evidence as to whether it is the thymic epithelium (99) or intrathymic bone marrow derived dendritic cells (104) which imprint MHC restriction, the bulk of the evidence favors the thymic epithelium.

The development of tolerance to self antigen may require contact of maturing T cells with specific cell types in the thymus. It seems likely that the thymic dendritic cells are the dominant stromal cell type involved in inducing self tolerance (74). It should be noted, however, that development of tolerance is unlikely to be solely an intrathymic process, and postthymic T cells probably play an important role in maintaining tolerance to some self antigens (29).

T cells exiting from the thymus are phenotypically and functionally mature, and self MHC restricted. In the peripheral blood, T cells comprise 70 to 80% of all lymphocytes and about 60 to 70% of the T cells are Th cells. In lymph nodes, T cells segregate in the paracortex, and in the spleen they segregate in the central region of the periarteriolar lymphoid sheath or white pulp.

Antigen Recognition by T cells

T cells, unlike B cells, do not directly bind antigen. Numerous studies, published since the mid-1970s, have clearly indicated that T cells recognize processed antigen which is complexed to MHC molecules (frequently called MHC antigens) (reviewed in references in 4 and 32). The T cell must recognize a foreign antigen and a self MHC molecule simultaneously in order to be activated. CTLs and Th cells can recognize antigen presented by either class I MHC molecules (HLA-A, HLA-B, and HLA-C in man; H-2K and H-2D in the mouse; RT1A in the rat), or class II molecules (HLA-DP, HLA-DQ, and HLA-DR in man; I-A and I-E in the mouse; and RT1B and RT1D in the rat). However, it appears that the vast majority of Th cells are restricted by class II MHC molecules (also called Ia antigens), whereas the majority of CTLs are restricted by class I MHC molecules (169).

In a Th cell response to a protein antigen (*e.g.*, egg-white lysozyme injected into a mouse (4)), the antigen must first be trapped and processed by an antigen-presenting cell (APC) which expresses class II MHC molecules. The APC may be a macrophage (4), a dendritic cell (171), a B cell (148), and under certain circumstances other cell types as well (103). The protein antigen is thought to be broken down into smaller peptides which are then returned to the cell surface complexed to a class II molecule. X-ray diffraction studies reveal that MHC molecules (at least class I molecules) have a cleft which probably represents the binding site for processed antigenic peptides (14). The mechanisms of antigen processing and antigen presentation, however, remain poorly understood.

Recent studies suggest that the T cell binds to the MHC + processed-antigen complex via a single receptor. The TCR for antigen consists of an α and a β chain (joined by a disulphide bridge), each with constant and variable regions resembling those of immunoglobulins (5, 87, 188). The variable portions of the TCR give rise to unique antigenic determinants which compose the clonotype of the T cell (*i.e.*, each T cell clone has a unique clonotype). The TCR is bound with the CD3 (T3) molecular complex on the membrane of T cells (188). A small subset of T cells uses a different receptor (γ/δ chains) (101), but the biologic significance of these T cells is unclear. The binding of the TCR to the MHC + processed-antigen complex appears to be strengthened or stabilized by the CD4 (T4) molecule (98). The CD4 molecule is a Th marker which has recently been shown to bind directly to class II MHC molecules (51), whereas the CD8 (T8) molecule of CTLs is thought to bind to class I MHC molecules. The formation of a molecular complex involving MHC class II, an antigenic peptide, the TCR, and the CD4 molecule results in the delivery of a first signal necessary for T cell activation. After this initial interaction, the APC secretes interleukin-1 (IL-1) which also promotes T cell activation (40). The activated Th cell then undergoes blastic transformation, proliferates, and secretes a number of soluble protein mediators collectively known as lymphokines or interleukins (IL). Activated Th cells express markedly increased amounts of IL-2 receptors (IL-2R) (56) and, unlike resting T cells, express Ia antigens (139).

Lymphokines Produced by Activated Th Cells

Activated Th cells can produce the following interleukins (Table 1): IL-2, also known as T cell growth factor (54); IL-3 (157); IL-4, formerly B cell stimulator factor 1 (125); IL-5, formerly T cell replacing factor, or B cell growth factor II (78); IL-6, formerly human B cell differentiation factor (BCDF), B cell stimulatory factor 2 (69), or interferon β-2 (50); γ-interferon (IFN) (39, 198); lymphotoxin (LT), also called tumor necrosis factor-β (TNF-β) (154, 198); as well as a number of less well characterized mediators.

Recently, it has been found that Th cells, at least in mice, fall into two subtypes depending on their pattern of lymphokine secretion (26, 27, 117). Thus, Th1 cells secrete IL-2, LT and γ-IFN, whereas Th2 cells secrete IL-4 and IL-5. Th1 cells produce higher amounts of granulocyte/monocyte colony-stimulating factor than Th2 cells, whereas IL-3 is produced equally by both cell types (27). In the rat, Th cells have been subdivided into two subsets based on the expression of the 0X22 antigen. 0X22+ Th cells secrete IL-2 but provide little or no help to B cells, while 0X22- Th cells do not secrete IL-2, but provide help to B cells (9). In humans, the $CD4^+$ subset of T cells can be divided into T helper cells ($2H4^-$ $4B4^+$ cells) and T suppressor/inducer cells ($2H4^+$, $4B4^-$ cells) (89, 153), but the spectrum of lymphokines secreted by these subsets is unknown. Interestingly, although IL-2 appears to be the main growth factor for both Th cells and CTLs, some T cells proliferate in response to IL-4 (93, 168). IL-2 and IL-4 have autocrine activity, since they can act on the same cells which produce these lymphokines.

TABLE 1. INTERLEUKINS PRODUCED BY Th CELLS

Name	Th Producer	TCGF[a]	CTDF[b]	BCGF[c]	BCDF[d]	Other functions
IL-2	Th1	+	+	+	+	Enhances NK growth and activity
IFN-γ	Th1	−	+	−	+	Inhibits viral replication Macrophage arming factor Induces Ia expression Inhibits IL-4 effects on B cells
LT	Th1	−	−	−	−	Cytotoxic lymphokine
IL-3	Th1/Th2	−	−	−	−	Multipotential CSF[e] Mast cell growth factor
IL-4	Th2	+	+	+	+	Mast cell growth factor Enhances IgE and IgG1 production Enhances Ia expression on B cell and macrophage Costimulates proliferation of hemopoietic progenitors
IL-5	Th2	−	−	+	+	Enhances IgA production Eosinophil differentiation factor
IL-6	Th2	−	+	−	+	Plasma cell growth factor inhibits viral replication

[a] T cell growth factor activity.
[b] Cytotoxic T lymphocyte differentiation factor activity.
[c] B cell growth factor activity.
[d] BCDF and/or B cell maturation factor activity.
[e] CSF, Colony-stimulating factor.

It is important to note that a single interleukin can have multiple activities (Table 1). The principal activities of the T cell-derived interleukins can be grouped as follows: pluripotential colony-stimulating activity (IL-3); T cell growth factor activity (IL-2, IL-4); B cell growth factor activity (IL-2, IL-4, IL-5); BCDF activity (IL-2, IL-4, IL-5, IL-6, γ-IFN, and B cell maturation factors (BMF); CTL differentiation factor activity (*e.g.*, IL-2, IL-4, γ-IFN); factors which act on macrophages (*e.g.*, γ-IFN and other macrophage arming factors); and lymphotoxin, a factor which is toxic to some tumor cells. IL-1, although probably not produced by T cells, often mediates effects similar to those of some T cell-derived interleukins.

The interplay of interleukins in inducing B cell, T cell, or macrophage responses is complex and incompletely understood. Consequently, the models described below must be considered tentative.

B CELL ACTIVATION, PROLIFERATION, AND DIFFERENTIATION

A number of excellent reviews have recently been written on this subject (61, 92, 128, 172, 185). B cells may be induced to maturation (differentiation) by two different pathways. Some lymphokines, known collectively as BMF, induce small resting B cells to mature directly (and secrete immunoglobulins), without proliferation. γ-IFN (163) and IL-5 (92), for example, mediate this type of activity. The significance of BMFs is unclear, as BMF activity is not likely to promote antigen-specific immunoglobulin (Ig) production. Perhaps, BMFs contribute to the maintenance of basal Ig secretion, as we will discuss later.

Antigen-specific antibody production, however, is likely to require interaction of a resting B cell clone with antigen, followed by activation, proliferation (clonal expansion), and differentiation. Activation may occur following cross-linking of the B cell receptor by some types of antigen (128), *e.g.*, T independent antigens with multiple repeating units. In many cases, the B cell not only binds the antigen, but also acts as an APC by processing and presenting the antigen (with MHC class II molecules) to Th cells (172, 185). This T cell-B cell cognate interaction results in antigen-specific MHC-restricted Th cell and B cell activation. The carrier effect, *i.e.*, the B cell and the T cell recognize a different portion of the same antigen, is thought to result from this type of T cell-B cell interaction. Studies of the immune response to hepatitis B surface antigen (HBsAg), for example, reveal that T cells and B cells respond to different synthetic peptides derived from HBsAg (112). Some polyclonal B cell activators, such as lipopolysaccharide (LPS), appear to mimic or replace T cell-mediated activation (200).

The activated B cell goes from the G0 to the G1 phase of the cell cycle, but requires B cell growth factors (IL-1, IL-2, IL-4, and IL-5) to progress further through the cell cycle (92, 128, 172, 185). B cells may proliferate extensively without secreting Ig (92). Differentiation depends on the presence of BCDFs such as IL-2, IL-4, IL-

5, and IL-6 (61, 92, 128, 185). However, IL-2, IL-4 and IL-5 promote both B cell proliferation and differentiation. IL-4 induces production of both IgG1 and IgE (125), IL-5 induces IgA secretion (185), while γ-IFN induces murine IgG2a secretion (166). Thus, T cell-derived factors influence the isotype of Ig produced.

The Effects of Lymphokines on CTL

IL-2 promotes both proliferation and differentiation of cytotoxic T-lymphocyte precursors (TCL-p). Recently, it has been proposed that IL-2 and γ-IFN are both necessary to induce CTL differentiation (58). A cytotoxic T cell differentiation factor has also been identified (186). IL-4 has potent cytotoxic T cell differentiation factor activity, and is possibly the most important lymphokine with this function (127).

In the mixed lymphocyte reaction, class II MHC-restricted responder Th cells are activated first, and secrete interleukins which stimulate CTL activity. These CTLs are primarily directed against the class I MHC molecules of target cells. It appears that the binding of modified or allogeneic class I MHC molecules delivers a first signal necessary for CTL-p activation, whereas IL-2, IL-4, and γ-IFN provide additional signals necessary for CTL proliferation and differentiation. Presumably, CTLs are activated by similar signals in viral infections, graft-*versus*-host disease (GVHD), allograft rejection, and some autoimmune diseases.

Th Cells and Delayed-Type Hypersensitivity (DTH)

The role of the Th cells as the initiators of DTH has been extensively documented. Recent studies suggest that DTH reactions are mediated primarily by the Th1 subset of Th cells (26).

Although Th cells initiate DTH, the response is highly dependent on the presence of macrophages. Activated Th cells secrete factors which act on macrophages (*e.g.*, γ-INF (39). The activated macrophages have increased phagocytic and killing activity and secrete a battery of mediators (e.g., IL-1, TNF-α, prostaglandins, superoxide ion) which promote a tissue response. In addition, during a DTH response TH1 cells produce IL-2 which promotes killing by natural killer (NK) cells (66). The role of NK cells in DTH responses is unclear, but NK cells may be involved in target cell killing in some autoimmune diseases (194). Activated Th1 cells also produce lymphotoxin which is cytotoxic to some cell types, and thus may contribute to tissue injury, as we will discuss later.

ORGAN-SPECIFIC AUTOIMMUNE DISEASES

Experimental Allergic Encephalomyelitis (EAE)

EAE was probably the first experimentally-induced autoimmune disease to be described. In 1933 Rivers *et al.* (145, 146) induced encephalomyelitis in monkeys with repeated injections of central nervous system (CNS) extracts. They reported that these CNS lesions were similar to the lesions found in patients who developed encephalomyelitis after rabies vaccination. In 1947, Freund, Stern, and Pisani (49), Kabat, Wolf and Bozer (75), Morgan (115), and Morrison (116) simultaneously reported that a single injection of homologous or heterologous CNS extracts emulsified in complete Freund's adjuvant (CFA) could induce EAE in guinea pigs, monkeys, and rabbits. Certain strains of rats, particularly Lewis rats, can be easily induced to develop EAE, and are now a preferred animal model for studies of this disease.

EAE in Lewis rats is characterized by inflammation of CNS white matter, usually 10 to 15 days after injecting a CNS extract in CFA (1, 8, 124, 189, 190). Mononuclear cells are seen surrounding postcapillary vessels, but demyelination is not prominent. The rats develop an ascending paralysis, sometimes with lethal brain stem lesions. However, the rats often recover, and are then markedly resistant to subsequent attempts to induce EAE (8, 29, 124). Immunohistochemical examination of tissues reveals that the earliest infiltrating cells are $CD4^+$ T cells (189). Later, macrophages and B cells accumulate in the lesions (190).

EAE can be transferred passively to normal rats with T cells, but not with serum (29, 120). A large body of evidence indicates that Th cells cause the disease, but not CTLs. For example, *in vivo* depletion of $CD4^+$ T cells with monoclonal antibodies abolishes susceptibility to disease, whereas depletion of $CD8^+$ T cells has no protective effect (170, 187). The target antigen in EAE is myelin basic protein (MBP). MBP has been sequenced and encephalitogenic peptides derived from this protein have been identified (65, 77). Ben-Nun, Wekerle, and Cohen (12) have isolated Th cell lines from rats which are specific for MBP, and which induce EAE when injected in normal rats. Remarkably small numbers of these T cells (10^5 or less) are sufficient to cause disease (12, 29). These MBP-specific Th lines require stimulation by Ia antigen-positive antigen-presenting cells and MBP, and can only produce EAE when injected into MHC compatible (at least at class II loci) recipient rats. Other investigators have isolated similar anti-MBP Th cell lines (190). In all cases, MBP-specific T cells lines must first be activated *in vitro*, with MBP/APC or a T cell mitogen (*e.g.*, concanavalin A (Con A)), in order to be able to induce EAE in recipient rats. Several other autoimmune diseases can be adoptively transferred with Th lymphocytes (Table 2).

Table 2. Examples of Experimental Autoimmune Diseases which have been Passively Transferred with Th Cells

Disease	References
Experimental allergic encephalomyelitis	12, 29, 68, 190
Experimental autoimmune thyroiditis	29, 147
Adjuvant arthritis	29, 183
Antigen-induced arthritis	81
Experimental autoimmune orchitis	105, 182
Insulin-dependent diabetes in the BB rat[a]	83, 84, 96, 100
Insulin-dependent diabetes in the NOD mouse[b]	7, 10, 113

[a] Con A-activated spleen cells contained both Th and non-T lymphoid cells.

[b] Both Th and CTLs are required for transfer of disease.

Several important findings have resulted from the study of MBP-specific Th cell lines. First, encephalitogenic MBP-specific Th cells can be isolated *in vitro* from the T cells of unimmunized Lewis rats (29, 190). Thus, autoreactive T cells are clearly part of the normal T cell repertoire. Second, MBP-specific Th cell lines can be isolated from EAE-resistant rat strains such as BS and BN (190). However, while BS-derived T cell lines are encephalitogenic, BN-derived MBP-specific T cell lines are not. Apparently, resistance to EAE occurs for different reasons in these two rat strains. Interestingly, BS rats have the same MHC haplotype as Lewis rats, *i.e.*, $RT1^l$, whereas BN rats carry the $RT1^n$ MHC haplotype. BN rats, possibly because of their MHC type, appear to lack encephalitogenic T cell clones, whereas in BS rats, encephalitogenic clones appear to be actively suppressed. Third, Ben-Nun and Cohen (11, 29) have demonstrated that the injection of inactivated (*e.g.*, with radiation) MBP-specific T cells in normal Lewis rats induces a state of resistance to EAE. Subsequently, these rats have a much lower incidence of EAE when injected with MBP in CFA. Despite resistance to disease, it is still possible to isolate MBP-specific T cells *in vitro* from these Lewis rats. It appears that the injection of inactivated MBP-specific T cells induces the generation of specific suppressor cells *in vivo* (29, 190). However, the nature of these suppressor cells remains unknown.

The mechanism by which MBP-specific Th cells home in to their CNS target is unclear. At least three distinct possibilities must be considered. Endothelial cells may express MHC class II antigens (*i.e.*, Ia antigens) (167), and MBP has been found in brain endothelial cells (164). Thus, endothelial cells may present MBP to Th cells. Alternatively, Th cells may cross the blood brain barrier and interact with Ia positive astrocytes. Under normal circumstances astrocytes express little or no Ia antigens; however, astrocytic Ia antigen expression increases dramatically in the presence of T cells, possibly through the action of T cell-derived γ-IFN. In fact, it is now clear that astrocytes can act as APCs (190). However, a recent study with bone marrow chimeras reveals that it is the MHC antigens of the bone marrow donors, and not those of the recipients, which determine the susceptibility to EAE (69). This suggests that the APC in EAE is of bone marrow origin.

Autoimmune Thyroiditis

The human and experimental thyroiditides represent a diverse group of diseases, where both thyroid antigen-specific autoantibodies and T cells have been identified. Unlike in EAE, there is clear evidence that autoantibodies contribute to the development of thyroid tissue lesions. These autoantibodies may modify thyrocyte function by binding to the thyrotropin receptor, or they may induce type II and III hypersensitivity responses by binding to thyroglobulin or other antigens. However, it is very likely that the production of these autoantibodies requires the participation of Th cells, and in some experimental models of thyroiditis autoantibodies appear to play only a minor role.

The obese strain (OS) chicken provides an interesting example of B cell-T cell cooperation in the development of thyroiditis. Bursectomy (on the day of hatching) of OS chickens protects against development of thyroiditis, and prevents the production of anti-thyroglobulin (anti-Tg) antibodies (192). Thymectomy, by contrast, increases the severity of thyroiditis, presumably by altering suppressive immunoregulatory pathways (193). However, when T cells are thoroughly depleted *in vivo* by injecting anti-T cell antibodies after thymectomy, OS chickens are protected from thyroiditis (129). Thus, autoantibody production is clearly T cell-dependent in OS chickens. The studies of Rose *et al.* (149) reveal that the development of thyroiditis in OS chickens is dependent on the coincidence of three independent genetic factors: the MHC, a malfunction of the thymic-dependent effector-suppressor T cell balance, and a defect in thyroid function. In fact, multigenic inheritance is a feature of almost all autoimmune diseases.

Experimental autoimmune thyroiditis (EAT) is induced by injecting mice with mouse thyroglobulin (Tg) in CFA (149). EAT, like EAE, can be transferred to recipient mice with T cells, but not with serum (34). Furthermore, Tg-specific Th cell lines have been isolated from mice, which can transfer thyroiditis (29, 147). The Tg-specific Th cell lines are restricted by class II MHC antigens, and share most of the properties of the MBP-specific Th cell lines described above (reviewed in reference 29). Mice can be rendered resistant to EAT by prior immunization with inactivated Tg-specific Th cells. These EAT-resistant mice still produce high titers of anti-Tg antibodies when injected with Tg/CFA, but they do not develop thyroiditis. This finding suggests that in EAT, tissue injury is mediated primarily by cell-mediated immunity, and not by autoantibodies. Furthermore, it appears that anti-Tg Th clones, like anti-MBP clones, are part of the normal T cell repertoire and are actively suppressed. Interestingly, thyroid antigen-specific T cell lines have recently been isolated from the thyroid gland of patients with autoimmune thyroiditis (102).

Normal thyroid epithelial cells do not express Ia antigens. However, Bottazzo and his colleagues (20, 62) have demonstrated that in glands with thyroiditis, thyrocytes do express Ia antigens. Thyrocytes can be induced to express Ia antigens *in vitro* by incubation with lectins or γ-IFN (reviewed in references 20 and 45). Thyrotropin synergizes with γ-IFN to induce Ia expression on thyrocytes (45). Ia-positive thyrocytes are effective antigen presenting cells (103). Moreover, in human autoimmune thyroiditis infiltrating T cells have been found to respond to Ia-positive thyrocytes (102).

These findings suggest that the "aberrant" expression of class II MHC molecules by endocrine cells may play a major role in the initiation of autoimmune disease. Conceivably, some cell surface molecules of endocrine cells only become immunogenic to Th cells when Ia antigens are coexpressed on the membrane. Interestingly, increased Ia antigen expression has been observed on target tissues in several immune-mediated diseases (Table 3), *e.g.*, Graves' disease, Hashimoto's thyroiditis, insulin-dependent diabetes, rheumatoid arthritis, Sjogren's syndrome, primary biliary cirrhosis, GVHD, and allograft

TABLE 3. IMMUNE-MEDIATED DISEASES WITH INCREASED IA ANTIGEN EXPRESSION ON TARGET TISSUES

Disease	References
Hashimoto's thyroiditis	3, 20, 45, 73
Graves' disease	3, 20, 45, 62, 73
Insulin-dependent diabetes	19, 20, 45, 48, 141
Primary biliary cirrhosis	45
Rheumatoid arthritis	25, 45, 80
GVHD	13, 90, 123
Allograft rejection	14, 60, 144

rejection (47). The activity of Ia antigens as the products of immune response genes (*i.e.* as restricting elements for Th cell responses) could readily explain disease associations with specific HLA class II antigens.

INSULIN-DEPENDENT DIABETES MELLITUS (IDDM)

Considerable evidence exists to suggest that IDDM is an autoimmune disease. Antibodies against islet cell cytoplasmic or cell membrane antigens can be identified in the serum of diabetic patients (20, 38). Nerup *et al.* (119), and later Boitard *et al.* (16–18), identified specific T cell responses to islet cell antigens *in vitro*, with T cells obtained from diabetic patients. Sibley *et al.* (162) reported rejection of syngeneic pancreatic transplants (*i.e.*, from identical twins) by long time diabetic patients.

SPONTANEOUS IDDM IN THE BIO-BREEDING (BB) RAT

The view that IDDM is an autoimmune disease has been considerably strengthened by the study of the BB rat and the nonobese diabetic (NOD) mouse, which both spontaneously develop IDDM. Since our own studies have been performed with BB rats, we will concentrate on this disease model. The BB rat is an excellent model of human IDDM (reviewed in references 110, 114, 118, 122, 131 and 150). Like the human disease, diabetes in the BB rat arises spontaneously during adolescence after an immune-mediated attack on the pancreatic islets. Disease is characterized by weight loss, hypoinsulinemia, hyperglycemia, ketonemia, glycosuria, and ketonuria. Death occurs if insulin therapy is not administered. Disease expression requires specific alleles of the MHC, as well as other genes. There are marked immune system abnormalities in the BB rat, which distinguish it from human IDDM in which immune abnormalities are more subtle. The incidence of diabetes reported in various BB rat colonies varies between about 20 and 60%. Diabetes-resistant strains of the BB rat also exist, and are frequently used as control animals.

The autoimmune nature of IDDM in BB rats is supported by the finding of an inflammatory infiltrate in islets of Langerhans (160), the identification of anti-islet cell antibodies in the serum (41), prevention of the disease with neonatal thymectomy (95) or other immunosuppressive treatments (91), passive transfer of disease with the Con A-activated lymphocytes of diabetic rats (83, 84, 96, 100), the isolation of islet cell-specific T cells from the pancreas of diabetic rats (131, 132, 134, 136), and the frequent association of thyroiditis with IDDM.

The onset of diabetes in BB rats coincides with the infiltration of islets of Langerhans by lymphoid cells. This lesion is referred to as insulitis, and has also been identified in recent onset diabetic patients (53). The islet infiltrate of BB rats consists of T cells, B cells, macrophages, NK cells, and less frequently eosinophils (160). β-islet cells are destroyed preferentially to other cell types, leading to severe insulinopenia and overt diabetes mellitus. In the BB rat (33), the lymphocytes infiltrating islets consist mainly of T helper cells ($0X19^+$, $W3/25^+$) with few T cytotoxic/suppressor cells ($0X19^+$, $0X8^+$). In a single case of human IDDM studied (19), the predominant subpopulation was cytotoxic/suppressor cells, but T helper cells and NK cells were also present in small numbers.

There is no evidence that viral or other infection is implicated in the causation of diabetes in the BB rat. BB rats raised under gnotobiotic conditions do not suffer a reduced incidence of diabetes (151), thus excluding horizontal transmission but not vertical transmission of an infectious agent. Viral particles have not been identified by electron microscopy in BB rat islet cells. A discussion of the putative role of viruses in human IDDM is beyond the scope of this review.

Islet cell surface antibodies, but not islet cell cytoplasmic antibodies, have been found in the BB rat (41), whereas in human IDDM, both islet cell surface antibodies and islet cell cytoplasmic antibodies are found.

Marked T cell lymphopenia, which is believed to be an autosomal recessive trait (59), is found in the peripheral blood, the lymph nodes, and the spleen of BB rats. T cell lymphopenia is an important predisposing factor for the development of IDDM in BB rats (59). $CD8^+$ T cell numbers are more severely depressed when $CD4^+$ T cells (137, 195). Furthermore, we found that the $CD8^+$ T cells of BB rats are not functional CTLs (137). CTL functional deficiency may explain, at least in part, the poor response of BB rats to allografts. BB rats also lack $RT6^+$ T cells, which are postulated to have important immunoregulatory functions (57). Interestingly, BB rats still generate delayed-type hypersensitivity responses to keyhole limpet hemocyanin (122).

The T cells of BB rats respond poorly to Con A and in mixed lymphocyte cultures (110, 114, 118, 122, 131, 150). We (135) found that Con A-induced IL-2 production by BB splenic T cells is markedly reduced. Production of IL-2, however, is restored when macrophages are depleted. Decreased IL-2 production has been described in human IDDM (199), in human and murine SLE (6, 97), in rheumatoid arthritis (30, 43) and other autoimmune conditions. The significance of this defect in lymphokine production remains to be determined. Potentially, decreased IL-2 production has adverse effects on suppressive immunoregulatory function.

Con-A activated spleen cells from acutely diabetic BB rats can induce diabetes in a large percentage of diabetes-prone BB rats which appears before 60 days *i.e.*, before the usual age of presentation (83, 84, 96, 100). Con-A activated spleen cells can also transfer diabetes to non-diabetes-prone strains that share the $RT1^{u-}$ haplotype (e.g., WF), but not to fully MHC-incompatible strains, on condition that the recipients are immunosuppressed by cyclophosphamide or neonatal thymectomy before cell transfer. These studies provide strong evidence that activated T cells can transfer diabetes and thus, by implication, that they are the immune cells which cause the disease. Furthermore, since our studies, and those of others (195), reveal that BB rats lack functional cytotoxic T lymphocytes the Th cell is the most likely initiator of islet cell injury in this rat strain.

The role of T cells in rat IDDM has also been studied by injecting monoclonal antibodies which react against specific subsets of lymphocytes. Injection of monoclonal antibodies 0X19 (pan-T cell), 0X8 (NK cells or CTLs), or W3/25 (Th cells) reduces the incidence of IDDM in BB rats (94). 0X19 also prevents insulitis but 0X8 does not. The injection of antisera to the NK marker asialo-GM1 also protects from diabetes (194). *In vitro* studies reveal that NK cells are directly toxic to β-islet cells (142). These findings are consistent with the hypothesis that T cells initiate insulitis, but that the islet destruction is mediated via NK cells. Macrophages, however, are also potential effector cells in insulitis, as we will discuss below.

We have provided further evidence of the involvement of T cells in diabetes by isolating Th cell lines specific for islet cell antigens from the spleen and pancreas of acutely diabetic BB or BB-derived (BBUF) rats (132, 134, 136). The cells grown express a T helper phenotype ($0X19^+$, $W3/13^+$, $W3/25^+$, $0X8^-$), and demonstrate T helper cell function by proliferating and producing IL-2 in the combined presence of islet cell antigen and MHC-compatible antigen-presenting cells. The activity of these Th cell lines is MHC-restricted, and can be inhibited by antibodies to the RT1D class II MHC antigens of the rat.

The mechanisms by which Th cells contribute to insulitis in BB rats are still unknown. Although Th cells could stimulate NK cells by producing IL-2 and γ-IFN, other possibilities must also be considered. There is evidence that cytokines produced by T cells or macrophages are toxic to islet cells. Supernatants of activated blood mononuclear cells from healthy human donors were reported to reduce glucose-induced insulin release from isolated Wistar rat islets, to decrease the islet content of insulin and glucagon, and to cause islet cell disintegration in a dose-dependent manner, as judged by both light microscopy and electron microscopy (107, 108). These effects were found to be due to IL-1 (106). Pukel *et al.* (143) found that γ-IFN inhibits induced insulin secretion of isolated rat islet cells and is cytotoxic to islet cells. They found that neither IL-1 nor TNF kill islet cells, but that the cytotoxic effects of γ-IFN are enhanced by the addition of IL-1 and even more so by the combination of IL-1 and TNF.

There is evidence that macrophages may be involved in islet cell injury. The insulitis lesions of BB rats contain macrophages as well as lymphocytes (160). Activated macrophages decrease glucose-induced insulin release (35) and are cytotoxic to syngeneic cultured mouse islets (159) and to syngeneic isolated rat islet cells (21). Macrophage injury could be mediated via cytokine production, *e.g.*, IL-1 and TNF-α. The only direct evidence that macrophages may be involved in islet cell destruction in diabetes is the demonstration that silica, which interferes with macrophage function, prevents diabetes in the BB rat (121).

As mentioned above, one hypothesis concerning the generation of endocrine autoimmunity suggests that the induction of MHC class II antigen expression on endocrine epithelial cells, possibly due to α-IFN after local viral infection, would enable these cells to present self antigens to autoreactive T cells. Normal endocrine islet cells express MHC class I antigens, but not class II antigens. The questions as to whether rat endocrine islet cells can be induced to express class II antigens and whether BB rat or human islet cells can constitutively express class II antigens have also been addressed with conflicting results (reviewed in reference 122).

In vitro, Ia antigen induction has been noted on the endocrine cells of isolated Lewis rat islets that are cultured without IFN for 7 days and then exposed to 500 units/ml of murine recombinant γ-IFN for 6 days (109). The combination of tumor necrosis factor or lymphotoxin synergizes with γ-IFN to induce Ia antigens on human islet cells (140). Aberrant expression of class II and hyperexpression of class I antigens have been reported on the β-cells in human recent-onset IDDM (19, 48, 141). Most islets in which class II positive endocrine cells are seen do not show insulitis, suggesting that the aberrant expression precedes the inflammatory infiltrates. Despite these interesting results, the importance of class II MHC antigen expression on islet cells is still unclear. Conceivably, islet cell antigens are processed by Ia^+ macrophages or dendritic cells, since macrophage-like cells containing phagocytosed endocrine cell granules have been identified in islets of Langerhans (70).

Spontaneous IDDM in the NOD Mouse

The NOD mouse develops a form of IDDM similar to the human and the BB rat (76). There are important differences, nevertheless, between the disease of NOD mice and BB rats. Although NOD mice have immunoregulatory defects, they do not develop the lymphopenia found in BB rats (22). The insulitis of NOD mice is characterized by a massive infiltration of islets of Langerhans by T cells which include both the $CD4^+$ and $CD8^+$ subtypes of T cells (76). Diabetes can be passively transferred to normal MHC-matched mice with the T cells of diabetic NOD mice (7, 10, 113). Both $CD4^+$ and $CD8^+$ T cells are required for transfer of IDDM. Recently, T cell lines have been derived directly from the islets of diabetic NOD mice (7). Only cell lines containing both $CD4^+$ and $CD8^+$ T cells could produce insulitis when injected into nondiabetic recipient mice. It thus appears that in the NOD mouse, the development of insulitis requires cooperation between Th cells and CTLs, where presumably the CTL is the actual effector cell. By contrast, the BB rat appears to lack functional CTLs. This difference suggests that there may be several pathways which lead to insulitis. However, the finding that IDDM can be transferred with T cells, and not with serum, in both NOD mice and BB rats suggests that antibodies are not required to induce insulitis.

SYSTEMIC AUTOIMMUNE DISEASE

Murine Models of SLE

SLE, or lupus is without doubt the most extensively studied autoimmune disease. One of the most important reasons is the availability of several mouse strains which spontaneously develop a form of SLE similar to the human disease. The genetic and immunologic characteristics of these mouse strains are described in detail in several recent reviews (36, 133, 165, 174–177) (Table 4). Three models of murine lupus have received the most attention: The New Zealand (NZB × NZW)F1 hybrids henceforth referred to as NZB/W), the BXSB strain, and the MRL/Mp-*lpr/lpr* strain henceforth referred to as MRL/lpr). The genetic origin and the immunologic abnormalities found in these three strains are quite different (Table 4). However, these mice share a number of pathologic features: severe polyclonal hypergammaglobulinemia; antinuclear antibodies (*e.g.*, anti-DNA); circulating immune complexes; anti-gp70 antibodies; and glomerulonephritis which is the principal cause of death. MRL/lpr mice frequently have rheumatoid factors (RF) in their serum and they develop a rheumatoid arthritis-like disease (64). Consequently, this mouse strain is also an interesting model for the study of rheumatoid arthritis (RA). MRL/lpr mice are also prone to develop necrotizing polyarteritis (174), and a Sjogren's disease-like inflammation of the salivary and lacrimal glands (72).

Genetic Aspects of Murine SLE

NZB/W, BXSB, and MRL mice can develop early onset (death in the 1st year of life) or late onset (death in the 2nd year of life) lupus, depending on the presence or absence of various accelerating factors. The disease of NZB/W mice is accelerated by female sex hormones and thus occurs much earlier in females. The disease of BXSB mice is accelerated by a Y-linked gene and occurs earlier in males (castration has no effect on this disease). Lupus is greatly accelerated in MRL mice by an autosomal recessive gene called *lpr*. MRL mice homozygous for this gene develop massive T cell hyperplasia which parallels the early onset of a SLE-like disease, as well as other manifestations of autoimmunity.

The inheritance of lupus in these mouse strains has been extensively studied. In all cases, the inheritance of severe early onset lupus is polygenic (28), although the *lpr* gene can induce a mild form of disease when transferred to mouse strains with no apparent predisposition to autoimmunity (174). The expression of lupus does not correlate with the presence of any well known genetic marker or with the MHC, since NZB, NZW, BXSB, and MRL mice each have a different MHC haplotype. Cell transfer experiments reveal that lupus can be transferred to lethally irradiated nonlupus-prone recipients with bone marrow stem cells obtained from lupus-prone mice. The thymus appears to play little role in the disease of NZB/W and BXSB mice, but is essential for disease expression in MRL/lpr mice (173, 175).

Cellular Immunology of Murine SLE

Many immunologic abnormalities have been described in murine lupus strains. These abnormalities affect B cell, T cell, and macrophage function. MRL/lpr mice develop massive T cell proliferation (polyclonal), BXSB mice have moderate B cell and monocytoid cell hyperplasia, whereas NZB/W mice have lymphocyte numbers which are closer to normal. Suppressor T cell function has been found to be decreased by some investigators (23, 86), but not by others (31, 178). Susceptibility to tolerance induction is decreased in lupus-prone mice, but the genetic studies of Dixon *et al.* (36) suggest that this abnormality is not associated with disease. The T cells of all lupus-prone mice have a decreased ability to produce IL-2 and several other lymphokines (6). This feature, as mentioned above, is found in other autoimmune diseases, and in human lupus. Polyclonal hypergammaglobulinemia and B cell hyperactivity are present in all the murine models of lupus (36, 133, 165, 174, 175, 177), as well as in patients with SLE (44). Thus, B cell hyperactivity is regarded by most investigators as a cardinal feature of SLE.

The work of Prud'homme, Theofilopoulos, Dixon and other investigators (reviewed in references 36, 133, 174, and 175) suggests that murine lupus can be divided into two immunologically distinct forms depending on the cause of B cell hyperactivity (Table 5). In NZB/W and BXSB mice, B cells (from a young age) hyper-respond when stimulated by a number of signals such as B cell mitogens (LPS, anti-μ antibodies), and lymphokines which induce B cell growth and differentiation (130). The B cells of MRL mice, however, do not show this type of hyperactivity. In MRL/lpr mice, abnormal proliferating T cells spontaneously produce a B cell differentiation factor which induces polyclonal B cell differentiation. This factor has been termed L-BCDF by Prud'homme *et al.* (138). More recently, Dobashi *et al.* (37) have described a similar factor. L-BCDF appears to act on both resting and activated B cells. With age, autoantibody production in lupus-prone mice switches from the IgM isotype, to predominantly IgG isotypes.

Table 4. Genetic and Immunopathologic Features of Lupus-Prone Mice[a]

Strain	MHC	Sex dominance	T cell hyperplasia	B cell hyperplasia	Protection by thymectomy	Accelerating factor
NZB/W	d/z	F	−	−	−	Female sex hormones
BXSB	b	M	−	+	−	Y-linked gene
MRL/lpr	k	M = F	++	−	+	lpr gene

[a] All the lupus-prone strains have polyclonal hypergammaglobulinemia, anti-dsDNA, anti-ssDNA, anti-gp70, circulating immune complexes, reduced complement levels, and glomerulonephritis which is the principal cause of death. MRL/lpr mice, unlike the other strains, have high titers of rheumatoid factors, arthritis, and high titers of anti-Sm antibodies.

TABLE 5. CELLULAR IMMUNE FUNCTION IN LUPUS-PRONE MICE

Strain	Increased IgSC[a]	Decreased IL-2 production[b]	Increased BCDF/BMF production[c]	B cell response to LPS	B cell response to BCGF and BCDF	Protection with anti-CD4
NZB/W	+	+	–	I[d]	I	+
BXSB	+	+	–	I	I	+
MRL/lpr	+	+	+	N[d]	N	?[e]

[a] Spontaneous Ig-secreting cells, *i.e.*, without mitogenic stimulation.
[b] Decreased IL-2 production in response to Con A or MLC.
[c] Spontaneous production of BCDF and BMF by unstimulated Th cells.
[d] I, increased; N, normal.
[e] Injection of anti-Thy1.2 antibodies prevents disease in MRL/lpr (196).

This switching event correlates with the appearance of tissue lesions. L-BCDF appears to induce switching from IgM to IgG secretion *in vitro* (138).

Studies performed over the last few years indicate that autoantibodies form part of the normal B cell repertoire. Thus, the polyclonal activation of normal B cells (from nonlupus-prone mice) *in vitro* with B cell mitogens results in the production of anti-DNA, RF, and other autoantibodies characteristic of systemic autoimmune diseases (42, 46). Hang *et al.* (63) demonstrated that the injection of lipid A (a polyclonal B cell activator derived from LPS) in normal mice, or young lupus-prone mice, resulted in the production of anti-DNA and other autoantibodies. Normal mice treated with lipid A developed only mild glomerulonephritis, while lupus-prone mice developed a markedly accelerated form of lupus-like disease. These results suggest that polyclonal activation is sufficient to induce autoantibody production, but the severity of resulting tissue lesions is genetically determined. In fact, the study of congenic recombinant lupus-prone mice indicates that multiple genes control autoantibody production (28).

Interestingly, a subset of B cells, *i.e.* Ly-1$^+$ B cells, appear to be responsible for most of the autoantibody production in lupus mice (67). The *xid* gene, which causes deletion of a subset of B cells, protects all lupus-prone mouse strains from disease (174, 175).

The role which specific autoantigens play in directing autoantibody production in systemic autoimmune diseases is unclear. First, anti-DNA, RFs, and other autoantibodies have a broad spectrum of reactivity. For example, anti-DNA antibodies may bind various combinations of dsDNA, ssDNA, synthetic polynucleotides, phospholipids, cytoskeletal proteins, polysaccharides, platelets, Raji cells, and lymphocytes (71, 158). It is likely that these multispecific autoantibodies react against microbial antigens, and cross-react only accidentally with DNA and other nuclear antigens. Second, the study of the variable gene segments of anti-DNA antibodies and RFs reveals that some autoantibodies are coded by unmutated germ line genes, whereas other autoantibodies appear to the products of gene segments which have undergone antigen-directed somatic mutations (24, 85, 156, 179). Third, the studies of Klinman and Steinberg (82), suggest that the proportion of autoantibody-producing B cells (*i.e.*, as a fraction of all B cells) is the same in normal and lupus-prone mice. This, and other evidence (85), suggests that the B cell repertoire of lupus-prone mice is normal.

The studies of the MRL/lpr mouse provide evidence that the secretion of a T cell-derived lymphokine can directly induce polyclonal B cell hyperactivity and autoantibody production. It is interesting that when the *lpr* gene is transferred into the background of nonlupus-prone mice, systemic autoimmunity results, but the severity of disease and the titers of the autoantibodies produced vary widely from one strain to another (174). Our results suggest that L-BCDF is produced by Th cells. The majority of the proliferating T cells of MRL/lpr mice have markers similar to those of early thymocytes (111). It is not clear if these thymocyte-like cells secrete L-BCDF, or if these cells differentiate further to generate mature Th cells in secondary lymphoid tissues, which then produce L-BCDF. Our studies, and those of Dobashi *et al.* (37), demonstrate that L-BCDF has B cell maturation factor activity. It is not known if L-BCDF is similar or identical with any of the known interleukins. However, IL-5 and IL-6 have activities similar to L-BCDF.

Some forms of chronic GVHD across Ia antigen incompatibilities (usually when there are no class I MHC antigenic differences) result in the production of antinuclear antibodies in the host, and a lupus-like disease (55, 184). In this case, it appears that donor Th cells respond to Ia antigens on host B cells. This results in mutual B cell and T cell activation. Furthermore, the activated T cells secrete B cell growth and differentiation factors which induce polyclonal Ig secretion (37). The production of autoantibodies in GVHD thus bears similarities with the disease of MRL/lpr mice. The GVHD model is the only well documented example of Ia-restricted T cell-B cell interactions in murine SLE; however, it has been proposed that the T cells of MRL/lpr mice may also react to self Ia antigens (191).

An attractive hypothesis is that B cell maturation factors (such as L-BCDF) normally contribute to the maintenance of basal immunoglobulin secretion. Surprisingly little is known of the mechanisms which regulate the rate of immunoglobulin secretion in body fluids. Clearly, plasma cells secrete large amounts of immunoglobulins on a continual basis, to maintain normal serum levels of Ig. Since plasma cells have a relatively short life, there must be a rapid turnover of these cells, and strict homeostatic mechanisms to maintain and control the generation of new Ig secreting cells. Since the action of BMFs is polyclonal and does not require activation of B cells with antigen, it is possible that the secretion of BMFs by Th cells plays an important role in the regulation of basal immunoglobulin production. In MRL/lpr mice, the excessive production of BMF would be expected to induce polyclonal hypergammaglobulinemia. In BXSB and NZB/W mice, due to genetically determined B cell hyperactivity, normal amounts of BMF may be sufficient to induce excessive Ig production.

Despite important B cell defects in BXSB and NZB/W mice, our results indicate that the B cells of these mice are still dependent on T cell-derived lymphokines for their activity (138). Thus, the B cells of these mice could not produce antigen-specific or polyclonal Ig *in vitro*, without the addition of appropriate T cell-derived lymphokines. Furthermore, the injection of anti-CD4 (*i.e.*, anti-L3T4) antibodies in NZB/W mice (197) and BXSB mice (196) depleted Th cells, and prevented development of lupus-like disease. This provides strong evidence that the production of autoantibodies in NZB/W mice is still T dependent. This finding may seem surprising in view of the fact that neonatally thymectomized or athymic (nude) lupus-prone mice develop disease (174). However, thymectomized and nude mice are not totally devoid of T cells, and develop increasing T cell function with age (175).

CONCLUSIONS

The experimental disease models described in this review demonstrate the diversity of autoimmune diseases, and illustrate some of the major differences between organ-specific and systemic autoimmune diseases.

In organ-specific autoimmune diseases, autoreactive Th clones are activated, which react to specific tissue antigens in an MHC-restricted way. These Th cells usually interact with B cells to induce the production of autoantibodies against target tissues. Autoantibodies, however, may or may not contribute to the development of tissue injury. For example, autoantibodies are essential for the development of thyroiditis in OS chickens, but play little or no role in the development of thyroiditis in EAT in mice. In EAE, CNS lesions appear to result entirely from a cell-mediated immune response.

Th clones specific for self antigens clearly form part of the normal T cell repertoire. These clones can be isolated *in vitro*, from both disease-susceptible or disease-resistant strains. Remarkably small numbers of cloned Th cells are capable of causing autoimmune disease when injected into normal recipient animals. These recipient animals, however, can develop resistance to autoimmunity under specific experimental conditions. For example, Lewis rats which have recovered from EAE are resistant to subsequent attempts to induce disease. Similarly, animals injected with inactivated autoreactive Th cells develop resistance to the type of autoimmunity produced by these Th cells. The immune mechanisms which maintain this type of resistance to autoimmunity are still unknown. It has been suggested that anti-clonotypic suppressor T cells are generated, but the existence of this type of suppressor cell has not been conclusively demonstrated.

EAE in Lewis rats and IDDM in BB rats are examples of diseases where tissue lesions appear to result from DTH-like immune responses. Presumably, specifically activated Th cells secrete lymphokines which act on macrophages and/or other effector cells to produce tissue injury. Furthermore, cytokines produced by Th cells and macrophages are known to be toxic to some cell types, *e.g*, pancreatic β cells. It is interesting to note that autoimmune diseases in different species which appear similar, can be mediated by different effector mechanisms. For example, diabetes-prone BB rats appear to lack functional CTLs and develop insulitis despite this defect, whereas the development of insulitis and IDDM in NOD mice is clearly dependent and a cooperative interaction between islet-cell-specific Th cells and CTLs.

In organ-specific autoimmunity, target tissues often aberrantly express Ia antigens. Bottazzo *et al.* (20) and Feldman (45) have popularized the theory that aberrant Ia expression, especially on endocrine cells, renders these cells immunogenic and may initiate autoimmune responses. Although attractive, this theory requires more extensive substantiation. Almost all tissues contain at least small numbers of constitutively Ia positive cells, *e.g.*, dendritic cells and macrophages, which may act as antigen-presenting cells for autoreactive Th cells.

The study of SLE in several mouse strains, and in humans, reveals major points of difference with the organ-specific autoimmune disease. For example, spontaneous murine SLE is not an MHC-restricted disease; T cells specific for DNA, RNA, and other nuclear antigens have not been identified; SLE cannot be passively transferred with T cells; the tissue lesions of SLE are primarily mediated by immune complexes; SLE, unlike most organ-specific autoimmune disease, is characterized by severe polyclonal B cell hyperactivity and polyclonal hypergammaglobulinemia; procedures which induce the production of antinuclear antibodies, *e.g.*, injection of B cell mitogens in mice or GVHD across class II MHC incompatibilities, do not induce production of organ-specific autoantibodies; procedures which induce development of organ-specific autoimmunity, *e.g.*, neonatal thymectomy in some strains of mice (180, 181) or rats (126), do not result in the production of SLE-like autoantibodies or disease. In fact, there is little clinical overlap between organ-specific and systemic autoimmune diseases.

Polyclonal B cell hyperactivity is a cardinal feature of human and murine SLE. It is apparent that the normal B cell repertoire contains numerous B cell clones which produce antibodies to DNA and other self antigens. Consequently, any process which polyclonally activates B cells results in the production of autoantibodies. These autoantibodies, however, do not necessarily cause tissue lesions, and several genes determine the susceptibility to systemic autoimmune diseases.

B cell hyperactivity may be secondary to genetically determined B cell defects (*e.g.*, in NZB/W and BXSB mice), or may result from Th cell hyperactivity (*e.g.*, MRL/lpr mice and chronic GVHD). IN MRL/lpr mice, T cells overproduce a B cell maturation factor which stimulates polyclonal Ig secretion. In chronic GVHD, Th cells respond to Ia antigens on B cells and secrete B cell stimulatory lymphokines. This process results in polyclonal B cell activation, proliferation, and differentiation and the generation of lupus-like autoantibodies and disease. In NZB/W and BXSB mice, B cells appear to overrespond to normal levels of T cell-derived B cell stimulatory lymphokines. In either case, hypergammaglobulinemia and autoantibody production results.

Our studies, as well as a review of the literature, lead us to believe that in many cases organ-specific autoimmunity results when Th cells respond to self antigens presented by Ia$^+$ target cells and induce local inflammatory reactions, whereas systemic autoimmunity (at least in SLE) results from the increased production of, or abnormal response to, Th cell-derived antigen-nonspecific B cell stimulatory factors. In all cases, multiple genes determine the susceptibility to autoimmune disease. The mechanisms which normally prevent or limit autoimmune responses remain poorly understood, and represent a challenging area for future studies.

This work was supported by the Medical Research Council of Canada, the Juvenile Diabetes Foundation International, and the Canadian Diabetes Association.

REFERENCES

1. Ackermann HP, Ulrich J, Heitz PU: Experimental allergic encephalomyelitis. Exudate and cellular infiltrate in the spinal cord of Lewis rats. Acta Neuropathol 54:149, 1981
2. Adkins B, Mueller C, Okada CY, Reichert RA, Weissman IL, Spangrude GJ: Early events in T-cell maturation. Ann Rev Immunol 5:325, 1987
3. Aichinger G, Fill H, Wick G: In situ immune complexes, lymphocyte populations and HLA-DR positive epithelial cells in Hashimoto thyroiditis. Lab Invest 52:132, 1985
4. Allen PM, Babbitt BP, Unanue ER: T cell recognition of lysozyme: the biochemical basis of presentation. Immunol Rev 98:171, 1987
5. Allison JP: Structure, function, and serology of the T-cell antigen receptor complex. Ann Rev Immunol 5:503, 1987
6. Altman A, Theofilopoulos AN, Weiner R, Katz DH, Dixon FJ: Analysis of T cell function in autoimmune murine strains. Defects in production of and responsiveness to interleukin 2. J Exp Med 154:791, 1981
7. Appel MC, O'Neil JJ, Wicker LB, Kurnick JT: Adoptive transfer of diabetes mellitus in NOD mice using islet derived T-lymphocyte cultures (abstr). Diabetes, in press 1988
8. Arnon R: Experimental allergic encephalomyelitis-susceptibility and suppression. Immunol Rev 58:5, 1981
9. Arthur RP, Mason D: T cells that help B cell responses to soluble antigen are distinguishable from those producing interleukin-2 on mitogenic or allogeneic stimulation. J Exp Med 163:774, 1986
10. Bendelac A, Carnaud C, Boitard C, Bach JF: Syngeneic transfer of autoimmune diabetes from diabetic NOD mice to healthy neonates. J Exp Med 166:823, 1987
11. Ben-Nun A, Cohen IR: Vaccination against autoimmune encephalomyelitis: attenuated autoimmune T cells confer resistance to induction of active EAE but not to EAE mediated by the intact T lymphocyte line. Eur J Immunol 11:949, 1981
12. Ben-Nun A, Wekerle H, Cohen IR: The rapid isolation of clonable, antigen-specific T lymphocyte lines capable of mediating autoimmune encephalomyelitis. Eur J Immunol 11:195, 1981
13. Beschorner WE, Farmer ER, Saral R, Stirling WL, Santos GW: Epithelial class II antigen expression in cutaneous graft versus host disease. Transplantation 44:237, 1987
14. Bjorkman PJ, Saper MA, Samraoui B, Bennett WS, Strominger JL, Wiley DC: The foreign antigen-binding site and T cell recognition regions of class I histocompatibility antigens. Nature 329:512, 1987
15. Bluestone JA, Pardoll D, Sharrow SO, Fowlkes BJ: Characterization of murine thymocytes with CD3-associated T cell receptor structures. Nature 326:82, 1987
16. Boitard C, Bach JF: Cell-mediated versus humoral immunity in autoimmune diseases and their pharmacologic control with particular reference to type 1 diabetes mellitus. In Concepts in Immunopathology, Vol 3, edited by Cruse JM, Lewis RE, p 193. Basel, Karger, 1986
17. Boitard C, Debray-Sachs M, Pouplard A, Assan R, Hamburger J: Lymphocytes from diabetics suppress insulin release in vitro. Diabetologia 21:41, 1981
18. Boitard C, Chatenoud LM, Debray-Sachs M: In vitro inhibition of pancreatic B cells by T lymphocytes in diabetes. J Immunol 129:2529, 1982
19. Bottazzo GF, Dean BM, McNally JM, McKay EH, Swift PGF, Gamble DR: In situ characterization of autoimmune phenomena and expression of HLA molecules in the pancreas in diabetic insulitis. N Engl J Med 313:353, 1985
20. Bottazzo GF, Todd I, Mirakian R, Belfiore A, Pujol-Borrell R: Organ-specific autoimmunity: a 1986 overview. Immunol Rev 94:137, 1986
21. Burkart V, Apples B, Kolb H: In vitro cytotoxic activity of macrophages against isolated islet cells (abstr). Diabetes 37 (Suppl):21A, 1988
22. Burkhardt K, Mandel T: Lymphocyte subsets, endocrine pancreatic function and periislet infiltration during ageing of the NOD mouse (abstr). Diabetes, in press 1988
23. Cantor H, McVay-Boudreau L, Hugenberger J, Naidorf K, Shen FW, Gershon RK: Immunoregulatory circuits among T cell sets. II. Physiological role of feedback inhibition in vivo: absence in NZB mice. J Exp Med 147:1116, 1978
24. Carson DA, Chen PP, Kipps TJ, Radoux V, Jirik F, Goldfien RD, Fox RI, Silverman GJ, Fong S: Molecular basis for the cross-reactive idiotypes on human anti-IgG autoantibodies (rheumatoid factors). In Autoimmunity and Autoimmune Disease, edited by Evered D, Whelan J, p 123. Chichester, John Wiley and Sons, 1987
25. Charron D, Teyton L: Autoimmunity in rheumatoid arthritis. In Concepts in Immunopathology, Vol 4, edited by Cruse JM, Lewis RE, p 200. Basel, Karger, 1987
26. Cher DJ, Mosmann TR: Two types of murine helper T cell clone. 2. Delayed -type hypersensitivity is mediated by Th1 clones. J Immunol 138:3688, 1987
27. Cherwinski HM, Schumaker JH, Brown KD, Mosmann TR: Two types of mouse helper T cell clone: J Exp Med 166:1229, 1987
28. Chused TM, McCoy KL, Lal RB, Brown EL, Bake PJ: Multigenic basis of autoimmune disease in New Zealand mice. In Concepts in Immunopathology, Vol 4, edited by Cruse JM, Lewis RE, p 129. Basel, Karger, 1987
29. Cohen IR: Regulation of autoimmune disease: physiological and therapeutic. Immunol Rev 94:5, 1986
30. Combe B, Pope RM, Fishbach M, Darnell B, Baron S, Talal N: Interleukin 2 in rheumatoid arthritis: production of and response to IL-2 in rheumatoid synovial fluid, synovial tissue and peripheral blood. Clin Exp Immunol 59:520, 1985
31. Creighton WD, Katz DH, Dixon FJ: Antigen-specific immunocompetency, B cell function and regulatory helper and suppressor T cell activities in spontaneously autoimmune mice. J Immunol 123:2627, 1979
32. Cresswell P: Antigen recognition by T lymphocytes. Immunol Today 8:67, 1987
33. Dean BM, Walker R, Boen AJ, Baird JD, Cooke A: Pre-diabetes in the spontaneously diabetic BB/E rat: lymphocyte subpopulations in the pancreatic infiltrate and expression of rat MHC class II molecules in endocrine cells: Diabetologia 28:614, 1985
34. De Baets MH: Autoimmune endocrine diseases. In Concepts in Immunopathology, Vol 2, edited by Cruse JM, Lewis RE, p 1. Basel, Karger, 1985
35. Debray-Sachs M, Boitard C, Assau R, Hamburger J: Are activated macrophages cytotoxic against normal cells. Transplant Proc 13:1111, 1981
36. Dixon FJ, Theofilopoulos AN, McConahey P, Prud'homme GJ: Murine systemic lupus erythematosus (SLE). In Progress in Immunology V, edited by Yamamura Y, Tada T, p 1115. Japan, Academic Press, 1983
37. Dobashi K, Ono S, Murakami S, Takahama Y, Katoh Y, Hamaoka T: Polyclonal B cell activation by a cell differentiation factor, B151-TRF2. III. B151-TRF2 as a B cell differentiation factor closely associated with autoimmune disease. J Immunol 138:780, 1987
38. Dobersen MJ: Humoral autoimmune aspects of insulin dependent

diabetes mellitus. In Concepts in Immunopathology, Vol 2, edited by Cruse JM, Lewis RE, p 32. Basel, Karger, 1985

39. Dolph OA, Hamilton TA: Molecular transductional mechanisms by which interferon gamma and other signals regulate macrophage development. Immunol Rev 97:5, 1987
40. Durum SK, Schmidt JA, Oppenheim JJ: Interleukin 1: an immunological perspective. Ann Rev Immunol 3:263, 1985
41. Dyrberg T, Nakhooda AF, Baekkeskov S, Lernmark A, Poussier P, Marliss EB: Islet cell surface antibodies and lymphocyte antibodies in the spontaneously diabetic BB Wistar rat. Diabetes 31:278, 1982
42. Dziarski R: Preferential induction of autoantibody secretion in polyclonal activation by peptidoglycan and lipopolysaccharide. J Immunol 128:1026, 1982
43. Emery P, Williamson DJ, Mackay IR: Role of cytokines in rheumatological inflammation. In Concepts in Immunopathology, Vol 4, edited by Cruse JM, Lewis RE, p 171. Basel, Karger, 1987
44. Fauci AS: Immunoregulation and autoimmunity: J Allergy Clin Immunol 66:5, 1980
45. Feldmann M: Regulation of HLA class II expression and its role in autoimmune disease. In Autoimmunity and Autoimmune Disease, edited by Evered D, Whelan J, p 88. Chichester, John Wiley and Sons, 1987
46. Fish F, Ziff M: The in vitro and in vivo induction of anti- double stranded DNA antibodies in normal and autoimmune mice. J Immunol 128:409, 1982
47. Forbes RDC, Parfrey NA, Gomersall M, Darden AG, Guttmann RD: Dendritic cell-lymphoid cell aggregation and major histocompatibility expression during rat cardiac allograft rejection. J Exp Med 164:1239, 1986
48. Foulis AK, Farquharson MA: Aberrant expression of HLA-DR antigens by insulin-containing beta cells in recent- onset type I diabetes mellitus: Diabetes 35:1215, 1986
49. Freund J, Stern ER, Pisani TM: Isoallergic encephalomyelitis in guinea pigs after one injection of brain and mycobacteria in water-in-oil emulsion. J Immunol 57:179, 1947
50. Garman RG, Jacobs KA, Clark SC, Raulet DH: BSF2 (beta2 interferon) functions as a second signal for IL-2 production by mature murine T cells. Proc Natl Acad Sci USA 84:7629, 1987
51. Gay D, Maddon P, Sekaly R, Talle MA, Godfrey M, Long E, Goldstein G, Chess L, Axel R, Kappler J, Marrack P: Functional interaction between human T cell protein CD4 and the major histocompatibility complex HLA-DR antigen. Nature 328:626, 1987
52. Gefler M, Marrack P: Development and modification of the lymphocyte repertoire. Nature 321:116, 1986
53. Gepts W: Pathologic anatomy of the pancreas in juvenile diabetes mellitus. Diabetes 14:619, 1965
54. Gillis S: Interleukin-2: biology and biochemistry. J Clin Immunol 3:1, 1983
55. Gleichmann E, VanElven EH, Vander Veen JPW: A systemic lupus erythematosus-like disease in mice induced by abnormal T-B cooperation. Preferential formation of autoantibodies characteristic of SLE. Eur J Immunol 12:152, 1982
56. Greene WC, Depper JM, Kronke M, Leonard WJ: The human interleukin 2 receptor: analysis of structure and function. Immunol Rev 92:29, 1986
57. Greiner DL, Mordes JP, Handler ES, Angelillo M, Nakamura N, Rossini AA: Depletion of RT6.1+ T lymphocytes induces diabetes in resistant BB/W rats. J Exp Med 166:461, 1987
58. Gromo G, Geller RL, Inverardi L, Bach FH: Signal requirements in a step-wise functional maturation of cytotoxic T lymphocytes. Nature 327:424, 1987
59. Guttmann RD, Colle E, Michel F, Seemayer T: Spontaneous diabetes mellitus syndrome in the rat. II. T lymphopenia and its association with clinical disease and pancreatic lymphocytic infiltration. J Immunol 130:1732, 1983
60. Hall BM, Bishop GA, Duggin GG, Horvath JS, Philips J, Tiller DJ: Increased expression of HLA-DR antigens on renal tubular cells in renal transplants: relevance to the rejection response. Lancet 2:247, 1984
61. Hamaoka T, Ono S: Regulation of B-cell differentiation. Ann Rev Immunol 4:167, 1986
62. Hanafusa T, Pujol-Borrell R, Chiovato L, Russell RCG, Doniach D, Bottazzo GF: Aberrant expression of HLA-DR antigen on thyrocytes in Grave's disease: relevance for autoimmunity. Lancet ii:1111, 1983
63. Hang L, Slack JH, Amundson C, Izui S, Theofilopoulos AN, Dixon FJ: Induction of murine autoimmune disease by chronic polyclonal B cell activation. J Exp Med 157:874, 1983
64. Hang LM, Theofilopoulos AN, Dixon FJ: A spontaneous rheumatoid arthritis-like disease in MRL/1 mice. J Exp Med 155:1690, 1982
65. Hashim GA: Myelin basic protein: structure, function and antigen determinants. Immunol Rev 39:60, 1978
66. Herberman RB: Multiple functions of natural killer cells, including immunoregulation as well as resistance to tumor growth. In Concepts in Immunopathology, Vol 1, edited by Cruse JM, Lewis RE, p 96, Basel, Karger, 1985
67. Herzenberg LA, Stall AM, Lalor PA, Sidman C, Moore WA, Parks DR, Herzenber LA: The Ly-1 B cell lineage. Immunol Rev 93:81, 1986
68. Hinrichs DJ, Wegmann KW, Dietsch GN: Transfer of experimental allergic encephalomyelitis to bone marrow chimeras. Endothelial cells are not a restricting element. J Exp Med 166:1906, 1987
69. Hirano T, Yasukawa K, Harada H, Taga T, Watanabe Y, Matsuda T, Kashiwamura S-I, Nakajima K, Koyama K, Iwamatsu A, Tsunasawa S, Sakiyama F, Matsui K, Takahara Y, Taniguchi T, Kishimoto T: Complementary DNA for a novel human interleukin (BSF-2) that induces B lymphocytes to produce immunoglobulin. Nature 324:73, 1986
70. In't Veld PA, Van De Winkel M, Markholst H, Rozing J, Gepts W, Pipeleers DG: Insulin-reactivity of non-endocrine Ia postive islet cells (abstr). Diabetes 37 (Suppl):6A, 1988
71. Isenberg D, Shoenfeld Y: The origin and significance of anti-DNA antibodies. Immunol Today 8:279, 1987
72. Jabs DA, Prendergast RA: Reactive lymphocytes in lacrimal gland and vasculitic renal lesions of autoimmune MRL/1pr mice express L3T4. J Exp Med 166:1198, 1987
73. Jansson R, Karlsson A, Forsum U: Intrathyroid HLA-DR expression and T lymphocyte phenotypes in Graves's thyrotoxicosis, Hashimoto's thyroiditis and nodular colloid goitre. Clin Exp Immunol 58:264, 1985
74. Jenkinson EJ, Jhittay P, Kingston R, Owen JJ: Studies of the role of the thymic microenvironment in the induction of tolerance to HMC antigens. Transplantation 39:331, 1985
75. Kabat EA, Wolf A, Bezer AE: Rapid production of acute disseminated encephalomyelitis in rhesus monkey by injection of heterologous and homologous brain tissue with adjuvants. J Exp Med 85:117, 1947
76. Katooka S, Stoh J, Fujiya H, Toyota T, Suzuki R: Immunologic aspects of the non-obese diabetic (NOD) mouse. Diabetes 32:247, 1983
77. Kibler RF, Fritz RB, Chou FC-H, Chou C-HJ, Peacocke NY, Brown NM, McFarlin DF: Immune response of Lewis rats to peptide C1 (residues 68–88) of guinea pig and rat myelin basic proteins. J Exp Med 146:1323, 1977
78. Kinashi T, Harada N, Severinson E, Tanabe T, Sideras P, Konishi M, Azuma C, Tominaga A, Bergstedt-Lindqvist S, Takahashi M, Matsuda F, Yaoita Y, Takatsu K, Honjo T: Cloning of complementary DNA encoding T-cell replacing factor and identity with B cell-growth factor II. Nature 324:70, 1986
79. Kingston R, Jenkinson EJ, Owen JJT: A single stem cell can recolonise an embryonic thymus producing phenotypically distinct T-cell populations. Nature 317:811, 1985
80. Klareskog L, Forsum U, Scheynius A, Kabelitz D, Wigzell H: Evidence in support of a self-perpetuating HLA-DR-dependent delayed-type cell reaction in rheumatoid arthritis. Proc Natl Acad Sci USA 72:3632, 1982
81. Klasen IS, Ladestein RMT, Donselaar IG, Van Den Berg WB, Tees R, Benner R: Joint inflammation in mice induced by a $MT4^+$ $Lyt2^-$ T cell clone. J Immunol 139:3275, 1987
82. Klinman DM, Steinberg AD: Systemic autoimmune disease arises from polyclonal B cell activation. J Exp Med 165:1755, 1987
83. Koevary S, Rossini AA, Stoller W, Chich W, Williams RM: Passive transfer of diabetes in the BB/W rat. Science 220:727, 1983
84. Koevary S, Williams RM, Stoller W, Chick W: Passive transfer of diabetes in BB/W and WF rats (abstr). Diabetes 32:200, 1983
85. Kofler R, Dixon FJ, Theofilopoulos AN: The genetic origin of autoantibodies. Immunol Today 8:374, 1987
86. Krakauer RS, Waldmann TA, Strober W: Loss of suppressor T cells in adult NZB/NZW mice. J Exp Med 144:662, 1976
87. Kronenberg M, Siu G, Hood LE, Shastri N: The molecular ge-

netics of the T-cell antigen receptor and T-cell antigen recognition. Ann Rev Immunol 4:529, 1986
88. Kruisbeek A, Mond J, Fowlkes BJ, Carmen J, Bridges S, Longo DL: Abscence of the Lyt-2^-, L3T4^+ lineage of T cells in mice treated neonatally with anti-I-A correlates with absence of intrathymic I-A bearing antigen-presenting cell. J Exp Med 161:1029, 1985
89. Kurt-Jones EA, Hamberg S, Ohara J, Paul WE, Abbas AK: Heterogeneity of helper/inducer T lymphocytes. J Exp Med 166:1774, 1987
90. Lampert IA, Suitters AJ, Chisholm PM: Expression of Ia antigen on epidermal keratinocytes in graft vs host disease. Nature 293:149, 1981
91. Laupacis A, Gardell C, Dupre J, Stiller CR, Keown P, Wallace AC: Cyclosporin prevents diabetes in BB Wistar rats. Lancet i:10, 1983
92. Lernhardt W, Karasuyama H, Rolind A, Melchers F: Control of the cell cycle of murine B lymphocytes: The nature of alpha and beta-B-cell growth factors and of B-cell maturation factors. Immunol Rev 99:241, 1987
93. Li JH, Shevach EM, Mizuguchi J, Ohara J, Mosmann T, Paul WE: B cell stimulatory factor 1 (IL-4) is a potent costimulant for normal resting T lymphocytes. J Exp Med 165:157, 1987
94. Like AA, Biron CA, Weringer EJ, Byman K, Sroczynski E, Guberski DL: Prevention of diabetes in BB rats with monoclonal antibodies that recognize T lymphocytes or natural killer cells. J Exp Med 164:1145, 1986
95. Like AA, Kislauskis E, Williams RM, Rossini AA: Neonatal thymectomy prevents spontaneous diabetes mellitus in the BB/W rat. Science 216:644, 1982
96. Like AA, Weringer EJ, Holdash A, McGill P, Atkinson D, Rossini AA: Adoptive transfer of autoimmune diabetes mellitus in BB/W inbred and hybrid rats. J Immunol 134:1583, 1985
97. Linker-Israeli M, Bakke AC, Kitridou RC, Gendler S, Gillis S, Horwitz DA: Defective production of IL-1 and IL-2 in patients with systemic lupus erythematosus. J Immunol 130:2651, 1983
98. Littman DR: The structure of the CD4 and CD8 genes. Ann Rev Immunol 5:561, 1987
99. Lo D, Sprent J: Identity of cells that imprint H-2-restricted T-cell specificity in the thymus. Nature 319:672, 1986
100. Logothetopoulos J, Valiquette N, MacGregor D, Hsia T: Transfer of Diabetes in neonatal rats: tissue localization of injected blasts. Diabetes 36:1116, 1987
101. Loh EY, Lanier LL, Turck CW, Littman DR, Davis MM, Chien Y-H, Weiss A: Identification and sequence of a fourth human T cell antigen receptor chain. Nature 330:569, 1987
102. Londei M, Bottazzo GF, Feldmann M: Human T cell clones from autoimmune thyroid glands: specific recognition of autologous thyroid cells. Science 228:85, 1985
103. Londei M, Lamb JR, Bottazzo GF, Feldmann M: Epithelial cells expressing aberrant MHC class II determinants can present antigen to cloned human T cells. Nature 312:639, 1984
104. Longo DL, Davis ML: Early appearance of donor-type antigen-presenting cells in the thymus of 1200 R radiation-induced bone marrow chimeras correlates with self-recognition of donor I region gene products. J Immunol 130:2525, 1983
105. Mahi-Brown CA, Yule TD, Tung KSK: Adoptive transfer of murine autoimmune orchitis to naive recipients with immune lymphocytes. Cell Immunol 106:408, 1987
106. Mandrup-Poulsen T, Bendtzen K, Nerup J, Dinarello CA, Svenson M, Nielsen JH: Affinity-purified human I 7 interleukin 1 is cytotoxic to isolated islets of Langerhans. Diabetologia 29:63, 1986
107. Mandrup-Poulsen T, Bendtzen K, Nerup J, Egeberg J, Nielsen JH: Mechanisms of pancreatic islet destruction: dose-dependent cytotoxic effect of soluble blood mononuclear cell mediators on isolated islet of Langerhans. Allergy 41:250, 1986
108. Mandrup-Poulsen T, Bendtzen, Nielsen JH, Bendenes G, Nerup J: Cytokines cause functional and structural damage to isolated islets of Langerhans. Allergy 40:424, 1985
109. Markmann JF, Hichey WF, Kimura H, Woehrle M, Barker CF, Naji A: Gamma interferon induces novel expression of Ia antigens by rat pancreatic islet endocrine cells. Pancreas 2:258, 1987
110. Marliss EB, Nakhooda AF, Poussier P, Sima AAF: The diabetic syndrome of the BB rat: possible relevance to type 1 (insulin-dependent) diabetes in man. Diabetologia 22:225, 1982
111. Miescher GC, Budd RC, Lees RK, MacDonald HR: Abnormal expression of T cell receptor genes in Lyt2^-, L3T4^+ lymphocytes of lpr mice: comparison with normal immature thymocytes. J Immunol 138:1959, 1987
112. Milich DR: Genetic and Molecular basis for T- and B-cell recognition of hepatitis B viral antigens. Immunol Rev 99:71, 1987
113. Miller BJ, Appel MC, O'Neil JJ, Wicker LS: Adoptive transfer of T cell subsets in NOD mice (abstr). Diabetes 37 (Suppl):4A, 1988
114. Mordes JP, Desemone J, Rossini AA: The BB rat: Diab Metab Rev 3:725, 1987
115. Morgan I: Allergic encephalomyelitis in monkeys in response to injection of normal monkey nervous tissue. J Exp Med 85:131, 1947
116. Morrison LR: Disseminated encephalomyelitis experimentally produced by use of homologous antigen. Arch Neurol Psychiatry 58:391, 1947
117. Mosmann TR, Coffman RL: Two types of mouse helper-T cell clone. Immunol Today 8:223, 1987
118. Naji A, Silvers WK, Barker CF: Autoimmunity and type I (insulin-dependent) diabetes mellitus. Transplantation 36:355, 1983
119. Nerup J, Andersen OO, Bendixen G, Egeverg J, Poulsen JE: Antipancreatic cellular hypersensitivity in diabetes mellitus. Diabetes 20:424, 1971
120. Ortiz-Ortiz L, Nakamura RM, Weigle WO: T cell requirement for experimental allergic encephalomyelitis induction in the rat. J Immunol 117:576, 1976
121. Oschilewski V, Kiesel V, Kolb H: Administration of silica prevents diabetes in BB rats. Diabetes 34:197, 1985
122. Parfrey NA, Prud'homme GJ, Colle E, Ono SJ, Fuks A, Seemayer TA, Guttmann RD: Immunologic and genetic studies of diabetes in the BB rat. CRC Critical Rev Immunol, in press 1988
123. Parfrey NA, Prud'homme GJ, Ste-Croix: Major histocompatibility complex induction in graft-*vs*-host disease (abstr). Lab Invest, in press 1988
124. Paterson, PY, Day ED, Whitacare CC: Neuroimmunologic Diseases: Effector cell responses and immunoregulatory mechanisms. Immunol Rev 55:89, 1981
125. Paul WE, Ohara J: B-cell stimulatory factor-1/interleukin 4. Ann Rev Immunol 5:429, 1987
126. Penhale WJ, Farmer A, Irvine WJ: Thyroiditis in T cell depleted rats. Clin Exp Immunol 21:362, 1975
127. Pfeifer JD, McKenzie DT, Swain SL, Dutton RW: B cell stimulatory factor 1 (IL-4) is sufficient for the proliferation and differentiation of lectin-stimulated CTL precursors. J Exp Med 166:1464, 1987
128. Pike BL, Alderson MR, Nossal GJV: T-independent activation of single B cells: an orderly analysis of overlapping stages in thee activation pathway. Immunol Rev 99:119, 1987
129. Pontes de Carvalho L, Wick G, Roitt IM: Requirement of T cells for the development of spontaneous autoimmune thyroiditis in obese strain chickens. J Immunol 126:750, 1981
130. Prud'homme GJ, Balderas RS, Dixon FJ, Theofilopoulos AN: B cell dependence on and response to accessory signals in murine lupus strains. J Exp Med 157:1815, 1983
131. Prud'homme, GJ, Colle E, Fuks A, Goldner-Sauve A, Guttmann RD: Cellular immune abnormalities and autoreactive T lymphocytes in insulin-dependent diabetes mellitus in rats. Immunol Today 6:160, 1985
132. Prud'homme GJ, Colle E, Fuks A, Guttmann RD: Major histocompatibility complex restriction of T lymphocyte responses to islet cell antigens in IDDM rats. Diabetes 36:237, 1987
133. Prud'homme GJ, Fieser TM, Dixon FJ, Theofilopoulos AN: B cell-tropic interleukins in murine systemic lupus erythematosus (SLE). Immunol Rev 78:159, 1984
134. Prud'homme GJ, Fuks A, Colle E, Guttmann RD: Isolation of T lymphocyte lines with specificity for islet cell antigens from spontaneously diabetic (insulin-dependent) rats. Diabetes 33:801, 1984
135. Prud'homme GJ, Fuks A, Colle E, Seemayer TA, Guttmann RD: Immune dysfunction in diabetes-prone BB rats. J Exp Med 159:463, 1984
136. Prud'homme GJ, Fuks A, Guttmann RD, Colle E: T cell hybrids with specificity for islet cell antigens. J Immunol 151:1535, 1986
137. Prud'homme GJ, Lapchak P, Parfrey NA, Colle E, Guttmann RD: Autoimmunity-prone BB rats lack functional cytotoxic T cells. Cell Immunol 114:198, 1988
138. Prud'homme GJ, Park CL, Feiser TM, Kofler R, Dixon FJ, Theofilopoulos AN: Identification of a B cell differentiation factor

(s) spontaneously produced by proliferating T cells in murine lupus strains of the lpr/lpr genotype. J Exp Med 157:730, 1983
139. Prud'homme GJ, Sohn U, Delovitch TL: The role of H-2 and Ia antigens in graft-vs-host reactions. J Exp Med 149:137, 1979
140. Pujol-Borrell R, Todd I, Doshi M, Bottazzo GF, Sutton R, Gray D, Adolf GR, Feldmann M: HLA class II induction in human islet cells by interferon gamma plus tumor necrosis factor or lymphotoxin: Nature 326:364, 1987
141. Pujol-Borrell R, Todd I, Doshi M, Gray D, Feldmann M, Bottazzo GF: Differential expression and regulation of MHC products in the endocrine and exocrine cells of the human pancreas. Clin Exp Immunol 65:128, 1986
142. Pukel C, Baquerizo, Rabinovitch A: Interleukin 2 activates BB/W diabetic rat lymphoid cells cytotoxic to islet cells. Diabetes 36:1217, 1987
143. Pukel C, Baquerizo H, Rabinovitch A: Leukocyte associated polypeptides (cytokines) involved in cytolysis of islet cells in vitro (abstr). Diabetes 37 (Suppl):7A, 1988
144. Rabin BS, Griffith BP, Hardesty RL: Vascular endothelial cell HLA-DR antigen and myocyte necrosis in human allograft rejection. Heart Transplant 4:293, 1985
145. Rivers TM, Schwentker FF: Encephalomyelitis accompanied by myelin destruction experimentally produced in monkeys. J Exp Med 61:689, 1935
146. Rivers TM, Sprunt DH, Berry GP: Observations on attempt to produce acute disseminated encephalomyelitis in monkeys. J Exp Med 58:39, 1933
147. Romball CG, Weigle WO: Transfer of experimental autoimmune thyroiditis with T cell clones. J Immunol 138:1092, 1987
148. Ron Y, Sprent J: T cell priming in vivo: a major role for B cells in presenting antigen to T cells in lymph nodes. J Immunol 138:2848, 1987
149. Rose NR, Bacon LD, Sundick RS, Kong YM, Esquivel P, Bigazzi PE: Genetic regulation in autoimmune thyroiditis. In Autoimmunity, edited by Talal N, p 63. New York, Academic Press, 1977
150. Rossini AA, Mordes JP, Like AA: Immunology of insulin dependent diabetes mellitus. Ann Rev Immunol 3:289, 1985
151. Rossini AA, Williams RM, Mordes JP, Appel MC, Like AA: Spontaneous diabetes in the gnotobiotic BB/W rat. Diabetes 28:1031, 1979
152. Royer HD, Ramarli D, Acuto O, Campen TJ, Reinherz EL: Genes encoding the T cell receptor Ti alpha and beta subunits are transcribed in an ordered manner during intrathymic ontogeny. Proc Natl Acad Sci USA 82:5510, 1985
153. Rudd CE, Morimoto C, Wong LL, Schlossman SF: The subdivision of the T4 (CD4) subset on the basis of the differential expression of L-C/T200 antigens. J Exp Med 166:1758, 1987
154. Ruddle NH: Lymphotoxin production in AIDS. Immunol Today 7:8, 1986
155. Samelson LE, Lindsten T, Fowlkes BJ, Van Den Elsen P, Terhorst C, Davis MM, Germain RN, Schwartz RH: Expression of genes of the T-cell antigen receptor complex in precursor thymocytes. Nature 315:765, 1985
156. Schlomchik MJ, Marshak-Rothstein, Wolfowicz CB, Rothstein TL, Weigert MG: The role of clonal selection and somatic mutation in autoimmunity. Nature 328:805, 1987
157. Schrader JW: The panspecific hemopoietin of activated T lymphocytes (interleukin 3). Ann Rev Immunol 4:205, 1986
158. Schwartz RS: Monoclonal lupus autoantibodies. Immunol Today 4:68, 1983
159. Schwizer RW, Leiter EH, Evans R: Macrophage mediated cytotoxicity against cultured pancreatic islet cells. Transplantation 37:539, 1984
160. Seemayer TA, Tannenbaum GS, Goldman H, Colle E: Dynamic time course studies of the spontaneously diabetic BB Wistar rat. Am J Pathol 106:237, 1982
161. Shortman K, Scollay R, Wilson A, Chen WF, Ewing T: Mature and immature thymocytes. In Progress in Immunology, Vol VI, edited by Cinader B, Miller RG, p 95. Orlando, Academic Press, 1986
162. Sibley R, Sutherland DER, Goetz F, Michael AK: Recurrent diabetes mellitus in the pancreas iso- and allograft. Lab Invest 53:132, 1985
163. Sidman CL, Marshall JD, Shultz LD, Gray PW, Johnson HM: Gamma interferon is one of several direct B cell maturing lymphokines. Nature 309:801, 1984
164. Simon J, Anzil AP: Immunohistological evidence of perivascular localization of basic protein in early development of EAE: Acta Neuropathol 27:33, 1974
165. Smith HR, Steinberg AD: Autoimmunity—a perspective. Ann Rev Immunol 1:175, 1983
166. Snapper CM, Paul WE: Interferon gamma and BSF-1 reciprocally regulated Ig isotype production. Science 236:944, 1987
167. Sobel RA, Blanchette BW, Bhan AK, Colvin RB: The immunopathology of experimental allergic encephalomyelitis. II. Endothelial cell Ia increases prior to inflammatory cell infiltration. J Immunol 132:2402, 1984
168. Spitz H, Yssel H, Takelve Y, Arai N, Yokota T, Lee F, Arai KI, Banchereau J, De Vries JE: Recombinant interleukin 4 promotes growth of human T cells. J Immunol 139:1142, 1987
169. Sprent J, Schaefer M, Lo D, Korngold R: Functions of purified L3T4$^+$ and Lyt-2$^+$ cells in vitro and in vivo. Immunol Rev 91:195, 1986
170. Sriram S, Ranges GE: Immunotherapy of autoimmune disease with T cell subset specific antibodies. In Concepts in Immunopathology, Vol 4, edited by Cruse JM, Lewis RE, p 275. Basel, Karger, 1987
171. Steiman RM, Inaba K, Schuler G, Witmer M: Stimulation of the immune response: contribution of dendritic cells. In Mechanisms of Host Resistance to Infectious Agents, Tumors, and Allografts, edited by Steiman RM, North RJ, p 71. New York, The Rockefeller Press, 1986
172. Swain SL, Dutton RW: Consequences of the direct interaction of helper T cells with B cells presenting antigen. Immunol Rev 99:263, 1987
173. Theofilopoulos AN, Balderas RS, Shawler DL, Lee S, Dixon FJ: Influence of the thymic genotype on the systemic lupus erythematosus-like disease of and T cell proliferation of MRL/lpr mice. J Exp Med 153:1405, 1981
174. Theofilopoulos AN, Dixon FJ: Murine models of systemic lupus erythematosus. Adv Immunol 37:269, 1985
175. Theofilopoulos AN, Prud'homme GJ, Dixon FJ: Autoimmune aspects of systemic lupus erythematosus. In Concepts in Immunopathology, Vol. 1, edited by Cruse JM, Lewis RE, p 190. Basel, Karger, 1985
176. Theofilopoulos AN, Prud'homme GJ, Feiser TM, Dixon FJ: B cell hyperactivity in murine lupus. I. Immunological abnormalities in lupus-prone strains and the activation of normal B cells. Immunology Today 4:287, 1983
177. Theofilopoulos AN, Prud'homme GJ, Feiser TM, Dixon FJ: B cell hyperactivity in murine lupus. II. Defects in response to and production of accessory signals in lupus-prone mice. Immunology Today 4:317, 1983
178. Theofilopoulos AN, Shawler DL, Eisenberg RA, Dixon FJ: Splenic immunoglobulin secreting cells and their regulation in autoimmune mice. J Exp Med 151:446, 1980
179. Trepecchio W, Maruya A, Barrett KJ: The heavy chain genes of a lupus anti-DNA autoantibody are encoded in the germ line of a nonautoimmune strain of mouse and conserved in strains of mice polymorphic for these gene locus. J Immunol 139:3139, 1987
180. Tung KSK, Smith S, Matzner P, Kasai K, Oliver J, Feuchter F, Anderson R: Murine autoimmune oophoritis. epididymoorchitis and gastritis induced by day 3 thymectomy: autoantibodies. Am J Pathol 126:303, 1987
181. Tung KSK, Smith S, Teuscher C, Chester C, Anderson RE: Murine autoimmune oophoritis, epididymoorchitis, and gastritis induced by day 3 thymectomy: immunopathology. Am J Pathol 126:293, 1987
182. Tung KSK, Yule TD, Mahi-Brown CA, Listrom MB: Distribution of histopathology and Ia positive cells in actively induced and passively transferred experimental autoimmune orchitis. J Immunol 138:752, 1987
183. Van Eden W, Holoshitz J, Cohen I: Antigen mimicry between mycobacteria and cartilage proteoglycans. In Concepts in Immunopathology, Vol 4, edited by Cruse JM, Lewis RE, p 144. Basel, Karger, 1987
184. Van Rappard-van der veen FM, Kiesel U, Poels L, Schuler W, Melief CJM, Lanckgent J, Gleichman E: Further evidence against random polyclonal antibody formation in mice with lupus-like graft-vs-host disease. J Immunol 132:1814, 1984
185. Vitetta ES, Bossie A, Fernandez-Botran R, Myers CD, Oliver KG, Sanders VM, Stevens TL: Interaction and activation of antigen-specific T and B cells. Immunol Rev 99:193, 1987
186. Wagner H, Hardt C, Rouse BT, Rollinghoff M, Schewich P,

Pfizemaier K: Dissection of the proliferative and differentiative signals controlling murine cytotoxic T lymphocyte responses. J Exp Med 155:1876, 1982

187. Waldor MK, Sriram S, Hardy R, Herzenberg LA, Lanier L, Lim M, Steiman L: Reversal of experimental allergic encephalomyelitis with monoclonal antibody to a T-cell subset marker. Science 227:415, 1985

188. Weiss A, Imboden J, Hardy K, Manger B, Terhorst C, Stobo J: The role of the T3/antigen receptor complex in T-cell activation. Ann Rev Immunol 4:593, 1986

189. Wekerle H: The lesion of acute experimental autoimmune encephalomyelitis: isolation and membrane phenotypes of lymphovascular complexes from encephalitic rat brain white matter. Lab Invest 51:199, 1984

190. Wekerle H, Fierz W: T lymphocyte autoimmunity in experimental autoimmune encephalomyelitis. In Concepts in Immunopathology, Vol 2, edited by Cruse JM, Lewis RE, p 102. Basel, Karger, 1985

191. Weston KM, Yeh ETH, Sy MS: Autoreactivity accelerates the development of autoimmunity and lymphoproliferation in MRL/lpr mice. J immunol 139:743, 1987

192. Wick G, Kite JF, Cole RK, Witebsky ES: Spontaneous autoimmune thyroiditis in the obese strain of chickens. III. The effect of bursectomy on the development of disease. J Immunol 104:45, 1970

193. Wick G, Kite JH, Witebsky E: Spontaneous thyroiditis in the obese strain of chickens IV. The effect of thymectomy and thymobursectomy on the development of disease. J Immunol 104:54, 1970

194. Woda BA, Handler ES, Padden C, Greiner DL, Reynolds C, Rossini AA: Anti-asialo GM1 prevents diabetes in diabetes prone but not RT6.1 depleted diabetes resistant BB rats (abstr). Diabetes 36 (Suppl 1):39, 1987

195. Woda BA, Like AA, Padden C, McFadden ML: Deficiency of phenotypic cytotoxic-suppressor T lymphocytes in the BB/W rat. J Immunol 136:856, 1986

196. Wofsy D: Administration of monoclonal anti-T cell antibodies retards murine lupus in BXSB mice. J Immunol 136:4554, 1986

197. Wofsy D, Seaman WE: Reversal of advanced murine lupus in NZB/NZW F1 mice by treatment with monoclonal antibody to L3T4. J Immunol 138:3247, 1987

198. Wong GHW, Goeddel DV: Tumor necrosis factors alpha and beta inhibit replication and synergize with interferons. Nature 323:819, 1987

199. Zier KS, Leo MR, Spielman RS, Baker L: Decreased synthesis of IL-2 in insulin dependent diabetes mellitus. Diabetes 33:552, 1984

200. Zubler RH, Glasebrook AL: Requirements for three signals in T-independent (lipopolysaccharide-induced) as well as T-dependent B cell responses. J Exp Med 155:666, 1982

Biology of Disease

Early Biochemical Events in Leukocyte Activation

REBECCA R. SANDBORG AND JAMES E. SMOLEN

Division of Pediatric Hematology-Oncology and Department of Pathology, University of Michigan Medical School, Ann Arbor, Michigan

INTRODUCTION

The neutrophil plays a key role in host defense by ingesting and destroying foreign cells and other infectious agents. During the inflammatory process, chemotactic factors generated by bacteria, damaged tissue, the complement system and other phagocytes serve as a signaling mechanism to recruit neutrophils to sites of infection and to stimulate the cell to exercise its destructive capabilities. These responses are initiated by the interaction of activating stimuli with specific cell surface receptors, resulting in directional movement of the neutrophil toward the chemotactic source. When the neutrophil encounters an ingestible particle, its pseudopod flows around it and fuses at the distal pole of the particle, thus forming a phagosome. Once ingestion occurs, there are two major mechanisms by which the particle is eliminated. Hydrolytic and bactericidal enzymes are released from cytoplasmic granules into the phagosomal compartment by the process of degranulation. Ingested material is also vulnerable to attack by reactive oxygen metabolites produced by the phagosomal membrane. The significance of these degradative processes to host defense is best illustrated in patients with various disorders of neutrophil function who suffer from severe and recurrent infections.

Activated neutrophils, like other secretory cells, undergo a number of biochemical changes which enable the cell to respond to surface stimulation. In recent years, significant progress has been made in identifying the molecular factors regulating these changes, as well as the temporal sequence in which they occur. However, our understanding is still incomplete and a considerable amount of research in this area remains to be conducted. The purpose of this review is to discuss the general mechanisms by which neutrophils transduce receptor-mediated stimuli into functional cellular responses. Attention has also been given to disorders of granule secretion since studies in defective neutrophils have expanded our knowledge of basic neutrophil physiology.

NEUTROPHIL GRANULES

In order to comprehend the roles neutrophils play in inflammation and host defense, it is useful to review the contents of the cytoplasmic granules. This section briefly describes the granules and their membranes.

Primary Granules

Neutrophil granules serves as reservoirs for digestive and hydrolytic enzymes before delivery into the phagosome. Based on their biochemical and morphologic properties and time of appearance during cell maturation, three major granule populations have been described. Azurophil or primary granules are synthesized first during granulocytopoiesis and contain myeloperoxidase, neutral proteases (elastase, cathepsin G, cathepsin D), acid hydrolases (β-glucuronidase, acid phosphatase, α-mannosidase, *N*-acetylglucosaminidase) and cationic proteins (122, 144, 152, 186, 223, 316, 354, 373, 422, 438). Two subpopulations of azurophil granules have been identified and differ in their distribution of several lysosomal enzymes (54, 120, 373, 422). Elastase can be preferentially released from the denser subpopulation (120), suggesting that these granule subpopulations may be under separate secretory control.

Azurophil granule proteins possess microbicidal activity and may additionally play a significant role in the tissue destruction observed during inflammatory reactions. Defensins are defined mcirobicidal peptides which are found in these granules (119, 316). These proteins are released concomitantly with other azurophil granule markers after stimulation (118). Bactericidal/permeability-increasing protein, a cationic protein which lyses Gram-negative bacteria, is also found in these granules (103, 421). Myeloperoxidase reacts with H_2O_2 and a halide to produce hypochlorous acid, a potent oxidant believed to significantly contribute to the killing of microorganisms (390). Myeloperoxidase may also play a modulating role in degranulation by its ability to inactivate chemotactic factors (65) and inhibit the mechanisms underlying the respiratory burst (180) and phagocytosis (99, 374). Deficiency of myeloperoxidase is an inherited condition and occurs relatively frequently among the general population (285). Some, but not all, individuals afflicted with this syndrome demonstrate a propensity toward certain opportunistic infections.

With respect to the tissue destruction observed during inflammatory reactions, the most important azurophil constituents are the proteases. Three of these proteases have been well characterized. The serine protease, elastase, hydrolyzes typical pancreatic elastase substrates and a variety of elastin preparations from several sources (268). Cathepsin G is a chymotrypsin-like neutral protease which hydrolyzes proteoglycans and insoluble collagen (402). Finally, cathepsin D can cleave leukokinogens to generate pharmacologically active leukokinins (231). It is also active against proteoglycans. Working in concert, these proteases can exacerbate existing inflammatory reactions by generating chemotactic factors from C5a (416).

Specific Granules

Specific or secondary granules are synthesized later during granulocytopoiesis. Proteins packaged within these granules include lysozyme, alkaline phosphatase, collagenase, vitamin B_{12}-binding protein, and lactoferrin (47, 176, 196, 233, 284, 346, 373). Lysozyme hydrolyzes cell wall proteoglycan of some bacterial species and is also found in azurophil granules. Lactoferrin is an iron-binding protein which appears to be necessary for hydroxyl radical formation (4) and cell adhesion (40). Like certain azurophil granule proteases, several specific granule proteins may contribute to inflammatory conditions. Collagenase, in the presence of a neutral protease hydrolyzes collagen fibrils; this enzyme may also be activated by oxidative metabolism (53). In addition, these granules also contain activators of the complement cascade (430). A modulatory role for these granules in cell locomotion is suggested by the observation that specific granule membranes contain receptors for chemoattractants *N*-formyl-methionyl-leucyl-phenylalanine (fMet-Leu-Phe) and C5a, and laminin (109, 264, 391, 436). These granule membranes also possess cytochrome *b* (35) and a flavin adenine dinucleotide containing flavoprotein (34) which appear to translocate to the plasma membrane upon cell stimulation, suggesting the potential for regulation of the respiratory burst. Individuals whose neutrophils are lacking in specific granule contents are susceptible to repeated staphylococcal skin and respiratory infections (46, 181, 382), emphasizing the importance of these proteins in host defense mechanisms. Neutrophils from these patients have impaired chemotaxis and adherence (115). The finding that these cells also do not increase expression of chemotactic receptors following activation is consistent with a role for these granules in locomotion and may underlie their defective chemotactic response.

Tertiary Granules

Although not well characterized, neutrophils also possess a granule population that cosediments with specific granules in most preparative schemes (95). These granules contain gelatinase (232, 368), an enzyme which bears many similarities to neutrophil collagenase (426). Tertiary granule membranes appear to have a pool of membrane glycoproteins which may participate in cell adhesion (289, 391). The C3bi receptor is essential to cell adhesiveness (6) and there is evidence to suggest that it is partially localized in tertiary granules (289).

As improved methods become available for the isolation and characterization of granules and their constituents, it is likely that other granule populations will be identified. For instance, "phosphasomes" which contain alkaline phosphatase have recently been isolated from neutrophils (36, 347). These granules are lighter in density than specific granules, but do not contain gelatinase. Their relationship to tertiary granules is unknown.

STIMULUS-RESPONSE COUPLING

The current model for the stimulus-response coupling pathway in the neutrophil is thought to involve the following intracellular sequence of events. The binding of a ligand with its receptor results in a conformational change in the receptor with the consequent activation of a membrane-bound guanine nucleotide-binding protein (G protein). Activation of the G protein leads to stimulation of a specific phospholipase C, which catalyzes the hydrolysis of phosphatidylinositol 4,5-bisphosphate to inositol 1,4,5-trisphosphate (IP_3) and 1,2-diacylglycerol. IP_3 induces the release of Ca^{2+} from intracellular membrane depots. 1,2-Diacylglycerol activates the Ca^{2+}-dependent enzyme, protein kinase C. Protein kinase C, through the phosphorylation of cellular proteins, may act alone or in concert with Ca^{2+} to elicit cell responses. Evidence for each event in the stimulus-response coupling pathway will be considered separately.

Receptors and Stimuli

fMet-Leu-Phe Receptors. Neutrophil responses can be evoked by a variety of particulate and soluble stimuli. Opsonized particles, immune complexes and chemotactic factors produced during the inflammatory process activate neutrophils by binding to specific cell surface receptors. Of the neutrophil chemotactic receptors, the *N*-formyl peptide receptor is the best characterized. *N*-Formyl peptides, the synthetic analogs of bacterial products, induce a variety of neutrophil responses and have been extensively employed as activating stimuli. Specific receptors for the chemotactic peptide, fMet-Leu-Phe, have been identified on the neutrophil surface (11, 251, 427) and binding of the formyl peptide to its receptor correlates with the ability of the cell to undergo chemotaxis and degranulation (307). The fMet-Leu-Phe receptor is stereospecific (307), appears to have both high and low affinity binding sites (209, 414), and has an apparent molecular weight of 50 to 70 kilodalton (kd) (3, 162, 249, 308). An intracellular location has also been suggested for the fMet-Leu-Phe receptor, since neutrophil activation results in enhanced fMet-Leu-Phe binding in normal cells (117), but not in egranulated neutrophil cytoplasts (116). These receptors have been identified on the membranes of specific granules and are biochemically similar to those on the cell surface (109, 121) suggesting that they are mobilized to the cell surface following cell activation and may thus serve a modulatory role.

The kinetics of ligand-receptor interactions have been studied using the *N*-formyl peptides. Binding of the chemotactic peptide, *N*-formyl-norleucyl-leucyl-phenylalanine to neutrophil plasma membranes is both time-dependent and saturable (321). *N*-formyl-norleucyl-leucyl-leucyl-phenylalanine, at saturating concentrations, occupies 50% of the available receptors on intact neutrophils within 30 seconds. Similar kinetics are observed by Sklar *et al.* (340), who employ a novel fluorometric technique for measuring the binding of chemotactic peptide. They estimate that no more than 20% of the receptors need to be occupied to evoke an optimal secretory response. However, most of the receptors need to be occupied for the response to be sustained (338).

Complement Receptors. Activation of the complement system generates several proteins with chemotactic activity. C5a, a derivative of C5, the most potent of the chemotactic proteins, induces neutrophil chemotaxis (417), degranulation (59), and superoxide generation (218). These responses result from the interaction of C5a with specific receptors on the cell surface (58). Binding of C5a to its receptor was shown to be reversible and saturable (304). The receptor was identified as a single polypeptide in the plasma membrane with an apparent molecular mass of 40 to 48 kd (165, 304). Binding studies have shown that there are 50,000 to 113,000 receptor sites/cell with a dissociation constant (Kd) of 2×10^{-9} M.

Neutrophils also express receptors for the complement-derived chemotactic factors C3b and C3bi. Receptors for C3b and C3bi (also known as CR1 and CR3, respectively) are sparse on resting neutrophils but significantly increase in number after activation with several stimuli (24, 25). Like fMet-Leu-Phe receptors, the stimulus-induced increase in surface expression of C3b and C3bi receptors appears to result from the mobilization of intracellular pools, although the subcellular locations for these receptors appear to be distinct (264). The C3b receptor is a glycoprotein with a molecular weight of 205 kd (104) and distributed on the plasma membrane within clusters (1).

Lipids. In addition to their participation as putative second messenger products in the stimulus-response coupling pathway, many lipid metabolites may be released from stimulated neutrophils and in turn modulate cell function by interacting with receptors on other neutrophils. Phospholipase A_2, present on both the granules and membranes of neutrophils (110, 112, 177, 345, 392, 393, 401), is activated during neutrophil stimulation (33, 64) yielding arachidonic acid as one of the major end products. Arachidonic acid is not only released from stimulated neutrophils (194, 405, 408, 410–412), but also serves as a stimulus for these cells (5, 240, 281). In addition to directly affecting cell function, metabolites of arachidonic acid, generated through either the cyclooxygenase or lipoxygenase pathways, may also stimulate neutrophils. The most potent cyclooxygenase product of activated neutrophils is thromboxane B_2, which in addition to its vasoconstrictor activity, may also enhance neutrophil chemotaxis (178), aggregation (387), and adhesiveness (370).

Arachindonic acid can also be metabolized by the lipoxygenase pathway to produce hydroxyeicosatetraenoic acids (HETEs), including 5-HETE, 12-HETE and 5,12-diHETE (31, 32). These compounds have also been shown to induce several neutrophil responses (30, 126–129, 239, 256, 260, 325, 376). Stimulated neutrophils also produce the diHETE leukotriene B_4 (LTB_4) through the lipoxygenase pathway. LTB_4 and other leukotrienes can be released in response to a variety of stimuli (2, 62, 63, 280, 299, 300, 306), even from neutrophil cytoplasts (143). Receptors for LTB_4 have been partially purified (108, 133, 134, 204, 205) and their activation serves as a potent stimulus for degranulation (236, 296, 329, 352), chemotaxis (90, 130, 172, 278, 279) and adherence (395).

Another potent mediator of inflammation produced by stimulated neutrophils is 1-O-alkyl-2-acetyl-*sn*-glyceryl-3-phosphorylcholine, also known as platelet-activating factor (PAF) (206, 386, 403, 404). Not only is PAF synthesized by neutrophils, but it has been shown to induce degranulation (61, 171, 257, 261, 262, 349, 350, 431), aggregation (91, 203, 257, 262) and superoxide generation (171). Ng and Wong (248) demonstrated that PAF receptors on neutrophil plasma membranes have a kd of 5×10^{-10} M.

Guanine Nucleotide Binding Proteins

Recent data strongly suggest that receptors for the chemotactic stimuli fMet-Leu-Phe, C5a, LTB_4, and PAF are coupled to cellular responses through a guanine nucleotide binding protein similar to the inhibitory protein, Gi, of the adenylate cyclase system. Evidence linking a G-protein to these receptors has been provided by studies demonstrating that guanine nucleotides can regulate the affinity of the fMet-Leu-Phe, PAF, and LTB_4 receptors (131, 248, 336, 337, 367). A high affinity GTPase located in neutrophil plasma membranes is stimulated by these same receptor-mediated stimuli, but not by the phorbol ester, phorbol 12-myristate 13-acetate (PMA) (106, 166). This enzymatic activity is likely to be involved in terminating the activation of the guanine nucleotide-binding protein.

Studies using pertussis toxin have proven instrumental in the understanding of G-protein involvement in the proposed stimulus-response coupling pathway. Pertussis toxin ADP-ribosylates the α-subunit of Gi of the adenylate cyclase system and also a 40,000 to 41,000 dalton protein in neutrophil plasma membranes (19, 29, 125, 272). Initial studies demonstrated a strong correlation between the ability of the toxin to catalyze the ADP-ribosylation of the membrane protein and to affect cellular responses initiated by surface receptors. However, pertussis toxin did not alter intracellular cyclic AMP levels, suggesting that the G-protein involved was distinct from Gi of the adenylate cyclase system (29). More recently, purification and characterization of a guanine nucleotide-binding protein in neutrophils have shown that this protein differs both structurally and immunochemically from previously reported guanine nucleotide-binding proteins (124, 125).

Not only can neutrophil responses be abolished by pertussis toxin, but stable guanine nucleotides can induce secretion in their own right as well as enhance Ca^{2+}-induced secretion in permeabilized neutrophils (15, 361). Whereas pertussis toxin inhibits fMet-Leu-Phe-induced secretion from intact cells, secretion in response to guanine nucleotides, PMA, and Ca^{2+} in not inhibited in the permeabilized cell system, suggesting that a second G-protein may be involved at more distal sites in secretion (15).

Phosphatidylinositol Metabolism

A membrane-associated phosphoinositide-specific phospholipase is activated upon stimulation with chemotactic stimuli. In particular, phospholipase C hydrolyzes phosphatidylinositol-4,5-bisphosphate (PIP_2) and phosphatidyl inositol-4-monophosphate (42, 69, 70, 98, 389) to the putative second messenger products, inositol 1,4,5-trisphosphate IP_3, and 1,2-diacylglycerol (42, 70, 98, 389). In permeabilized neutrophils, IP_3 has been shown to interact with a specific intracellular receptors (371) and stimulate the release of Ca^{2+} (43, 295). Evidence has been presented that the Ca^{2+} is not derived from either mitochondria (295) or the endoplasmic reticulum (187), but rather from a distinct organelle which has been termed "calciosome" (188). Receptor stimulation also elicits the production of inositol 1,3,4-trisphosphate and inositol 1,3,4,5-tetrakisphosphate, but these compounds do not appear to have significant functional consequences with regard to Ca^{2+} release (43).

It is believed that guanine nucleotide-binding proteins are involved in the receptor-mediated activation of phospholipase C. Chemotactic factors stimulate reductions in PIP_2 levels, and increase inositol phosphate levels (234, 400). These changes are not observed if cells are pretreated with pertussis toxin (344, 400). Fluoride treatment, which stimulates G-proteins, also directly stimulates the accumulation of inositol lipids (383), while stimuli which do not interact with cell surface receptors, such as PMA and A23187, do not induce IP_3 formation (42, 389). It has been suggested that G-proteins regulate phospholipase C activity by lowering the Ca^{2+} requirement necessary for activation to resting Ca^{2+} levels (10, 44). Guanine nucleotides have been shown to stimulate IP_3 production in permeabilized neutrophils (44). This effect is enhanced by fMet-Leu-Phe and inhibited by pertussis toxin. Calcium is also effective in inducing inositol phosphate production, but guanine nucleotides reduce the calcium requirements from millimolar to micromolar levels (44). Similar results have been reported using plasma membranes from HL60 cells (10), although in this study, pertussis toxin was ineffective in abolishing guanine nucleotide-induced inositol phosphate production. The existence of second G-protein, distinct from that linked to the fMet-Leu-Phe receptors, was thus proposed (10).

Recent data indicate that protein kinase C may be important in regulating phospholipase C activity. The protein kinase C activator, PMA inhibits stimulus-induced GTPase activity (214), chemotaxis, capping, Ca^{2+} mobilization, and inositol phosphate production (191, 234, 344), and stimulates the pertussis toxin-mediated ADP-ribosylation of a 41,000 dalton membrane protein (214). Although pertussis toxin treatment results in similar inhibition of these stimulus-induced responses, the mechanism underlying the two effects appears to be different. Pertussis toxin prevents formyl-peptide-stimulated binding of guanine nucleotides to membrane fractions, whereas nucleotide binding is unaffected by pretreatment with PMA (344). In contrast, the hydrolysis of PIP_2 by guanine nucleotides is inhibited by PMA, but not pertussis toxin. It has thus been suggested that phorbol esters acting through protein kinase C modulate the coupling of G-proteins to phospholipase C (344). Pertussis toxin presumably exerts its inhibitory effects through uncoupling of the receptors from the G-protein.

CALCIUM

The importance of Ca^{2+} as an effector of cellular function has received widespread attention in recent years. Like other cell types, the intracellular Ca^{2+} concentration in resting neutrophils is maintained at submicromolar levels by a plasma membrane-bound Ca^{2+}-ATPase pump (193, 265, 266). There is substantial evidence that intracellular Ca^{2+} levels rise in stimulated neutrophils and that these increments may directly or indirectly bring about cell responses.

Elevations in intracellular free Ca^{2+} levels have been directly demonstrated using the fluorescent probes, quin-2 and fura-2 (132, 185, 190, 198, 201, 235, 294, 302, 406, 424). Studies employing quin-2 as the Ca^{2+} probe indicate that after stimulation with fMet-Leu-Phe, intracellular Ca^{2+} rises almost immediately from a resting level of 0.1 to 1 μM (185, 294, 424). Increases in intracellular Ca^{2+} have also been reported using the photoprotein, obelin (348), as well as the Ca^{2+}-sensitive intracellular enzyme, phosphorylase *a* (343). While quantitation of Ca^{2+} levels may be underestimated using quin-2, levels as high as 6 μM have been reported using obelin as the Ca^{2+} indicator (343).

There appear to be two separate pools involved in regulating the stimulus-induced rise in intracellular Ca^{2+} levels; there is an initial mobilization of Ca^{2+} from intracellular depots, followed by an influx of extracellular Ca^{2+}. Studies using chlortetracycline have provided evidence that Ca^{2+} is mobilized from intracellular stores. Neutrophils pretreated with chlortetracycline exhibit a reduction in fluorescence when exposed to any number of stimuli, suggesting that Ca^{2+} is being released from membrane-bound stores (68, 236, 241, 353, 359). 8-(N, N-diethylamido)-octyl 3, 4, 5 trimethoxybenzoate hydrochloride inhibits mobilization of intracellular Ca^{2+} and completely blocks neutrophil responses (351, 357), indicating that mobilization is important in eliciting cellular responses. Although quin-2 and chlortetracycline have been used to monitor changes in intracellular Ca^{2+}, these probes also inhibit cellular responses by their ability to chelate intracellular Ca^{2+} (101, 102, 142, 201, 341, 379). A23187, which, in addition to acting as an ionophore, displaces membrane-bound Ca^{2+} (253), renders cells unresponsive to subsequent stimulation (57, 238). These observations are consistent with the notion that Ca^{2+} derived from intracellular stores is essential to cell activation.

As discussed above, the mechanism by which Ca^{2+} is released after cell activation appears to involve the breakdown of membrane phospholipids (98, 189, 200). In permeabilized neutrophils, IP_3 binds to a specific, saturable receptor (371) and induces the specific release of intracellular Ca^{2+} (295). However, the precise location of the storage pool contributing to observed increases in Ca^{2+} has not been unequivocally identified. The fluorescence of chlortetracycline in labeled neutrophils has been reported to be localized in the plasma membrane and perinuclear region of the cell (68). In this study, fluorescence was observed only from the plasma membrane of neutrophil cytoplasts, suggesting that Ca^{2+} located in the endoplasmic reticulum contributes to the increase in intracellular Ca^{2+}. Such a location has not been verified. In subcellular fractions of neutrophil homogenates, IP_3 only stimulated Ca^{2+} release from microsomes (187). Secretory granules did not release Ca^{2+} although they have been reported to possess Ca^{2+}-pumping activity (179). Further separation of microsomal components suggested that neither the plasma membrane nor the endoplasmic reticulum is involved in sequestering IP_3-sensitive Ca^{2+} (187). An unidentified microsomal component capable of pumping and releasing Ca^{2+} awaits further characterization.

Several lines of evidence suggest that the stimulus-induced rise in intracellular Ca^{2+} also results from an increase in plasma membrane permeability to extracellular Ca^{2+}. Radioisotope studies have demonstrated that Ca^{2+} is taken up from the extracellular medium in response to a variety of stimuli (20, 184, 227). The ability of the ionophores A23187 and ionomycin to stimulate neutrophil responses also suggests that an influx of extracellular Ca^{2+} is important in affecting cell function. It has also been demonstrated that La^{3+}, which blocks both Ca^{2+} and Mn^{2+} uptake, attenuates the fMet-Leu-Phe-induced increase in intracellular Ca^{2+} to levels observed in the absence of extracellular Ca^{2+} (8). However, other Ca^{2+} channel blockers had no effect on stimulus-induced Ca^{2+} increments (8) and appear to exert their inhibitory actions on neutrophils through mechanisms not involving Ca^{2+} fluxes (167, 287). The permeability changes to Ca^{2+} appeared to be independent of the activation of voltage-dependent Ca^{2+} channels because depolarization with high potassium or gramicidin affected neither resting nor stimulated Ca^{2+} levels (8).

The initial mobilization of intracellular Ca^{2+} liberated in response to IP_3 appears to directly regulate the permeability changes to Ca^{2+} across the plasma membrane. In a recent study using both quin-2 and fura-2, it was shown that the rate of intracellular calcium increase after fMet-Leu-Phe stimulation was attenuated in the absence of extracellular Ca^{2+} (407). Patch clamp experiments revealed that calcium channels in the plasma membrane were insensitive to both fMet-Leu-Phe and IP_3, but opened if Ca^{2+} in the bathing medium was raised above 10^{-7} M Ca^{2+} (407). These findings are consistent with the previously reported observation that enhanced Ca^{2+} permeability during activation is dependent on mobilization of intracellular Ca^{2+}, since TMB-8 inhibited the Ca^{2+} permeability changes (184). However, degranulation is not blocked by ethylene glycol *bis* (β-aminoethyl ether)-*N,N'*-tetraacetic acid (EGTA), suggesting that extracellular Ca^{2+} and a Ca^{2+} influx are not absolute requirements for cellular response (357).

In an effort to directly demonstrate Ca^{2+}-dependent secretion, neutrophils have been permeabilized with the cholesterol-complexing agents saponin (360) and digitonin (295, 362), and exposed to Ca^{2+} in an EGTA-containing medium. Azurophil granule markers could not be released from saponin-permeabilized neutrophils. In contrast, micromolar levels of Ca^{2+} alone were sufficient to induce the release of both specific and azurophil granule constituents from digitonin-permeabilized cells, although specific granule secretion required lower Ca^{2+} concentrations. Granule secretion from neutrophils permeabilized with Sendai virus (15, 16, 136) also displays differential sensitivity to Ca^{2+}. The implication that azurophil and specific granule exocytosis differ in their Ca^{2+} requirements is supported by intact cell studies using quin-2 and ionomycin to establish the desired intracellular Ca^{2+} concentrations (199).

Although not yet reported in permeabilized cells, it has been further demonstrated in intact cells that specific granules themselves may contain subpopulations with different Ca^{2+} sensitivities (288). Secretion from granules bearing vitamin B_{12}-binding protein were more sensitive to elevations in intracellular Ca^{2+} than those enriched in lactoferrin. A similar conclusion can be drawn from morphologic data. The two lysosomal probes, sulforhodamine and fluorescein-dextran were initially sequestered together in specific granules to the same extent, but entered phagosomes at different rates, suggesting that subpopulations of specific granules exist and are released differentially (415).

The significance of stimulus-induced elevations in intracellular Ca^{2+} in signal transduction is at present unclear. Several investigators have reported that inducing optimal increments in intracellular Ca^{2+} levels is ineffective in evoking some neutrophil responses (185, 200, 294, 319). In addition, C3bi-mediated phagocytosis occurs independently of a measurable rise in intracellular Ca^{2+} (197) as do responses to PMA (320). These observations indicate that Ca^{2+} is not a sufficient or mandatory signal in the proposed activation pathway. Elucidation of the role of this cation in signal transduction awaits further investigation.

Protein Kinase C

The phorbol ester, PMA, has been used extensively as an activating stimulus to investigate the stimulus-response coupling pathways operative in neutrophils. The phosphorylation state of a wide variety of intracellular proteins changes upon stimulation with PMA (9, 273, 309, 423). These changes occur in parallel with the induction of neutrophil functional responses and have also been observed with chemotactic peptide stimulation (164, 309), suggesting the involvement of a protein kinase in the activation pathway. The ability of PMA to elicit neutrophil responses has been attributed to the activation of a Ca^{2+}-sensitive, phospholipid-dependent protein kinase (protein kinase C or PKC). High levels of PKC have been detected in neutrophils (147, 163). In other cell types, it has been demonstrated that the intracellular receptor for PMA is PKC (250, 398). In neutrophils, receptors for PMA are located in the cytoplasm of resting cells and redistributed to the plasma membrane after cell activation (252). A similar stimulus-induced shift in PKC activity was also reported, suggesting that PKC is the receptor for PMA in this cell type (252). Immunocytochemical data suggest that this shift in activity represents translocation from the cytosol to the membrane in both neutrophils (93) and HL60 cells (328).

It is generally believed that activation of the kinase is achieved physiologically by 1,2-diacylglycerol which is derived from the hydrolysis of phosphatidylinositols after receptor activation (42, 70, 98, 389). Consistent with this notion is the observation that synthetic diacylglycerols also activate neutrophils by interacting with the same intracellular receptor as PMA (259). The mobilization of diacylglycerol after receptor activation may activate PKC by sensitizing the enzyme to resting levels of intracellular Ca^{2+} because PMA reduces the K_m for its putative receptor, PKC, into the submicromolar range (250).

There is evidence to suggest that other signals generated during neutrophil activation may also regulate PKC activity. PMA and the synthetic diacylglycerol, 1-oleoyl-2-acetylglycerol potentiate the stimulatory actions of several chemotactic peptides and the ionophores, A23187 and ionomycin, on O_2^- generation and degranulation (96, 97, 255, 286, 384, 423). In addition, it has been suggested that arachidonate liberated concomitantly with diacylglycerol after cell activation may also regulate PKC because arachidonate and other unsaturated fatty acids can activate PKC in neutrophils (216). 1-oleoyl-2-acetylglycerol also potentiates the actions of arachidonate (258). Phospholipase A_2 eliminates the stimulatory effects of PMA on O_2^- generation and protein phosphorylation, further supporting a regulatory role for arachidonate on PKC activity (273).

Intracellular mechanisms which negatively modulate PKC may also exist. It has been reported that neutrophil specific granules contain a potent inhibitor of PKC which may serve to dampen or at least regulate its activity in intact cells (13). Pretreatment of cells with PMA can inhibit Ca^{2+} mobilization as well as the subsequent response to several stimuli (15, 192, 234). These effects may be related to the ability of phorbol ester to prevent PIP_2 hydrolysis (344).

The close correlation between the activation of PKC and neutrophil functions (26, 75, 252, 258, 259, 423) and the synergy between the activation of PKC agonists and other stimuli (26, 96, 258, 286) has suggested a role for this enzyme in stimulus-response coupling. While PKC has been implicated in the phosphorylation changes occurring after cell activation (9, 147, 163, 273, 423), neutrophils also contain other kinases in addition to PKC which may also be involved in cell activation (173–175, 243, 394). The inability of the PKC inhibitors, H-7 and H-9 (123, 429) to block neutrophil activation in response to several stimuli supports this possibility and suggests that PKC activation is not a necessary requirement for cell activation.

pH

Changes in intracellular pH are thought to play an important role in activating or regulating various neutrophil responses. Stimulation of neutrophils with fMet-Leu-Phe, phospholipase C, or phorbol esters, is associated with a biphasic pH change which is characterized by an initial acidification followed by an alkalinization (137–139, 141, 226, 228, 318, 420, 437). These changes may reflect stimulus-induced metabolic responses within the cell and their compensatory mechanisms or may serve to regulate subsequent neutrophil responses.

A number of lines of evidence suggest that the initial acidification of the cytosol which is associated with the extrusion of protons is the result of stimulus-induced activation of the plasma membrane NADPH oxidase and/or the hexose monophosphate shunt. Activators of the respiratory burst stimulate proton secretion, whereas inhibitors of alkalinization have been shown to attenuate secretion (139, 140, 388, 420). Cytoplasmic acidification is not observed in patients with chronic granulomatous disease, who lack a functional NADPH oxidase (141). Activation of the oxidase with oxidizing agents causes acidification. Another study showed that the protons are in fact derived from carbonic acid generated by activation of the hexose monophosphate shunt (37) rather than direct activation of the oxidase.

Due to their inherent acidity (224, 358, 385), secretory granules have also been considered potential candidates for cytoplasmic acidification. However, acidification has been observed in neutrophil cytoplasts as well, which are devoid of granules and nuclei. Thus, it is unlikely that secretory granules are the source of protons in this response.

It is well established that alkalinization of the cytosol results from proton extrusion. Most evidence suggests that hydrogen ions are exchanged for sodium ions with an apparent stoichiometry of 1:1 (330). Alkalinization is sodium-dependent and amiloride-sensitive (138, 141, 318, 331, 333), suggesting the involvement of a sodium-hydrogen antiport. 4,4-Diisothiocyano-2,2′-disulphonic acid stilbene, a disulfonic stilbene and inhibitor of anion fluxes, had no effect on alkalinization or acidification, suggesting that pH changes are not mediated by a Cl^-/HCO_3^- exchange mechanism.

Cyclic Nucleotides

Exposure of neutrophils to phagocytizable particles results in a rapid doubling of cyclic adenosine 3′,5′-monophosphate (cAMP) levels (149). This increment is prompt (maximal within 15 seconds) and brief (returning to basal levels in 1 to 2 minutes). Such a rapid response, which is comparable to the earliest changes in neutrophil biochemistry and physiology, could possibly play a role in stimulus-response coupling. Stimulated increments in cAMP levels were also reported in rabbit (169) and human (148, 158, 213, 242, 334, 356) neutrophils. The observations that changes in cAMP levels correlate closely with chemotaxis and degranulation (242), display specific desensitization after repeated exposures to the same stimulus, and that this desensitization is accompanied by a parallel decrease in O_2^- generation (332), suggest that changes in cyclic nucleotide levels may be of mechanistic significance. In addition, several substrates for the cAMP-dependent protein kinase have been detected in neutrophil cytosol which could potentially mediate the actions of cAMP (163).

However, a number of lines of evidence suggest that changes in cAMP are not important in stimulus-response coupling in neutrophils. First, cAMP increases can be induced by low concentrations of fMet-Leu-Phe without accompanying degranulation or O_2^- generation (356), suggesting that the former events are not sufficient for the latter. Second, generation of O_2^- and secretion of lysozyme, but not β-glucuronidase, can be induced by concanavalin A and PMA, stimuli which do not provoke any changes in cAMP levels (366). Similar observations were reported for other stimuli (242). Thus, increments in cAMP do not appear to be necessary for discharge of specific granules or O_2^- generation. Finally, Simchowitz showed that an inhibitor of adenylate cyclase, which blocks the stimulated increase in cAMP, does not impair neutrophil responses (335). These findings seem to rule out cAMP in a second messenger role. However, redistribution of cAMP (without concomitant elevated levels) could still be of mechanistic significance, as immunochemical observations of cAMP show it to be localized near forming phagosomes (298).

The Cytoskeleton

Microfilaments. The neutrophil cytoskeleton has been implicated in pseudopod formation and cell movement. The cytoplasm of the neutrophil is a highly filamentous 3-dimensional network predominantly composed of the contractile protein actin (247, 297, 369). Actin comprises 10% of the protein of the neutrophil and exists either as a globular monomer (G-actin) or as a double helical polymer (F-actin). The distribution between these two actin states shifts dramatically after cell activation. Neutrophil stimulation with chemotactic peptides causes a decrease in the amount of G-actin (14) with an accompanying increase in F-actin (23, 105, 159–161, 378, 409). The rate of polymerization is rapid and is initiated within the first few seconds after stimulation, suggesting that these changes play a role in the stimulus-response coupling pathway. These changes have also been related to an increase in the amount of actin associated with the detergent-insoluble cytoskeleton (317, 425, 432) and a biphasic right angle light scattering response (341, 342). Cytoskeletal rearrangements also occur in response to phorobol esters and the ionophore A23187, although at a slower rate and to a lesser extent than with chemotactic peptides (207, 326, 432).

Neutrophils also contain the contractile protein myosin, which is concentrated with actin in the pseudopods of migrating neutrophils (397, 428). Myosin represents about 10% of the cytoplasmic protein of neutrophils (41). Like striated muscle, neutrophil myosin is a hexamer composed of two heavy polypeptide chains and four light polypeptide chains. The heavy chains contain globular heads which bind actin and also possess ATPase activity (369). Myosin contracts the actin gel by hydrolysis of ATP which provides energy for contraction (327, 381). The ability of myosin to modulate contraction may be regulated by the phosphorylation of myosin light chains (369). Stimulation with chemotactic peptide leads to the phosphorylation of myosin light chains in neutrophils (105). It has been suggested that in nonmuscle cells, phosphorylation of myosin light chains is regulated by a calmodulin-dependent myosin light chain kinase (369). The interaction between actin and myosin could explain how force is generated by movement and the dependence of phagocytosis on metabolic energy.

In addition to actin and myosin, neutrophils contain several actin-binding proteins which regulate the polymerization state of actin in the cell. These regulatory proteins may in turn be regulated by signals generated during cell activation. Actin in psueodpods exists as a gel due to an actin-binding protein of high molecular weight which cross-links actin filaments (41). Calcium concentrations greater than 2×10^{-7} M dissolve the actin gel by activating a protein called gelsolin (434) which shortens actin filaments between the cross-linking proteins (435). When the calcium concentration falls below the critical level, gelsolin becomes inactive and reannealing and gelation of actin filaments occur (433, 435). Control of directional movement can be shown experimentally to arise from regulation of the network consistency by gelsolin and Ca^{2+} (375). Polymerization can also be regulated by the protein profilin which binds actin monomers and inhibits polymerization of G-actin (369).

There is some evidence that chemotactic peptides initiate cytoskeleton changes through a guanine nucleotide-binding protein. fMet-Leu-Phe and LTB_4 cause an increase in F-actin and the amount of actin associated with the cytoskeleton, both of which are totally abolished by pretreatment of cells with pertussis toxin (23, 317). These observations are consistent with the finding that pretreatment with pertussis toxin also inhibits peptide induced chemotaxis (18). However, several signal transduction pathways may exist because phorbol ester-induced cytoskeletal rearrangements are insensitive to pertussis toxin pretreatment (317).

Several reports suggest that a rise in intracellular free Ca^{2+} levels is not an absolute requirement for the initiation of actin polymerization. Cytoskeletal rearrangements are not dependent on extracellular Ca^{2+} in the medium (55, 161, 425). Abolishing stimulus-induced Ca^{2+} transients attenuates, but does not completely eliminate these changes (23, 432), suggesting a modulatory role for Ca^{2+}. A modulatory role for this cation is also indicated by the finding that this cation disrupts the stimulus-induced association of actin with the detergent-insoluble cytoskeleton (425). In addition, phorbol esters elicit effects indepedently of intracellular Ca^{2+} changes (326).

It has also been shown that the interaction of actin binding proteins with actin may also be regulated by PIP_2. PIP_2 has been reported to disassociate profilin-actin complexes (195) and also strongly inhibit gelsolin activity (170). The inhibitory effect of PIP_2 on gelsolin activity was independent of Ca^{2+} and eliminated by treatment with phospholipase A_2 and phospholipase C (170).

Microtubules. Another important cytoskeletal structure in neutrophils is the microtubule, which is a hollow fiber, 24 nm in diameter. Microtubules assemble as cylindrical polymers of the 55,000 dalton protein tubulin, which is found as a heterodimer of α- and β subunits. Soluble tubulin dimers in the cytopolasm appear to be in equilibrium with the assembled form, permitting ready "growth" or "dissolution" of these structures by shifting of the equilibrium. In many systems, microtubules can serve as "skeletal" support for the cell and perhaps for microfilaments and other contractile systems.

Microtubule assembly can be controlled in a variety of ways, both *in vivo* and *in vitro*. Agents which increase cGMP levels promote the assembly of tubulin. Ca^{2+} promotes dissolution of polymerized tubulin, as do agents which elevate cAMP levels; however, in neutrophils it also appears that the state of microtubule assembly also controls cAMP levels (210, 237). Tubulin polymerization can also be controlled by redox conditions *in vitro* (21, 220). In neutrophils, redox conditions are a function of glutathione oxidation; indeed, the amount of oxidized glutathione, which increases as a consequence of oxidative metabolism in stimulated neutrophils, appears to regulate microtubule disassembly (52, 276, 322, 323). There is some evidence that oxidation increases the tyrosinolation of tubulin, which directly favors microtubule disassembly (245, 246, 324, 399); tubulin tyrosinolation is found largely in the plasma membrane fraction of stimulated neutrophils (92, 247).

Microtubules may play a role in stimulus-response coupling in neutrophils. The number of these structures increases following exposure to a number of stimuli and correlates closely with secretion (69, 135, 153–155, 221, 419). No significant changes in microtubule numbers have been reported for chemotactic activation (7, 67). The fact that colchicine, which promotes microtubule disassembly, can inhibit phagocytosis, chemotaxis, surface adhesion, and degranulation, suggests that these structures are important in all of these processes. Microtubules have been implicated in more subtle phenomena in that they can govern the planar disposition of plasma membrane components (27, 100, 275, 277, 355, 396).

FUSION

It is generally believed that the process of degranulation involves the fusion of granule membranes with the phagosome membrane followed by the discharge of granule contents into the phagosome compartment. While morphologic and biochemical data support this hypothesis, this area of research has, in general, received little attention and a direct demonstration that neutrophil membrane fusion takes place is lacking. In other secretory cells, recent studies have been directed toward reconstructing an *in vitro* correlate of the fusion process through the use of artificial lipid membranes or reconstitution of the pertinent subcellular components. In such attempts, microscopic, fluorimetric, and electrophysiologic methods have largely been employed. The goal of these investigations is to definitively establish that secretory processes such as degranulation occur as the result of fusion of granule membranes with the plasma membrane and ultimately to discern the molecular mechanisms governing these processes. Results from these studies may provide valuable insights into mechanisms potentially operative in the neutrophil as well.

Calcium

As discussed above, the importance of elevated levels of free Ca^{2+} in degranulation has been directly demonstrated in permeabilized neutrophils (15, 136, 295, 360–364). In the adrenal chromaffin cell model, *in vitro* fusion events have been studied and appear to require Ca^{2+}. The release of chromaffin granule contents can be stimulated by low micromolar concentrations of Ca^{2+} in the presence of isolated membranes (182, 183), perhaps providing a model system for exocytosis. It has also been reported that the rate and extent of cortical vesicle fusion in sea urchin eggs is Ca^{2+}-dependent (78, 440).

Ca^{2+} may promote membrane fusion intracellularly through its interactions with negatively charged head groups of membrane phospholipids (267, 413). Electrostatic interactions might otherwise prevent their association. Polylysine and other metal cations have been shown to induce aggregation and fusion of phospholipid vesicles in a pH-dependent fashion (267, 413). The pH dependence of fusion may be related to the ability of hydrogen ions to provide a charge neutralizing effect. Thus, Ca^{2+} may change the physical properties of granules and membranes in such a way as to allow them to come into close apposition.

Ca^{2+} may alone induce membrane interactions or may initiate other Ca^{2+}-dependent processes responsible for fusion. Freeze fracture analysis of the exocytotic process has revealed that the patterns produced when granules fuse with the plasma membrane depend on whether Ca^{2+} is derived from an intracellular or extracellular source (56). It was suggested that fusion involves reorganization of the cytoskeleton and that such reorganization is influenced by source of Ca^{2+} (56).

Ca^{2+} may play a role in the fusion by regulating proteins participating in the fusion process. For instance, phospholipase A_2, the enzyme responsible for the liberation of arachidonic acid, is present in both granule and neutrophil membranes (110, 112, 177, 345, 393, 401). The membrane-bound enzyme is activated during stimulation (33, 64) and is Ca^{2+}-dependent (111). Phospholipase A_2-treated plasma membranes have been shown to induce the release of chromaffin granule contents, suggesting that arachidonic acid or one of its metabolites may participate in membrane fusion processes (168). Further support for a role for these lipids in fusion comes from studies demonstrating that inhibition of phospholipase A_2 or the cyclooxygenase and lipoxygenase pathways of arachidonate metabolism also inhibits degranulation (244, 254, 348, 365).

Synexins

Ca^{2+} may likewise interact with other proteins to regulate fusion. Synexins belong to a class of Ca^{2+}-binding proteins found in adrenal chromaffin cells called chromobindins (81), some of which are phosphorylated after stimulation (222). At low micromolar concentrations of Ca^{2+}, synexin binds to chromaffin granules (83) and can undergo self-aggregation in the presence of *cis*-unsaturated fatty acids (377). At high concentrations of Ca^{2+} (200 μM), it can induce the granules to aggregate and then fuse (82, 290). Recently, three synexin-like proteins have been isolated from human neutrophils with properties similar to the synexins found in adrenal chromaffin cells (219). These proteins not only demonstrate the ability to aggregate specific granules in the presence of Ca^{2+} but also induce the rapid fusion of granules with liposomes. Rapid fusion was highly dependent on the presence of Ca^{2+} and arachidonic acid.

Osmotic Forces

Observations from several laboratories suggest that osmotic forces may also play a role in membrane fusion. Hyperosmotic solutions have been shown to inhibit secretion in a variety of cell types, including adrenal chromaffin cells (51, 145, 290, 291, 441). *In vitro* studies using artificial membranes have further illustrated the importance of osmotic forces in affecting exocytosis (107, 418). Secretory granules of sea urchin eggs have been observed to swell irreversibly during Ca^{2+}-induced degranulation (441). In addition, hyperosmotic conditions both shrink cortical vesicles and inhibit exocytosis suggesting that vesicle swelling is crucial to membrane fusion (440).

Whereas these observations support the notion that membrane fusion involves osmotic forces, there are data which, in contrast, indicate that these changes are inconsequential. In adrenal chromaffin cells rendered permeable with digitonin, exocytosis was relatively insensitive to hyperosmotic solutions (157). Furthermore, exocytosis could be inhibited by raising the ionic strength of the medium, suggesting that inhibition of secretion in intact cells occurs as a result of alterations in intracellular ionic strength rather than increased osmolarity. Hypotonic solutions are likewise ineffective in eliciting secretion from this cell type (156), which is contrary to what one would expect if osmotic forces were to have a substantial impact on fusion. Analogous results have recently been reported for permeabilized neutrophils (380). In mast cells, electrical and microscopic measurements have demonstrated that large membrane capacitance increases, indicative of membrane fusion, always precede granule swelling, further questioning whether osmotic forces are a prerequisite for granule membrane fusion *in vivo* (45, 439).

Protein Phosphorylation

Protein phosphorylation and dephosphorylation reactions occur in stimulated neutrophils and appear to be important in a number of cellular responses (9, 150, 273, 309, 423). There is also evidence that membrane fusion requires the dephosphorylation of an as yet unidentified cellular protein(s). Microinjection of alkaline phosphatase or calcineurin in paramecium cells induces exocytosis as well as the dephosphorylation of a 65 kd phosphoprotein (207, 229). Microinjection of anti-calcineurin strongly inhibits membrane fusion, suggesting that dephosphorylation induced by this protein may affect fusion. The importance of protein dephosphorylation in exocytotic secretion from other cell types has been demonstrated (372).

OXIDATIVE METABOLISM

Activated neutrophils produce several microbicidal oxygen metabolites, including superoxide anion (O_2^-), H_2O_2, hydroxyl radicals (OH·) hypochlorous acid (HOCl), and singlet oxygen. Substantial evidence indicates that these reactive metabolites are generated by a nicotinamide adenine dinucleotide phosphate(NADPH)-dependent oxidase, located on the plasma membrane, which reduces molecular oxygen to O_2^-. The oxidase is quiescent in resting neutrophils and is stimulated following neutrophil activation. The importance of the NADPH-oxidase to the bactericidal capacity of the cell is demonstrated in individuals with chronic granulomatous disease whose neutrophils fail to generate O_2^- and related metabolites.

Components of the NADPH-Dependent Oxidase

The NADPH-oxidase appears to be a composite of cytochrome *b*-245 (38, 84, 114, 202), a flavin adenine dinucleotide-dependent flavoprotein (86, 202), and a ubiquinone (79, 80, 87, 225), although evidence against a ubiquinone component has also been reported (208). These constituents are believed to be assembled as an electron transport chain serving to ferry electrons from NADPH to oxygen. NADPH is subsequently regenerated through the hexose monophosphate shunt (22, 34). That these constituents may indeed be intrinsic to the oxidase has been recognized in studies utilizing neutrophils from individuals with the genetic disorder, chronic granulomatous disease. Patients with the X-linked form of the disease lack cytochrome *b* (28, 34, 86, 269, 301, 311) and contain reduced levels of flavoprotein (34, 86, 269). Levels of both oxidase components are normal in patients with the autosomally transmitted form (28, 86, 269), but the enzyme cannot be activated (311, 313).

The subcellular localization of the NADPH-oxidase as well as its mechanism of activation have been disputed. Cytochrome *b* consists of a 23 kd protein subunit and a 76 to 92 kd glycoprotein subunit (310), both of which are missing in X-linked chronic granulomatous disease. This cytochrome has been reported to be distributed between the plasma membrane and the membranes of cytoplasmic granules in resting cells (35, 84, 208, 225, 270, 283, 312). Stimulation results in the translocation of the cytochrome from granule fractions to the plasma membrane (35, 270, 283, 312). The flavoprotein contains a polypeptide of 45 kd (85). Evidence for a similar subcellular distribution (283) and stimulus-induced translocation of the flavoprotein has also been reported (34, 39). Based on these observations, several investigators have advanced the hypothesis that the granules are involved in activation of the oxidase (34, 35, 151). However, the relevance of the translocation phenomenon to oxidase activation is obscure. Translocation has not been universally reported (208) and does not correlate with the level of O_2^- production after activation with varied stimuli (270). Stimulation of neutrophils with chemotactic peptides produce maximal levels of O_2^- generation without the translocation of the flavoprotein (283). However, under the same conditions, significant translocation of cytochrome *b* is observed. In addition, lysosomal enzyme secretion can be inhibited without concomitant inhibition of the oxidase activation (225). In support of this notion is the observation that in the cell-free system, all the oxidase activity is located in the plasma membrane-enriched fraction and neither azurophil nor specific granules are required for activation (89). Thus, although translocation of specific oxidase components may occur, its significance is not understood.

The Cell-Free NADPH-Dependent Oxidase System

Considerable attention has been given to the molecular factors underlying activation of the NADPH-oxidase and multiple pathways appear to exist. Stimulation of the oxidase enzyme results in the generation of O_2^- after a lag period of several seconds (71, 72, 74, 215, 339), thus allowing sufficient time for the intervention of many of the aforementioned biochemical events in the activation pathway. Studies conducted in intact cells have been extended to broken cells. Cell-free oxidase activity was first reported in homgenates from resting guinea pig peritoneal macrophages (49, 50). Activation of the NADPH-oxidase required both a particulate and soluble fraction, and certain unsaturated fatty acids and anionic detergents. Cell-free oxidase activity has also been obtained from neutrophil homogenates and appears to have similar requirements (89, 217). The oxidase has also recently been fully solubilized from neutrophil membranes and displays kinetic properties similar to the oxidase of intact cells (88). Studies employing this system may prove valuable in characterizing the mechanism(s) underlying activation of the NADPH-dependent oxidase.

Stimulus-Response Coupling

Evidence for a guanine nucleotide binding protein in the stimulus-response coupling pathway has been presented. Pertussis toxin treatment of neutrophils inhibits fMet-Leu-Phe-induced O_2^- generation in intact cells, supporting the involvement of Gi-like proteins in signal transduction (113, 150, 274). In the cell-free system, the stable guanine nucleotides GTP-γ-S and Gpp(NH)p as well as fluoride stimulate the oxidase (113, 314, 315). Enzyme activation has also been reported to be Mg^{2+}-dependent in the cell-free system, further supporting a role for a G-protein in the process (89, 113). However, basal and guanine nucleotide-stimulated NADPH-oxidase activity is not diminished in the membranes of neutrophils pretreated with either pertussis toxin (113, 314) or cholera toxin (113). Thus, although Gi-like proteins are implicated in the transduction pathway in intact cells, these studies suggest that a guanine nucleotide-binding protein distinct from Gi or Gs is involved in the activation pathway in the broken cell preparation.

Some evidence indicates that phosphatidylinositol turnover is also not a central feature of the oxidoreductase activation pathway. In Ca^{2+}-depleted cells, fMet-Leu-Phe and concanavalin A stimulate O_2^- production without inducing phosphatidylinositol hydrolysis (305). Similarly, neutrophils pretreated with nonstimulatory doses of PMA generate O_2^- upon stimulation, without an accompanying liberation of inositol phosphates (94), suggesting that phospholipase C is not involved in activation.

Stimulation of the neutrophil is associated with the phosphorylation of cellular proteins thought to be involved in the activation of the NADPH-oxidase (146, 271, 292, 293). PMA, the PKC activator (250), stimulates O_2^- production in intact cells and results in the phosphorylation of a 90 kd membrane protein, which precedes the appearance of O_2^- (292). Treatment of neutrophils with an antibody directed against a 90 kd macrophage surface antigen delays the onset of both phosphorylation and O_2^- generation, but phosphorylation always precedes the onset of O_2^- production (292). The phosphorylation of two 46 kd proteins has also been reported (271).

Stimulus-induced phosphorylation is enhanced by the addition of PKC and inhibited by the PKC inhibitor H-7, suggesting a role for PKC in protein phosphorylation and oxidase activation. Furthermore, a stimulus-induced increase in diacylglycerol levels, which parallels O_2^- production and demonstrates the same concentration dependency as O_2^-, has been reported (303). Arachidonate and other *cis*-unsaturated fatty acids elicit production of O_2^- in intact cells (12, 73, 230) and also activate PKC (216), suggesting that their effects are mediated through a PKC-dependent pathway. In addition, reconstitution of partially purified PKC in the arachidonate-activated cell-free system is reported to result in activation of the NADPH-oxidase (77).

It has thus been proposed that the cytosolic cofactor of the cell-free oxidase is PKC. Several lines of evidence argue against this hypothesis. In whole neutrophils (17, 150, 212) and in the reconstituted system (66, 315), several PKC inhibitors are ineffective in abolishing stimulus-induced activation of the oxidase. In addition, translocation of PKC, considered by some to be a prerequisite for activation, was reported not to occur in cells at concentrations of fMet-Leu-Phe which are sufficient to prime cells (17). No cofactor activity has been identified in the cytosols of several tissues, indicating that the presence of the oxidase cofactor is neutrophil-specific, whereas the presence of PKC is not (282, 315). In addition, in the cell-free system, arachidonate activation is achieved in the absence of PKC cofactors and ATP (76). Recently, the cytosolic cofactor has been partially purified and appears to exist in two forms, neither of which is PKC (89). In addition, a patient with chronic granulomatous disease was reported to have normal levels of PKC, but generated only 3% of normal O_2^- when stimulated with PMA.

It has been proposed that arachidonate-induced activation might involve a phospholipase A_2-mediated release of arachidonic acid and its subsequent metabolism through either the lipoxygenase or cyclooxygenase pathways. Some support for this hypothesis has been obtained with intact cells. Phospholipase A_2 inhibition suppresses the release of arachidonate acid as well as the production of O_2^- (211, 212). Likewise, cyclooxygenase and lipoxygenase inhibitors suppress O_2^- production (48) and hydroxyl radical formation (60), while soybean lipoxygenase stimulates hydroxyl radical formation (60). The phospholipase A_2-mediated pathway does not appear to involve PKC because stimulation with opsonized zymosan is not inhibited by H-7 (212). Inhibition of phospholipase A_2 results in the inhibition of O_2^- generation induced by opsonized zymosan, but not PMA, suggesting different activation pathways. Like the proposed PKC-mediated pathway, observations in intact cells are not easily extended to the cell-free system because arachidonic acid activation in the cell-free system appears to be independent of phospholipase A_2 activation (211).

CONCLUSIONS

This review has attempted to dissect several early events in stimulated neutrophils and relate the significance of these changes to various biologic activities of the cell. It is apparent from studies in this area that signal transduction in the *in vivo* situation reflects a complex sequence of interrelated events. Depending on the experimental conditions employed, the requirements for a putative second messenger product can be directly demonstrated or completely eliminated. To account for these seemingly disparate observations, it is likely that, in addition to the proposed mechanisms which have been described, auxiliary or regulatory signals are generated in parallel and participate in mediating functional responses. It is also possible that divergent pathways exist.

In order to better resolve many discrepancies encountered during *in vivo* studies, the ultimate goal is to reconstitute the activation process *in vitro*. In this regard, the development of the cell-free NADPH-dependent oxidase system may be a useful paradigm. Investigations utilizing this system may not only contribute to the discernment of general stimulus-secretion coupling mechanisms in neutrophils, but also have particular relevance to understanding the biochemical basis of chronic granulomatous disease, a disorder which appears to represent a breakdown of the activation pathway at either of two locations.

REFERENCES

1. Abrahamson DR, Fearon DT: Endocytosis of the C3b receptor of complement within coated pits in human polymorphonuclear leukocytes and monocytes. Lab Invest 48:162, 1983
2. Aehringhaus U, Wolbling RH, Konig W, Patrono C, Peskar BM, Peskar BA: Release of leukotriene C_4 from human polymorphonuclear leucocytes as determined by radioimmunoassay. FEBS Lett 146:111, 1982
3. Allen RA, Jesaitis AJ, Sklar LA, Cochrane CG, Painter RG: Physicochemical properties of the N-formyl peptide receptor on human neutrophils. J Biol Chem 261:1854, 1986
4. Ambruso DR, Johnston RB Jr: Lactoferrin enhances hydroxyl radical production by human neutrophils, neutrophil particulate fractions, and an enzymatic generating system. J Clin Invest 67:352, 1981
5. Andersen BR, Amirault HJ, LeBreton GC: The effects of arachidonic acid and other fatty acids on canine neutrophil metabolism. Prostaglandins 22:469, 1981
6. Anderson DC, Schmalstieg FC, Arnaout MA, Hughes BJ, Tosi MF, Buffone GJ, Brinkley BR, Dickey WD, Abramson JS, Springer TA, Boxer LA, Hollers JM, Smith CW: Abnormalities of polymorphonuclear leukocyte function associated with a heritable deficiency of high molecular weight surface glycoproteins (GP138): common relationship to diminished cell adherence. J Clin Invest 74:536, 1984
7. Anderson DG, Wible LJ, Hughes BJ, Smith CW, Brinkley BR: Cytoplasmic microtubules in polymorphonuclear leukocytes: effects of chemotactic stimulation and colchicine. Cell 31:719, 1982
8. Andersson T, Dahlgren C, Pozzan T, Stendahl O, Lew PD: Characterization of fMet-Leu-Phe receptor-mediated Ca^{2+} influx across the plasma membrane of human neutrophils. Mol Pharmacol 30:437, 1986
9. Andrews PC, Babior BM: Endogenous protein phosphorylation by resting and activated human neutrophils. Blood 61:333, 1983
10. Anthes JC, Billah MM, Cali A, Egan RW, Siegel MI: Chemotactic peptide, calcium and guanine nucleotide regulation of phospholipase C activity in membranes from DMSO-differentiated HL60 cells. Biochem Biophys Res Commun 145:825, 1987
11. Aswanikumar S, Corcoran B, Schiffmann E, Day AR, Freer RJ, Showell HJ, Becker EL, Pert CB: Demonstration of a receptor on rabbit neutrophils for chemotactic peptides. Biochem Biophys Res Commun 74:810, 1977
12. Badwey JA, Curnutte JT, Karnovsky ML: *cis*-Polyunsaturated fatty acids induce high levels of superoxide production by human neutrophils. J Biol Chem 256:12640, 1981
13. Balazovich KJ, Smolen JE, Boxer LA: Endogenous inhibitor of

protein kinase C: association with human peripheral blood neutrophils but not with specific granule-deficient neutrophils or cytoplasts. J Immunol 137:1665, 1986

14. Barrett S, Garratty E, Garratty G: Cell surface heterogeneity of human blood neutrophils and monocytes. Br J Haematol 43:575, 1979
15. Barrowman MM, Cockcroft S, Gomperts BD: Two roles of guanine nucleotides in the stimulus-secretion sequence of neutrophils. Nature 319:504, 1986
16. Barrowman MM, Cockcroft S, Gomperts BD: Differential control of azurophilic and specific granule exocytosis in sendai-virus-permeabilized rabbit neutrophils. J Physiol 383:115, 1987
17. Bass DA, Gerard C, Olbrantz P, Wilson J, McCall CE, McPhail LC: Priming of the respiratory burst of neutrophils by diacylglycerol. Independence from activation or translocation of protein kinase C. J Biol Chem 262:6643, 1987
18. Becker EL, Kermode JC, Naccache PH, Yassin R, Marsh ML, Munoz JJ, Sha'afi RI: The inhibition of neutrophil granule enzyme secretion and chemotaxis by pertussis toxin. J Cell Biol 100:1641, 1985
19. Becker EL, Kermode JC, Naccache PH, Yassin R, Munoz JJ, Marsh ML, Huang CK, Sha'afi RI: Pertussis toxin as a probe of neutrophil activation. Fed Proc 45:2151, 1986
20. Becker EL, Showell HJ, Naccache PH, Sha'afi RI: The role and interrelationships of Ca^{2+} and arachidonic acid metabolism in stimulated neutrophil functions. In Biochemistry of Acute Allergic Reactions, edited by Becker EL, Simon AS, Austen KF, p 257. New York, Alan R. Liss, 1981
21. Beckman JK, Gay JC, Brash AR, Lukens JN, Oates JA: Investigations of the biological activity of leukotriene A4 in human polymorphonuclear leukocytes. Biochem Biophys Res Commun 133:23, 1985
22. Bender JG, Van Epps DE: Inhibition of human neutrophil function by 6-aminonicotinamide: the role of the hexose monophosphate shunt in cell activation. Immunopharmacology 10:191, 1985
23. Bengtsson T, Stendahl O, Andersson T: The role of the cytosolic free Ca^{2+} transient for fMet-Leu-Phe induced actin polymerization in human neutrophils. Eur J Cell Biol 42:338, 1986
24. Berger M, Cross AS: Lymphoblastoid cell supernatants increase expression of C3b receptors on human polymorphonuclear leucocytes: direct binding studies with 125I-C3b. Immunology 51:431, 1984
25. Berger M, O'Shea J, Cross AS, Folks TM, Chused TM, Brown EJ, Frank MM: Human neutrophils increase expression of C3bi as well as C3b receptors upon activation. J Clin Invest 74:1566, 1984
26. Berkow RL, Kraft AS: Bryostatin, a non-phorbol macrocyclic lactone, activates intact human polymorphonuclear leukocytes and binds to the phorbol ester receptor. Biochem Biophys Res Commun 131:1109, 1985
27. Berlin RD, Oliver JM: Control of cell surface topography. Nature 247:45, 1974
28. Bohler MC, Seger RA, Mouy R, Vilmer E, Fischer A, Griscelli C: A study of 25 patients with chronic granulomatous disease: a new classification by correlating respiratory burst, cytochrome b, and flavoprotein. J Clin Immunol 6:136, 1986
29. Bokoch GM, Gilman AG: Inhibition of receptor-mediated release of arachidonic acid by pertussis toxin. Cell 39:301, 1984
30. Bokoch GM, Reed RW: Effect of various lipoxygenase metabolites of arachidonic acid on degranulation of polymorphonuclear leukocytes. J Biol Chem 256:5317, 1981
31. Borgeat P, Hamberg M, Samuelsson B: Transformation of arachidonic acid and homogamma-linoleic acid by rabbit polymorphonuclear leukocytes. Monohydroxy acids from novel lipoxygenases. J Biol Chem 251:7816, 1976
32. Borgeat P, Samuelsson B: Transformation of arachidonic acid by rabbit polymorphonuclear leukocytes. Formation of a novel dihydroxyeicosatetraenoic acid. J Biol Chem 254:2643, 1979
33. Bormann BJ, Huang CK, Mackin WM, Becker EL: Receptor-mediated activation of a phospholipase A_2 in rabbit neutrophil plasma membrane. Proc Natl Acad Sci USA 81:767, 1984
34. Borregaard N: The respiratory burst of phagocytosis: biochemistry and subcellular localization. Immunol Lett 11:165, 1985
35. Borregaard N, Heiple JM, Simons ER, Clark RA: Subcellular localization of the b cytochrome component of the human neutrophil microbicidal oxidase: translocation during activation. J Cell Biol 97:52, 1983
36. Borregaard N, Miller LJ, Springer TA: Chemoattractant-regulated mobilization of a novel intracellular compartment in human neutrophils. Science 237:1204, 1987
37. Borregaard N, Schwartz JH, Tauber AI: Proton secretion by stimulated neutrophils. Significance of hexose monophosphate shunt activity as a source of electrons and protons for the respiratory burst. J Clin Invest 74:455, 1984
38. Borregaard N, Simons ER, Clark RA: Involvement of cytochrome b-245 in the respiratory burst of human neutrophils. Infect Immun 38:1301, 1982
39. Borregaard N, Tauber AI: Subcellular localization of human neutrophil NADPH oxidase; b-cytochrome and associated flavoprotein. J Biol Chem 259:47, 1984
40. Boxer LA, Haak RA, Yang HH, Wolach JB, Whitcomb JA, Butterick CJ, Baehner RL: Membrane-bound lactoferrin alters the surface properties of polymorphonuclear leukocytes. J Clin Invest 70:1049, 1982
41. Boxer LA, Stossel TP: Interactions of actin, myosin, and an actin-binding protein in chronic myelogenous leukemia leukocytes. J Clin Invest 57:964, 1976
42. Bradford PG, Rubin RP: Characterization of formylmethionyl-leucyl-phenylalanine stimulation of inositol trisphosphate accumulation in rabbit neutrophils. Mol Pharmacol 27:74, 1985
43. Bradford PG, Rubin RP: Quantitative changes in inositol 1,4,5-trisphosphate in chemoattractant-stimulated neutrophils. J Biol Chem 261:15644, 1986
44. Bradford PG, Rubin RP: Guanine nucleotide regulation of phospholipase C in permeabilized rabbit neutrophils. Inhibition by pertussis toxin and sensitization to submicromolar calcium concentrations. Biochem J 239:97, 1986
45. Breckenridge LJ, Almers W: Final steps in exocytosis observed in a cell with giant secretory granules. Proc Natl Acad Sci USA 84:1945, 1987
46. Breton-Gorius J, Mason DY, Buriot D, Vilde JL, Griscelli C: Lactoferrin deficiency as a consequence of a lack of specific granules in neutrophils from a patient with recurrent infections. Detection by immunoperoxidase staining for lactoferrin and cytochemical electron microscopy. Am J Pathol 99:413, 1980
47. Bretz U, Baggiolini M: Biochemical and morphological characterization of azurophil and specific granules of human neutrophil polymorphonuclear leukocytes. J Cell Biol 63:251, 1974
48. Bromberg Y, Pick E: Unsaturated fatty acids as second messengers of superoxide generation by macrophages. Cell Immunol 79:240, 1983
49. Bromberg Y, Pick E: Unsaturated fatty acids stimulate NADPH-dependent superoxide production by cell-free system derived from macrophages. Cell Immunol 88:213, 1984
50. Bromberg Y, Pick E: Activation of NADPH-dependent superoxide production in a cell-free system by sodium dodecyl sulfate. J Biol Chem 260:13539, 1985
51. Brown EM, Pazoles CJ, Creutz CE, Aurbach GD, Pollard HB: Role of anions in parathyroid hormone release from dispersed bovine parathyroid cells. Proc Natl Acad Sci USA 75:876, 1978
52. Burchill BR, Oliver JM, Pearson CB, Leinbach ED, Berlin RD: Microtubule dynamics and glutathione metabolism in phagocytizing human polymorphonuclear leukocytes. J Cell Biol 76:439, 1978
53. Burkhardt H, Hartmann F, Schwingel ML: Activation of latent collagenase from polymorphonuclear leukocytes by oxygen radicals. Enzyme 36:221, 1986
54. Calamai EG, Spitznagel JK: Characterization of rat polymorphonuclear leukocyte subcellular granules. Lab Invest 46:597, 1982
55. Carson M, Weber A, Zigmond SH: An actin-nucleating activity in polymorphonuclear leukocytes is modulated by chemotactic peptides. J Cell Biol 103:2707, 1986
56. Chandler DE, Kazilek CJ: Chemotactic peptide-induced exocytosis in neutrophils: granule fusion patterns depend on the source of messenger calcium. J Cell Sci 83:293, 1986
57. Chandler D, Meusel G, Schumaker E, Stapleton C: FMLP-induced enzyme release from neutrophils: a role for intracellular calcium. Am J Physiol 245:C196, 1983
58. Chenoweth DE, Hugli TE: Demonstration of specific C5a receptor on intact human polymorphonuclear leukocytes. Proc Natl Acad

Sci USA 75:3943, 1978

59. Chenoweth DE, Hugli TE: Human C5a and C5a analogs as probes of the neutrophil C5a receptor. Mol Immunol 17:151, 1980
60. Cheung K, Lark J, Robinson MF, Pomery PJ, Hunter S: The production of hydroxyl radical by human neutrophils stimulated by arachidonic acid-measurements by ESR spectroscopy. Aust J Exp Biol Med Sci 64:157, 1986
61. Chilton FH, O'Flaherty JT, Walsh CE, Thomas MJ, Wykle RL, DeChatelet LR, Waite BM: Platelet activating factor. Stimulation of the lipoxygenase pathway in polymorphonuclear leukocytes by 1-O-alkyl-2-O-acetyl-sn-glycero-3-phosphocholine. J Biol Chem 257:5402, 1982
62. Claesson HE, Lindgren JA, Gustafsson B: Opsonized bacteria stimulate leukotriene synthesis in human leukocytes. Biochim Biophys Acta 836:361, 1985
63. Claesson HE, Lundberg U, Malmsten C: Serum-coated zymosan stimulates the synthesis of leukotriene B_4 in human polymorphonuclear leukocytes. Inhibition by cyclic AMP. Biochem Biophys Res Commun 99:1230, 1981
64. Clancy RM, Dahinden CA, Hugli TE: Arachidonate metabolism by human polymorphonuclear leukocytes stimulated by N-formyl-Met-Leu-Phe or complement component C5a is independent of phospholipase activation. Proc Natl Acad Sci USA 80:7200, 1983
65. Clark RA: Chemotactic factors trigger their own oxidative inactivation by human neutrophils. J Immunol 129:2725, 1982
66. Clark RA, Leidal KG, Pearson DW, Nauseef WM: NADPH oxidase of human neutrophils. Subcellular localization and characterization of an arachidonate-activatable superoxide-generating system. J Biol Chem 262:4065, 1987
67. Clay LKL, Murphy RC, Andres JL, Lynch J, Henson PM: Structure elucidation of platelet activating factor derived from human neutrophils. Biochem Biophys Res Commun 121:815, 1984
68. Coates TD, Torres M, Harman J, Williams V: Localization of chlorotetracycline fluorescence in human polymorphonuclear neutrophils. Blood 69:1146, 1987
69. Cockcroft S: Ca^{2+}-dependent conversion of phosphatidylinositol to phosphatidate in neutrophils stimulated with fMet-Leu-Phe or ionophore A23187. Biochim Biophys Acta 795:37, 1984
70. Cockcroft S, Baldwin JM, Allan D: The Ca^{2+}-activated polyphosphoinositide phosphodiesterase of human and rabbit neutrophil membranes. Biochem J 221:477, 1984
71. Cohen HJ, Chovaniec ME: Superoxide production by digitonon-stimulated guinea pig granulocytes. The effects of N-ethyl maleimide, divalent cations and glycolytic and mitochondrial inhibitors on the activation of the superoxide generating system. J Clin Invest 61:1088, 1978
72. Cohen HJ, Chovaniec ME: Superoxide generation by digitonin-stimulated guinea pig granulocytes. A basis for a continuous assay for monitoring superoxide production and for the study of the activation of the generating system. J Clin Invest 61:1081, 1978
73. Cohen HJ, Chovaniec ME, Takahashi K, Whitin JC: Activation of human granulocytes by arachidonic acid: its use and limitations for investigating granulocyte functions. Blood 67:1103, 1986
74. Cohen HJ, Newburger PE, Chovaniec ME, Whitin JC, Simons ER: Opsonized zymosan-stimulated granulocytes. Activation and activity of the superoxide-generating system and membrane potential changes. Blood 58:975, 1981
75. Cooke E, Hallett MB: The role of C-kinase in the physiological activation of the neutrophil oxidase. Evidence from using pharmacological manipulation of C-kinase activity in intact cells. Biochem J 232:323, 1985
76. Cox JA, Jeng AY, Blumberg PM, Tauber AI: Comparison of subcellular activation of the human neutrophil NADPH-oxidase by arachidonic acid, sodium dodecyl sulfate (SDS), and phorbol myristate acetate (PMA). J Immunol 138:1884, 1987
77. Cox JA, Jeng AY, Sharkey NA, Blumberg PM, Tauber AI: Activation of the human neutrophil nicotinamide adenine dinucleotide phosphate (NADPH)-oxidase by protein kinase C. J Clin Invest 76:1932, 1985
78. Crabb JH, Jackson RC: *In vitro* reconstitution of exocytosis from plasma membrane and isolated secretory vesicles. J Cell Biol 101:2263, 1985
79. Crawford DR, Schneider DL: Identification of ubiquinone-50 in human neutrophils and its role in microbicidal events. J Biol Chem 257:6662, 1982
80. Crawford DR, Schneider DL: Ubiquinone content and respiratory burst activity of latex-filled phagolysosomes isolated from human neutrophils and evidence for the probable involvement of a third granule. J Biol Chem 258:5363, 1983
81. Creutz CE, Dowling LG, Sando JJ, Villar-Palasi C, Whipple JH, Zaks WJ: Characterization of the chromobindins. Soluble proteins that bind to the chromaffin granule membrane in the presence of Ca^{2+}. J Biol Chem 258:14664, 1983
82. Creutz CE, Scott JH, Pazoles CJ, Pollard HB: Further characterization of the aggregation and fusion of chromaffin granules by synexin as a model for compound exocytosis. J Cell Biochem 18:87, 1982
83. Creutz CE, Sterner DC: Calcium dependence of the binding of synexin to isolated chromaffin granules. Biochem Biophys Res Commun 114:355, 1983
84. Cross AR, Higson FK, Jones OTG, Harper AM, Segal AW: The enzymic reduction and kinetics of oxidation of cytochrome b-245 of neutrophils. Biochem J 204:479, 1982
85. Cross AR, Jones OT: The effect of the inhibitor diphenylene iodonium on the superoxide-generating system of neutrophils. Specific labelling of a component polypeptide of the oxidase. Biochem J 237:111, 1986
86. Cross AR, Jones OTG, Garcia R, Segal AW: The association of FAD with the cytochrome b-245 of human neutrophils. Biochem J 208:759, 1982
87. Cunningham CC, DeChatelet LT, Spach PI, Parce JW, Thomas MJ, Lees CJ, Shirley PS: Identification and quantitation of electron-transport components in human polymorphonuclear leukocytes. Biochim Biophys Acta 682:430, 1982
88. Curnutte JT, Kuver R, Babior BM: Activation of the respiratory burst oxidase in a fully soluble system from human neutrophils. J Biol Chem 262:6450, 1987
89. Curnutte JT, Kuver R, Scott PJ: Activation of neutrophil NADPH oxidase in a cell-free system. Partial purification of components and characterization of the activation process. J Biol Chem 262:5563, 1987
90. Dahinden CA, Clancy RM, Hugli TE: Stereospecificity of leukotriene B_4 and structure-function relationships for chemotaxis of human neutrophils. J Immunol 133:1477, 1984
91. Dahl ML: Aggregating and prostanoid-releasing effects of platelet-activating factor and leukotrienes on human polymorphonuclear leukocytes and platelets. Int Arch Allergy Appl Immunol 76:145, 1985
92. Dahl ML, Puustinen T, Uotila P: U-60,257 has no effect on the metabolism of arachidonic acid in nonstimulated human polymorphonuclear leukocytes. Res Commun Chem Pathol Pharmacol 44:355, 1984
93. Deli E, Kiss Z, Wilson E, Lambeth JD, Kuo JF: Immunocytochemical localization of protein kinase C in resting and activated human neutrophils. FEBS Lett 221:365, 1987
94. Della-Bianca V, Grzeskowiak M, Cassatella MA, Zeni L, Rossi F: Phorbol 12, myristate 13, acetate potentiates the respiratory burst while inhibits phosphoinositide hydrolysis and calcium mobilization by formyl-methionyl-leucyl-phenylalanine in human neutrophils. Biochem Biophys Res Commun 135:556, 1986
95. Dewald B, Bretz U, Baggiolini M: Release of gelatinase from a novel secretory compartment of human neutrophils. J Clin Invest 70:518, 1982
96. Dewald B, Payne, TG, Baggiolini M: Activation of NADPH oxidase of human neutrophils. Potentiation of chemotactic peptide by a diacylglyercol. Biochim Biophys Acta 125:367, 1984
97. Di Virgilio FD, Lew DP, Pozzan T: Protein kinase C activation of physiological processes in human neutrophils at vanishingly small cytosolic Ca^{2+} levels. Nature 310:691, 1984
98. Dougherty RW, Godfrey PP, Hoyle PC, Putney JW Jr, Freer RJ: Secretagogue-induced phosphoinositide metabolism in human leucocytes. Biochem J 222:307, 1984
99. Dri P, Soranzo MR, Cramer R, Menegazzi R, Miotti V, Patriarca P: Role of myeloperoxidase in respiratory burst of human polymorphonuclear leukocytes. Studies with myeloperoxidase-deficient subjects. Inflammation 9:21, 1985
100. Dunham PB, Goldstein IM, Weissmann G: Potassium and amino acid transport in human leukocytes exposed to phagocytic stimuli. J Cell Biol 63:215, 1974
101. Elferink JGR, Deierkauf M: The effect of verapamil and other

calcium antagonists on chemotaxis of polymorphonuclear leukocytes. Biochem Pharmacol 33:35, 1984

102. Elferink JGR, Deierkauf M: The effect of quin2 on chemotaxis by polymorphonuclear leukocytes. Biochim Biophys Acta 846:364, 1985

103. Elsbach P, Weiss J: Oxygen-dependent and oxygen-independent mechanisms of microbicidal activity of neutrophils. Immunol Lett 11:159, 1985

104. Fearon DT: Identification of the membrane glycoprotein that is the C3b receptor of the human erythrocyte, polymorphonuclear leukocyte, B lymphocyte, and monocyte. J Exp Med 152:20, 1980

105. Fechheimer M, Zigmond SH: Changes in cytoskeletal proteins of polymorphonuclear leukocytes induced by chemotactic peptides. Cell Motility 3:349, 1983

106. Feltner DE, Smith RH, Marasco WA: Characterization of the plasma membrane bound GTPase from rabbit neutrophils. I. Evidence for an Ni-like protein coupled to the formyl peptide, C5a, and leukotriene B_4 chemotaxis receptors. J Immunol 137:1961, 1986

107. Fisher LR, Parker NS: Osmotic control of bilayer fusion. Biophys J 46:253, 1984

108. Fleisch JH, Rinkema LE, Marshall WS: Pharmacologic receptor for the leukotrienes. Biochem Pharmacol 33:3919, 1984

109. Fletcher MP, Gallin JI: Human neutrophils contain an intracellular pool of putative receptors for the chemoattractant N-formyl-methionyl-leucyl-phenylalanine. Blood 62:792, 1983

110. Franson R, Patriarca P, Elsbach P: Phospholipid metabolism by phagocytic cells. Phospholipases A_2 associated with rabbit polymorphonuclear leukocyte granules. J Lipid Res 15:380, 1974

111. Franson R, Waite M: Relation between calcium requirement, substrate charge, and rabbit polymorphonuclear leukocyte phospholipase A_2 activity. Biochemistry 17:4029, 1978

112. Franson R, Weiss J, Martin L, Spitznagel JK, Elsbach P: Phospholipase A activity associated with the membranes of human polymorphonuclear leukocytes. Biochem J 167:839, 1977

113. Gabig TG, English D, Akard LP, Schell MJ: Regulation of neutrophil NADPH oxidase activation in a cell-free system by guanine nucleotides and fluoride. Evidence for participation of a pertussis and cholera toxin-insensitive G protein. J Biol Chem 262:1685, 1987

114. Gabig TG, Schervish EW, Santinga JT: Functional relationship of the cytochrome b to the superoxide-generating oxidase of human neutrophils. J Biol Chem 257:4114, 1982

115. Gallin JI, Fletcher MP, Seligmann BE, Hoffstein S, Cehrs K, Mounessa N: Human neutrophil-specific granule deficiency: a model to assess the role of neutrophil-specific granules in the evolution of the inflammatory response. Blood 59:1317, 1982

116. Gallin JI, Metcalf JA, Roos S, Seligmann B, Friedman MM: Organelle-depleted human neutrophil cytoplasts used to study fMet-Leu-Phe receptor modulation and cell function. J Immunol 133:415, 1984

117. Gallin JI, Wright DG, Schiffmann E: Role of secretory events in modulating human neutrophil chemotaxis. J Clin Invest 62:1364, 1978

118. Ganz T: Extracellular release of antimicrobial defensins by human polymorphonuclear leukocytes. Infect Immun 55:568, 1987

119. Ganz T, Selsted ME, Szklarek D, Harwig SSL, Daher K, Bainton DF, Lehrer RI: Defensins. Natural peptide antibiotics of human neutrophils. J Clin Invest 76:1427, 1985

120. Garcia RC, Peterson CG, Segal AW, Venge P: Elastase in the different primary granules of the human neutrophil. Biochem Biophys Res Commun 132:1130, 1985

121. Gardner JP, Melnick DA, Malech HL: Characterization of the formyl peptide chemotactic receptor appearing at the phagocytic cell surface after exposure to phorbol myristate acetate. J Immunol 136:1400, 1986

122. Gennaro R, Dolzani L, Romeo D: Potency of bactericidal proteins purified from the large granules of bovine neutrophils. Infect Immun 40:684, 1983

123. Gerard C, McPhail LC, Marfart A, Stimler-Gerard NP, Bass DA, McCall CE: Role of protein kinases in stimulation of human polymorphonuclear leukocyte oxidative metabolism by various agonists. Differential effects of a novel protein kinase inhibitor. J Clin Invest 77:61, 1986

124. Gierschik P, Falloon J, Milligan G, Pines M, Gallin JI, Spiegel A: Immunochemical evidence for a novel pertussis toxin substrate in human neutrophils. J Biol Chem 261:8058, 1986

125. Gierschik P, Sidiropoulos D, Spiegel A, Jakobs KH: Purification and immunochemical characterization of the major pertussis-toxin-sensitive guanine-nucleotide-binding protein of bovine-neutrophil membranes. Eur J Biochem 165:185, 1987

126. Goetzl EJ: A role for endogenous mono-hydroxy-eicosatetraenoic acids (HETEs) in the regulation of human neutrophil migration. Immunology 40:709, 1980

127. Goetzl EJ, Brash AR, Tauber AI, Oates JA, Hubbard WC: Modulation of human neutrophil function by monohydroxyeicosatetraenoic acids. Immunology 39:491, 1980

128. Goetzl EJ, Hill HR, Gorman RR: Unique aspects of the modulation of human neutrophil function by 12-L-hydroperoxy-5,8,10,14-eicosatetraenoic acid. Prostaglandins 19:71, 1980

129. Goetzl EJ, Pickett WC: The human PMN leukocyte chemotactic activity of complex hydroxy-eicosatetraenoic acids (HETEs). J Immunol 125:1789, 1980

130. Goetzl EJ, Pickett WC: Novel structural determinants of the human neutrophil chemotactic activity of leukotriene B. J Exp Med 153:482, 1981

131. Goldman DW, Chang FH, Gifford LA, Goetzl EJ, Bourne HR: Pertussis toxin inhibition of chemotactic factor-induced calcium mobilization and function in human polymorphonuclear leukocytes. J Exp Med 162:145, 1985

132. Goldman DW, Gifford LA, Olson DM, Goetzl EJ: Transduction by leukotriene B_4 receptors of increases in cytosolic calcium in human polymorphonuclear leukocytes. J Immunol 135:525, 1985

133. Goldman DW, Goetzl EJ: Specific binding of leukotriene B_4 to receptors on human polymorphonuclear leukocytes. J Immunol 129:1600, 1982

134. Goldman DW, Goetzl EJ: Heterogeneity of human polymorphonuclear leukocyte receptors for leukotriene B_4. Identification of a subset of high affinity receptors that transduce the chemotactic response. J Exp Med 159:1027, 1984

135. Goldstein I, Hoffstein S, Gallin J, Weissmann G: Mechanisms of lysosomal enzyme release from human leukocytes: microtubule assembly and membrane fusion induced by a component of complement. Proc Natl Acad Sci USA 70:2916, 1973

136. Gomperts BD, Barrowman MM, Cockcroft S: Dual role for guanine nucleotides in stimulus-secretion coupling. Fed Proc 45:2156, 1986

137. Grinstein S, Cohen S: Cytoplasmic [Ca^{2+}] and intracellular pH in lymphocytes. Role of membrane potential and volume-activated Na^+/H^+ exchange. J Gen Physiol 89:185, 1987

138. Grinstein S, Elder B, Furuya W: Phorbol ester-induced changes of cytoplasmic pH in neutrophils: role of exocytosis in Na^+-H^+ exchange. Am J Physiol 248:C379, 1985

139. Grinstein S, Furuya W: Cytoplasmic pH regulation in phorbol ester-activated human neutrophils. Am J Physiol 251:C55, 1986

140. Grinstein S, Furuya W: Cytoplasmic pH regulation in activated human neutrophils: effects of adenosine and pertussis toxin on Na^+/H^+ exchange and metabolic acidification. Biochim Biophys Acta 889:301, 1986

141. Grinstein S, Furuya W, Biggar WD: Cytoplasmic pH regulation in normal and abnormal neutrophils. Role of superoxide generation and Na^+/H^+ exchange. J Biol Chem 261:512, 1986

142. Grzeskowiak A, Della-Bianca V, Cassatella MA, Rossi F: Complete dissociation between the activation of phosphoinositide turnover and of NADPH oxidase by formyl-methionyl-leucyl-phenylalanine in human neutrophils depleted of Ca^{2+} and primed by subthreshold doses of phorbol 12,myristate 13,acetate. Biochem Biophys Res Commun 135:785, 1986

143. Haines KA, Giedd KN, Weissmann G: Leukotriene B_4 synthesis and metabolism by neutrophils and granule-free cytoplasts. Biochem J 233:583, 1986

144. Hallgren R, Venge P: Cationic proteins of human granulocytes: enhancement of phagocytosis of Staphylococcus protein a-IgG complexes. Inflammation 1:237, 1976

145. Hampton RY, Holz RW: Effects of changes in osmolality on the stability and function of cultured chromaffin cells and the possible role of osmotic forces in exocytosis. J Cell Biol 96:1082, 1983

146. Hayakawa T, Suzuki K, Suzuki S, Andrews PC, Babior BM: A possible role for protein phosphorylation in the activation of the respiratory burst in human neutrophils. Evidence from studies

with cells from patients with chronic granulomatous disease. J Biol Chem 261:9109, 1986

147. Helfman DM, Applebaum BD, Volger WR, Kuo JF: Phospholipid-sensitive Ca^{2+}-dependent protein kinase and its substrates in human neutrophils. Biochem Biophys Res Commun 111:847, 1983
148. Herlin T, Borregaard N: Early changes in cyclic AMP and calcium efflux during phagocytosis by neutrophils from normals and patients with chronic granulomatous disease. Immunology 48:17, 1983
149. Herlin T, Petersen CS, Esmann V: The role of calcium and cyclic adenosine 3′,5′-monophosphate in the regulation of glycogen metabolism in phagocytozing human polymorphonuclear leukocytes. Biochim Biophys Acta 542:63, 1978
150. Heyworth PG, Segal AW: Further evidence for the involvement of a phosphoprotein in the respiratory burst oxidase of human neutrophils. Biochem J 239:723, 1986
151. Higson FK, Durbin L, Pavlotsky N, Tauber AI: Studies of cytochrome b-245 translocation in the PMA stimulation of the human neutrophil NADPH-oxidase. J Immunol 135:519, 1985
152. Hodinka RL, Modrzakowski MC: Bactericidal effect of granule contents from rat polymorphonuclear leukocytes. Infect Immun 40:139, 1983
153. Hoffstein S, Goldstein IM, Weissmann G: Role of microtubule assembly in lysosomal enzyme secretion from human polymorphonuclear leukocytes. J Cell Biol 73:242, 1977
154. Hoffstein S, Soberman R, Goldstein I, Weissmann G: Concanavalin A induces microtubule assembly and specific granule discharge in human polymorphonuclear leukocytes. J Cell Biol 68:781, 1976
155. Hoffstein S, Weissmann G: Microfilaments and microtubules in calcium ionophore-induced secretion of lysosomal enzymes from human polymorphonuclear leukocytes. J Cell Biol 78:769, 1978
156. Holz RW: The role of osmotic forces in exocytosis from adrenal chromaffin cells. Ann Rev Physiol 48:175, 1986
157. Holz RW, Senter RA: Effects of osmolality and ionic strength on secretion from adrenal chromaffin cells permeabilized with digitonin. J Neurochem 46:1835, 1986
158. Hopkins NK, Lin AH, Gorman RR: Evidence for mediation of acetyl glyceryl ether phosphorylcholine stimulation of adenosine 3′,5′-(cyclic)monophosphate levels in human polymorphonuclear leukocytes by leukotriene B_4. Biochim Biophys Acta 763:276, 1983
159. Howard TH, Oresajo CO: A method for quantifying F-actin in chemotactic peptide activated neutrophils: study of the effect of tBOC peptide. Cell Motility 5:545, 1985
160. Howard TH, Oresajo CO: The kinetics of chemotactic peptide-induced change in F-actin content, F-actin distribution, and the shape of neutrophils. J Cell Biol 101:1078, 1985
161. Howard TH, Wang D: Calcium ionophore, phorbol ester, and chemotactic peptide-induced cytoskeleton reorganization in human neutrophils. J Clin Invest 79:1359, 1987
162. Huang CK: Partial purification and characterization of formyl-peptide receptor from rabbit peritoneal neutrophils. J Leukocyte Biol 41:63, 1987
163. Huang CK, Hill JM Jr, Bormann BJ, Mackin WM, Becker EL: Endogenous substrates for cyclic AMP-dependent and calcium-dependent protein phosphorylation in rabbit peritoneal neutrophils. Biochim Biophys Acta 760:126, 1983
164. Huang CK, Hill JM Jr, Bormann BJ, Mackin WM, Becker EL: Chemotactic factors induced vimentin phosphorylation in rabbit peritoneal neutrophil. J Biol Chem 259:1386, 1984
165. Huey R, Hugli TE: Characterization of a C5a receptor on human polymorphonuclear leukocytes (PMN). J Immunol 135:2063, 1985
166. Hyslop PA, Oades ZG, Jesaitis AJ, Painter RG, Cochrane CG, Sklar LA: Evidence for N-formyl chemotactic peptide-stimulated GTPase activity in human neutrophil homogenates. FEBS Lett 166:165, 1984
167. Irita K, Fujita I, Takeshige K, Minakami S, Yoshitake J: Calcium channel antagonist induced inhibition of superoxide production in human neutrophils. Mechanisms independent of antagonizing calcium influx. Biochem Pharmacol 35:3465, 1986
168. Izumi F, Yanagihara N, Wada A, Toyohira Y, Kobayashi H: Lysis of chromaffin granules by phospholipase A_2-treated plasma membranes. A cell-free model for exocytosis in adrenal medulla. FEBS Lett 196:349, 1986
169. Jackowski S, Sha'afi RI: Response of adenosine cyclic 3′,5′-monophosphate level in rabbit neutrophils to the chemotactic peptide formyl-methionyl-leucyl-phenylalanine. Mol Pharmacol 16:473, 1979
170. Janmey PA, Stossel TP: Modulation of gelsolin function by phosphatidylinositol 4,5-bisphosphate. Nature 325:362, 1987
171. Jouvin-Marche E, Poitevin B, Benveniste J: Platelet-activating factor (PAF-acether), an activator on neutrophil functions. Agents Actions 12:716, 1982
172. Jubiz W: A reevaluation of the chemotactic potency of leukotriene B_4 (LTB_4). Biochem Biophys Res Commun 110:842, 1983
173. Juhl H: Phosphorylation of glycogen synthase i from human polymorphonuclear leukocytes. Mol Cell Biochem 35:77, 1981
174. Juhl H, Esmann V: Phosphorylation of rabbit skeletal muscle glycogen synthase I by the cAMP dependent protein kinase, the cAMP independent synthase kinase and the phosvitin kinase from human polymorphonuclear leukocytes. Mol Cell Biochem 30:131, 1980
175. Juhl H, Esmann V: Phosphorylation of glycogen synthase in a homogenate of human polymorphonuclear leukocytes. Mol Cell Biochem 35:93, 1981
176. Kane SP, Peters TJ: Analytical subcellular fractionation of human granulocytes with reference to the localization of vitamin B_{12}-binding proteins. Clin Sci Mol Med 49:171, 1975
177. Kaplan L, Weiss J, Elsbach P: Low concentration of indomethacin inhibit phospholipase A_2 of rabbit polymorphonuclear leukocytes. Proc Natl Acad Sci USA 75:2955, 1978
178. Kitchen EA, Root JR, Dawson W: Chemotactic activity of thromboxane B_2, prostaglandins and their metabolites for polymorphonuclear leukocytes. Prostaglandins 16:239, 1978
179. Klempner MS: An adenosine triphosphate-dependent calcium uptake pump in human neutrophil lysosomes. J Clin Invest 76:303, 1985
180. Kobayashi M, Tanaka T, Usui T: Inactivation of lysosomal enzymes by the respiratory burst of polymorphonuclear leukocytes. Possible involvement of myeloperoxidase-H_2O_2-halide system. J Lab Clin Med 100:896, 1982
181. Komiyama A, Morosawa H, Nakahata T, Miyagawa Y, Akabane T: Abnormal neutrophil maturation in a neutrophil defect with morphologic abnormality and impaired function. J Pediatr 94:19, 1979
182. Konings F, De Potter W: Calcium-dependent *in vitro* interaction between bovine adrenal medullary cell membranes and chromaffin granules as a model for exocytosis. FEBS Lett 126:103, 1981
183. Konings F, De Potter W: The chromaffin granule-plasma membrane interaction as a model for exocytosis: quantitative release of granular content. Biochem Biophys Res Commun 104:254, 1982
184. Korchak HM, Rutherford LE, Weissmann G: Stimulus response coupling in the human neutrophil. I. Kinetic analysis of changes in calcium permeability. J Biol Chem 259:4070, 1984
185. Korchak HM, Vienne K, Rutherford LE, Wilkenfeld C, Finkelstein MC, Weissmann G: Stimulus response coupling in the human neutrophil. II. Temporal analysis of changes in cytosolic calcium and calcium influx. J Biol Chem 259:4076, 1984
186. Korn ED, Weisman RA: Phagocytosis of latex beads by Acanthamoeba. II. Electron microscopic study of the initial events. J Cell Biol 34:219, 1967
187. Krause KH, Lew PD: Subcellular distribution of Ca^{2+} pumping sites in human neutrophils. J Clin Invest 80:107, 1987
188. Krause KH, Lew PD: Calciosomes: evidence for a new type of organelle regulating intracellular Ca^{2+} in phagocytes (abstr). Clin Res 35:480, 1987
189. Krause KH, Schlegel W, Wollheim CB, Andersson T, Waldvogel FA, Lew PD: Chemotactic peptide activation of human neutrophils and HL-60 cells. Pertussis toxin reveals correlation between inositol trisphosphate generation, calcium ion transients, and cellular activation. J Clin Invest 76:1348, 1985
190. Kruskal BA, Shak S, Maxfield FR: Spreading of human neutrophils is immediately preceded by a large increase in cytoplasmic free calcium. Proc Natl Acad Sci USA 83:2919, 1986
191. Lad PM, Olson CV, Grewal IS: A step sensitive to pertussis toxin and phorbol ester in human neutrophils regulates chemotaxis and capping but not phagocytosis. FEBS Lett 200:91, 1986
192. Lad PM, Olson CV, Grewal IS: Role of a pertussis toxin substrate in the control of lectin-induced cap formation in human neutrophils. Biochem J 238:29, 1986

193. Lagast H, Pozzan T, Lew PD, Waldvogel FA: Phorbol myristate acetate stimulated the plasma membrane calcium pump without raising cytoplasmic free calcium, $(Ca^{++})_i$. Clin Res 31:410a, 1983
194. Lapetina EG, Billah MM, Cuatrecasas P: Rapid acylation and deacylation of arachidonic acid into phosphatidic acid of horse neutrophils. J Biol Chem 255:966, 1980
195. Lassing I, Lindberg U: Specific interaction between phosphatidylinositol 4,5-bisphosphate and profilactin. Nature 314:472, 1985
196. Leffell MS, Spitznagel JK: Association of lactoferrin with lysoszyme in granules of human polymorphonuclear leukocytes. Infect Immun 6:761, 1972
197. Lew PD, Andersson T, Hed J, Di Virgilio F, Pozzan T, Stendahl O: Ca^{2+}-dependent and Ca^{2+}-independent phagocytosis in human neutrophils. Nature 315:509, 1985
198. Lew PD, Dayer JM, Wollheim CB, Pozzan T: Effect of leukotriene B_4, prostaglandin E_2 and arachidonic acid on cytosolic-free calcium in human neutrophils. FEBS Lett 166:44, 1984
199. Lew PD, Monod A, Waldvogel FA, Dewald B, Baggiolini M, Pozzan T: Quantitative analysis of the cytosolic free calcium dependency of exocytosis from three subcellular compartments in intact human neutrophils. J Cell Biol 102:2197, 1986
200. Lew PD, Monod A, Waldvogel FA, Pozzan T: Role of cytosolic free calcium and phospholipase C in leukotriene-B_4-stimulated secretion in human neutrophils. Comparison with the chemotactic peptide formyl-methionyl-leucyl-phenylalanine. Eur J Biochem 162:161, 1987
201. Lew PD, Wolheim CB, Waldvogel FA, Pozzan T: Modulation of cytosolic-free calcium transients by changes in intracellular calcium-buffering capacity: correlation with exocytosis and O_2^- production in human neutrophils. J Cell Biol 99:1212, 1984
202. Light DR, Walsh C, O'Callaghan AM, Goetzl EJ, Tauber AI: Characteristics of the cofactor requirements for the superoxide-generating NADPH oxidase of human polymorphonuclear leukocytes. Biochemistry 20:1468, 1981
203. Lin AH, Morton DR, Gorman RR: Acetyl glyceryl ether phosphorylcholine stimulates leukotriene B_4 synthesis in human polymorphonuclear leukocytes. J Clin Invest 70:1058, 1982
204. Lin AH, Ruppel PL, Gorman RR: Leukotriene B_4 binding to human neutrophils. Prostaglandins 28:837, 1984
205. Lin AH, Ruppel PL, Gorman RR: Detergent solubilization of human neutrophil leukotriene B_4 receptors. Biochem Biophys Res Commun 128:878, 1985
206. Ludwig JC, McManus LM, Clark PO, Hanahan DJ, Pinckard RN: Modulation of platelet-activating factor (PAF) synthesis and release from human polymorphonuclear leukocytes (PMN): role of extracellular Ca^{2+}. Arch Biochem Biophys 232:102, 1984
207. Lumpert CJ, Kersken H, Gras U, Plattner H: Screening of enzymatic mechanisms possible involved in membrane fusion during exocytosis in paramecium cells. Cell Biol Int Rep 11:405, 1987
208. Lutter R, van Zwieten R, Weening RS, Hamers MN, Roos D: Cytochrome b, flavins, and ubiquinone-50 in enucleated human neutrophils (polymorphonuclear leukocyte cytoplasts). J Biol Chem 259:9603, 1984
209. Mackin WM, Huang CK, Becker EL: The formylpeptide chemotactic receptor on rabbit peritoneal neutrophils. I. Evidence for two binding sites with different affinities. J Immunol 129:1608, 1982
210. Malawista SE, Oliver JM, Rudolph SA: Microtubules and cyclic AMP in human leukocytes: on the order of things. J Cell Biol 77:881, 1978
211. Maridonneau Parini I, Tauber AI: Activation of NADPH-oxidase by arachidonic acid involves phospholipase A_2 in intact human neutrophils but not in the cell-free system. Biochem Biophys Res Commun 138:1099, 1986
212. Maridonneau Parini I, Tringale SM, Tauber AI: Identification of distinct activation pathways of the human neutrophil NADPH-oxidase. J Immunol 137:2925, 1986
213. Marx RS, McCall CE, Bass DA: Chemotaxin-induced changes in cyclic adenosine monophosphate levels in human neutrophils. Infect Immun 29:284, 1980
214. Matsumoto T, Molski TFP, Volpi M, Pelz C, Kanaho Y, Becker EL, Feinstein MB, Naccache PH, Sha'afi RI: Treatment of rabbit neutrophils with phorbol esters results in increased ADP-ribosylation catalyzed by pertussis toxin and inhibition of the GTPase stimulated by fMet-Leu-Phe. FEBS Lett 198:295, 1986
215. McNeil PL, Kennedy AL, Waggoner AS, Taylor DL, Murphy RF: Light-scattering changes during chemotactic stimulation of human neutrophils: kinetics followed by flow cytometry. Cytometry 6:7, 1985
216. McPhail LC, Clayton CC, Snyderman R: A potential second messenger role for unsaturated fatty acids: activation of Ca^{2+}-dependent protein kinase. Science 224:622, 1984
217. McPhail LC, Shirley PS, Clayton CC, Snyderman R: Activation of the respiratory burst enzyme from human neutrophils in a cell-free system. Evidence for a soluble cofactor. J Clin Invest 75:1735, 1985
218. McPhail LC, Synderman R: Activation of the respiratory burst enzyme in human polymorphonuclear leukocytes by chemoattractants and other soluble stimuli. Evidence that the same oxidase is activated by different transductional mechanisms. J Clin Invest 72:192, 1983
219. Meers P, Ernst JD, Duzgunes N, Hong KL, Fedor J, Goldstein IM, Papahadjopoulos D: Synexin-like proteins from human polymorphonuclear leukocytes. Identification and characterization of granule-aggregating and membrane-fusing activities. J Biol Chem 262:7850, 1987
220. Mellon MG, Rebhun LI: Sulfhydryls and the *in vitro* polymerization of tubulin. J Cell Biol 70:226, 1976
221. Meuller HW, O'Flaherty JT, Wykle RL: The molecular species distribution of platelet-activating factor synthesized by rabbit and human neutrophils. J Biol Chem 259:14554, 1984
222. Michener ML, Dawson WB, Creutz CE: Phosphorylation of a chromaffin granule-binding protein in stimulated chromaffin cells. J Biol Chem 261:6548, 1986
223. Miyasaki KT, Wilson ME, Cohen E, Jones PC, Genco RJ: Evidence for and partial characterization of three major and three minor forms of human neutrophil myeloperoxidase. Arch Biochem Biophys 246:751, 1986
224. Mollinedo F, Manara FS, Schneider DL: Acidification activity of human neutrophils. Tertiary granules as a site of ATP-dependent acidification. J Biol Chem 261:1077, 1986
225. Mollinedo F, Schneider DL: Subcellular localization of cytochrome b and ubiquinone in a tertiary granule of resting human neutrophils and evidence for a proton pump ATPase. J Biol Chem 259:7143, 1984
226. Molski TFP, Ford C, Weisman SJ, Sha'afi RI: Cell alkalinization is not necessary and increased sodium influx is not sufficient for stimulated superoxide production. FEBS Lett 203:267, 1986
227. Molski TFP, Naccache PH, Sha'afi RI: Stimulus-dependent changes in calcium metabolism in rabbit neutrophils. Cell Calcium 4:57, 1983
228. Molski TFP, Naccache PH, Volpi M, Wolpert LM, Sha'afi RI: Specific modulation of the intracellular pH of rabbit neutrophils by chemotactic factors. Biochem Biophys Res Commun 94:508, 1980
229. Momayezi M, Lumpert CJ, Kersken H, Gras U, Plattner H, Krinks MH, Klee CB: Exocytosis induction in Paramecium tetraurelia cells by exogenous phosphoprotein phosphatase *in vivo* and *in vitro*: possible involvement of calcineurin in exocytotic membrane fusion. J Cell Biol 105:181, 1987
230. Morimoto YM, Sato E, Nobori K, Takahashi R, Utsumi K: Effect of calcium ion on fatty acid-induced generation of superoxide in guinea pig neutrophils. Cell Struct Funct 11:143, 1986
231. Movat HZ, Steinberg SG, Flavio M, Habal FM, Ranadive NS: Demonstration of a kinin-generating enzyme in the lysosomes of human polymorphonuclear leukocytes. Lab Invest 29:669, 1973
232. Murphy G, Bretz U, Baggiolini M, Reynolds JJ: The latent collagenase and gelatinase of human polymorphonuclear neutrophil leucocytes. Biochem J 192:517, 1980
233. Murphy G, Reynolds JJ, Bretz U, Baggiolini M: Collagenase as a component of the specific granules of human neutrophil leukocytes. Biochem J 162:195, 1977
234. Naccache PH, Molski MM, Volpi M, Becker EL, Sha'afi RI: Unique inhibitory profile of platelet activating factor induced calcium mobilization, polyphosphoinositide turnover and granule enzyme secretion in rabbit neutrophils towards pertussis toxin and phorbol ester. Biochem Biophys Res Commun 130:677, 1985
235. Naccache PH, Molski MM, Volpi M, Shefcyk J, Molski TF, Loew L, Becker EL, Sha'afi RI: Biochemical events associated with the stimulation of rabbit neutrophils by platelet-activating factor. J

Leuk Biol 40:533, 1986
236. Naccache PH, Molski TFP, Borgeat P, Sha'afi RI: Mechanism of action of leukotriene B_4: intracellular calcium redistribution in rabbit neutrophils. J Cell Physiol 118:13, 1984
237. Naccache PH, Molski TFP, Borgeat P, Sha'afi RI: Association of leukotriene B_4 with the cytoskeleton of rabbit neutrophils. Effect of chemotactic factor and phorbol esters. Biochem Biophys Res Commun 124:963, 1984
238. Naccache PH, Molski TFP, Borgeat P, Sha'afi RI: Intracellular calcium redistribution and its relationship to fMet-Leu-Phe, leukotriene B_4, and phorbol ester induced rabbit neutrophil degranulation. J Cell Physiol 122:273, 1985
239. Naccache PH, Sha'afi RI, Borgeat P, Goetzl EJ: Mono- and dihydroxyeicosatetraenoic acids alter calcium homeostasis in rabbit neutrophils. J Clin Invest 67:1584, 1981
240. Naccache PH, Showell HJ, Becker EL, Sha'afi RI: Arachidonic acid induced degranulation of rabbit peritoneal neutrophils. Biochem Biophys Res Commun 87:292, 1979
241. Naccache PH, Volpi M, Showell HJ, Becker EL, Sha'afi RI: Chemotactic factor-induced release of membrane calcium in rabbit neutrophils. Science 203:461, 1979
242. Naef A, Damerau B, Keller HU: Relationship between the transient cAMP increase, exocytosis from specific and azurophil granules and chemotaxis in neutrophil granulocytes. Agents Actions 14:63, 1984
243. Nahas N, Juhl H, Esmann V: Chromatographic characteristics and subcellular localization of synthase phosphatase, phosphorylase phosphatase and histone phosphatase in human polymorphonuclear leukocytes. Mol Cell Biochem 58:147, 1984
244. Nakanishi M, Goto K: Inhibitory effects of anti-inflammatory drugs on enzyme release from rabbit polymorphonuclear leukocyte lysosomes. Biochem Pharmacol 24:421, 1975
245. Nath J, Flavin M, Gallin JI: Tubulin tyrosinolation in human polymorphonuclear leukocytes: studies in normal subjects and in patients with the Chediak-Higashi syndrome. J Cell Biol 95:519, 1982
246. Nath J, Gallin JI: Studies in normal and chronic granulomatous disease neutrophils indicate a correlation of tubulin tyrosinolation with the cellular redox state. J Clin Invest 71:1273, 1983
247. Nath J, Gallin JI: Ionic requirements and subcellular localization of tubulin tyrosinolation in human polymorphonuclear leukocytes. J Immunol 136:628, 1986
248. Ng DS, Wong K: GTP regulation of platelet-activating factor binding to human neutrophil membranes. Biochem Biophys Res Commun 141:353, 1986
249. Niedel J, Davis J, Cuatrecasas P: Covalent affinity labelling of the formyl peptide chemotactic receptor. J Biol Chem 255:7063, 1980
250. Niedel JE, Kuhn LJ, Vandenbark GR: Phorbol diester receptor copurifies with protein kinase C. Proc Natl Acad Sci USA 80:36, 1983
251. Niedel J, Wilkinson S, Cuatrecasas P: Receptor-mediated uptake of 125I-chemotactic peptide by human neutrophils. J Biol Chem 254:10700, 1979
252. Nishihira J, O'Flaherty JT: Phorbol myristate acetate receptors in human polymorphonuclear neutrophils. J Immunol 135:3439, 1985
253. Northover AM: The effects of some non-steroidal anti-inflammatory agents on membrane-associated calcium in rabbit peritoneal neutrophils. Biochem Pharmacol 34:3123, 1985
254. Northover BJ: Effect of indomethacin and related drugs on the calcium ion-dependent secretion of lysosomal and other enzymes by neutrophil polymorphonuclear leukocytes *in vitro*. Br J Pharmacol 59:253, 1977
255. Nourshargh S, Hoult JR: Divergent effects of co-carcinogenic phorbol esters and a synthetic diacylglycerol on human neutrophil chemokinesis and granular enzyme secretion. Br J Pharmacol 91:557, 1987
256. O'Flaherty JT, Hammett MJ, Shewmake TB, Wykle RL, Love SH, McCall CE, Thomas MJ: Evidence for 5,12-dihydroxy-6-8-10,14-eicosatetraenoate as a mediator of human neutrophil aggregation. Biochem Biophys Res Commun 103:552, 1981
257. O'Flaherty JT, Salzer WL, Cousart S, McCall CE, Paintadosi C, Surles JR, Hammett MJ, Wykle RL: Platelet-activating factor and analogues: comparative studies with human neutrophils and rabbit platelets. Res Commun Chem Pathol Pharmacol 39:291, 1983
258. O'Flaherty JT, Schmitt JD, Wykle RL: Interactions of arachidonate metabolism and protein kinase C in mediating neutrophil function. Biochem Biophys Res Commun 127:916, 1985
259. O'Flaherty JT, Schmitt JD, Wykle RL, Redman JF Jr, McCall CE: Diacylglycerols and mezerein activate neutrophils by a phorbol myristate acetate-like mechanism. J Cell Physiol 125:192, 1985
260. O'Flaherty JT, Thomas MJ: Effect of 15-lipoxygenase-derived arachidonate metabolites on human neutrophil degranulation. Prostaglandins Leukotrienes Med 17:199, 1985
261. O'Flaherty JT, Wykle RL, Lees CJ, Shewmake T, McCall CE, Thomas MJ: Neutrophil-degranulating action of 5,12-dihydroxy-6,8,10,14-eicosatetraenoic acid and 1-O-alkyl-2-O-acetyl-*sn*-glycero-3-phosphocholine. Comparison with other degranulating agents. Am J Pathol 105:264, 1981
262. O'Flaherty JT, Wykle RL, Miller CH, Lewis JC, Waite M, Bass DA, McCall CE, DeChatelet LR: 1-O-alkyl-*sn*-glyceryl-3-phosphorylcholines. A novel class of neutrophil stimulants. Am J Pathol 103:70, 1981
263. O'Flaherty JT, Wykle RL, Thomas MJ, McCall CE: Neutrophil degranulation responses to combinations of arachidonate metabolites and platelet-activating factor. Res Commun Chem Pathol Pharmacol 43:3, 1984
264. O'Shea JJ, Brown EJ, Seligmann BE, Metcalf JA, Frank MM, Gallin JI: Evidence for distinct intracellular pools of receptors for C3b and C3bi in human neutrophils. J Immunol 134:2580, 1985
265. Ochs DL, Reed PW: ATP-dependent calcium transport in plasma membrane vesicles from neutrophil leukocytes. J Biol Chem 258:10116, 1983
266. Ochs DL, Reed PW: Ca^{2+}-stimulated, Mg^{2+}-dependent ATPase activity in neutrophil plasma membrane vesicles. Coupling to Ca^{2+} transport. J Biol Chem 259:102, 1984
267. Ohki S, Duax J: Effects of cations and polyamines on the aggregation and fusion of phosphatidylserine membranes. Biochim Biophys Acta 861:177, 1986
268. Ohlsson K: Granulocyte collagenase and elastase and their interactions with a1-antitrypsin and a2-macroglobulin. In Proteases and Biological Control, edited by Reich D, Rifkin DB, Shaw E, p 591. Cold Spring Harbor, Cold Spring Harbor Laboratories, 1975
269. Ohno Y, Buescher ES, Roberts R, Metcalf JA, Gallin JI: Reevaluation of cytochrome b and flavin adenine dinucleotide in neutrophils from patients with chronic granulomatous disease and description of a family with probable autosomal recessive inheritance of cytochrome b deficiency. Blood 67:1132, 1986
270. Ohno Y, Seligmann BE, Gallin JI: Cytochrome b translocation to human neutrophil plasma membranes and superoxide release. Differential effects of N-formylmethionylleucylphenylalanine, phorbol myristate acetate, and A23187. J Biol Chem 260:2409, 1985
271. Ohtsuka T, Okamura N, Ishibashi S: Involvement of protein kinase C in the phosphorylation of 46 kDa proteins which are phosphorylated in parallel with activation of NADPH oxidase in intact guinea-pig polymorphonuclear leukocytes. Biochim Biophys Acta 888:332, 1986
272. Okajima F, Ui M: ADP-ribosylation of the specific membrane protein by islet-activating protein, pertussis toxin, associated with inhibition of a chemotactic peptide-induced arachidonate release in neutrophils. Possible role of the toxin substrate in Ca^{2+}-mobilizing biosignaling. J Biol Chem 259:13863, 1984
273. Okamura N, Ohashi S, Nagahisa N, Ishibashi S: Changes in protein phosphorylation in guinea pig polymorphonuclear leukocytes by treatment with membrane-perturbing agents which stimulate superoxide anion production. Arch Biochem Biophys 228:270, 1984
274. Okamura N, Uchida M, Ohtsuka T, Kawanishi M, Ishibashi S: Diverse involvements of Ni protein in superoxide anion production in polymorphonuclear leukocytes depending on the type of membrane stimulants. Biochem Biophys Res Commun 130:939, 1985
275. Oliver JM, Berlin RD: Surface and cytoskeletal events regulating leukocyte membrane topography. Semin Hematol 20:282, 1983
276. Oliver JM, Spielberg SP, Pearson CB, Schulman JD: Microtubule assembly and function in normal and glutathione synthetase-

deficient polymorphonuclear leukocytes. J Immunol 120:1181, 1978

277. Oliver JM, Ukena TE, Berlin RD: Effects of phagocytosis and colchicine on the distribution of lectin-binding sites of the cell surface. Proc Natl Acad Sci USA 71:394, 1974
278. Palmblad J, Malmsten CL, Uden AM, Radmark O, Engstedt L, Samuelsson B: Leukotriene B_4 is a potent and stereospecific stimulator of neutrophil chemotaxis and adherence. Blood 58:658, 1981
279. Palmblad J, Uden AM, Lindgren JA, Radmark O, Hansson G, Malmsten CL: Effects of novel leukotrienes on neutrophil migration. FEBS Lett 144:81, 1982
280. Palmer RMJ, Salmon JA: Release of leukotriene B_4 from human neutrophils and its relationship to degranulation induced by N-formyl-methionyl-leucyl-phenylalanine, serum-treated zymosan and the ionophore A23187. Immunology 50:65, 1983
281. Panus PC, Eddy LJ, Longenecker GL: Measurement of malonyldialdehyde production during sodium arachidonate-induced polymorphonuclear leukocyte aggregation. J Pharmacol Methods 13:179, 1985
282. Parkinson JR, Akard JP, Schell MJ, Gabig TG: Cell-free activation of phagocyte NADPH-oxidase; tissue and differentiation-specific expression of cytosolic cofactor activity. Biochem Biophys Res Commun 145:1198, 1987
283. Parkos CA, Cochrane CG, Schmitt M, Jesaitis AJ: Regulation of the oxidative response of human granulocytes to chemoattractants. No evidence for stimulated traffic of redox enzymes between endo and plasma membranes. J Biol Chem 260:6541, 1985
284. Parmley RT, Takagi M, Barton JC, Boxer LA, Austin RL: Ultrastructural localization of lactoferrin and iron-binding protein in human neutrophils and rabbit heterophils. Am J Pathol 109:343, 1982
285. Parry MF, Root RK, Metcalf JA, Delaney KK, Kaplow LS, Richar WJ: Myeloperoxidase deficiency. Prevalence and clinical significance. Ann Int Med 95:293, 1981
286. Penfield A, Dale MM: Synergy between A23187 and 1-oleoyl-2-acetyl-glycerol in superoxide production by human neutrophils. Biochem Biophys Res Commun 125:332, 1984
287. Pennington JE, Kemmerich B, Kazanjian PH, Marsh JD, Boerth LW: Verapamil impairs human neutrophil chemotaxis by a non-calcium-mediated mechanism. J Lab Clin Med 108:44, 1986
288. Perez HD, Marder S, Elfman F, Ives HE: Human neutrophils contain subpopulations of specific granules exhibiting different sensitivities to changes in cytosolic free calcium. Biochem Biophys Res Commun 145:976, 1987
289. Petrequin PR, Todd RF III, Devall LJ, Boxer LA, Curnutte JT III: Association between gelatinase release and increased plasma membrane expression of the Mol glycoprotein. Blood 69:605, 1987
290. Pollard HB, Creutz CE, Fowler V, Scott J, Pazoles CJ: Calcium-dependent regulation of chromaffin granule movement, membrane contact, and fusion during exocytosis. Cold Spring Harbor Symp Quant Biol 46:819, 1982
291. Pollard HB, Tack Goldman K, Pazoles CJ, Creutz CE, Shulman NR: Evidence for control of serotonin secretion from human platelets by hydroxyl ion transport and osmotic lysis. Proc Natl Acad Sci 74:5295, 1977
292. Pontremoli E, Melloni E, Salamino F, Sparatore B, Michetti M, Sacco O, Horecker BL: Activation of NADPH oxidase and phosphorylation of membrane proteins in human neutrophils: coordinate inhibition by a surface antigen-directed monoclonal antibody. Biochem Biophys Res Commun 140:1121, 1986
293. Pontremoli S, Melloni E, Salamino F, Sparatore B, Michetti M, Sacco O, Horecker BL: Activation of NADPH oxidase and phosphorylation of membrane proteins in human neutrophils: coordinate inhibition by a surface antigen-directed monoclonal antibody. Biochem Biophys Res Commun 140:1121, 1986
294. Pozzan T, Lew DP, Wollheim CB, Tsein RY: Is cytosolic ionized calcium regulating neutrophil activation? Science 221:1413, 1983
295. Prentki M, Wollheim CB, Lew PD: Ca^{2+} homeostasis in permeabilized human neutrophils. Characterization of Ca^{2+}-sequestering pools and the action of inositol 1,4,5-trisphosphate. J Biol Chem 259:13777, 1984
296. Prescott SM, Zimmerman GA, Seeger AR: Leukotriene B_4 is an incomplete agonist for the activation of human neutrophils. Biochem Biophys Res Commun 122:535, 1984
297. Pryzwansky KB, Schliwa M, Porter KR: Comparison of the three-dimensional organization of unextracted and Triton-extracted human neutrophilic polymorphonuclear leukocytes. Eur J Cell Biol 30:112, 1983
298. Pryzwansky KB, Steiner AL, Spitznagel JK, Kapoor CL: Compartmentalization of cyclic AMP during phagocytosis of human neutrophilic granulocytes. Science 211:407, 1981
299. Radmark O, Malmsten C, Samuelsson B, Clark DA, Goto G, Marfat A, Corey EJ: Leukotriene A: stereochemistry and enzymatic conversion to leukotriene B. Biochem Biophys Res Commun 92:954, 1980
300. Radmark O, Malmsten C, Samuelsson B, Goto G, Marfat A, Corey EJ: Leukotriene A. Isolation from human polymorphonuclear leukocytes. J Biol Chem 255:11828, 1980
301. Riccardi S, Giordano D, Schettini F, De Mattia D, Lovecchio T, Santoro N, Fumarulo R: Cytochrome b and FAD content in polymorphonuclear leucocytes in a family with X-linked chronic granulomatous disease. Scand J Haematol 37:333, 1986
302. Rickard JE, Sheterline P: Evidence that phorbol ester interferes with stimulated Ca^{2+} redistribution by activating Ca^{2+} efflux in neutrophil leucocytes. Biochem J 231:623, 1985
303. Rider LG, Niedel JE: Diacylglycerol accumulation and superoxide anion production in stimulated human neutrophils. J Biol Chem 262:5603, 1987
304. Rollins TE, Springer MS: Identification of the polymorphonuclear leukocytes C5a receptor. J Biol Chem 260:7157, 1985
305. Rossi F, Grzeskowiak M, Della-Bianca V: Double stimulation with FMLP and Con A restores the activation of the respiratory burst but not of the phosphoinositide turnover in Ca^{2+}-depleted human neutrophils. A further example of dissociation between stimulation of the NADPH oxidase and phosphoinositide turnover. Biochem Biophys Res Commun 140:1, 1986
306. Salari H, Braquet P, Naccache P, Borgeat P: Characterization of effect of N-formyl-methionyl-leucyl-phenylalanine on leukotriene synthesis in human polymorphonuclear leukocytes. Inflammation 9:127, 1985
307. Schiffman E, Aswanikumar S, Venkatasubramanian K, Corcoran BA, Pert CB, Brown J, Gross E, Day AR, Freer RJ, Showell AH, Becker EL: Some characteristics of the neutrophil receptor for chemotactic peptides. FEBS Lett 117:1, 1980
308. Schmitt M, Painter RG, Jesaitis AJ, Preissner K, Sklar LA, Cochrane CG: Photoaffinity labeling of the N-formyl peptide receptor binding site of intact human polymorphonuclear leukocytes. A label suitable for following the fate of the receptor-ligand complex. J Biol Chem 258:649, 1983
309. Schneider C, Zanetti M, Romeo D: Surface-reactive stimuli selectively increase protein phosphorylation in human neutrophils. FEBS Lett 127:4, 1981
310. Segal AW: Absence of both cytochrome b-245 subunits from neutrophils in X-linked chronic granulomatous disease. Nature 326:88, 1987
311. Segal AW, Cross AR, Garcia RC, Borregaard N, Valerius NH, Soothill JF, Jones OTG: Absence of cytochrome b-245 in chronic granulomatous disease. A multicenter European evaluation of its incidence and relevance. N Engl J Med 308:245, 1983
312. Segal AW, Jones OTG: The subcellular distribution and some properties of the cytochrome b component of the microbicidal oxidase system of human neutrophils. Biochem J 182:181, 1979
313. Segal AW, Jones OTG: Absence of cytochrome b reduction in stimulated neutrophils from both female and male patients with chronic granulomatous disease. FEBS Lett 110:111, 1980
314. Seifert R, Rosenthal W, Schultz G: Guanine nucleotides stimulate NADPH oxidase in membranes of human neutrophils. FEBS Lett 205:161, 1986
315. Seifert R, Schultz G: Fatty-acid-induced activation of NADPH oxidase in plasma membranes of human neutrophils depends on neutrophil cytosol and is potentiated by stable guanine nucleotides. Eur J Biochem 162:563, 1987
316. Selsted ME, Harwig SSL, Ganz T, Schilling JW, Lehrer RI: Primary structures of three human neutrophil defensins. J Clin Invest 76:1436, 1985
317. Sha'afi RI, Molski TFP: Signalling for increased cytoskeletal actin in neutrophils. Biochem Biophys Res Commun 145:934, 1987
318. Sha'afi RI, Naccache PH, Molski TFP, Volpi M: Chemotactic stimuli-induced changes in pHi of rabbit neutrophils. In Intracel-

lular pH: its Measurement Regulation, and Utilization in Cellular Functions, p 513. New York, Alan R. Liss, 1982
319. Sha'afi RI, Shefcyk J, Yassin R, Molski TFP, Volpi M, Naccache PH, White JR, Feinstein MB, Becker EL: Is a rise in intracellular concentration of free calcium necessary or sufficient for stimulated cytoskeletal-associated actin? J Cell Biol 102:1459, 1986
320. Sha'afi RI, White JR, Molski TFP, Shefcyk J, Volpi M, Naccache PH, Feinstein MB: Phorbol 12-myristate 13-acetate activates rabbit neutrophils without an apparent rise in the level of intracellular free calcium. Biochem Biophys Res Commun 114:638, 1983
321. Sha'afi RI, Williams K, Wacholtz MC, Becker EL: Binding of the chemotactic synthetic peptide (^{3}H)formyl-norleu-leu-phe to plasma membrane of rabbit neutrophils. FEBS Lett 91:305, 1978
322. Shak S, Goldstein IM: Carbon monoxide inhibits w-oxidation of leukotriene B_4 by human polymorphonuclear leukocytes: evidence that catabolism of leukotriene B_4 is mediated by a cytochrome P-450 enzyme. Biochem Biophys Res Commun 123:475, 1984
323. Shak S, Goldstein IM: w-Oxidation is the major pathway for the catabolism of leukotriene B_4 in human polymorphonuclear leukocytes. J Biol Chem 259:10181, 1984
324. Shak S, Goldstein IM: Leukotriene B_4 w-hydroxylase in human polymorphonuclear leukocytes. Partial purification and identification as a cytochrome P-450. J Clin Invest 76:1218, 1985
325. Shak S, Perz HD, Goldstein IM: A novel dioxygenation product of arachidonic acid possesses potent chemotactic activity for human polymorphonuclear leukocytes. J Biol Chem 258:14948, 1983
326. Sheterline P, Rickard JE, Boothroyd B, Richards RC: Phorbol ester induces rapid actin assembly in neutrophil leucocytes independently of changes in $[Ca^{2+}]_i$ and pHi. J Muscle Res Cell Motil 7:405, 1986
327. Shibata N, Tatsumi N, Tanaka K, Okamura Y, Senda N: A contractile protein possessing Ca^{2+} sensitivity (natural actomysin) from leucocytes. Its extraction and some of its properties. Biochim Biophys Acta 256:565, 1972
328. Shoji M, Girard PR, Mazzei GJ, Vogler WR, Kuo JF: Immunochemical evidence for phorbol ester-induced protein kinase C translocation in HL60 cells. Biochem Biophys Res Commun 135:1144, 1986
329. Showell HJ, Otterness IG, Marfar A, Corey EJ: Inhibition of leukotriene B_4-induced neutrophil degranulation by leukotriene B_4-dimethylamide. Biochem Biophys Res Commun 106:741, 1982
330. Simchowitz L: Chemotactic factor-induced activation of Na^+/H^+ exchange in human neutrophils. II. Intracellular pH changes. J Biol Chem 260:13248, 1985.
331. Simchowitz L: Chemotactic factor-induced activation of Na^+/H^+ exchange in human neutrophils. I. Sodium fluxes. J Biol Chem 260:13237, 1985
332. Simchowitz L, Atkinson JP, Spilberg I: Stimulus-dependent deactivation of chemotactic factor-induced cyclic AMP response and superoxide generation by human neutrophils. J Clin Invest 66:736, 1980
333. Simchowitz L, Cragoe EJ Jr: Regulation of human neutrophil chemotaxis by intracellular pH. J Biol Chem 261:6492, 1986
334. Simchowitz L, Fischbein LC, Spilberg I, Atkinson JP: Induction of a transient elevation in intracellular levels of adenosine-3′,5′-monophosphate by chemotactic factors: an early event in human neutrophil activation. J Immunol 124:1482, 1980
335. Simchowitz L, Spilberg I, Atkinson JP: Evidence that the functional responses of human neutrophils occur independently of transient elevations in cyclic AMP levels. J Cyclic Nucleotide Protein Phosphor Res 9:35, 1983
336. Sklar LA, Bokoch GM, Button D, Smolen JE: Regulation of ligand-receptor dynamics by guanyl nucleotides: rapidly interconverting states for the neutrophil formyl peptide receptor (abstr). Fed Proc 45:5705, 1986
337. Sklar LA, Bokoch GM, Button D, Smolen JE: Regulation of ligand-receptor dynamics by guanine nucleotides. Real-time analysis of interconverting states for the neutrophil formyl peptide receptor. J Biol Chem 262:135, 1987
338. Sklar LA, Hyslop PA, Oades ZG, Omann GM, Jesaitis AJ, Painter RG, Cochrane CG: Signal transduction and ligand-receptor dynamics in the human neutrophil. Transient responses and occupancy-response relations at the formyl peptide receptor. J Biol Chem 260:11461, 1985
339. Sklar LA, Jesaitis AJ, Painter RG, Cochrane CG: The kinetics of neutrophil activation. The response to chemotactic peptides depends upon whether ligand-receptor interaction is rate-limiting. J Biol Chem 256:9909, 1981
340. Sklar LA, McNeil VM, Jesaitis AJ, Painter RG, Cochrane CG: A continuous, spectroscopic analysis of the kinetics of elastase secretion by neutrophils. The dependence of secretion upon receptor occupancy. J Biol Chem 257:5471, 1982
341. Sklar LA, Oades ZG: Signal transduction and ligand-receptor dynamics in the neutrophil. Ca^{2+} modulation and restoration. J Biol Chem 260:11468, 1985
342. Sklar LA, Omann GM, Painter RG: Relationship of actin polymerization and depolymerization to light scattering in human neutrophils: dependence on receptor occupancy and intracellular Ca^{2+}. J Cell Biol 101:1161, 1985
343. Slonczewski JL, Wilde MW, Zigmond SH: Phosphorylase a activity as an indicator of neutrophil activation by chemotactic peptide. J Cell Biol 101:1191, 1985
344. Smith CD, Uhing RJ, Snyderman R: Nucleotide regulatory protein-mediated activation of phospholipase C in human polymorphonuclear leukocytes is disrupted by phorbol esters. J Biol Chem 262:6121, 1987
345. Smith DM Jr, Waite M: Phospholipid metabolism in human neutrophil subfractions. Arch Biochem Biophys 246:263, 1986
346. Smith GP, Peters TJ: The release of granule components from human polymorphonuclear leukocytes in response to both phagocytic and chemical stimuli. Biochim Biophys Acta 719:304, 1982
347. Smith GP, Sharp G, Peters TJ: Isolation and characterization of alkaline phosphatase-containing granules (phosphasomes) from human polymorphonuclear leucocytes. J Cell Sci 76:167, 1985
348. Smith RJ: Nonsteroid anti-inflammatory agents: regulators of the phagocytic secretion of lysosomal enzymes from guinea pig neutrophils. J Pharmacol Exp Ther 207:618, 1978
349. Smith RJ, Bowman BJ: Stimulation of human neutrophil degranulation with 1-O-octadecyl-2-O-acetyl-*sn*-glyceryl-3-phosphorylcholine: modulation by inhibitors of arachidonic acid metabolism. Biochem Biophys Res Commun 104:1495, 1982
350. Smith RJ, Bowman BJ, Iden SS: Characteristics of 1-O-hexadecyl- and 1-*O*-octadecyl-2-O-acetyl-*sn*-glyceryl-3-phosphorylcholine-stimulated granule enzyme release from human neutrophils. Clin Immunol Immunopathol 28:13, 1983
351. Smith RJ, Iden SS: Phorbol myristate acetate-induced release of granule enzymes from human neutrophils: inhibition by the calcium antagonist 8-(N,N-diethylamido)-octyl 3,4,5 trimethoxybenzoate hydrochloride. Biochem Biophys Res Commun 91:263, 1979
352. Smith RJ, Iden SS, Bowman BJ: Activation of the human neutrophil secretory process with 5(S), 12(R)-dihydroxy-6,14-*cis*-8,10-trans-eicosatetraenoic acid. Inflammation 8:365, 1984
353. Smolen JE: The fluorescence response of chlortetracycline-loaded human neutrophils is modulated by prostaglandin E_1, but not by cyclic nucleotides. FEBS Lett 163:119, 1983
354. Smolen JE: Secretion from neutrophils: a critique of modern *in vitro* techniques. In *In Vitro* Methods for Studying Secretion, edited by Poisner AM, Trifaro JM, p 29. Amsterdam, Elsevier 1987
355. Smolen JE, Karnovsky ML: The effect of phagocytosis on guinea pig granulocyte membrane markers. J Cell Physiol 102:71, 1980
356. Smolen JE, Korchak HM, Weissmann G: Increased levels of cyclic adenosine-3′,5′-monophosphate in human polymorphonuclear leukocytes after surface stimulation. J Clin Invest 65:1077, 1980
357. Smolen JE, Korchak HM, Weissmann G: The roles of extracellular and intracellular calcium in lysosomal enzyme release and superoxide anion generation by human polymorphonuclear leukocytes. Biochim Biophys Acta 677:512, 1981
358. Smolen JE, Korchak HM, Weissmann G: The kinetics of lysosomal degranulation of human neutrophils as measured by 9-aminoacridine quenching. Biochim Biophys Acta 762:145, 1983
359. Smolen JE, Noble P, Freed R, Weissmann G: Metabolic requirements for maintenance of the chlortetracycline-labeled pool of membrane-bound calcium in human neutrophils. J Cell Physiol 117:415, 1983
360. Smolen JE, Stoehr SJ: Micromolar concentrations of free calcium provoke secretion of lysozyme from human neutrophils permeabilized with saponin. J Immunol 134:1859, 1985

361. Smolen JE, Stoehr SJ: Guanine nucleotides reduce the free calcium requirement for secretion of granule constituents from permeabilized human neutrophils. Biochim Biophys Acta 889:171, 1986
362. Smolen JE, Stoehr SJ, Boxer LA: Human neutrophils permeabilized with digitonin respond with lysosomal enzyme release when exposed to micromolar levels of free calcium. Biochim Biophys Acta 886:1, 1986
363. Smolen JE, Stoehr SJ, Traynor AE, Sklar LA: The kinetics of secretion from permeabilized human neutrophils: release of elastase and correlations with other granule constituents and right angle light scatter. J Leukocyte Biol 41:8, 1987
364. Smolen JE, Todd RF III, Boxer LA: Expression of a granule membrane marker on the surface of neutrophils permeabilized with digitonin. Correlations with Ca^{2+}-induced degranulation. Am J Pathol 124:281, 1986
365. Smolen JE, Weissmann G: Effects of indomethacin, 5,8,11,14-eicosatetraynoic acid, and p-bromophenacyl bromide on lysosomal enzyme release and superoxide. Biochem Pharmacol 29:533, 1979
366. Smolen JE, Weissmann G: Stimuli which provoke secretion of azurophil granules induce increments in adenosine cyclic 3′,5′-monophosphate. Biochim Biophys Acta 672:197, 1981
367. Snyderman R, Pike MS, Edge S, Lane B: A chemoattractant receptor on macrophages exists in two affinity states regulated by guanine nucleotides. J Biol Chem 98:444, 1984
368. Sopata I, Dancewicz AM: Presence of a gelatin-specific proteinase and its latent form in human leucocytes. Biochim Biophys Acta 370:510, 1974
369. Southwick FS, Stossel TP: Contractile proteins in leukocyte function. Semin Hematol 20:305, 1983
370. Spagnuolo PJ, Ellner JJ, Hassid A, Dunn MJ: Thromboxane A_2 mediates augmented polymorphonuclear leukocyte adhesiveness. J Clin Invest 66:406, 1980
371. Spat A, Bradford PG, McKinney JS, Rubin RP, Putney JW Jr: A saturable receptor for 32P-inositol-1,4,5-trisphosphate in hepatocytes and neutrophils. Nature 319:514, 1986
372. Spearman TN, Hurley KP, Olivas R, Ulrich RG, Butcher FR: Subcellular location of stimulus-affected endogenous phosphoproteins in the rat parotid gland. J Cell Biol 99:1354, 1984
373. Spitznagel JK, Dalldorf FG, Leffel MS, Folds JD, Welsh IRH, Cooney MH, Martin LE: Character of azurophil and specific granules purified from human polymorphonuclear leukocytes. Lab Invest 30:744, 1974
374. Stendahl O, Coble BI, Dahlgren C, Hed J, Molin L: Myeloperoxidase modulates the phagocytic activity of polymorphonuclear neutrophil leukocytes. Studies with cells from a myeloperoxidase-deficient patient. J Clin Invest 73:366, 1984
375. Stendahl OI, Stossel TP: Actin-binding protein amplifies actomyosin contraction, and gelsolin confers calcium control on the direction of contraction. Biochem Biophys Res Comm 92:675, 1980
376. Stenson WF, Parker CW: Monohydroxytetraenoic acids (HETEs) induce degranulation of human neutrophils. J Immunol 124:2100, 1980
377. Sterner DC, Zaks WJ, Creutz CE: Stimulation of the Ca^{2+}-dependent polymerization of synexin by *cis*-unsaturated fatty acids. Biochem Biophys Res Commun 132:505, 1985
378. Stewart DIH, Crawford N: Redistribution of membrane-bound and cytosolic actin in rabbit polymorphonuclear leucocytes during phagocytosis. Biochem J 225:807, 1985
379. Stickle DF, Daniele RP, Holian A: Cytosolic calcium, calcium fluxes, and regulation of alveolar macrophage superoxide anion production. J Cell Physiol 121:458, 1984
380. Stoehr SJ, Smolen JE: Osmotic forces are not critical for Ca^{2+}-induced secretion from permeabilized human neutrophils. J Cell Physiol 135:169, 1988
381. Stossel TP, Pollard TD: Myosin in polymorphonuclear leukocytes. J Biol Chem 248:8288, 1973
382. Strauss RG, Bove KE, Jones JF, Mauer AM, Fulginiti VA: An anomaly of neutrophil morphology with impaired function. N Engl J Med 290:478, 1974
383. Strnad CF, Parente JE, Wong K: Use of fluoride ion as a probe for the guanine nucleotide-binding protein involved in the phosphoinositide-dependent neutrophil transduction pathway. FEBS Lett 206:20, 1986
384. Strnad CF, Wong K: Effect of the calcium ionophore A23187 on superoxide generation in phorbol ester human neutrophils. Can J Physiol Pharmacol 63:1543, 1985
385. Styrt B, Klempner MS: Internal pH of human neutrophil lysosomes. FEBS Lett 149:113, 1982
386. Sugiura T, Onuma Y, Sekigichi N, Waku K: Ether of phospholipids in guinea pig polymorphonuclear leukocytes and macrophages. Occurrence of high levels of 1-O-alkyl-2-acyl-*sn*-glycero-3-phosphocholine. Biochim Biophys Acta 712:515, 1982
387. Tahamont MV, Gee MH, Flynn JT: Aggregation and thromboxane synthesis and release in isolated sheep neutrophils and lymphocytes in response to complement stimulation. Prostaglandin Leukotrienes Med 16:181, 1984
388. Takanaka K, O'Brien PJ: Proton release by polymorphonuclear leukocytes during phagocytosis or activation by digitonin or fluoride. Biochem Int 11:127, 1985
389. Takenawa T, Ishitoya J, Homma Y, Kato M, Nagai Y: Role of enhanced inositol phospholipid metabolism in neutrophil activation. Biochem Pharmacol 34:1931, 1985
390. Tauber AI, Borregaard N, Simons E, Wright J: Chronic granulomatous disease: A syndrome of phagocyte oxidase deficiencies. Medicine 62:286, 1983
391. Todd RF III, Arnaout MA, Rosin RE, Crowley CA, Peters WA, Babior BM: Subcellular localization of the large subunit of Mo1, a surface glycoprotein associated with neutrophil adhesion. J Clin Invest 74:1280, 1984
392. Tou JS: Activation of the metabolism of the fatty acyl group in granulocyte phospholipids by phorbol myristate acetate. Biochim Biophys Acta 665:491, 1981
393. Traynor JR, Authi KS: Phospholipase A_2 activity of lysosomal origin secreted by polymorphonuclear leukocytes during phagocytosis or treatment with calcium. Biochim Biophys Acta 665:571, 1981
394. Tsung PK, Sakamoto T, Weissmann G: Protein kinase and phosphatases from human polymorphonuclear leukocytes. Biochem J 145:437, 1975
395. Tuy FPD, Henry J, Rosenfeld C, Kahn A: Protein kinases in normal human blood cells. Am J Hematol 15:105, 1983
396. Ukena TE, Berlin RD: Effect of colchicine and vinblastine on the topographical separation of membrane functions. J Exp Med 136:1, 1972
397. Valerius NH, Stendahl O, Hartwig JH, Stossel TP: Distribution of actin-binding protein and mysoin in polymorphonuclear leukocytes during locomotion and phagocytosis. Cell 24:195, 1981
398. Vandenbark GR, Kuhn LJ, Niedel JE: Possible mechanism of phorbol diester-induced maturation of human promyelocytic leukemia cells. Activation of protein kinase C. J Clin Invest 73:448, 1984
399. Vanderhoek JY, Ekborg SL, Bailey JM: Nonsteroidal anti-inflammatory drugs stimulate 15-lipoxygenase/leukotriene pathway in human polymorphonuclear leukocytes. J Allergy Clin Immunol 74:412, 1984
400. Verghese MW, Charles L, Jakoi L, Dillon SB, Snyderman R: Role of a guanine nucleotide regulatory protein in the activation of phospholipase C by different chemoattractants. J Immunol 138:4374, 1987
401. Victor M, Weiss J, Klempner MS, Elsbach P: Phospholipase A_2 activity in the plasma membrane of human polymorphonuclear leukocytes. FEBS Lett 136:298, 1981
402. Virca GD, Metz G, Schnebli HP: Similarities between human and rat leukocyte elastase and cathepsin G. Eur J Biochem 144:1, 1984
403. Virella G, Espinoza A, Patrick H, Colwell JA: Polymorphonuclear leucocytes release a factor(s) that induces platelet aggregation and ATP release after interaction with insoluble and surface-fixed immune complexes. Clin Exp Immunol 49:684, 1982
404. Virella G, Lopes-Virella MFL, Shuler C, Sherwood T, Espinoza GA, Winocour P, Colwell JA: Release of PAF by human polymorphonuclear leucocytes stimulated by immune complexes bound to Sepharose particles and human erythrocytes. Immunology 50:43, 1983
405. Volpi M, Molski TFP, Naccache PH, Feinstein MB, Sha'afi RI: Phorbol 12-myristate, 13-acetate potentiates the action of the calcium ionophore in stimulating arachidonic acid release and production of phosphatidic acid in rabbit neutrophils. Biochem

Biophys Res Commun 128:594, 1985

406. Volpi M, Yassin R, Tao W, Molski TFP, Naccache PH, Sha'afi RI: Leukotriene B_4 mobilizes calcium without the breakdown of polyphosphoinositides and the production of phosphatidic acid in rabbit neutrophils. Proc Natl Acad Sci USA 81:5966, 1984
407. von Tscharner V, Prod'hom B, Baggiolini M, Reuter H: Ion channels in human neutrophils activated by a rise in free cytosolic calcium concentration. Nature 324:369, 1986
408. Waite M, DeChatelet LR, King L, Shirley PS: Phagocytosis-induced release of arachidonic acid from human neutrophils. Biochem Biophys Res Commun 90:984, 1978
409. Wallace PJ, Wersto RP, Packman CH, Lichtman MA: Chemotactic peptide-induced changes in neutrophil actin conformation. J Cell Biol 99:1060, 1984
410. Walsh CE, DeChatelet LR, Chilton FH, Wykle RL, Waite M: Mechanism of arachidonic acid release in human polymorphonuclear leukocytes. Biochim Biophys Acta 750:32, 1983
411. Walsh CE, DeChatelet LR, Thomas MJ, O'Flaherty JT, Waite M: Effect of phagocytosis and ionophores on release and metabolism of arachidonic acid from human neutrophils. Lipids 16:120, 1981
412. Walsh CE, Waite BM, Thomas MJ, DeChatelet LR: Release and metabolism of arachidonic acid in human neutrophils. J Biol Chem 256:7228, 1981
413. Walter A, Steer CJ, Blumenthal R: Polylysine induces pH-dependent fusion of acidic phospholipid vesicles: a model for polycation-induced fusion. Biochim Biophys Acta 861:319, 1986
414. Walter RJ, Marasco WA: Direct visualization of formylpeptide receptor binding on rounded and polarized human neutrophils: Cellular and receptor heterogeneity. J Leukocyte Biol 41:377, 1987
415. Wang YL, Goren MB: Differential and sequential delivery of fluorescent lysosomal probes into mouse peritoneal macrophages. J Cell Biol 104:1749, 1987
416. Ward PA, Hill JH: C5 chemotactic fragments produced by an enzyme in lysosomal granules of neutrophils. J Immunol 104:535, 1970
417. Webster RO, Zanolari B, Henson PM: Neutrophil chemotaxis in response to surface-bound C5a. Exp Cell Res 129:55, 1980
418. Weening RS, Schoorel ER, Roos D, VanSchaik ML, Voetman AA, Bot AA, Batenburg Plenter AM, Willems C, Zeijhemaker WP, Astaldi A: Effect of ascorbate on abnormal neutrophil, platelet, and lymphocyte function in a patient with the Chediak-Higashi syndrome. Blood 57:856, 1981
419. Weintraub ST, Ludwig JC, Mott GE, McManus LM, Lear C, Pinckard RN: Fast atom bombardment-mass spectrometric identification of molecular species of platelet-activating factor produced by stimulated polymorphonuclear leukocytes. Biochem Biophys Res Commun 129:868, 1985
420. Weisman SJ, Punzo A, Ford C, Sha'afi RI: Intracellular pH changes during neutrophil activation: Na^+/H^+ antiport, J Leukocyte Biol 41:25, 1987
420. Weiss J, Olsson I: Cellular and subcellular localization of the bactericidal/permeability-increasing protein of neutrophils. Blood 69:652, 1987
422. West BC, Rosenthal AS, Gelb NA, Kimball HR: Separation and characterization of human neutrophil granules. Am J Pathol 77:41, 1974
423. White JR, Huang CK, Hill JM Jr, Naccache PH, Becker EL, Sha'afi RI: Effect of phorbol 12-myristate 13-acetate and its analogue 4a-phorbol 12,13-didecanoate on protein phosphorylation and lysosomal enzyme release in rabbit neutrophils. J Biol Chem 259:8605, 1984
424. White JR, Naccache PH, Molski TFP, Borgeat P, Sha'afi RI: Direct demonstration of increased intracellular concentration of free calcium in rabbit and human neutrophils following stimulation with chemotactic factor. Biochem Biophys Res Commun 113:44, 1983
425. White JR, Naccache PH, Sha'afi RI: Stimulation by chemotactic factor of actin association with the cytoskeleton in rabbit neutrophils. Effects of calcium and cytochalasin B. J Biol Chem 258:14041, 1983
426. Williams HR, Lin TY: Human polymorphonuclear leukocyte collagenase and gelatinase. Comparison of certain enzymatic properties. Int J Biochem 16:1321, 1984
427. Williams LT, Snyderman R, Pike MC, Lefkowitz RJ: Specific receptor sites for chemotactic peptides on human polymorphonuclear leukocytes. Proc Natl Acad Sci USA 74:1204, 1977
428. Wolosewick JJ: Distribution of actin in migrating leukocytes *in vivo*. Cell Tissue Res 236:517, 1984
429. Wright CD, Hoffman MD: The protein kinase C inhibitors H-7 and H-9 fail to inhibit human neutrophil activation. Biochem Biophys Res Commun 135:749, 1986
430. Wright DG, Gallin JI: A functional differentiation of human neutrophil granules: generation of C5a by a specific (secondary) granule product and inactivation of C5a by azurophil (primary) granule products. J Immunol 119:1068, 1977
431. Wykle RL, Miller CH, Lewis JC, Schmitt JD, Smith JA, Surles JR, Piantadosi C, O'Flaherty JT: Stereospecific activity of 1-O-alkyl-2-O-acetyl-*sn*-glycero-3-phosphocholine and comparison of analogs in the degranulation of platelets and neutrophils. Biochem Biophys Res Commun 100:1651, 1981
432. Yassin R, Shefcyk J, White JR, Tao W, Volpi M, Molski TFP, Naccache PH, Feinstein MB, Sha'afi RI: Effects of chemotactic factors and other agents on the amounts of actin and a 65,000-mol-wt protein associated with the cytoskeleton of rabbit and human neutrophils. J Cell Biol 101:182, 1985
433. Yin HL, Hartwig JH, Maruyama K, Stossel TP: Ca^{2+} control of actin filament length. Effects of macrophage gelsolin on actin polymerization. J Biol Chem 256:9693, 1981
434. Yin HL, Stossel TP: Control of cytoplasmic actin gel-sol transformation by gelsolin, a calcium-dependent regulatory protein. Nature 281:583, 1979
435. Yin HL, Zaner KS, Stossel TP: Ca^{2+} control of actin gelation. Interaction of gelsolin with actin filaments and regulation of actin gelation. J Biol Chem 255:9494, 1980
436. Yoon PS, Boxer LA, Mayo LA, Young AY, Wicha MS: Human neutrophil laminin receptors: activation-dependent receptor expression. J Immunol 138:259, 1987
437. Yuli I, Oplatka A: Cytosolic acidification as an early transductory signal in human neutrophil chemotaxis. Science 235:340, 1987
438. Zeya HI, Spitznagel JK: Cationic protein-bearing granules of polymorphonuclear leukocytes: separation from enzyme-rich granules. Science 163:1069, 1972
439. Zimmerberg J, Curran M, Cohen FS, Brodwick M: Simultaneous electrical and optical measurements show that membrane fusion precedes secretory granule swelling during exocytosis of beige mouse mast cells. Proc Natl Acad Sci USA 84:1585, 1987
440. Zimmerberg J, Sardet C, Epel D: Exocytosis of sea urchin egg cortical vesicles *in vitro* is retarded by hyperosmotic sucrose: kinetics of fusion monitored by quantitative light-scattering microscopy. J Cell Biol 101:2398, 1985
441. Zimmerberg J, Whitaker M: Irreversible swelling of secretory granules during exocytosis caused by calcium. Nature 315:581, 1985

Biology of Disease

Nonimmunologic Mechanisms of Glomerular Injury

JEAN L. OLSON, AND ROBERT H. HEPTINSTALL

Department of Pathology, The Johns Hopkins University School of Medicine, Baltimore, Maryland

BACKGROUND

The importance of immunologic processes in the pathogenesis of glomerulonephritis has long been recognized, and over the past 30 years considerable progress has been made. However, the importance of nonimmunologic factors in causing glomerular damage has only recently been emphasized in spite of many older studies on the effects of reduction of functioning renal mass, manipulation of diet, and induction of high blood pressure. Furthermore, the possibility that these factors might be important in the pathogenesis of chronic renal disease in general has received little attention.

A model of partial nephrectomy, in which one kidney and a portion of the other were removed, had been used to study renal failure as early as 1899 (19), but, Chanutin and co-workers (27, 28) were the first to use it to explore chronic renal insufficiency in detail. They noted (27) that rats deprived of much of their renal substance developed hypertension, polyuria, albuminuria, nitrogen retention, and renal and cardiac hypertrophy, further observing (28) that the severity of renal insufficiency depended on the diet provided and that increased protein accentuated impairment. The partial renal ablation model was used only sparingly for the next 30 years except for a scattering of articles briefly describing glomerular and vascular injury (70, 96, 121), but in 1960 a more complete description of the morphologic changes was provided by Koletsky and Goodsit (66). They reduced renal mass by approximately 75% and studied various organs including the kidney between 7 to 10 months after operation. Most of the animals developed hypertension, proteinuria, and uremia; this was accompanied by necrotizing arteritis in the mesentery, gastrointestinal tract, adrenal glands, testes, and remnant kidney. Glomerular injury, focal at first but eventually becoming diffuse, was manifest by thickening of capillary loops, formation of adhesions, epithelial cell swelling, and fibrinoid necrosis. The inevitable result was obliteration of glomeruli. Tubular loss and interstitial fibrosis, which was commensurate with the degree of glomerular damage, was further noted. A group of rats provided with 1% sodium chloride as their drinking water all developed sustained hypertension which was accompanied by accelerated and more severe vascular and glomerular lesions.

To this point no satisfactory explanation had been advanced for the mechanism of glomerular injury induced by reduction of renal mass. Addis, Myers, and Oliver (1) had shown that unilateral nephrectomy produced increased glomerular filtration rate (GFR) in the remaining kidney as a functional adaptation, and this idea was extended to reduction in nephron number regardless of the type of injury by Bricker *et al.* (22). They proposed that such a loss must lead to increased function in the remaining nephrons and that the degree of that hyperfunction would depend on the total number of surviving nephrons (22). This idea, in the context of the partial renal ablation model, was addressed by Morrison and Howard (84). They first (84) determined inulin clearance, as a measure of GFR, in rats with ablation of approximately ⅚ of renal mass at various intervals ranging from 4 to 50 weeks after operation. As expected, clearance was decreased when compared with control animals, but when calculations were made for clearance/single nephron by dividing total clearance by the number of surviving glomeruli, it was found that single nephron GFR was doubled compared with control animals. Similar calculations were made for paraminohippurate clearance, but although the results were more difficult to interpret, it was considered that plasma flow through individual nephrons was also increased. It was further noted that with increasing time there was a progressive decrease in inulin clearance which on the basis of a previous study (83) was regarded as due to progressive glomerular obliteration. This was confirmed by Shimamura and Morrison (108) who studied the morphologic sequence of the glomerular injury for 10 to 50 weeks after ⅚ reduction in renal mass. They found progressive glomerulosclerosis. By light microscopy, this was characterized by an initial increase in glomerular size with prominence of the visceral epithelial cells, and gradual accumulation of hyaline material within the glomeruli. Ultrastructural studies revealed that the earliest lesions occurred within epithelial cells and included effacement of foot processes, appearance of protein reabsorption droplets and vacuoles, and increased cytoplasmic filaments. Separation of both endothelial and epithelial cells from the glomerular basement membrane (GBM) was documented, and with continuing injury the mesangial matrix increased in amount and obliterated the capillary lumina. Coupling these observations with those made previously (83), the authors proposed that glomerular hyperfiltration may be responsible for the progressive glomerular injury found in this model of partial renal ablation. Furthermore, they suggested that a similar situation may obtain in chronic renal disease in humans. As nephrons are lost, the remaining nephrons are exposed to hyperfiltration resulting in progressive glomerular injury regardless of the original insult.

Additional interest in the use of the model of severe renal ablation to elucidate possible mechanisms of nonimmunologic glomerular injury was stimulated by the work of Purkerson, Hoffsten, and Klahr (98). They reduced renal mass to approximately ⅛ of normal and examined the rats from 14 to 90 days later. Hypertension, proteinuria, and progressive renal dysfunction developed and were accompanied by severe glomerular injury consisting of deposition of serum proteins in the mesangium and in the subendothelial space, mesangial sclerosis, microaneurysm formation, and capillary thrombi. At 4 weeks after operation, approximately 33% of the glomeruli were involved, and at 90 days, this percentage had increased to 90%. The amount of injury could be lessened by various manipulations. Antihypertensive agents given as triple therapy (hydrochlorothiazide, reserpine, and hydralazine) diminished but did not abolish the glomerular damage, whereas heparin, which lowered blood pressure and prevented azotemia, almost completely abrogated glomerular injury. The authors concluded that increased glomerular permeability, manifest by serum protein leakage into the mesangium and the subendothelial space, led to eventual capillary occlusion and was important in the pathogenesis of this form of renal damage.

Studies in various models of experimental hypertension also provided valuable information on nonimmunologic glomerular injury. Wilson and Byrom (117, 118) showed that glomerular damage was confined to the nonclipped kidney in rats made hypertensive by the application of a silver clip to one renal artery, the other kidney and its artery being untouched (2K1C model). Thus, glomerular changes were regarded as being the result of exposure to the high blood pressure; the glomeruli in the clipped kidney were unaffected because the silver clip afforded protection against the effects of the raised pressure. Glomerular changes included focal or complete necrosis of the tuft, adhesions of the tuft to Bowman's capsule, increased cellularity of the tuft, and complete hyalinization. Further evidence for the injurious effects of direct transmittal of increased pressure came from studies in which saline was injected forcibly into the arterial system (24, 49, 120), from the steroid-hypertension model in which additional partial constriction of one renal artery considerably reduced glomerular injury in the constricted kidney (48), and from studies in which removal of the silver clip from the renal artery in clip-hypertension gave rise to acute glomerular changes in the once-clipped kidney (23). Other early experiments recorded increased blood flow through glomeruli in steroid hypertension (50), and demonstrated endothelial and mesangial cell injury in the glomeruli as a result of exposure to increased pressure (113). These changes were similar to those described after ablation of renal mass and included lifting of endothelial cells from the GBM with accumulation of material in the subendothelial space, platelet and fibrin thrombi, eventual capillary occlusion, mesangial cell swelling, increase in mesangial matrix, and generalized epithelial cell injury.

FACTORS INFLUENCING PROGRESSION OF NONIMMUNOLOGIC GLOMERULAR INJURY

Many factors work together to influence the progression of glomerular injury, and their interrelations are complex. In the following discussion the effects of each are considered separately although it is recognized that this separation is artificial. Because most of the experiments described in this section have used the model of renal ablation, it is important for the reader to know that various degrees of ablation have been used by different investigators. The convention used in this review is to relate the extent of ablation to total renal mass so that $^5/_6$ nephrectomy indicates that one kidney plus $^2/_3$ of the other kidney have been rendered functionless either by removal or infarction. Variations in amount of renal mass reduced and the use of different sexes may account for some of the apparent inconsistencies between groups of investigators.

Hemodynamic Factors

Glomerular Hemodynamics. The presence of superficial glomeruli in the Munich-Wistar rat and the development of micropuncture techniques to study these glomeruli allowed Hostetter *et al.* (53) to directly examine hemodynamic alterations in individual nephrons induced by $^{11}/_{12}$ renal ablation. At 7 days after operation, the rats had significant proteinuria, polyuria, and mild blood pressure elevation. Results from micropuncture supported the finding of Morrison and Howard (84) that hyperfiltration was present in the remaining nephrons. This augmentation in the single nephron glomerular filtration rate (SNGFR) was due to increase in both glomerular plasma flow rate (Q_A) and in glomerular capillary pressure (P_{GC}). In addition, there was decreased resistance in both the afferent and efferent arterioles. Morphologic examination of the glomeruli confirmed that these physiologic adaptations were accompanied by structural alterations. Small blebs such as are seen in membrane injury appeared in endothelial cells, which became detached from the GBM, with subsequent accumulation of electron-dense material in the subendothelial space. Epithelial cells contained numerous protein reabsorption droplets, had increased pinocytotic activity at the base of the pedicels, formed blebs secondary to the attenuation of cytoplasm, and showed focal foot process effacement and microvillous transformation. Slight increase in mesangial matrix accompanied by mild increase in numbers of mesangial cells was also noted. Additional support for the idea that these hemodynamic alterations might be responsible for the structural injury was garnered from an additional group of rats with $^{11}/_{12}$ renal ablation fed a low protein diet. In these animals, there was a return of the glomerular hemodynamic measurements to normal and a lessening of the degree of injury to the glomeruli such that they were indistinguishable from those of control animals. This confirmed the much earlier observations that dietary manipulation could modify this kind of injury (28), and provided a possible explanation for the mechanism involved, namely, that alterations in glomerular hemodynamics were responsible for the morphologic changes observed. Alteration in vascular resistance is important in the pathogenesis of glomerular injury in the renal ablation model, and the decreased afferent arteriolar resistance present in it permits increased transmission of pressure and flow to the glomeruli. Additional support for this concept is found in the demonstration of loss of autoregulation by rats with renal ablation before the appearance of glomerular injury (16).

Attention, should however be paid to a very recent study which concluded that altered hemodynamics do not completely explain glomerular injury (123). Repeated micropuncture measurements were made in superficial glomeruli at 2-week intervals up to 6 weeks after $^5/_6$ or $^7/_8$ nephrectomy. Values of SNGFR and P_{GC} for individual superficial glomeruli were compared with the sclerosis index, a measure of glomerular damage, derived from serial sections of the same glomeruli that were punctured. Since degree of sclerosis showed no relationship to the highest level of SNGFR or P_{GC}, the authors concluded that the altered hemodynamics, rather than causing direct damage, may act as a trigger for other injurious processes. These results are interesting but some caution must be observed in interpreting the results since the authors demonstrated great variability in SNGFR or P_{GC} within the same glomerulus. Therefore, it is not possible to be certain that the highest values that they obtained represented the maximum values experienced by that glomerulus.

Systemic Hypertension. The adverse effects of hypertension were briefly referred to earlier and it is well-known that systemic hypertension may accelerate the progression of renal disease in many experimental as well as clinical situations (9). Since the renal ablation model is complicated by varying degrees of hypertension depending on the extent of kidney substance removed, it is appropriate to provide some background on the renal injury induced by various forms of hypertension. All experimental models of hypertension produce injury to small arteries and arterioles within the kidney (8, 38, 50, 91, 94, 117, 119) and these occur to a more or less equal degree for a given height and duration of hypertension (94). However, the degree of glomerular injury varies from one type of experimental model to another and in a general way depends on the resistance of the afferent arterioles (94). In the case of the Okamoto spontaneously hypertensive rat in which the afferent arterioles are characterized by markedly increased resistance (6, 8, 10, 31), little glomerular injury is noted (38). The same is true for the stroke-prone variant of the spontaneously hypertensive rat (94), although the juxtamedullary glomeruli do show severe changes presumably because autoregulation is not so efficient for this population of glomeruli. When afferent arteriolar resistance is decreased as in the case of deoxycorticosterone (DOC)-salt hypertension (35), glomerular injury is extensive (50, 94). Thus, preglomerular vasoconstriction appears to protect glomeruli from the effects of systemic hypertension, whereas dilation of preglomerular vessels, by virtue of permitting transmission of systemic pressures to glomerular capillaries, leads to glomerular injury (94). Further evidence for the importance of preglomerular resistance is provided by a study in which saline was forcibly injected into the renal arterial system. When the preglomerular vessels were relaxed by injection of aminophylline before injecting saline, the degree of glomerular damage was considerably increased compared with rats not so treated (49). Changes in vascular resistance are reflected in alterations in autoregulation in certain hypertensive models; loss of autoregulation is found in rats with DOC-salt hypertension (81) and a milder degree of loss is present in the nonclipped kidney of the 2K1C hypertensive rat (104).

Glomerular Hypertension. It is clear from what has been said that increased pressure and/or flow to the glomeruli is important in determining glomerular injury, thus in both the renal ablation model (53) and in various models of experimental hypertension (35, 106) there is an increase in SNGFR, Q_A, and importantly P_{GC}. This is reinforced by experiments using antihypertensive agents. When a combination of hydrochlorothiazide, reserpine, and hydralazine (triple therapy) was used to treat the hypertension in renal ablation or DOC-salt hypertension, there was only slight decrease in the degree of glomerular injury in spite of reduction of systemic blood pressure (5, 34, 98, 100). In both models triple therapy failed to reduce P_{GC} (5, 34). It was suggested that the diuretic, in combination with the vasodilation present in both models, stimulated the production of renin resulting in efferent arteriolar constriction and elevated P_{GC} (5). In contrast, when converting enzyme inhibitor (CEI), was used to lower systemic blood pressure in the renal ablation model, there was a sharp decrease in the percentage of glomeruli involved by sclerosis (4, 5, 76, 100), accompanied by a lesser degree of proteinuria (4, 76, 100). Micropuncture studies demonstrated that in addition to a decrease in systemic blood pressure there was a decrease in P_{GC} but no change in either SNGFR or Q_A. Thus, the difference between triple therapy and administration of CEI was that the latter caused a decrease in efferent arteriolar resistance with consequent lowering of P_{GC}. These studies emphasize the role of increased pressure in the glomerular capillaries as a cause of glomerular injury and at the same time minimize the part played by increased blood flow through the glomeruli. Meyer *et al.* (75) have extended studies on CEI by administering it as late as 2 months after $^5/_6$ nephrectomy, a time at which some glomerular injury had already occurred. Glomerular injury had stabilized in the treated group when the animals were examined 10 weeks later. Micropuncture assessment showed reduction in P_{GC} with preservation of elevated SNGFR and Q_A.

Role of Prostaglandins and Angiotensin II. The studies cited above have demonstrated that renal ablation results in hemodynamic alterations accompanied by glomerular injury, and that increased glomerular capillary pressure seems to be an important determinant of this injury. Before proceeding to analyze other factors which may be important in the pathogenesis of progressive glomerular injury, it would be useful to consider possible mechanisms which may account for the production of this increased glomerular pressure. Control of renal hemodynamics is a complicated subject and full consideration of this topic is beyond the scope of this review. Interested readers are referred to a complete discussion of this subject by Navar and Rosivall (87). In a general way, alterations in flow and pressure are dictated by the interaction of many polypeptides and other substances, which in normal circumstances act through a careful system of checks and balances. The principal components include the prostanoids and renin-angiotensin system. Vasodilation is controlled by prostaglandins (PG) E_2 and I_2, and vasoconstriction is governed by angiotensin II (AII) and thromboxane A_2.

When renal mass is reduced, excretion of prostaglandin E_2 (PGE_2), the major vasodilatory PG of the rat (110), is increased (69, 109) suggesting heightened formation of prostanoids. Since afferent arteriolar dilation is an almost immediate response to renal ablation (85), increased PGE_2 is probably available rapidly. That such a process occurs and is important in the maintenance of glomerular function after renal ablation has been tested by several authors using either inhibitors or stimulators of PG synthesis. Nath, Chmielewski, and Hostetter (85) studied the effects of acute administration of indomethacin, a nonspecific PG synthesis inhibitor, on rats with $^5/_6$ ablation 3 to 4 weeks after operation. They found that GFR and SNGFR were reduced owing to a decrease in Q_A and the ultrafiltration coefficient (K_f) which is the product of the filtration surface area and the hydraulic conductivity, but no change was recorded in P_{GC}. It was concluded that the hemodynamic effects of prostaglandins on afferent and efferent arteriolar resistance, and on K_f, account for the increase in flow and filtration after renal ablation. Furthermore, it was stated that maintenance of GFR in this model is critically dependent on the increased synthesis of vasodilatory PGs. Clinical investigations also support the idea that PGs are required to sustain renal function in humans with chronic renal failure (29). The essential role of increased PGs in the maintenance of GFR is further documented by using dietary manipulation to alter PG synthesis in rats with renal ablation (103). Scharschmidt *et al.* (103) found that decrease in the synthesis of PGs in such rats was accompanied by a worsening of renal function and increased glomerulosclerosis. Other possible consequences of alteration of PG metabolism will be discussed below in the section on the effects of dietary factors.

An increase in PGE_2 after renal ablation is likely to stimulate increase in AII which modulates the vasodilation due to PGE_2 (4, 5, 76, 100) and causes constriction of efferent arterioles (25) resulting in increased P_{GC}. The results of administration of CEI to rats with partial renal ablation referred to earlier indirectly supports the idea that this sequence of events occurs in renal ablation (4, 5, 76). The decline in resistance of the efferent arteriole is proportionately greater than that in the afferent arteriole, an effect that would be expected after the inhibition of AII production (105).

Summary. Rats with renal ablation develop progressive glomerular injury which is due, at least in part, to altered glomerular hemodynamics, namely increased P_{GC}. The increase in P_{GC} is related to a decrease in afferent arteriolar resistance which is greater than the decrease in efferent arteriolar resistance. These changes in glomerular hemodynamics are controlled by increased synthesis of PGE_2 which stimulates increased AII, and are necessary in order to maintain GFR. Experiments using CEI indicate that reduction of P_{GC} is associated with lessening of glomerular damage.

Coagulation

As described briefly in the introductory paragraphs, Purkerson, Hoffsten, and Klahr (98) noted the presence of capillary occlusions, sometimes containing fibrin, in studies on the natural progression of glomerular lesions resulting from renal ablation. It was noted that administration of heparin to rats with 7/8 nephrectomy resulted in almost complete prevention of glomerular lesions 4 weeks after operation; the only abnormality recorded was the presence of "droplets" in the mesangium. Although treatment with heparin also lowered blood urea nitrogen and systemic blood pressure, it was concluded that capillary occlusion played an important role in the progression of this type of glomerular injury. Olson (90) confirmed that administration of heparin to rats with 11/12 nephrectomy prevented the development of glomerular sclerosis up to 14 days postoperation. Since heparin has many biologic activities (57), it was concluded that any one, or several, of these working alone or in concert might have conferred this protection. Those activities which seem most likely to play a role include: anticoagulation, lowering of blood pressure, alterations in glomerular hemodynamics, and possibly an inhibition of cellular proliferation which is responsible for increased production of mesangial matrix.

Another facet of the part played by coagulation in the pathogenesis of progressive glomerular sclerosis in renal ablation is the role of the platelet and its products, particularly since platelet thrombi are present as an early component of the injury (92, 93, 98). Because thromboxane A_2 is a potent stimulator of platelet aggregation as well as being a vasoconstricting agent, Purkerson *et al.* (99) examined the effects of thromboxane synthetase antagonists. When rats with 7/8 nephrectomy were treated with such antagonists and compared 5 weeks later with rats subjected to this degree of nephrectomy only, there was a reduction in glomerular injury, lowering of blood pressure, decrease in urinary protein excretion, and decrease in blood urea nitrogen. The view was advanced that the increased glomerular pressure known to occur in renal ablation (53) results in endothelial injury which stimulates platelet aggregation and the release of products such as platelet-derived growth factor (PDGF). These in turn alter capillary permeability and induce proteinuria. It was speculated that the protective effect of thromboxane synthetase antagonist resulted from an interruption in this sequence with decreased platelet aggregation and prevention of release of potentially injurious platelet products. Similar results were obtained using thromboxane synthesis inhibitors in the Dahl salt-sensitive rat, another experimental model of glomerular injury (122). In both of these studies the authors demonstrated that the antagonists lowered the levels of thromboxane without affecting the levels of PGE_2 or prostaglandin I_2 (99, 122).

Dietary Factors

Protein. Diet has a profound effect on the progression of renal injury (63). An early demonstration of an adverse effect of increased dietary protein on renal function was provided in 1927 (80), and as mentioned earlier Chanutin and Ludewig (28) confirmed this in rats with more severe renal ablation. When given to rats with partial nephrectomy for prolonged periods (52), high protein diets lead to increased GFR and accelerated renal failure accompanied by glomerular injury. The increased GFR occurring with increased dietary protein is attended by rises in serum PGE_2 and AII (95). Indomethacin attenuates the increase in GFR induced by high dietary protein in human beings, further supporting the idea that PGE_2 is important in causing the rise in GFR (67). Rats with 2K1C hypertension fed high dietary protein show a complete loss of autoregulation, whereas similar rats on a control diet show only a slight upward adjustment in autoregulation (104).

As referred to earlier, Hostetter *et al.* (53) showed that a low protein diet in rats with 11/12 nephrectomy lessened the glomerular injury. This protection was accompanied by decreases in systemic blood pressure and P_{GC} to control levels. Similar results have been documented by others in the ablation model (86). Low protein diet also conferred protection from further injury in rats with established glomerular damage (75); in this experiment the low protein diet was not introduced until 8 weeks after 5/6 renal ablation. As a further part of this study the effects of a low protein diet were compared with those of CEI in rats with established renal ablation. With both procedures there was a stabilizing of proteinuria, a limitation of glomerular injury and a return of P_{GC} to control levels. This confirms that a principal effect of a low protein diet is reduction of glomerular hypertension. A further effect of a low protein diet is to lessen the loss of autoregulation after 5/6 nephrectomy (16); a similar effect was shown in rats with 2K1C hypertension (104). It should be noted that recent work suggests that many of the effects produced by low protein diets may be secondary to low-calorie intake. A careful examination of all the possible dietary factors in closely controlled studies is clearly needed in order to determine which of them are important in producing the beneficial effect on glomerular injury (56, 73).

Lipids. The role of dietary lipids and the progression of renal disease is more controversial. Stemming from the observation that the nephrotic syndrome is accompanied by abnormalities in lipid metabolism, including decreased catabolism of lipoproteins (82), Moorhead, Chan, and Varghese (82) in a recent review offer the hypothesis that lipids may be directly toxic to endothelial cells and may stimulate mesangial cell proliferation. Additional suggestive evidence that abnormalities in lipid metabolism are capable of producing glomerular injury is derived from several sources which include the following: studies in obese Zucker rats (89); the effects of lowering hyperlipidemia in obese and in partially nephrectomized rats (59, 60); and the finding of focal glomerular sclerosis in morbidly obese humans (58). The first two of these will be discussed here but the third will be considered in the section on relationship to human disease.

The obese Zucker rat has an autosomal recessive disorder characterized by elevated serum levels of both cholesterol and triglycerides, mild glucose intolerance due to insulin resistance, and the occurrence of focal glomerular sclerosis. No abnormalities have been found in glomerular hemodynamics in this strain (89). Lowering of both cholesterol and triglycerides, using either clofibric acid or mevinolin, resulted in a reduction in the number of sclerotic glomeruli in both the Zucker rat (59) and in the Sprague-Dawley rat with reduction in renal mass (60). Mevinolin is a specific inhibitor of 3-hydroxy-3-methylglutaryl-coenzyme A reductase, the rate-limiting step in cholesterol synthesis. In the study using the Zucker rat, it was found that lowering of serum cholesterol was more important than the decline in serum triglycerides in ameliorating the glomerular lesions. It was speculated that lowering serum cholesterol may lessen cholesterol deposition in mesangial cells and reduce mesangial cell proliferation, although it was admitted that the precise mechanisms remain to be determined. In the study using lipid-lowering agents in Sprague-Dawley rats with 5/6 nephrectomy, similar results were obtained (60). In these experiments the rats were treated with clofibric acid for 10 weeks after 5/6 nephrectomy; this resulted in a decrease in serum cholesterol level, in urinary albumin excretion, and in percentage of glomeruli affected by glomerulosclerosis. A slight but not statistically significant lowering of blood pressure was noted. Micropuncture, using stop-flow techniques 4 weeks after operation, revealed no differences in SNGFR, P_{GC}, Q_A, or K_f between the treated and untreated groups. Clofibric acid has many actions including the inhibition of hepatic release of lipoproteins, interference with albumin binding of free fatty acids, inhibition of cholesterol biosynthesis, and enhancement of lipoprotein lipase activity. Which of these specific events is involved in the glomerular sparing effect is not understood. Mevinolin was also employed in this study, lowering both serum cholesterol and triglycerides and affording a similar degree of protection of the glomeruli. It was concluded that lipid abnormalities may play an important role in the pathogenesis of glomerular sclerosis.

Numerous studies have recently appeared concerning the effect of dietary manipulation of PG synthesis both in rats with renal ablation and in other models of kidney disease. As discussed earlier, it is clear that the increased synthesis of PGE_2 seen in rats after renal ablation is an adaptive response by the kidney to maintain glomerular function (85). When menhaden oil, which inhibits the cyclooxygenase arm of prostanoid synthesis and produces an increase in the lipoxygenase products, was given to rats with 2/3 nephrectomy, decreased urinary PGE_2, greater proteinuria, and more glomerulosclerosis were found, despite lowering of serum cholesterol and triglycerides (103). It was suggested that the decrease in PGE_2 far outweighed the benefits of reducing thromboxane and was detrimental to the survival of the animals that required increased PGE_2 to maintain renal function.

The consequences of increasing PG synthesis has also been examined. Barcelli, Weiss, and Pollak (12) fed increased linoleic acid, a PG precursor, for 20 weeks to rats with 3/4 nephrectomy. They found that rats with high dietary linoleic acid had lower levels of serum creatinine, less proteinuria, and a decreased proportion of sclerotic glomeruli. Another group of investigators (47) has confirmed the protective effect of linoleic acid when fed to rats with 7/8 nephrectomy. When rats on this diet were examined 5 weeks after operation they were found to have lower systemic blood pressure, less urinary protein excretion, and fewer glomeruli with sclerosis. They also had increased urinary excretion of thromboxane B_2, GFR, and renal plasma flow. Thromboxane B_2 is the stable metabolite of thromboxane A_2 and its increase in the urine reflects an increase in production of thromboxane A_2. The interpretation of the results concerning GFR and renal plasma flow is uncertain as the changes may reflect preservation of glomeruli rather than true increases in flow and pressure within individual glomeruli. The mechanism for this improvement in renal function is not yet understood although it has been suggested that membrane fluidity may be altered by changes in composition of tissue polyunsaturated fatty acid. Additional experiments have been performed in rats with 3/4 nephrectomy using three different oils rich in polyunsaturated fatty acids in the diet (11). When renal histology was studied 21 weeks later it was found that only one of the three oils, salmon oil, had a salutary effect. Animals exposed to this particular oil had reduction in serum creatinine, decrease in thromboxane A_2 production by platelets, and an increase in urinary prostaglandin E_3. The other two oils, evening primrose and safflower, produced a similar reduction in serum creatinine levels but no difference in the number of sclerotic glomeruli, platelet production of thromboxane A_2 or urinary PGE_3 (the stable metabolite of PGE_2) as compared with the control group. The implications of changes in thromboxane have been discussed in the section on coagulation and will not be repeated. The interpretation of the effects of altering PG synthesis awaits a better understanding of the manner in which these different oils alter PG metabolism. More complete studies of these different diets with careful analysis and perhaps longer experimental periods will be required to sort out all the various factors which are implicated.

Phosphate. Changes in dietary phosphate may also affect the progression of glomerular sclerosis. Earlier studies which examined this question did not properly take into account the unpalatable nature of the diet when phosphate is restricted (68), so that most of the beneficial effects could have been explained by malnutrition. However, a more recent study in which the effect of phosphate depletion was examined in rats with 5/6 nephrectomy suggests that low serum phosphate may provide protection from glomerular injury in this model independent of dietary protein levels (71). Use was made of dihydroxyaluminum aminoacetate, a potent phosphate binder, which decreased phosphate without decreasing dietary intake of protein. The rats were given this phosphate binder 1 month after the nephrectomy at a time when renal injury had been initiated. The treated rats had hypophosphatemia, hypercalcemia, decreased urinary protein excretion, decreased serum cholesterol and triglycerides, lower serum creatinine, and improved survival. Blood pressure and body weight did not differ from phosphate replete animals. Both glomerular and tubulointerstitial disease showed less severe progression in the phosphate-depleted rats.

Other dietary factors which have been studied in the model of renal ablation include: total caloric intake (56, 73, 114), carbohydrates (65), and sodium (66). These have been reviewed by Kleinknecht and Laouari (65) and will not be considered further.

Hypertrophic and Hormonal Factors

Structural Hypertrophy. Reduction in renal mass in rats produces structural (4, 107) as well as functional hypertrophy. Evidence that this structural hypertrophy is important in the pathogenesis of glomerular sclerosis was first suggested by the observation that glomerular volume was increased in the model of renal ablation (4) and in DOC-salt hypertension (35). Both of these models are associated with severe glomerular injury. Most recent evidence for the importance of hypertrophy has been provided in an examination of differences in susceptibility to glomerular injury between two strains of rats, and in two additional studies presently published only in abstract form. Grond *et al.* (45) found that PVG/c rats had more glomeruli than did Wistar rats. When both strains were subjected to nephrectomy, glomerular volume was smaller in the PVG/c rats and there was no evidence of injury. In fact glomeruli in PVG/c rats with one kidney were smaller than those of Wistar rats with two kidneys. Recently, Ichikawa, Yoshida, and Fogo (55) combined partial nephrectomy on the right side with ureteral diversion (UD), nephrectomy, or sham operation on the left. Both the UD and nephrectomy groups showed similar degrees of glomerular hypertension, hyperfiltration, and hyperperfusion, but the UD group did not demonstrate structural hypertrophy; glomerular volumes were identical with those of the sham operation group. Despite the presence of alterations in glomerular hemodynamics, the UD group had fewer sclerotic glomeruli than the nephrectomy group. The authors concluded that hypertrophy must precede the development of sclerosis and that hyperfunction does not necessarily lead to sclerosis. Fries *et al.* (42) produced adriamycin nephrosis in Munich-Wistar rats and 4 weeks later performed 4/5 nephrectomy in some of them. They found that the combination of increased P_{GC} and hypertrophy was associated with the most severe injury. They invoked Laplace's Law which states that wall tension is equal to the product of radius and pressure. Thus, for a given increase in P_{GC}, the tension will be greater in capillary loops that are dilated as part of the hypertrophy. The exact mechanisms of injury secondary to wall tension are likely to be mechanical but further study is required.

Factors Controlling Hypertrophy. The factors which control compensatory renal hypertrophy are not entirely understood. However, several factors which seem to play a role in causing hypertrophy have also been associated with the progression of glomerular sclerosis. No investigator has yet been able to identify and isolate a kidney-specific renotropic growth factor despite innumerable attempts to do so. It has been suggested that a reasonable alternative to such a factor might be increased tissue sensitivity to normally circulating growth factors (40). Several growth factors have been implicated; they include retinoids (7), PDGF (64), growth hormone (GH) (32), thyroxine (2), ACTH (112) and a variety of other hormones. Argiles *et al.* (7) found increased amounts of retinol-binding protein and cellular retinoic acid-binding protein in the urine of living-related kidney donors immediately after surgery. The retinoids carried in the blood by retinol-binding protein were also increased in these donors and have been shown to have metabolic properties related to hypertrophy. Doi *et al.* (32) have recently examined mice transgenic for GH, growth hormone-releasing factor or insulin-like growth factor-1. All three had increased serum levels of insulin-like growth factor-1 and enlarged glomeruli, but only the two (GH and growth hormone-releasing factor) with elevated circulating serum levels of GH showed an increased frequency of glomerulosclerosis. The authors suggested that the insulin-like growth factor-1, which has been shown to be increased after unilateral nephrectomy (37), may play a role in the hypertrophy and increased glomerular size, but that the addition of other factors such as GH may be necessary to provoke cellular proliferation.

Miscellaneous Factors

Several miscellaneous factors also affect the rate of progression of nonimmunologic glomerular injury including anemia, calcium, and strain or species differences. Patients with chronic renal failure are frequently anemic and it is possible that this anemia may help to protect their glomeruli from additional damage. In a preliminary study Garcia *et al.* (43) have shown that inducing anemia by an iron-deficient diet in rats with renal ablation resulted in lowered blood pressure, decreased P_{GC}, increased Q_A, and lessened proteinuria. Although no histology was reported, the authors concluded that anemia reduced glomerular hypertension in this model and thus prevented glomerular injury. Furthermore, the finding of increased Q_A in association with probable decreased glomerular injury still further weakens the case for increased blood flow causing glomerular injury, a point that was made earlier in this review when describing studies using CEI (5). Increased dietary calcium causes rapid deterioration of renal failure in DOC-salt hypertension rats. When such rats are given the calcium channel blocker, nifedipine, systemic blood pressure is lowered, proteinuria is reduced, and glomerular sclerosis is prevented despite no reduction in P_{GC} (33). It was concluded that calcium entry into cells may play a role in the development of glomerulosclerosis in this model of hypertension.

Strain Differences. It has become apparent that different strains of rats and diverse species of animals manifest varying susceptibility to glomerular injury (20, 41, 45, 72, 89, 102). Strain differences were first noted in the glomerular lesion in the aging rat, with Sprague-Dawley (17, 30), Lewis (13), and Wistar (51) strains showing the most severe alterations. As referred to briefly in the section dealing with hypertrophy, Grond *et al.* (45) compared the development of glomerular injury over a 1-year period after removal of 1 kidney in Wistar and PVG/c rats. Whereas the Wistar rats developed progressive glomerular injury after ablation, the PVG/c rats did not. This resistance to damage was accompanied by decreased urinary excretion of protein. It was found that PVG/c rats had 20% more glomeruli than did Wistar rats and that the glomerular volume in PVG/c rats after nephrectomy was smaller than that of even sham-operated Wistar rats. It seems likely that the smaller size of glomeruli in this strain of rats may play an important role in affording protection after renal ablation. The Milan hypertensive rat strain shows less susceptibility to the glomerulosclerosis of aging than does the Milan normotensive rat (20). In this case "protection" of the glomeruli was afforded by the increased afferent arteriolar resistance secondary to an enhanced autoregulatory capability in the hypertensive rats. As mentioned previously, the obese Zucker rat has an increased propensity to develop focal glomerulosclerosis which is associated with elevated serum lipids and is independent of any alterations in glomerular hemodynamics (59, 89). Strain differences have also been shown in the glomerular lesions of diabetic nephropathy with the Munich-Wistar rat showing focal glomerular sclerosis (54) and Lewis rats manifesting diffuse mesangiosclerosis (111).

Species Differences. Different species of animals also manifest varying vulnerability to glomerular injury. Rats develop glomerulosclerosis with increasing age (30, 44) whereas dogs do not (18). There are also differences, at least in degree, in response to reduction of renal mass. Several groups of investigators have examined the effect of reducing renal mass in the dog (18, 97, 102). In general, the dog shows less tendency to develop glomerulosclerosis than the rat, but it should be emphasized that if sufficient renal mass is removed, and the dogs followed for several years, many will develop progressive glomerulosclerosis (18, 97). Bourgoignie (18) suggested that the difference in susceptibility to the development of glomerulosclerosis between dogs and rats may lie in different feeding patterns. Since dogs are fed only once a day, GFR is elevated only during that one postprandial period. In contrast, rats have access to food all day so that GFR may remain raised throughout the day. A similar mechanism has been proposed by Brenner (21).

These strain and species differences in susceptibility to renal disease are likely to have a genetic basis. Although little is known at the molecular level, a recent publication is of interest. MacKay *et al.* (72) examined mice transgenic for the transforming gene encoding large T-antigen in the early region of simian virus 40, and found progressive glomerulosclerosis accompanied by the appearance of tubular proliferative lesions. Possible pathogenetic factors such as age, hypertension, diabetes mellitus, decreased glomerular number, and immune complexes were excluded. Because expression of large T-antigen *in vitro* alters production of collagen, proteoglycans, and PDGF (72), it was suggested that dysregulation of genes might be responsible for the changes encountered. Thus, it is possible that modification of the availability of these substances may also be important in the pathogenesis of glomerulosclerosis.

STRUCTURAL BASIS FOR MECHANISMS OF INJURY

The glomerular lesions seen in experimental hypertension and after renal ablation appear identical and probably arise through similar mechanisms. Since more is known about the changes after ablation the following account will confine itself to this model. In order to assess the role of various factors in the pathogenesis of the glomerular lesions after reduction of renal mass, most of the studies cited above used light microscopic evaluation of either a simple percentage of damaged glomeruli or a glomerular damage index which stratified the severity of glomerular injury. Several of these articles did not clearly define the glomerular abnormalities which were counted when using percentages. It is now reasonable to return to a more detailed consideration of the morphologic alterations in order to see how the factors discussed above including P_{GC}, hypertrophy, coagulation, lipid abnormalities, and cellular proliferation might act to produce the lesions which have been described. The time course of the appearance and severity of lesions varies according to the strain of rat used and the amount of renal tissue reduced. However, with the possible exception of the appearance of microaneurysms, most changes described are qualitatively similar despite differences of strain or extent of ablation.

Light microscopic examination of remnant kidneys reveals focal segmental glomerulosclerosis appearing as early as 7 days after operation (53, 66, 92, 93, 98, 108). Adhesions commonly form between portions of the glomerular tuft and Bowman's capsule (66, 92, 93, 108), and are frequently associated with increased prominence of epithelial cells containing protein reabsorption droplets. Platelet thrombi are noted as an early alteration (90, 92, 98). Some capillary lumina become occluded by the appearance of fibrin thrombi or formation of hyalinosis lesions (Fig. 1) (92, 98) containing lipid (66, 92). Capillaries are dilated (108) with formation of microaneurysms in extreme cases (98), and glomerular volume increased (107). Simultaneously, an increase in mesangial matrix accompanied by an increase in mesangial cell number develops (Fig. 2), and rats with greater degrees of ablation occasionally show accumulation of hyalinosis-like material within the mesangium (92, 98). With increasing time after operation, these changes progress to involve entire glomeruli which become solidified. At the same time, greater numbers of glomeruli become affected. Glomeruli in superficial and juxtamedullary cortex are affected equally (92, 94) although it should be noted that in certain models of experimental hypertension the juxtamedullary population is unduly involved (94). The tubular epithelium becomes hypertrophied to a degree similar to the glomerular hypertrophy. Other changes in the tubules and interstitium are secondary to glomerular alterations. Vascular alterations including fibrinoid necrosis and medial hypertrophy (66, 90, 93) are for the most part restricted to arterioles and interlobular arteries

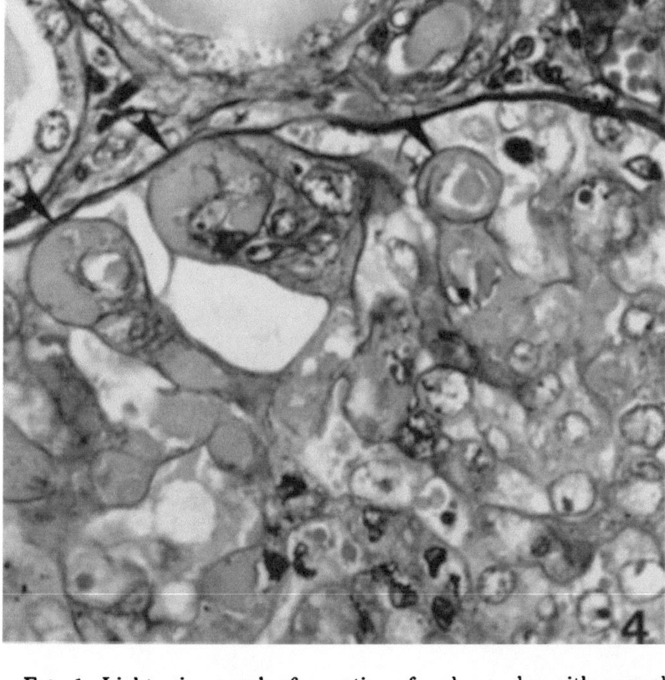

FIG. 1. Light micrograph of a portion of a glomerulus with several hyalinosis lesions (*arrowheads*). There is loss of epithelial cells from GBM. Methenamine silver; ×650.

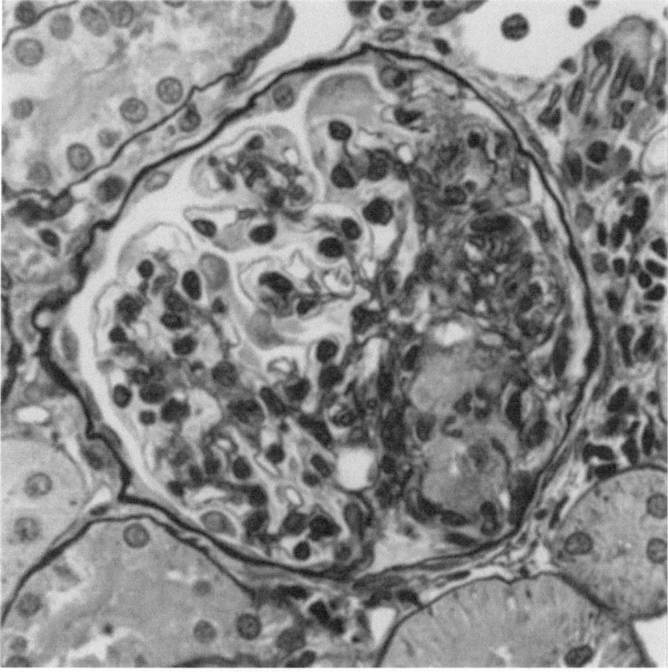

FIG. 2. Light micrograph of a glomerulus with segmental sclerosis and adhesion of glomerular tuft to Bowman's capsule. Methenamine silver; ×330.

and are almost certainly a consequence of the hypertension which develops.

One of the early physiologic indicators of glomerular injury after reduction of renal mass is the occurrence of increased urinary excretion of albumin which coincides with the appearance of the earliest morphologic alterations noted on ultrastructural examination. Studies of glomerular permeability, after reduction of renal mass using anionic, neutral, and cationic forms of horseradish peroxidase, demonstrated that there is an effective loss of charge in the filtration barrier allowing increased passage of albumin across the capillary wall (93). Additional experiments in the same study also detected a size-defect in the glomerular barrier to filtration for molecules greater than 52 Å. A recent study using rats with unilateral nephrectomy and nephrotoxic serum nephritis examined the effect of altering perfusion pressure by aortic ligature on glomerular permeability (88). Such rats are hypertensive and have increased urinary excretion of protein. When they were acutely subjected to aortic ligature at a time when they had established glomerular injury and proteinuria, there was a decrease in perfusion pressure, P_{GC}, and urinary protein. Since there was an immediate and direct response of protein excretion to the changes in P_{GC}, the authors suggested that the alterations in glomerular permeability were mediated directly by increased P_{GC}.

Electron microscopy has been used to examine the cellular elements of the glomerular filter. Both endothelial and epithelial cells manifest evidence of injury after renal ablation. Endothelial cells become separated from the GBM, and flocculent material as well as fibrin begins to accumulate in the subendothelial space (92, 93). Additional evidence for endothelial injury is the appearance of platelet thrombi (Fig. 3), particularly in areas where the endothelial cells are lifted away from the basement membrane, and the presence of small membrane blebs. What are presumed to be plasma proteins accumulate in the subendothelial space, gradually encroaching on the capillary lumina and leading to the formation of hyalinosis lesions (Fig. 4) which often contain lipid and foamy macrophages. At the same time, numerous alterations in epithelial cells take place including coarsening of the foot processes, increase in microfilaments in the cytoplasm, accumulation of protein reabsorption droplets, and bleb formation. In addition, as the severity of epithelial cell injury progresses, the foot processes separate from the GBM leaving bare areas as potential sites for large defects in the filtration barrier (Fig. 4). Hemodynamic alterations, hypertrophic factors, coagulation and lipid abnormalities may contribute to this sequence of injury. Initially, increased P_{GC} may cause direct mechanical stress to endothelial cells. Increased caliber of capillaries as a part of hypertrophy would magnify such an effect secondary to further increase in wall tension according to the law of Laplace (78). The identification of stress fibers in the endothelial cells of arterioles and capillaries near the hilus of the glomerulus (90) suggests that this hypothesis has some merit. The presence of platelet thrombi has been well documented at early stages by both light and electron microscopy. Furthermore, such thrombi have been shown to be associated with damaged endothelium especially near areas of bare GBM. These findings suggest that endothelial damage is an important early alteration which may produce a cascade of other effects. The presence of foamy macrophages in relation to hyalinosis lesions suggests a potential role of serum lipid abnormalities, but alternatively may simply reflect the occurrence of cell death with the lipid arising from

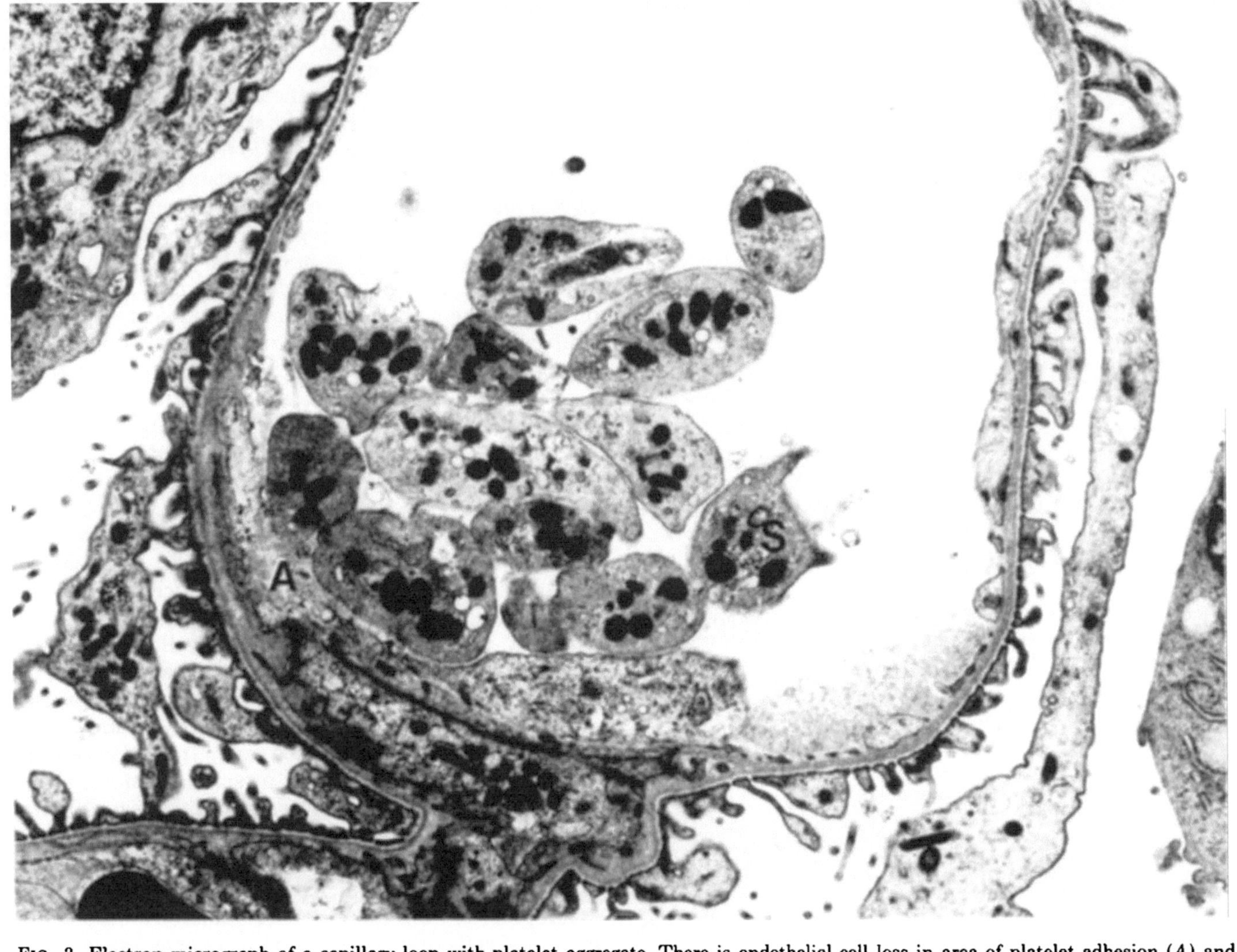

FIG. 3. Electron micrograph of a capillary loop with platelet aggregate. There is endothelial cell loss in area of platelet adhesion (*A*) and change of shape (*S*) in some of the platelets. Uranyl acetate and lead citrate; ×11,900.

the cell membranes. Epithelial cells become enlarged and may also increase in number, but the mechanism for this proliferation is not clarified by morphologic examination. Possible factors involved in the pathogenesis of the epithelial injury include increase in flow across the capillary wall, mechanical distension of the capillary wall, and the hypertrophy itself (101).

The mesangium also undergoes severe alterations simultaneously with the changes observed in the peripheral capillary loop. Increased traffic of macromolecules through the mesangium has been demonstrated by an accumulation of native ferritin within the matrix (93). This change is accompanied by an increase in the matrix material as well as by a mild increase in the number of cells. Some of the cells are extrinsic to the glomerulus, are foamy, and probably represent macrophages. In experiments in which marked degrees of ablation are accompanied by severe hypertension, mesangiolysis and the accumulation of hyalinosis-like material have been observed (92, 98). The two major factors which affect the mesangium are likely to be the increased P_{GC} and release of factors from platelets such as PDGF. Administration of heparin to rats with renal ablation virtually eliminates the occurrence of glomerular sclerosis, at least up to 4 weeks after operation. In addition to its anticoagulant properties, heparin has many different physiologic effects and actions (57). In this situation it could be beneficial by interfering with the release of platelet factors or by inhibiting proliferation of mesangial cells (26). Such antiproliferative effects could contribute to the improved outcome of treatment with heparin in this model.

RELATIONSHIP TO HUMAN DISEASE

The discussion to this point has been confined to experimental models, but several interesting parallels have been demonstrated in humans. It has been proposed that any renal disease which results in loss of a critical number of nephrons may progress to end-stage by the mechanisms discussed earlier (21), and the similar morphologic changes seen in many end-stage kidneys, regardless of the original disease, give some support to this. Furthermore, the rate of progression of renal disease to occurrence of renal failure is hastened by the presence of hypertension (9), and the demonstration that adequate

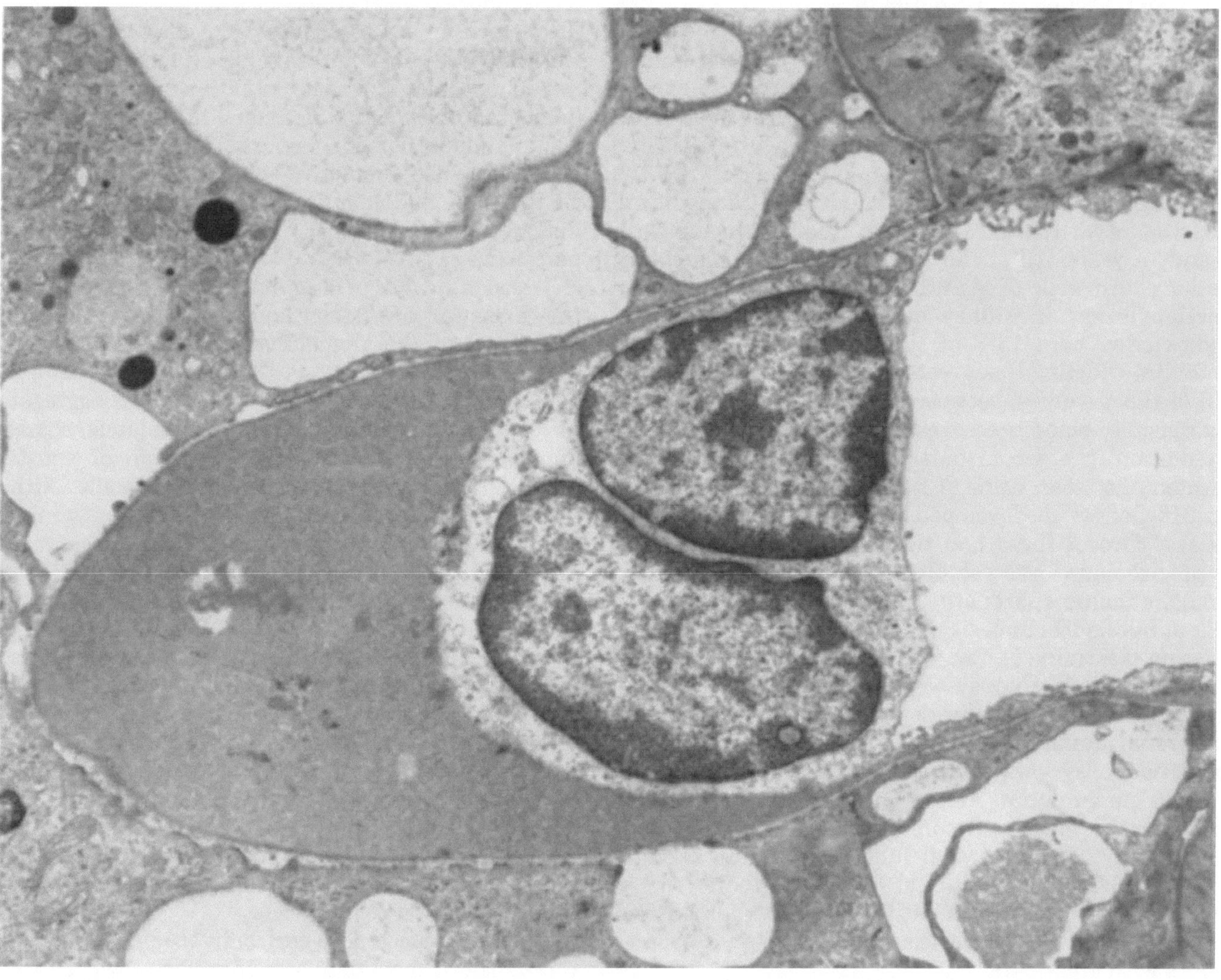

FIG. 4. Electron micrograph of crescent-shaped hyalinosis lesion between endothelial cell and GBM. Extensive effacement of foot processes and focal areas (*arrowhead*) where epithelial cells have detached from GBM are apparent. Uranyl acetate and lead citrate; ×9,400.

control of hypertension in diabetes mellitus slows the development of diabetic nephropathy (79) is an example of this.

The important glomerular lesions found in the renal ablation model are focal sclerosis and hyalinosis. Such lesions have been described in a variety of human conditions which include morbid obesity (58), oligomeganephronia (39), reflux nephropathy (15, 36, 61), unilateral renal agenesis (14, 62, 115), and after nephrectomy for unilateral renal disease (14, 62, 124). These will be described in turn and parallels drawn with causative factors derived from animal stuides. When morbidly obese patients develop the nephrotic syndrome, focal glomerular sclerosis is the most common lesion identified on biopsy (58). Of 17 such patients, 9 (53%) had focal glomerular sclerosis compared with 2 of 6 (33%) of a group of nonobese patients with similar presentation. The situation is similar to the occurrence of focal glomerular sclerosis in the Zucker obese rat (89). The other 4 conditions listed have a common link to the renal ablation model in that there is a loss of functioning renal mass with the likelihood of changed glomerular hemodynamics and hypertrophy. Oligomeganephronia is a condition in which patients are born with reduced numbers of nephrons; those that are present are increased in size (39) and sometimes show changes of focal sclerosis (74). Reflux nephropathy is attended by severe scarring of the renal parenchyma, and focal sclerosis, accompanied by proteinuria, sometimes occurs in the surviving glomeruli (61). Morphometric studies have been carried out and have shown increase in glomerular diameter and surface area (36). It has been suggested that the advent of focal sclerosis provides an explanation for the progressive renal failure that occurs in certain patients whose renal function deteriorates in spite of the correction of reflux (61). Unilateral renal agenesis was shown to be attended by focal glomerular sclerosis in two out of seven cases studied by Kiprov, Colvin, and McCluskey (62), and additional cases have been described by others (14, 115). Morphometric assessment of glomeruli showed a great increase in glomerular size (14). Unilateral nephrectomy in adult patients with disease confined to that kidney has given equivocal results. One group of workers (124) found that 9 of 24 patients so treated developed proteinuria and 4 of these had focal glomerular sclerosis in the remaining kidney. Another group (62) failed to find glomerular lesions in 10 patients who had undergone removal of 1 kidney 8 to 46 years earlier.

Transplant donors represent one final group of human subjects that should be discussed in view of the experimental evidence that glomerular injury ensues after reduction of renal mass. Many authors have investigated long-term renal function in transplant donors (3, 46, 77, 116) (Table 1). The follow-up periods have ranged from 2 to 28 years with the mean in most studies being between 10 and 15 years. All of the authors have concluded that the long-term risk of significant deterioration of renal function is low in kidney donors. However, in the 4 studies cited here 13% of the donors developed mild proteinuria (defined as greater than 200 mg/24 hours). In 3 of the 4 studies, between 19 and 50% of the donors had diastolic blood pressures > 90 mm Hg at follow-up. In addition, the serum creatinine level was uniformly elevated to a mean value of 1.2 mg/dl in all 4 studies. Of the 218 donors, 5 developed clinical evidence of renal disease. Two of these had the nephrotic syndrome but no precise cause was established (77). Another patient had light chain nephropathy on biopsy (3) while a fourth patient had morbid obesity, hypertension, elevated level of serum creatinine (1.4 mg/dl), and proteinuria (1.3 gm/24 hours), but no biopsy was performed (3). The fifth patient developed insulin-dependent diabetes 7 years after renal donation and had proteinuria of 1 gm/24 hours; no biopsy was performed (46). These compilations of follow-up on donors are certainly encouraging that in most case no harm will come to the living donor of a kidney with regard to renal function. Yet at the same time it is clear that additional follow-up studies will be required to examine the effects for longer periods of time. Furthermore, it is evident that it is necessary to screen donors with great care.

SUMMARY

From the above discussion it is clear that many factors have been invoked in the pathogenesis of progressive glomerular injury. Those which are most important include increased P_{GC}, coagulation, serum lipid abnormalities, and hypertrophy. Although many hemodynamic alterations have been identified, increased P_{GC} was noted most constantly. Furthermore, the loss of autoregulatory capability which was observed in some models with progressive glomerulosclerosis usually resulted in increased P_{GC}. Increased P_{GC} has been associated with augmented dietary protein and is seen in the Munich-Wistar rat made diabetic. Such an increase in P_{GC} could cause direct mechanical injury to endothelial and epithelial cells, as well as be responsible for increased mesangial traffic of macromolecules with the potential for stimulating cellular proliferation and mesangial matrix increase. Additional support for the importance of increased P_{GC} is provided by the protective effect of decreasing P_{GC} with CEI therapy and anemia, and by the enhanced autoregulatory capability in both the Milan and Okamoto hypertensive rats.

The significance of coagulation factors is confirmed by the formation of platelet and fibrin thrombi in the development of the glomerular lesions. The sequence of glomerular injury suggests that endothelial damage occurs with subsequent formation of platelet aggregates as a response to this injury. Formation of platelet aggregates may be associated with the production of substances potentially injurious to the endothelial cells. Although blocking the appearance of such thrombi by administration of heparin or thromboxane synthetase inhibitor prevents glomerular injury, the blood pressure lowering effect of these agents complicates the interpretation of the studies.

Serum lipid abnormalities are also important factors in the progression of nonimmunologic glomerular injury. Such abnormalities are observed with increased dietary phosphorus or lipid, in the obese Zucker rat, and in rats with diabetes mellitus. Reduction in serum cholesterol by administration of clofibric acid or mevinolin diminishes glomerular injury independent of alterations in glomerular hemodynamics. The possible link between increased serum lipids and augmentation of glomerular injury is at present indirect.

The importance of hypertrophy as a contributing factor to the progression of nonimmunologic glomerular injury is suggested by several lines of evidence. Hypertrophy, with increase in glomerular size and caliber of capillary loops, may amplify the effect of increased P_{GC} by further intensifying the tension and mechanical stress on all elements of the capillary wall. The association of increased glomerular injury and the ability of glomeruli to enlarge in response to nephrectomy in certain strains of rats emphasizes the importance of hypertrophy. Various hormonal and genetic factors which cause glomerular hypertrophy are also associated with glomerulosclerosis.

In conclusion, many factors have been shown to influence progressive and glomerular damage. It is unlikely

TABLE 1. LONG-TERM RENAL FUNCTION IN TRANSPLANT DONORS

Author	Number of donors	Follow-up (years) mean (range)	Serum creatinine (mg/dl) mean (range)	Urinary protein (mg/24 h) mean (range)	Percentage with diastolic pressure > 90 mm Hg
Vincenti *et al.* (116)	20	15.8 (14.5–18.5)	1.16 NA[a]	141 (40–448)	15
Anderson *et al.* (100)	100	12.6 (10–20)	1.2 (0.1–1.8)	89 (3–1,334)	19
Miller *et al.* (77)	46	6 (2–15)	1.2 (0.3–2.0)	140 (33–418)	31
Hakim *et al.* (46)	52	15 (10–28)	1.28 (0.65–2.2)	188 (30–1,000)	48

[a] NA, Not available.

that one of them is solely responsible and the injury is probably the result of their considerable interplay.

Acknowledgment: We would like to thank Mrs. Mary Swaner for secretarial assistance.

Address reprint requests to: Jean L. Olson, M.D., Department of Pathology, The Johns Hopkins Hospital, 600 North Wolfe Street, Baltimore, MD 21205.

REFERENCES

1. Addis TB, Myers BA, Oliver J: The regulation of renal activity. IX. The effect of unilateral nephrectomy on the function and structure of the remaining kidney. Arch Intern Med 34: 243, 1924
2. Alfrey AC: Thyroid and parathyroid hormones in experimental renal failure. In The Progressive Nature of Renal Disease, edited by Mitch WE, Brenner BM, Stein JH, p 37. New York. Churchill Livingstone, 1986
3. Anderson CF, Velosa JA, Frohnert PP, Torres VE, Offord KP, Vogel JP, Donadio JV Jr, Wilson DM: The risks of unilateral nephrectomy: status of kidney donors 10 to 20 years postoperatively. Mayo Clin Proc 60:367, 1985
4. Anderson S, Meyer TW, Rennke HG, Brenner BM: Control of hypertension limits glomerular injury in rats with reduced renal mass. J Clin Invest 76:612, 1985
5. Anderson S, Rennke HG, Brenner BM: Therapeutic advantage of converting enzyme inhibitors in arresting progressive renal disease associated with systemic hypertension in the rat. J Clin Invest 77:1993, 1986
6. Arendshorst WJ, Beierwaltes WH: Renal and nephron hemodynamics in spontaneously hypertensive rats. Am J Physiol 236:F246, 1979
7. Argiles A, Mourad G, Basset N, Axelrud-Cavadore C, Haiech J, Mion C, Cavadore JC, Demaille JG: Acute adaptive changes to unilateral nephrectomy in humans. Kidney Int 32:714, 1987
8. Azar S, Johnson MA, Scheinman J, Bruno L, Tobian L: Regulation of glomerular capillary pressure and filtration rate in young Kyoto hypertensive rats. Clin Sci 56:203, 1979
9. Baldwin DS, Neugarten J: Blood pressure control and progression of renal insufficiency. In The Progressive Nature of Renal Disease, edited by Mitch WE, Brenner BM, Stein JH, p 81. New York, Churchill Livingstone, 1986
10. Bank N, Alterman L, Aynedjian HS: Selective deep nephron hyperfiltration in uninephrectomized spontaneously hypertensive rats. Kidney Int 24:185, 1983
11. Barcelli UO, Miyata J, Ito Y, Gallon L, Laskarzewski P, Weiss M, Hitzemann R, Pollak VE: Beneficial effects of polyunsaturated fatty acids in partially nephrectomized rats. Prostaglandins 32:211, 1986
12. Barcelli UO, Weiss M, Pollak VE: Effects of dietary prostaglandin precursor on the progression of experimentally induced chronic renal failure. J Lab Clin Med 100:786, 1982
13. Bell RH Jr, Borjesson BS, Wolf PL, Fernández-Cruz L, Brimm JE, Lee S, Sayers HJ, Orloff MJ: Quantitative morphological studies of aging changes in the kidney of the Lewis rat. Renal Physiol 7:176, 1984
14. Bhathena DB, Julian BA, McMorrow RG, Baehler RW: Focal sclerosis of hypertrophied glomeruli in solitary functioning kidneys of humans. Am J Kidney Dis 5:226, 1985
15. Bhathena DB, Weiss JH, Holland NH, McMorrow RG, Curtis JJ, Lucas BA, Luke RG: Focal and segmental glomerular sclerosis in reflux nephropathy. Am J Med 68:886, 1980
16. Bidani AK, Schwartz MM, Lewis EJ: Renal autoregulation and vulnerability to hypertensive injury in remnant kidney. Am J Physiol 252:F1003, 1987
17. Bolton WK, Benton FR, Maclay BA, Sturgill BC: Spontaneous glomerular sclerosis in aging Sprague-Dawley rats. I. Lesions associated with mesangial IgM deposits. Am J Pathol 85:277, 1976
18. Bourgoignie JJ, Gavellas G, Martinez E, Pardo V: Glomerular function and morphology after renal mass reduction in dogs. J Lab Clin Med 109:380, 1987
19. Bradford JR: The results following partial nephrectomy and the influence of the kidney upon metabolism. J Physiol 23:415, 1899
20. Brandis A, Bianchi G, Reale E, Helmchen U, Kuhn K: Age-dependent glomerulosclerosis and proteinuria occurring in rats of the Milan normotensive strain and not in rats of the Milan hypertensive strain. Lab Invest 55:234, 1986
21. Brenner BM: Nephron adaptation to renal injury or ablation. Am J Physiol 249:F324, 1985
22. Bricker NS, Klahr S, Lubowitz H, Rieselbach RE: Renal function in chronic renal disease. Medicine 44:263, 1965
23. Byrom FB: The Hypertensive Vascular Crisis: An Experimental Study. New York, Grune and Stratton, 1969
24. Byrom FB, Dodson LF: The causation of acute arterial necrosis in hypertensive disease. J Pathol Bact 60:357, 1948
25. Carmines PK, Morrison TK, Navar LG: Angiotensin II effects on microvascular diameters of *in vitro* blood-perfused juxtamedullary nephrons. Am J Physiol 251:F610, 1986
26. Castellot JJ, Hoover RL, Harper PA, Karnovsky MJ: Heparin and glomerular epithelial cell-secreted heparinlike species inhibit mesangial cell proliferation. Am J Pathol 120:427, 1985
27. Chanutin A, Ferris EB: Experimental renal insufficiency produced by partial nephrectomy I. Control diet. Arch Int Med 49:767, 1932
28. Chanutin A, Ludewig S: Experimental renal insufficiency produced by partial nephrectomy: V. Diets containing whole dried meat. Arch Int Med 58:60, 1936
29. Clive DM, Stoff JS: Renal syndromes associated with nonsteroidal antiinflammatory drugs. N Engl J Med 310:563, 1984
30. Couser WG, Stilmant MM: Mesangial lesions and focal glomerular sclerosis in the aging rat. Lab Invest 33:491, 1975
31. DiBona GF, Rios LL: Mechanism of exaggerated diuresis in spontaneously hypertensive rats. Am J Physiol 235:F409, 1978
32. Doi T, Striker LJ, Quaife C, Conti FG, Palmiter R, Behringer R, Brinster R, Striker GE: Progressive glomerulosclerosis develops in transgenic mice chronically expressing growth hormone and growth hormone releasing factor but not in those expressing insulinlike growth factor-1. Am J Pathol 131:398, 1988
33. Dworkin LD, Benstein J, Feiner HD, Parker M: Nifedipine prevents glomerular injury without reducing glomerular pressure in rats with DOCA salt hypertension (abstr). Kidney Int 33:374, 1988
34. Dworkin LD, Feiner HD, Randazzo J: Glomerular hypertension and injury in deoxycorticosterone-salt rats on antihypertensive therapy. Kidney Int 31:718, 1987
35. Dworkin LD, Hostetter TH, Rennke HG, Brenner BM: Hemodynamic basis for glomerular injury in rats with desoxycorticosterone-salt hypertension. J Clin Invest 73:1448, 1984
36. El-Khatib MT, Becker GJ, Kincaid-Smith PS: Morphometric aspects of reflux nephropathy. Kidney Int 32:261, 1987
37. Fagin JA, Melmed S: Relative increase in insulin-like growth factor I messenger ribonucleic acid levels in compensatory renal hypertrophy. Endocrinology 120:718, 1987.
38. Feld LG, Van Liew JB, Galaske RG, Boylan JW, Chang H: Selectivity of renal injury and proteinuria in the spontaneously hypertensive rat. Kidney Int 12:332, 1977
39. Fetterman GH, Habib R: Congenital bilateral oligonephronic renal hypoplasia with hypertrophy of nephrons (oligoméganéphronie). Am J Clin Pathol 52:199, 1969
40. Fine LG: The biology of renal hypertrophy. Kidney Int 29:619, 1986
41. Fine LG: Preventing the progression of human renal disease: have rational therapeutic principles emerged? Kidney Int 33:116, 1988
42. Fries JU, Sandstrom D, Meyer TW, Rennke HG: Glomerular hypertrophy and epithelial cell injury are determinants of progressive glomerulosclerosis in the rat (abstr). Kidney Int 33:374, 1988
43. Garcia DL, Anderson S, Sandquist KJ, Rennke HG, Brenner BM: Anemia lessens systemic/glomerular hypertension and proteinuria in renal ablation (abstr). Kidney Int 33:375, 1988
44. Goldstein RS, Tarloff JB, Hook JB: Age-related nephropathy in laboratory rats. FASEB J 2:2241, 1988
45. Grond J, Beukers JYB, Schiltjuis MS, Weening JJ, Elema JD: Analysis of renal structural and functional features in two rat strains with a different susceptibility to glomerular sclerosis. Lab Invest 54:77, 1986
46. Hakim RM, Goldszer RC, Brenner BM: Hypertension and proteinuria: long-term sequelae of uninephrectomy in humans. Kidney Int 25:930, 1984
47. Heifets M, Morrissey JJ, Purkerson ML, Morrison AR, Klahr S:

Effect of dietary lipids on renal function in rats with subtotal nephrectomy. Kidney Int 32:335, 1987

48. Heptinstall RH, Hill GS: Steroid-induced hypertension in the rat. A study of the effects of renal artery constriction in hypertension caused by desoxycorticosterone. Lab Invest 16:751, 1967
49. Hill GS: Studies on the pathogenesis of hypertensive vascular disease: effect of high-pressure intra-arterial injections in rats. Circ Res 27:657, 1970
50. Hill GS, Heptinstall RH: Steroid-induced hypertension in the rat: a microangiographic and histologic study on the pathogenesis of hypertensive vascular and glomerular lesions. Am J Pathol 52:1, 1968
51. Hirokawa K: Characterization of age-associated kidney disease in Wistar rats. Mech Ageing Dev 4:301, 1975
52. Hostetter TH, Meyer TW, Rennke HG, Brenner BM: Chronic effects of dietary protein in the rat with intact and reduced renal mass. Kidney Int 30:509, 1986
53. Hostetter TH, Olson JL, Rennke HG, Venkatachalam MA, Brenner BM: Hyperfiltration in remnant nephrons: a potentially adverse response to renal ablation. Am J Physiol 241:F85, 1981
54. Hostetter TH, Troy JL, Brenner BM: Glomerular hemodynamics in experimental diabetes mellitus. Kidney Int 19:410, 1981
55. Ichikawa I, Yoshida Y, Fogo A: Glomerular hyperfiltration, hyperperfusion or hypertension does not mediate the hypertrophy of glomeruli which predisposes to sclerosis (abstr). Kidney Int 33:377, 1988
56. Iwasaki K, Gleiser CA, Masoro EJ, McMahan CA, Seo E-J, Yu BP: Influence of the restriction of individual dietary components on longevity and age-related disease of Fischer rats: the fat component and the mineral component. J Gerontol 43:B13, 1988
57. Jaques LB: Heparin: an old drug with a new paradigm. Science 206:528, 1979
58. Kasiske BL, Crosson JT: Renal disease in patients with massive obesity. Arch Intern Med 146:1105, 1986
59. Kasiske BL, O'Donnell MP, Cleary MP, Keane WF: Treatment of hyperlipidemia reduces glomerular injury in obese Zucker rats. Kidney Int 33:667, 1988
60. Kasiske BL, O'Donnell MP, Garvis WJ, Keane WF: Pharmacologic treatment of hyperlipidemia reduces glomerular injury in rat 5/6 nephrectomy model of chronic renal failure. Circ Res 62:367, 1988
61. Kincaid-Smith P: Glomerular and vascular lesions in chronic atrophic pyelonephritis and reflux nephropathy. In Advances in Nephrology, vol 5, edited by Hamburger J, Crosnier J, Maxwell MH, p 3. Chicago, Chicago Year Book Medical Publishers, 1975
62. Kiprov DD, Colvin RB, McCluskey RT: Focal and segmental glomerulosclerosis and proteinuria associated with unilateral renal agenesis. Lab Invest 46:275, 1982
63. Klahr S, Buerkert J, Purkerson ML: Role of dietary factors in the progression of chronic renal disease. Kidney Int 24:579, 1983
64. Klahr S, Purkerson ML, Heifets M: Factors that may retard the progression of renal disease. Kidney Int 32(Suppl 22):S35, 1987
65. Kleinknecht C, Laouari D: The influence of dietary components on experimental renal disease. In The Progressive Nature of Renal Disease, edited by Mitch WE, Brenner BM, Stein JH, p 17. New York, Churchill Livingstone, 1986
66. Koletsky S, Goodsit, AM: Natural history and pathogenesis of renal ablation hypertension. Arch Pathol 69:654, 1960
67. Krishna GG, Newell G, Miller E, Heeger P, Smith R, Polansky M, Kapoor S, Hoeldtke R: Protein-induced glomerular hyperfiltration: role of hormonal factors. Kidney Int 33:578, 1988
68. Laouari D, Kleinknecht C, Cournot-Witmer G, Habib R, Mounier F, Broyer M: Beneficial effect of low phosphorus diet in uraemic rats: a reappraisal. Clin Sci 63:539, 1982
69. Logan JL, Lee SM, Benson B, Michael UF: Inhibition of compensatory renal growth by indomethacin. Prostaglandins 31:253, 1986
70. Loomis D: Hypertension and necrotizing arteritis in the rat following renal infarction. Arch Pathol 41:231, 1946
71. Lumlertgul D, Burke TJ, Gillum DM, Alfrey AC, Harris DC, Hammond WS, Schrier RW: Phosphate depletion arrests progression of chronic renal failure independent of protein intake. Kidney Int 29:658, 1986
72. MacKay K, Striker LJ, Pinkert CA, Brinster RL, Striker GE: Glomerulosclerosis and renal cysts in mice transgenic for the early region of SV40. Kidney Int 32:827, 1987
73. Maeda H, Gleiser CA, Masoro EJ, Murata I, McMahan CA, Yu BP: Nutritional influences on aging of Fischer 344 rats: II. Pathology. J Gerontol 40:671, 1985
74. McGraw M, Poucell S, Sweet J, Baumal R: The significance of focal segmental glomerulosclerosis in oligomeganephronia. Int J Pediatr Nephrol 5:67, 1984
75. Meyer TW, Anderson S, Rennke HG, Brenner BM: Reversing glomerular hypertension stabilizes established glomerular injury. Kidney Int 31:752, 1987
76. Meyer TW, Anderson S, Rennke HG, Brenner BM: Converting enzyme inhibitor therapy limits glomerular injury in rats with renal insufficiency. Am J Med 79(Suppl C):31, 1985
77. Miller IJ, Suthanthiran M, Riggio RR, Williams JJ, Riehle RA, Vaughan ED, Stubenbord WT, Mouradian J, Cheigh JS, Stenzel KH: Impact of renal donation: long-term clinical and biochemical follow-up of living donors in a single center. Am J Med 79:201, 1985
78. Miller PL, Rennke HG, Meyer TW: Dietary protein restriction reduces glomerular volume and proteinuria in rats with established adriamycin nephrosis (abstr). Kidney Int 33:380, 1988
79. Mogensen CE: Progression of nephropathy in long-term diabetics with proteinuria and effect of initial antihypertensive treatment. Scand J Clin Lab Invest 36:383, 1976
80. Moise TS, Smith AH: The effect of high protein diet on the kidneys. Arch Pathol 4:530, 1927
81. Moore LC, Schnermann J, Yarimizu S: Feedback mediation of SNGFR autoregulation in hydropenic and DOCA- and salt-loaded rats. Am J Physiol 237:F63, 1979
82. Moorhead JF, Chan MK, Varghese Z: The role of abnormalities of lipid metabolism in the progression of renal disease. In The Progressive Nature of Renal Disease, edited by Mitch WE, Brenner BM, Stein JH, p 133. New York, Churchill Livingstone, 1986
83. Morrison AB: Experimentally induced chronic renal insufficiency in the rat. Lab Invest 11:321, 1962
84. Morrison AB, Howard RM: The functional capacity of hypertrophied nephrons: effect of partial nephrectomy on the clearance of inulin and PAH in the rat. J Exp Med 123:829, 1966
85. Nath KA, Chmielewski DH, Hostetter TH: Regulatory role of prostanoids in glomerular microcirculation of remnant nephrons. Am J Physiol 252:F829, 1987
86. Nath KA, Kren SM, Hostetter TH: Dietary protein restriction in established renal injury in the rat: selective role of glomerular capillary pressure in progressive glomerular dysfunction. J Clin Invest 78:1199, 1986
87. Navar LG, Rosivall L: Contribution of the renin-angiotensin system to the control of intrarenal hemodynamics. Kidney Int 25:857, 1984
88. Neugarten J, Alfino P, Langs C, Schact RG, Baldwin DS: Nephrotoxic serum nephritis with hypertension: perfusion pressure and permselectivity. Kidney Int 33:53, 1988
89. O'Donnell MP, Kasiske BL, Cleary MP, Keane WF: Effects of genetic obesity in renal structure and function in the Zucker rat II. Micropuncture studies. J Lab Clin Med 106:605, 1985
90. Olson JL: The role of heparin as a protective agent following reduction of renal mass. Kidney Int 25:376, 1984
91. Olson JL, Boitnott JK, Heptinstall RH: Clip-ablation: a model of experimental hypertension in the rat. Lab Invest 57:291, 1987
92. Olson JL, de Urdaneta AG, Heptinstall RH: Glomerular hyalinosis and its relation to hyperfiltration. Lab Invest 52:387, 1985
93. Olson JL, Hostetter TH, Rennke HG, Brenner BM, Venkatachalam MA: Mechanisms of altered glomerular permselectivity and progressive glomerulosclerosis following extensive ablation of renal mass. Kidney Int 22:112, 1982
94. Olson JL, Wilson SK, Heptinstall RH: Relation of glomerular injury to preglomerular resistance in experimental hypertension. Kidney Int 29:849, 1986
95. Paller MS, Hostetter TH: Dietary protein increases plasma renin and reduces pressor reactivity to angiotensin II. Am J Physiol 251:F34, 1986
96. Pappenheimer AM: The effect of experimental reduction of kidney substance upon parathyroid glands and skeletal tissue. J Exp Med 64:965, 1936
97. Polzin DJ, Leininger JR, Osborne CA, Jeraj K: Development of renal lesions in dogs after 11/12 reduction of renal mass. Lab Invest 58:172, 1988

98. Purkerson ML, Hoffsten PE, Klahr S: Pathogenesis of the glomerulopathy associated with renal infarction in rats. Kidney Int 9:407, 1976
99. Purkerson ML, Joist JH, Yates J, Valdes A, Morrison A, Klahr S: Inhibition of thromboxane synthesis ameliorates the progressive kidney disease of rats with subtotal ablation. Proc Natl Acad Sci USA 82:193, 1985
100. Raij L, Chiou XC, Owens R, Wrigley B: Therapeutic implications of hypertension-induced glomerular injury: comparison of enalapril and a combination of hydralazine, reserpine, and hydrochlorothiazide in an experimental model. Am J Med 79(Suppl C):37, 1985
101. Rennke HG: Structural alterations associated with glomerular hyperfiltration. In The Progressive Nature of Renal Disease, edited by Mitch WE, Brenner BM, Stein JH, p 111. New York, Churchill Livingstone, 1986
102. Robertson JL, Goldschmidt M, Kronfeld DS, Tomaszewski JE, Hill GS, Bovee KC: Long-term renal responses to high dietary protein in dogs with 75% nephrectomy. Kidney Int 29:511, 1986
103. Scharschmidt LA, Gibbons NB, McGarry L, Berger P, Axelrod M, Janis R, Ko YH: Effects of dietary fish oil on renal insufficiency in rats with subtotal nephrectomy. Kidney Int 32:700, 1987
104. Schnermann J, Gokel M, Weber PC, Schubert G, Briggs JP: Tubuloglomerular feedback and glomerular morphology in Goldblatt hypertensive rats on varying protein diets. Kidney Int 29:520, 1986
105. Schor N, Ichikawa I, Brenner BM: Mechanism of action of various hormones and vasoactive substances on glomerular ultrafiltration in the rat. Kidney Int 20:442, 1981
106. Schwietzer G, Gertz K-H: Changes of hemodynamics and glomerular ultrafiltration in renal hypertension of rats. Kidney Int 15:134, 1979
107. Shea SM, Raskova J, Morrison AB: A stereologic study of glomerular hypertrophy in the subtotally nephrectomized rat. Am J Pathol 90:201, 1978
108. Shimamura T, Morrison AB: A progressive glomerulosclerosis occurring in partial five-sixths nephrectomized rats. Am J Pathol 79:95, 1975
109. Stahl RAK, Kudelka S, Paravincini M, Schollmeyer P: Prostaglandin and thromboxane formation in glomeruli from rats with reduced renal mass. Nephron 42:252, 1986
110. Stahl RAK, Thaiss F: Eicosanoids: biosynthesis and function in the glomerulus. Renal Physiol 10:1, 1987
111. Steffes MW, Mauer SM: Diabetic glomerulopathy in man and experimental animal models. Int Rev Exp Pathol 26:147, 1984
112. Stephan F, de Laharpe F, Reviele P, Parmentier C, Kole-Back MH, Turlot J, Le Minor J, Stahl A: Histomorphometric study of the enhancement of renal compensatory hypertrophy by ACTH in the rat. Horm Metab Res 16:366, 1984
113. Still WJS, Dennison SM: The pathogenesis of the glomerular changes in steroid-induced hypertension in the rat. Lab Invest 20:249, 1969
114. Tapp D, Wortham W, Addison J, Barnes J, Venkatachalam MA: Calorie restriction retards the progression of chronic renal failure in rats (abstr). Kidney Int 33:386, 1988
115. Thorner PS, Arbus GS, Celermajer DS, Baumal R: Focal segmental glomerulosclerosis and progressive renal failure associated with a unilateral kidney. Pediatrics 73:806, 1984
116. Vincenti F, Amend WJC Jr, Kaysen G, Feduska N, Birnbaum J, Duca R, Salvatierra O: Long-term renal function in kidney donors. Transplantation 36:626, 1983
117. Wilson C, Byrom FB: Renal changes in malignant hypertension: experimental evidence. Lancet 1:136, 1939
118. Wilson C, Byrom FB: The vicious cycle in chronic Bright's disease. Experimental evidence from the hypertensive rat. Q J Med 10:65, 1941.
119. Wilson SK, Solez K, Boitnott JK, Heptinstall RH. The effects of heparin treatment on hypertension and vascular lesions in stroke-prone spontaneously hypertensive rats. Am J Pathol 102:62, 1981
120. Wolfgarten M, Mogarey FR: Vascular fibrinoid necrosis in hypertension. J Pathol Bact 77:597, 1959
121. Wood JE Jr, Ethridge C: Hypertension with arteriolar and glomerular changes in the albino rat following subtotal nephrectomy. Proc Soc Exp Biol Med 30:1039, 1933
122. Yamashita W, Ito Y, Weiss MA, Ooi BS, Pollak VA: A thromboxane synthetase antagonist ameliorates progressive renal disease of Dahl-S rats. Kidney Int 33:77, 1988
123. Yoshida Y, Fogo A, Shiraga H, Glick AD, Ichikawa I: Serial micropuncture analysis of single nephron function in subtotal renal ablation. Kidney Int 33:855, 1988
124. Zucchelli P, Cagnoli L, Casanova S, Donini U, Pasquali S: Focal glomerulosclerosis in patients with unilateral nephrectomy. Kidney Int 24:649, 1983

Biology of Disease

The Pathogenesis of Atherosclerosis: Atherogenesis and Inflammation

J. MICHAEL MUNRO AND RAMZI S. COTRAN

Departments of Pathology, Brigham and Women's Hospital and Harvard Medical School, Boston, Massachusetts

INTRODUCTION

Atherosclerosis and its complications, such as myocardial infarction, stroke, and peripheral vascular disease, remain major causes of morbidity and mortality in the Western World; coronary heart disease alone accounts for over half a million deaths in the United States annually (4). Because atherosclerosis is a slowly progressive disease, which begins in childhood and does not become manifest until middle-age or later, its etiology and pathogenesis have been difficult to elucidate. Yet in the past decade or two, cellular and molecular approaches to the study of the cells of the vascular wall, as well as innovative methods for examination of abnormalities in lipid metabolism, have provided numerous insights into the pathogenesis of atherosclerosis. One of these insights is the resurgent appreciation that atherosclerosis is a response of the vascular wall to injury (117–119), having many of the features of the inflammatory response in other tissues (81, 119). Atherosclerosis was likened to inflammation by Rayer in 1823 (112), and this concept was extended by Virchow (145) a few decades later; in 1950, Saphir and Gore (124) spoke of the evidence for an inflammatory basis of coronary arteriosclerosis in the young, and most recently Joris and Majno (81) stressed the similarities between the two processes. That atherosclerosis has similarities to inflammation will be apparent from the considerations which follow, as will be the implications of these concepts to future work on the pathogenesis of atherosclerosis and its prevention and treatment.

This overreview will not cover the serum lipid abnormalities, relation to thrombosis, or complications of atherosclerosis, nor review all the various controversies concerning its etiology and pathogenesis, but rather focus on work that links atherogenesis to the inflammatory process.

THE LESIONS OF ATHEROSCLEROSIS

Human atherosclerosis involves medium-sized muscular arteries, such as the coronary, carotid, basilar, and vertebral arteries, as well as the aorta and the arteries supplying the lower extremities (iliac, femoral). Although a number of variants of atherosclerotic lesions have been described, the two most studied are the fatty streak and the fibro-fatty plaque.

Classical intimal fatty streaks are grossly visible, slightly raised, yellow areas which are narrow and longitudinally-oriented. Microscopically, they consist of subendothelial aggregates of foam cells, which are cells whose cytoplasm is filled with lipid droplets, mostly cholesteryl esters and free cholesterol. Recent studies in which monoclonal antibodies were used as markers of macrophages and smooth muscle cells have shown that a significant majority of the foam cells in fatty streaks are macrophages, the rest being of smooth muscle derivation (3, 143). T lymphocytes are also present (101). Fatty streaks characteristically have little extracellular lipid.

The fundamental lesion of atherosclerosis is the atheromatous or fibrofatty plaque. This is the lesion that causes narrowing of the artery, predisposes to thrombosis, calcifies, and leads to weakening of the muscle and aneurysmal dilation. Atheromatous plaques are approximately rounded, raised lesions, usually off-white to white in color superficially, and perhaps a centimeter in diameter. The center of larger plaques may exude a yellow, grumous fluid, hence the name atheroma (Greek for gruel). Plaques exhibit histologic variability, but a typical cellular plaque (Fig. 1) consists of: a fibrous cap, composed mostly of smooth muscle cells with a few leukocytes, and relatively dense connective tissue containing elastin, collagen fibrils, proteoglycans, and basement membrane (85, 102, 154); a cellular area beneath and to the side of the cap consisting of a mixture of macrophages, smooth muscle cells, and T lymphocytes (79); and a deeper "necrotic core" which contains cellular debris, extracellular lipid droplets, cholesterol crystals, and calcium deposits. This necrotic core often contains numerous large foam cells of both the macrophage and smooth muscle type. Finally, one can sometimes see, particularly around the periphery of the lesions, proliferating small blood vessels, which are evidence of neovascularization from the direction of the adventitia. The relative content of fibrous tissue and lipid within a plaque is variable; coronary artery lesions are often largely fibrous. Thus, on a straightforward histologic level, it can be seen that plaques and sites of inflammation have common features, including leukocytic infiltration, mesenchymal cell proliferation, fibrosis, calcification, and angiogenesis.

The distribution of plaques is important to explain. The most common site is the lower descending aorta, predominantly around the ostia of the major branches, followed by the coronary arteries, usually within the first six centimeters, the arteries of the lower extremities, descending thoracic aorta, the internal carotids, and the Circle of Willis. Some of this localization can be explained by hemodynamic factors, such as shear stress or disturbed flow (59, 86), but certainly not all of it. Particularly vexing is the problem of determining the reason behind the heterogeneous distribution between and within individual subjects. Why, for example, do some patients have disease only in the coronaries and not in the brain or vice versa, and some have severe aortic atherosclerosis with clear coronaries?

The relationship of fatty streaks to atheromatous plaques is controversial (98). Fatty streaks occur early in life, and by the age of 10 years, have covered approximately 10% of the aortic intimal surface, but this 10% includes areas which are not particularly susceptible to developing fibrous plaques later in life (97). In addition, fatty streaks frequently affect individuals in parts of the globe where plaques are relatively infrequent (96). However, fatty streaks do occur in coronary arteries at the same anatomic sites which are later prone to develop plaques (99, 133). Such fatty streaks in the coronaries continue to occupy increasing surface areas and seem to precede the formation of advanced lesions. Finally, some experimental evidence supports the concept of evolution of fatty streaks into plaques. For example, in a hypercholesterolemic non-human primate model, Faggiotto and Ross (43) showed that fatty-streak-like lesions were the earliest to develop, and that many of the advanced lesions of atherosclerosis in the species under study occurred at sites where fatty streaks were originally present. On balance, it appears that fatty streaks are of universal occurrence and distribution, and most, especially those in the aorta, either disappear or remain harmless. In certain locations (*e.g.*, in coronary arteries) and especially in the predisposed individual, these streaks may conceivably evolve into fibrous plaques.

An additional "lesion" which may bear a material relationship to atherosclerosis is diffuse intimal thickening. In infancy, the endothelium of large and medium-sized arteries is generally directly apposed to the underlying media, but as the individual grows, these two structures become separated by accumulating extracellular matrix and cells. The matrix contains collagen, elastin, proteoglycans, and fibronectins. Smooth muscle cells, macrophages, and T lymphocytes are present within the matrix, presumably having arrived from the media and arterial lumen. The smooth muscle cells can then be regarded as an intrinsic intimal population, and

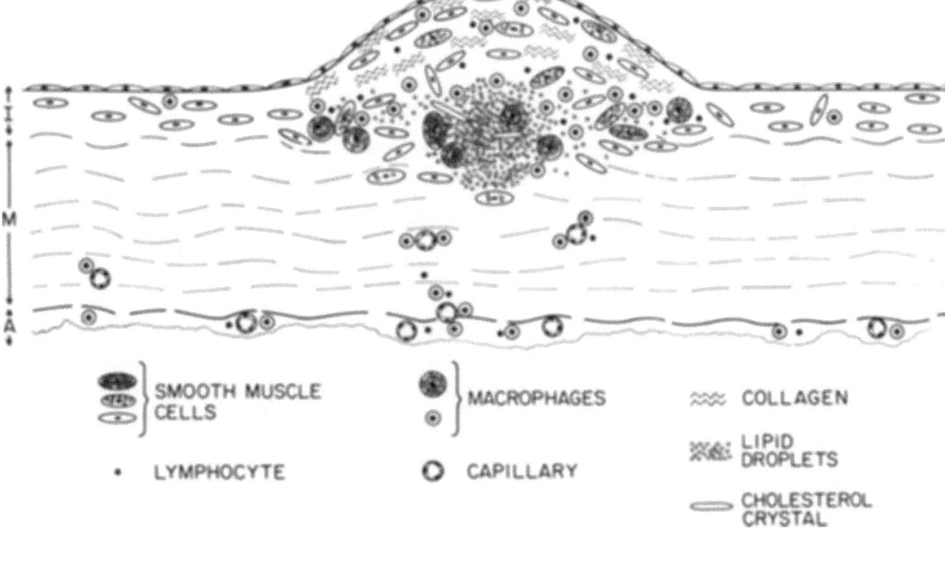

FIG. 1. Schematic representation of a cross-section through an atherosclerotic plaque (*I*, intima; *M*, media; *A*, adventitia, medial smooth muscle cells not drawn in). Overlying endothelium is intact in this example. Note "cap" with smooth muscle cells and collagenous bands. Underneath this is the core region with abundant extracellular lipid and foam cells. Macrophages are widely distributed, and lymphocytes can be seen in the cap and to the sides of the core. Adventitial capillaries are gravitating toward the intimal lesion.

are often designated myointimal cells. After a few years of life the intima, now being composed of endothelium and underlying cells and matrix, continues to increase in height and is said to show diffuse intimal thickening. In general, this thickening can be taken as normal, presumably the result of hemodynamic or other stresses to the artery wall over time. However, it has been noted that in certain anatomic sites, this thickening can be focal (133), forming "cushions" which predate plaques, thus suggesting that the latter may be causally related to the former. In contrast, some of these anatomic sites are locations which are always spared lesions (*e.g.*, flow dividers).

THE PATHOGENESIS OF ATHEROSCLEROSIS

Any theory or concept of atherogenesis must account for: (a) the mechanism of smooth muscle proliferation, which is a fundamental process in the development of the plaque; (b) the presence of lipid in most lesions; (c) the focal nature of the lesions and their general distribution; and (d) the role of the major risk factors, particularly hyperlipidemia, hypertension and smoking, in the development of atheromatous plaques.

Although there are investigators who argue for the primacy of one pathogenetic mechanism, or necessary sequence of events in atherogenesis, the current trend is to consider atherosclerosis as a response of the vascular wall to a variety of initiating agents, and that multiple pathogenetic mechanisms contribute to the formation of the plaques (119, 134).

The Response to Injury Hypothesis

The best-studied current hypothesis of atherosclerosis is the response to injury hypothesis, based on the early proposals made by Virchow. A modern version of this hypothesis, formulated by Ross and Glomset in 1976 (118), was based on two important experimental observations: (a) that smooth muscle proliferation and lesions resembling atheromatous plaques can be induced in experimental animals by endothelial denudation (such as with a balloon catheter), the development of lesions being accentuated by hypercholesterolemia; and (b) that a factor derived from platelets can induce smooth muscle growth *in vitro* (this substance being platelet-derived growth factor, PDGF, see below). The initial hypothesis postulated that injury to arterial endothelium by mechanical, chemical, toxic, viral, or immunologic agents caused endothelial denudation, and was followed by platelet adhesion and aggregation, with consequent release of PDGF, in turn leading to migration into and proliferation of smooth muscle cells in the intima and secretion of connective tissue components. With repeated insults, the typical atheromatous plaque could form. The response to injury hypothesis has been instrumental in stimulating research on various aspects of endothelial and smooth muscle cell biology and on the mechanisms by which various risk factors precipitate atherosclerosis. It soon became apparent, however, that actual denudation was not a consistent early feature of an important form of atherosclerosis, that initiated by hypercholesterolemia alone (35); and that platelet adhesion is neither necessary nor sufficient to cause the lesions (126). Over the years, the hypothesis (119) has had to be modified in the following three ways: (a) as is now clear, the endothelium can respond to a variety of stimuli, not simply by undergoing necrosis and denudation, but by subtle changes in function (endothelial dysfunction), or by the induction of new endothelial properties; thus, non-denuding injury may be as important in initiating the lesions of atherosclerosis as frank denudation; (b) platelets are not the sole initiators of smooth muscle proliferation, since growth promoting (and growth inhibitory) factors derived from other cell types, such as macrophages, may regulate smooth muscle growth; (c) monocytes and macrophages are major cellular components of lesions and are likely to play a role in its initiation and evolution. We will now review the various components of the response to injury hypothesis.

ENDOTHELIUM AND ENDOTHELIAL INJURY

Recent research on vascular endothelium, sparked to a considerable degree by the response to injury hypothesis, has established endothelial cells as active cells which perform a variety of critical functions, including modulating permeability characteristics of tissues, transferring metabolic substances between blood and tissues, maintaining hemostasis and thromboresistance, synthesizing and metabolizing a variety of biologically active molecules, and regulating vascular tone, inflammatory and immune functions and vascular cell growth (31, 58, 77, 148). It has also become clear that the endothelium responds to various stimuli, not simply as a passive target sustaining cellular injury or death, but by undergoing specific alterations in function, metabolism, and structure which directly influence the evolution of the response to the injurious stimuli. Some of these alterations are increases and decreases in normal constitutive functions, and others are due to induction of new functions and molecules (148). For example, hemodynamic changes, such as altered shear stress, induce shape changes and increased fluid pinocytosis, and turbulent flow increases endothelial replication without causing endothelial necrosis (34, 36). Platelets become adherent to apparently intact endothelium treated with chemicals, or transformed by SV40 virus in culture (58). The cytokines, interleukin 1 (IL-1, produced by various cells) and tumor necrosis factor (TNF), produced by macrophages, induce increased procoagulant activity of endothelium (12, 13), increased adhesion of leukocytes to endothelium (16), and the synthesis of new surface protein molecules (107). Hypercholesterolemia or hypercholesterolemic serum lipoproteins promote monocyte adhesion to endothelium *in vivo* (53, 82) and *in vitro* (1, 41). Hypertension and hyperlipidemia may focally increase endothelial replication (47, 126) possibly resulting from transient foci of denudation. Reidy and Schwartz (113, 113a) have made a good case for so-called "nondenuding" injury. They showed detachment of single endothelial cells caused by endotoxin, quickly followed by replacement from adjacent cells without denudation. These transient foci of injury may not cause significant platelet adhesion, but can be associated with local increased permeability. Heparin-like proteoglycan molecules, derived from endothelium, cause smooth muscle growth inhibition, and their loss may promote proliferation (22, 24). These are but a few examples of the multitude of possible ways in which the endothelium may theoretically influence the arterial response to injury without undergoing necrosis. Some of the above phenomena may well initiate a sequence of events which contributes to the development of an atheromatous lesion. Further data regarding endothelium, particularly relating to growth factor production, are discussed below.

PLATELETS IN ATHEROGENESIS

The earliest and most consistent consequence of denuding endothelial injury is the adhesion of platelets to the subendothelial connective tissue (117). In experimental animals this begins within seconds after denudation, and although greater numbers of leukocytes subsequently become attached, platelets are the predominant cell type in the first 24 hours. Adhesion is followed by the platelet release reaction. Goldberg, Stemerman, and Handin (61) used immunofluorescence microscopy to demonstrate the presence of platelet factor 4 in the subendothelium after denudation. Presumably other biologically important molecules are also released from platelets, including β-thromboglobulin, vasoconstrictive amines, arachidonic acid metabolites, and, of most relevance to atherogenesis, mitogenic factors. Platelets secrete PDGF, epidermal growth factor, transforming growth factor-β (TGF-β), and other less well-characterized mitogens. As will be detailed later, PDGF induces both migration and proliferation of smooth muscle cells (64, 116).

Platelets are excellent candidates as the initiators of intimal plaque formation after denuding injury. In almost all models studied, the major burst of smooth muscle mitotic activity occurs within 48 hours of denudation, consistent with the presence of adherent activated platelets at these early time periods. Mitotic activity declines considerably thereafter, as platelets disappear. Platelet products gain access into the intima and PDGF is highly cationic, potentially adsorbing to the glycosaminoglycan-rich anionic intima. Several studies have shown that experimentally-induced thrombocytopenia inhibits the intimal proliferation after balloon-de-endothelialization or catheter injury (*e.g.*, 50). In a model of endothelial injury induced by homocystinemia, Harker, Harlan, and Ross (68) showed that sulfinpyrazone, an inhibitor of the platelet release reaction, suppressed the smooth muscle mitogenic response. In humans, it is highly likely that platelets are involved in early lesion formation in catheter-induced injury, in peri-anastomotic lesions of vascular grafts, and in other traumatic vascular lesions. The role of platelets after nondenuding injury is less certain, as is their role in experimental atherosclerosis related to hyperlipidemia. Recently, however, Faggiotto, Ross, and Harker (44) found that platelets are also abundant at sites of fatty streaks in their study involving hypercholesterolemic non-human primates, about 5 months after initiation of the relevant diet, in areas where the endothelium had lifted from the underlying mass of foam cells. They suggested that platelets may contribute to the subsequent smooth muscle proliferation in this model.

MONOCYTES AND MACROPHAGES

Of the cells visible in atherosclerotic lesions, those which have attracted particular attention are the foam cells. Early investigators generally held that those arose from resident cells, such as endothelial or smooth muscle cells. However, in 1933 Anitschkow (2) described monocytes and foam cells in aortic lesions of rabbits, as well as cells with microscopic features interpreted as intermediate between the two. He concluded that foam cells could develop from small monocytes and stated that monocytes seemed to invade the aortic wall directly from the lumen. Later, it was acknowledged that the foam cells of human atherosclerotic lesions could be macrophages (40), and early electron microscopic surveys illustrated leukocytes adherent to the endothelium and in the intima in both experimental and human atherosclerosis (135, 136). Confirmation of the importance of the macrophage foam cell followed careful morphologic studies in animals such as those of Gerrity and Associates (52–54). Using Yorkshire pigs subjected to high lipid diets, he demonstrated monocytes adherent to the luminal endothelium, migrating between endothelial cells, and forming macrophage foam cells in atherosclerotic lesions. Likewise, experiments on rabbits (151), rats (82), pigeons (88), and monkeys (44) have shown that one of the earliest events in experimental atherosclerosis, induced by hypercholesterolemia, is increased adhesion of monocytes to what appears to be intact arterial endothelium, a phenomenon which can be well-demonstrated using scanning electron microscopy. In a study on pigtail monkeys, Faggiotto, Ross and Harker (44) showed that within 12 days of a high fat, high cholesterol diet, groups of monocytes attached to the surface of the arterial endothelium, often in junctional areas between endothelial cells. It is inferred that these monocytes then migrated subendothelially where they accumulated lipid and transformed into foam cells. The general pattern in various animal models seems to be that all or most foam cells in the early experimental lesions are macrophages by morphologic, immunohistochemical, or other criteria; smooth muscle-derived foam cells are a relatively minor or late feature.

Recent work indicates that fatty streak foam cells in humans are also predominantly macrophages (3, 143), suggesting a cellular sequence of events similar to that found in animal studies. Using immunohistochemical techniques on carotid plaques, it has been shown that 40 to 70% of the cells may be leukocytes, depending on the precise area within the lesion (79). Most of these are macrophages, although not necessarily foam cells. In a recent study using both macrophage and smooth muscle markers, Gown, Tsukada, and Ross (63) found that macrophages were numerically dominant in fibro-fatty lesions. In fibrous plaques, smooth muscle cells predominated, though variable numbers of macrophages were present. "Advanced" plaques (which may have undergone complications) were most heterogeneous, but still contained macrophages. It should be noted that in association with both fatty streaks and advanced atherosclerosis, there may be an inflammatory infiltrate in the adventitia (84, 125, 137).

The possible mechanisms of increased monocyte adhesion to endothelium in hypercholesterolemia are just beginning to be examined. Rogers *et al.* (114) found that macrophages from hypercholesterolemic rats show increased adhesion to cultured endothelial cells. Alderson *et al.* (1) showed that exposure of cultured bovine aortic endothelial cells to certain human low density lipoproteins (LDLs), β-very low density lipoprotein (β-VLDL) from cholesterol-fed rabbits, or VLDL from cholesterol/saturated fat-fed monkeys increased the subsequent adherence of monocytes (1, 41). The increased adhesion in these studies was modest and the mechanisms involved were not examined.

Recent studies have also shown that a variety of non-lipid factors can induce increased adhesion of leukocytes to endothelium *in vitro* by acting primarily on leukocytes (*e.g.*, complement components), primarily on endothelial cells (*e.g.*, IL-1) or on both cell types (*e.g.*, TNF) (16, 69). Adhesion molecules on leukocytes (*e.g.*, the CD 11/18 antigen complex) (123, 148) and endothelium (*e.g.*, endothelial-leukocyte adhesion molecule, E-LAM 1) (14) are involved in these interactions. Whether these mechanisms have a role in the monocyte adhesion consequent to hypercholesterolemia deserves to be investigated.

Once monocytes have adhered to arterial endothelium, what is the stimulus for them to emigrate into the intima? Electron microscopic studies in experimental animals clearly show that monocytes pass between endothelial cells. Frequently, in association with monocyte emigration, there is focal increased permeability to macromolecules (52). The factors that favor leukocyte emigration into the arterial wall in atherosclerosis are starting to be examined. Mazzone, Jensen and Chait (95) reported factors derived from cultured smooth muscle cells which were chemotactic for monocytes *in vitro.* Gerrity showed that extracts from plaque-prone areas (of hypercholesterolemic swine aorta) contained at least one monocyte chemotactic factor which was active only against monocytes from hypercholesterolemic animals. Others have published several related reports, including data on chemotactic substance production by cultured endothelial cells (11, 37, 110, 142). These factors have not as yet been well-characterized. After monocyte emigration into the intima has occurred, a variety of macrophage-derived factors may be involved in the recruitment of additional monocytes into the lesions (see below). It can thus be seen that many of the mechanisms in atherosclerosis, such as leukocyte adhesion and emigration, and increased endothelial permeability, are similar to or even identical with those which occur in inflammation. A key question concerns the precise mechanistic relationship between ambient lipids and these cellular events *in vivo.*

The mechanisms of foam cell formation by macrophages have been investigated in numerous studies. In early studies, Brown, Goldstein and their associates incubated macrophages with high concentrations of LDL, but were not able to convert them into foam cells, presumably because the resident peritoneal macrophages they used had few or no functional receptors for native (*i.e.*, unmodified) LDL (19). Other monocyte/macrophage sources are, however, known to have LDL receptors, but nevertheless foam cells do not form when such cells are incubated with native LDL alone. However, if the LDL is modified by acetylation, acetoacetylation, or conjugation with malondialdehyde, it is taken up rapidly and actively by macrophages which readily become foam cells in culture. These chemically-modified forms can be internalized because of the presence on the surface of macrophages of a specific receptor, termed the acetyl-LDL or scavenger receptor. It must be said, however, that despite the ease by which foam cells can be produced using the above modified LDL's *in vitro*, there is to date no evidence that these LDL forms are present *in vivo*; it is nevertheless *theoretically* possible that malondialdehyde is produced during platelet aggregation in amounts sufficient to achieve appreciable local concentrations of malondialdehyde-modified LDL (48). Another modification of LDL that leads to its uptake by macrophages occurs after incubation of LDL with cultured endothelial cells (74). This uptake also occurs by way of the acetyl-LDL receptor and is saturable, as is the case for any receptor-mediated uptake. The endothelial cell effect is now known to be due to peroxidation of the LDL, and is dependent on the presence of metal ions in the culture medium. Smooth muscle cells and macrophages are also capable of modifying LDL in a similar manner, *i.e.*, by peroxidation (111). In the presence of high metal ion concentrations, direct chemical oxidation of LDL may lead to its uptake by macrophages. Not only could oxidized LDL be taken up by macrophages, but it has additionally been shown by Steinberg and his colleagues that these products are chemotactic for human monocytes (111). Some supportive evidence for the potential *in vivo* importance of oxidized LDL is provided by a study showing reduced arterial lesion formation in atherosclerosis-prone rabbits treated with the antioxidant drug probucol (83). Perhaps the most important mechanism of foam cell formation occurs via the β-VLDL receptor (currently considered to be genetically distinct from the LDL receptor). It has been shown that β-VLDL from animals fed cholesterol and VLDL from hypertriglyceridemic humans bind to the β-VLDL receptor, resulting in internalization, hydrolysis, and re-esterification of cholesterol, and its storage in lipid droplets, thus producing the foam cell (57).

Given that macrophages are present in the atheromatous plaque, what role do they play in the initiation or evolution of lesions? In view of the large number of secretory products and biologic activities of macrophages (104), a great number of functions can be ascribed to them in plaques, but these would be no different from their activities in other inflammatory processes. Of possible specific relevance in atherosclerosis, however, are the following observations. As previously noted, IL-1 and TNF, both produced by activated macrophages, are capable of inducing a molecule on endothelial cells which increases leukocyte adhesion, including the adhesion of monocytes (15, 107). Leukotriene B_4, complement fragment C5a, transforming growth factor-β (5, 146), IL-1 (90a), TNF (149), granulocyte-macrophage colony stimulating factor (150) and PDGF (38) are examples of macrophage products that are chemotactic for leukocytes. These two activities, inducing increased endothelial adhesiveness and leukocyte chemotaxis, may form an amplification mechanism for the recruitment of further leukocytes into the atheromatous plaque. Macrophages may produce toxic substances, such as reduced oxygen species and proteases. The production of these is enhanced by modified LDL (70, 71). They may injure neighboring mesenchymal cells and connective tissue (153), and may alter LDL in a way that allows foam cell formation (105). Oxygen metabolites may also cause endothelial injury and indeed, in the studies of Faggiotto and Ross (44) in pigtail monkeys, endothelial denudation was described in the vicinity of large foam-laden macrophages, about 5 months after the induction of hypercholesterolemia. This denudation has, however, not generally been identified in other animal models (82). Oxidized LDL not only can be taken up by macrophages as stated, but along with native LDL may have cytotoxic effects on cultured smooth muscle cells, fibroblasts, and endothelial cells (25, 73, 75). Thus reduced oxygen species, oxidized LDL, or proteases could be responsible for the central necrosis which regularly occurs in large atheromatous plaques. Along with platelets, macrophages can produce 12-hydroxyeicosatetraenoic acid, an eicosanoid which is chemokinetic for smooth muscle cells (103). The formation of this compound is increased when macrophages are incubated with acetyl-LDL (94). Macrophages secrete factors that induce the proliferation of fibroblasts, smooth muscle cells, and endothelium (60, 87, 93). Recent studies suggest that the principal fibroblast and smooth muscle cell growth activity in macrophages is PDGF-like, the PDGF is additionally chemotactic for smooth muscle cells (64) (see below). Macrophages or activated macrophages also secrete IL-1, which is a mitogen for fibroblasts, fibroblast growth factor (FGF), (17), which is also a mitogen for vascular endothelial cells; TGF-α (91), which causes endothelial and fibroblast proliferation, and angiogenesis factors, which may induce the neovascularization characteristic of plaques (108). The angiogenic effect may be mediated by TNF (49, 87a) or FGF. There is some evidence that the TNF gene is expressed by cells of atherosclerotic lesions (7a). Macrophages may also produce potential growth inhibitory or modulatory substances, such as prostaglandin E_2, interferon-α, and TGF-β (5, 6, 104). Macrophages may stimulate matrix production by smooth muscle cells, for example via TGF-β production (5, 26). Finally, it has been suggested that macrophages may have a role in the apparent regression of atheromatous plaques which can occur experimentally. Studies have shown that compared to lipid-fed control animals, those earlier maintained on high lipid diets and then switched to low lipid diets have a decreased amount of stainable lipid in their arteries (92, 121). The work of Daoud *et al.* (32) has demonstrated abundant macrophages in such regressing lesions, and it is at least theoretically possible that macrophages could ferry lipid out of the intima. Indeed, Gerrity (54) and Faggiotto and Ross (44) interpreted some of their electron micrographs in hypercholesterolemic animals as showing macrophage foam cells in the process of returning to the arterial lumen. Whether this form of *regression* occurs to an important degree in human atherosclerosis is controversial.

Lymphocytes and Their Interactions

Although it has long been known that perivascular lymphocyte infiltrates are often seen in the adventitia of arteries with atherosclerosis (84, 125, 137), recent immunocytochemical studies show that T cells are also present in both early and advanced intimal lesions. Jonasson *et al.* (79) studied internal carotid arteries removed at surgery with a panel of monoclonal antibodies in order to identify various cell types. They found that, in addition to macrophages being present in plaques, about 20% of the cell population in the fibrous cap expressed the T3 (CD3) antigen, indicating that they were T lymphocytes. T cells were also isolated from the plaques and detected by a rosetting assay; many of the T cells were activated as indicated by the expression of HLA-DR (80). Recently T lymphocytes have also been found in early lesions of atherosclerosis, in the form of fatty streaks (101). T cells in lesions, together with activated macrophages, could conceivably represent a cell-mediated, delayed type hypersensitivity form of immune response, and the question arises as to whether the lymphocytes present in atherosclerotic lesions recognize or are directed against specific antigens in the arterial wall. One study demonstrated that lymphocytes of patients with atherosclerotic disease were capable of recognizing an antigen contained within human arterial wall, as indicated by a migration inhibition assay (90). HLA-DR expression has been demonstrated on smooth muscle cells (80) in atheromatous plaques but not in uninvolved artery, and there is some evidence that class II antigen expression by smooth muscle cells is an important event in the pathogenesis of an experimental model of auto-immune vasculitis involving lymphocytes (100). While the relevance of these phenomena to atherogenesis is unclear, the role of a local immune reaction in atherosclerosis deserves further study.

MECHANISMS OF SMOOTH MUSCLE PROLIFERATION

Inflammation outside of arteries is often characterized by proliferation of fibroblasts, which then deposit collagen and other substances. In the arterial intima, it is the smooth muscle cell which serves this role. Smooth muscle proliferation is a critical event in the development of an atheromatous plaque. Smooth muscle cells are present in fatty streaks, although they are overshadowed by macrophage-derived foam cells; in the fibrous cap of the well-developed fibro-fatty plaque they appear to be the predominant cell type. It is evident that the smooth muscle cells synthesize the bulk of the connective tissue matrix, including collagen, elastic tissue, and the proteoglycans (85, 102, 154). In addition, they can accumulate lipid and become foam cells.

Experimental studies after balloon endothelial denudation indicate that the source of intimal smooth muscle cells is the media. There is very early replication of smooth muscle cells within the media, followed by migration into the intima and further replication (28, 152). The same sequence of events probably occurs in humans, although there is no *a priori* reason why the early proliferation may not be in the cells of diffuse intimal thickening (see above), and indeed, in swine there is some evidence that myointimal cells may be a source of the proliferating smooth muscle cells within plaques (140).

One of the most important issues in atherosclerosis is the determination of the kinds of biochemical signals which underlie smooth muscle proliferation. PDGF (120), the first postulated growth factor in atherogenesis, remains one of the most likely candidates as it is produced by most cell types involved in lesions-platelets, macrophages, endothelial and smooth muscle cells—and because it can induce both smooth muscle migration and proliferation (64, 116). PDGF is thought to be involved in inflammation in various sites, and its actions are not confined to growth control (120, 132). It is a highly cationic protein composed of two chains (A and B) with molecular weights of approximately 17,000 daltons. It is present in the α granules of platelets and megakaryocytes and is released after platelet aggregation in combination with platelet factor 4 and β-thromboglobulin. PDGF binds to smooth muscle cells and other mesenchymal cells (but not to most endothelia) via-high-affinity receptors, resulting in a multitude of biologic events, in addition to the induction of migration and proliferation. For example, PDGF causes increased endocytosis, cholesterol synthesis, and LDL receptor expression in mesenchymal cells (35), and is also a potent vasoconstrictive agent (10).

PDGF, or PDGF-like molecules, are now known to be secreted by a number of different cell types, including tumor cells. The presence of PDGF mRNA in human artery has been reported as preliminary data (7, 7a). Of particular relevance to atherosclerosis is the secretion of PDGF by macrophages (128) and endothelial cells (39). Macrophages from a variety of sites have been known to secrete factors that stimulate the proliferation of fibroblasts, smooth muscle cells, and endothelium (60, 87, 93). Production of these factors is enhanced by activation of macrophages with lipopolysaccharide, immune complexes, and other substances. It has recently been shown that a significant proportion of this growth promoting activity is similar, if not identical, to PDGF, based on competitive binding to the same receptor, the ability to be recognized by anti-PDGF antibody, and by Northern blot analysis of mRNA (128). Endothelial cells in culture also produce a PDGF-like molecule, whose release is stimulated by endotoxin, phorbol esters, and TNF (65). Both the A and B chain of PDGF are synthesized by cultured endothelial cells (29, 30). Although *in vivo* intact arteries generally have very low levels of mRNA for PDGF, it could be that synthesis and release can be induced *in vivo* by certain stimuli, with consequent induction of smooth muscle proliferation. Thus, it is at least theoretically possible that some component of hypercholesterolemic serum may trigger secretion of PDGF by intact endothelium, accounting for the initiation of smooth muscle proliferation under these circumstances.

Smooth muscle cells also secrete a growth factor that is PDGF-like (127). Whereas aortic smooth muscle cells from adult rats have receptors for PDGF, they do not secrete it, while similar smooth muscle cells from newborn rats secrete a PDGF-like molecule, but lack PDGF receptors. Atherosclerotic lesions of rats have the same characteristics as smooth muscle from newborn rats, that is they secrete PDGF, and have decreased numbers of receptors compared to uninjured smooth muscle (147). Such findings suggest that regulation of PDGF expression by the smooth muscle cells themselves may be a determinant of their proliferative state, and may be involved in the intimal cellular proliferation which follows endothelial injury.

There are other potential smooth muscle growth factors, apparently distinct from PDGF, which are produced by endothelium, smooth muscle and macrophages, but these have not been well-characterized (33, 67). TGF-β can be produced by endothelium and macrophages, and is present in platelets; it has been reported to cause growth inhibition of subconfluent smooth muscle cells and proliferation of such cells in agar (6). Hyperlipidemic serum has been reported to cause smooth muscle proliferation in culture (46). Smooth muscle proliferation could, on the other hand, be theoretically ascribed to the loss of an inhibitory molecule present in the vascular wall. Such molecules have been described, including heparin-like molecules secreted by endothelial cells (22, 24), and by smooth muscle cells (51). An endoglycosidase enzyme which can liberate the growth inhibitory activity is present in platelets and is also available within the vessel wall (23, 115).

One further concept relating to smooth muscle proliferation in atherosclerosis merits attention. This is the monoclonal hypothesis of Benditt and Benditt (9). The background to their experimental data is that certain individuals are heterozygous for a particular enzyme, specifically glucose-6-phosphate dehydrogenase, in that they possess both A and B isoenzymes. Since glucose-6-phosphate dehydrogenase is X-linked, roughly half the cells of a female heterozygote will contain only isoenzyme A and the other half only isoenzyme B. Thus, if a tumor develops in one of these subjects, and originates from a single cell, the entire tumor should contain either isoenzyme A or B only (*i.e.*, the tumor can be seen to be monoclonal in origin). Benditt and Benditt (9) found that some atherosclerotic plaques of heterozygotes contained only one of the isoenzymes, which was interpreted as indicating a monoclonal proliferation of smooth muscle cells. Atherosclerosis could thus be viewed as a phenomenon similar to a benign neoplastic process, one implication being that a mutation may have been induced in the original cells by an as yet unknown agent. The monoclonal hypothesis has been questioned on the basis of later studies showing less clearcut results and on theoretical grounds, principally that monoclonality or oligoclonality could develop as a consequence of the selection of a subpopulation of cells during the course of lesion development (45, 141).

Several pieces of evidence, however, are consistent with Benditt's concepts. Benditt's group has shown herpes virus mRNA by *in situ* hybridization in cells of human atheromatous lesions (8). Focal fibromuscular plaques have been induced in the abdominal aorta of cockerels by repeated injections of the carcinogen dimethylbenz[a]-anthracene and benzo[a]pyrene. Dimethylbenz[a]-anthracene and methoxamine administered to chickens in an initiation-promotion protocol also induce small focal mounds of cells in the thoracic aorta (91a). Repeated injections of the oncogenic Marek's disease virus in cockerels results in microscopic plaques in the thoracic aorta not found in controls (42). And finally, transforming genes have been extracted from DNA samples of human coronary artery plaques (106). While all of these findings do not make a case for Benditt's original hypothesis, they do open the question of autonomous smooth muscle proliferation as an event in some forms of atherosclerosis.

In summary, there is no dearth of mechanisms to account for smooth muscle proliferation in the vessel wall in atherosclerosis. In the case of denuding endothelial injury, as can be induced experimentally, or clearly occurs in humans at peri-anastomotic areas of vascular grafts, platelets and macrophages can release PDGF and potentially other growth factors. In non-denuding injury, factors from adherent macrophages (which occur in hypercholesterolemia), or possibly endothelial cells, may cause smooth muscle proliferation. It must be admitted, however, that it is difficult to be certain of mechanisms which are relevant *in vivo*. Pharmacologic agents which inhibit platelet adhesion or platelet function, and antiplatelet antibodies, have been shown to inhibit the acute smooth muscle proliferation which occurs after endothelial denudation (50, 68), but these agents have other confounding effects. To date it has not been possible to suppress proliferation with anti-PDGF antisera. Clowes and Karnovsky (27) have been able to suppress the acute proliferative response after air-induced endothelial injury with heparin, including non-anticoagulant heparin, suggesting that growth regulation by the endothelial and smooth muscle heparin-like molecules may play a role *in vivo*.

RISK FACTORS AND LIPIDS IN ATHEROGENESIS

Despite our increased understanding of the basic lesions of atherosclerosis, and the cellular events that lead to lesion development, the precise mechanisms by which the various risk factors initiate or contribute to atherogenesis are unclear. It is likely that the important risk factors—hyperlipidemia, hypertension, and smoking (109), affect more than one step in atherogenesis, including the function of any of the cell types involved and the constituents of the plasma which interact with the vessel wall. Smoking, for example, or some component of cigarette smoke, has effects on platelets and platelet function, plasma lipoprotein levels, macrophage responses, and hemodynamic regulation and has been claimed to cause endothelial injury (66, 72, 78, 129). As well as causing an increased extent of atherosclerosis (138), smoking may accelerate the progression of individual lesions. A variety of endothelial abnormalities has been described in hypertensive animals and some of these may be important determinants in atherogenesis. Hypertension could cause mechanical injury, or conceivably an alteration of metabolic function of endothelial or other arterial cells. Hemodynamic factors (59), leading to endothelial and platelet events, almost certainly contribute to the iatrogenic atherosclerosis occurring in venous grafts used in coronary bypass surgery. Endothelial injury and dysfunction have also been shown to occur in experimental animals subjected to manipulations that are associated with increased risk of atherosclerosis, such as diabetes mellitus and stressful stimulation (62).

The clinical, epidemiologic, and experimental evidence linking hyperlipidemia to atherogenesis is well-established (134) and will not be reviewed. A number of mechanisms have been postulated, on theoretical grounds and from experimental studies, to account for the role of lipids in lesion formation. Most of these link LDL and β-VLDL to atherogenesis. LDL is the major carrier of cholesterol in plasma and is the molecule which is most tightly linked to the risk of coronary heart disease in epidemiological studies (20, 89); β-VLDL is a β fraction derived from chylomicrons and VLDL, but which contains more cholesterol than VLDL and has a β rather than a pre-β mobility on electrophoresis.

In the first place, increases in plasma levels of LDL or other lipids may *increase the rate of their penetration* into the artery wall and its subsequent uptake and degradation by vascular smooth muscle cells and infiltrating macrophages (18, 130, 131). The local conditions in the intima exposed to increased LDL concentrations may cause the cellular accumulation of cholesterol esters and the formation of foam cells. It has been shown for example, that LDL complexes to intimal proteoglycans and that such proleoglycan-LDL complexes are taken up by macrophages with the resulting formation of foam cells (122, 144). Modification of LDL, perhaps by high concentrations of malondialdehyde (48), or by oxidation (105) also promote foam cell formation. Secondly, there is both *in vivo* and *in vitro* evidence that certain lipoproteins may affect endothelial cells directly, without causing denudation. Foci of increased permeability (52, 55a), increased replication (47), altered anionic sites (56, 88), and increased monocyte adhesion (see above) have been shown in experimental hypercholesterolemia. *In vitro*, increased monocyte adhesion appears to be, at least in part, an endothelial-dependent effect (1, 41). Monocyte adhesion itself is associated with foci of increased permeability *in vivo*, and it has been shown that monocyte migration leads to increased LDL transport across aortic endothelial cell monolayers in culture (139). LDL causes endothelial injury *in vitro* (73, 75). It has also been postulated that chronically elevated levels of LDL may increase the number of cholesterol molecules in the plasma membranes of cells, including endothelial cells, affecting endothelial cell malleability and causing endothelial cell retraction (76). Thirdly, lipoproteins may have direct effects on smooth muscle. LDL can clearly cause smooth muscle injury (75). Fisher-Dzoga, Frazer, and Wissler (46) have reported that smooth muscle cell proliferation is stimulated by components of hyperlipidemic serum. Platelet aggregation, with subsequent re-

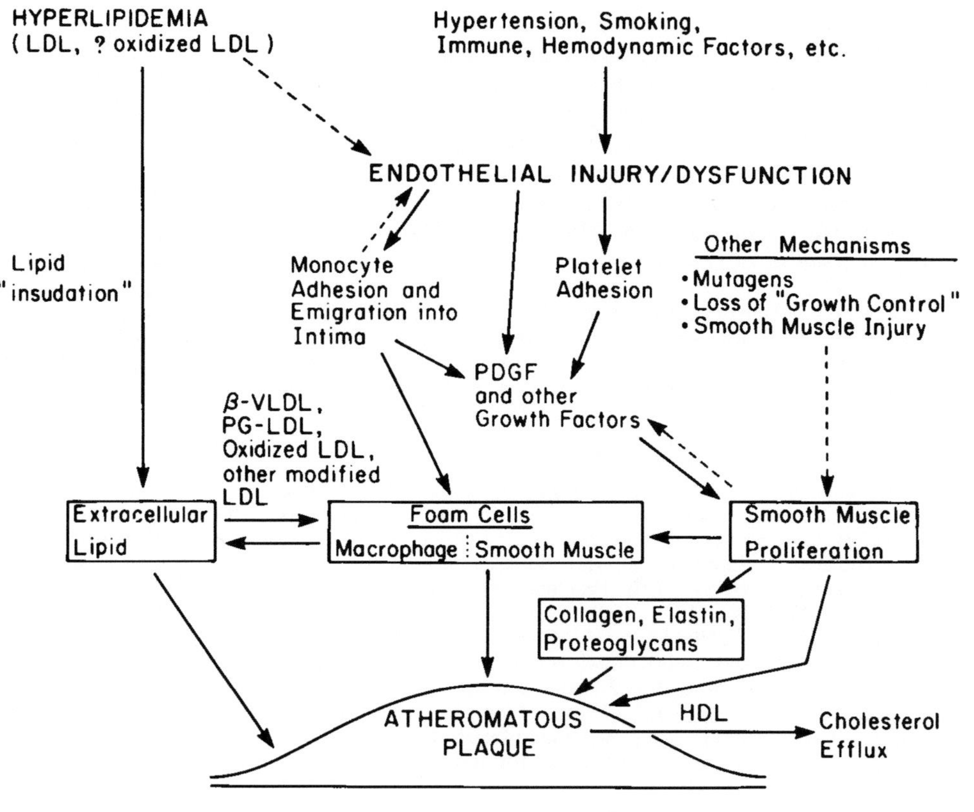

FIG. 2. Schematic diagram of a hypothetical sequence of events and cellular interactions in atherogenesis (PG-LDL, proteoglycan-low density lipoprotein; HDL, high density lipoprotein, see text). From Cotran R. S., and Munro J. M.: Pathogenesis of atherosclerosis: recent concepts. In Grundy S. M. amd Bearn A. G. (eds.) The role of cholesterol in atherosclerosis: New therapeutic opportunites. Philadelphia, Hanley and Belfus, 1988, p. 5).

lease of PDGF and smooth muscle replication, is favored by higher LDL levels (21). Finally, cellularly modified LDL causes monocyte recruitment by chemotactic mechanisms, inhibition of macrophage motility, and the formation of foam cells (110, 111).

SUMMARY AND CONCLUSIONS

Current concepts of the pathogenesis of atherosclerosis have been reviewed, emphasizing some of the similarities of the mechanisms and events involved to those in inflammation. Figure 2 is a schematic summary of these events. Hyperlipidemia, or some component of hyperlipidemic serum, as well as other risk factors, are thought to cause endothelial injury, resulting in adhesion of platelets and/or monocytes and release of PDGF (and other growth factors), which leads to smooth muscle migration and proliferation. It is clear that endothelial injury need not be denuding, and in fact may consist of altered endothelial function (dysfunction); adhesion of monocytes, increased permeability of endothelium, and disturbances in growth control can occur without morphologically obvious endothelial injury. Hyperlipidemia, hypertension, smoking, immune injury, and other risk factors may contribute to this endothelial dysfunction in different ways and sometimes in combination. Smooth muscle cells produce large amounts of collagen, elastin, and proteoglycans and these form part of the atheromatous plaque. Hyperlipidemia contributes in a number of ways (as discussed earlier), and indeed, in the severely hypercholesterolemic patient, such as one with familial hypercholesterolemia, is alone sufficient to cause atherosclerosis in the absence of other risk factors. Foam cells of atheromatous plaques are derived both from macrophages and from smooth muscle cells; from macrophages via the β-VLDL receptor and also possibly by way of LDL modification, recognized by the acetyl-LDL receptor (such as oxidized LDL); and from smooth muscle cells by less certain mechanisms. Extracellular lipid is derived from insudation from the lumen, particularly in the presence of hypercholesterolemia, and also from degenerating foam cells. Cholesterol accumulation in the plaque should be viewed as reflecting imbalance between influx and efflux, and it is possible that high-density lipoprotein is the molecule which helps clear the cholesterol from these accumulations (134). The diagram (*right*) also depicts the possibility that smooth muscle proliferation may occur without endothelial injury at all. There are several postulated mechanisms for such an occurrence: loss of growth control, direct smooth muscle injury (such as by LDL), and autonomous proliferation by the mechanisms suggested by Benditt.

The theoretical scheme presented is based largely on *in vitro* work, only partly substantiated by experimental and human studies, and does not explain the precise mechanisms by which all risk factors increase the susceptibility to atherosclerosis. However, the similarities of the cellular interactions in lesion formation to those in inflammation have important implications for future study of atherosclerosis, and potentially for its prevention and therapy.

Acknowledgments: The authors would like to thank Dr. Peter F. Davies for helpful criticism of the manuscript, and Ms. Julie Smith for assistance in its preparation.

Excerpts from this review appear in Cotran R. S. and Munro J. M.: Pathogenesis of atherosclerosis: Recent concepts. In Grundy S. M. and Bearn A. G. (eds). The role of cholesterol in atherosclerosis: New therapeutic opportunities. Philadelphia, Hanley and Belfus, 1988, with permission of the publisher.

This work was supported by Grant #HL 22602 from the National Heart, Lung, and Blood Institute, and NIH Training Grant #5T32 HL07627-03.

Address reprint requests to: Ramzi S. Cotran, M.D., Department of Pathology, Brigham and Women's Hospital, 75 Francis Street, Boston, MA 02115.

REFERENCES

1. Alderson LM, Endemann G, Lindsey S, Pronczuk A, Hoover RL, Hayes KC: LDL enhances monocyte adhesion to endothelial cells *in vitro*. Am J Pathol 123:334, 1986
2. Anitschkow N: Experimental arteriosclerosis in animals. In Arteriosclerosis: A Survey of the Problem, edited by Cowdry EV, p. 271. New York, MacMillan, 1933
3. Aqel NM, Ball RY, Waldmann H, Mitchinson MJ: Identification of macrophages and smooth muscle cells in human atherosclerosis using monoclonal antibodies. J Pathol 146:197, 1985
4. Arteriosclerosis: Report of the Working Group on Arteriosclerosis of the National Heart, Lung, and Blood Institute: Vol. 2, Washington, D.C., U.S. Department of Health and Human Services, Washington, D.C., 1981
5. Assoian RK, Fleurdelys BE, Stevenson HC, Miller PJ, Madtes DK, Raines EW, Ross R, Sporn MB: Expression and secretion of type β transforming growth factor by activated human macrophages. Proc Natl Acad Sci USA 84:6020, 1987
6. Assoian RK, Sporn MB: Transforming growth factor-beta acts on aortic smooth muscle cells. In Atherosclerosis VII, edited by Fidge NH, Nestel PJ, p. 459. Amsterdam, Excerpta Medica, 1986
7. Barrett TB, Benditt EP: *Sis* (PDGF-β chain) gene transcript levels are elevated in human atherosclerotic lesions compared to normal artery. Proc Natl Acad Sci USA 84:1099, 1987

7a. Barrett TB, Benditt EP: Expression of growth factors and other genes in atherosclerotic plaques and in normal artery, (abstr). J Mol Cell Cardiol 19 (suppl IV):S.3, 1987

8. Benditt EP, Barrett T, McDougall JK: Viruses in the etiology of atherosclerosis. Proc Natl Acad Sci USA 80:6386, 1983
9. Benditt EP, Benditt JM: Evidence for a monoclonal origin of human atherosclerotic plaques. Proc Natl Acad Sci (USA) 70:1753, 1973
10. Berk BC, Alexander RW, Brock T, Gimbrone MA Jr, Webb CR: Vasoconstriction: a new activity for platelet-derived growth factor. Science 232:87, 1986
11. Berliner JA, Territo M, Almada L, Carter A, Shafonsky E, Fogelman AM: Monocyte chemotactic factor produced by large vessel endothelial cells *in vitro*. Arteriosclerosis 6:254, 1986
12. Bevilacqua MP, Pober JS, Majeau GR, Cotran RS, Gimbrone MA Jr: Interleukin 1 (IL-1) induces biosynthesis and cell surface expression of procoagulant activity in human vascular endothelial cells. J Exp Med 160:618, 1984
13. Bevilacqua MP, Pober JS, Majeau GR, Fiers W, Cotran RS, Gimbrone MA Jr: Recombinant tumor necrosis factor induces procoagulant activity in cultured human vascular endothelium: Characterization and comparison with the actions of interleukin 1. Proc Natl Acad Sci USA 83:4533, 1986
14. Bevilacqua MP, Pober JS, Mendrick DL, Cotran RS, Gimbrone MA, Jr: Identification of an inducible endothelial-leukocyte adhesion molecule, E-LAM 1. Proc Natl Acad Sci USA 84:9238, 1987
15. Bevilacqua MP, Pober JS, Wheeler ME, Cotran RS, Gimbrone MA Jr: Interleukin-1 activation of vascular endothelium: Effects on procoagulant activity and leukocyte adhesion. Am J Pathol 121:394, 1985
16. Bevilacqua MP, Pober JS, Wheeler ME, Cotran RS, Gimbrone MA Jr: Interleukin 1 acts on cultured human vascular endothelium to increase the adhesion of polymorphonuclear leukocytes, monocytes, and related leukocyte cell lines. J Clin Invest 76:2003, 1985
17. Bitterman PB, Wewers MD, Rennard SI, Adelberg S, Crystal RG: Modulation of alveolar macrophage-driven fibroblast proliferation by alternative macrophage mediators. J Clin Invest 77:700, 1986
18. Bremmelgaard A, Stender S, Lorentzen J, Kjeldsen K: *In vivo* flux of plasma cholesterol into human abdominal aorta with advanced therosclerosis. Arteriosclerosis 6:442, 1986
19. Brown MS, Goldstein JL: Lipoprotein metabolism in the macrophage: implications for cholesterol deposition in atherosclerosis. Annu Rev Biochem 52:223, 1983
20. Carlson LA, Ericsson M: Quantitative and qualitative serum lipoprotein analysis. Part 2. Studies in male survivors of myocardial infarction. Atherosclerosis 21:435, 1975
21. Carvalho ACA, Colman RW, Lees RS: Platelet function in hyperlipoproteinemia. N Engl J Med 290:434, 1974
22. Castellot JJ Jr, Addonizio ML, Rosenberg R, Karnovsky MJ: Cultured endothelial cells produce a heparin-like inhibitor of smooth muscle cell growth. J Cell Biol 90:372, 1981
23. Castellot JJ Jr, Favreau LV, Karnovsky MJ, Rosenberg RD: Inhibition of vascular smooth muscle cell growth by endothelial cell-derived heparin. J Biol Chem 257:11256, 1982
24. Castellot JJ Jr, Rosenberg RD, Karnovsky MJ: Endothelium, heparin and the regulation of vascular smooth muscle cell growth. In Biology of Endothelial Cells, edited by Jaffe E, p 118. Boston, Martinus Nijhoff Publishers, 1974
25. Cathcart MK, Morel DW, Chisolm GM III: Monocytes and neutrophils oxidize low density lipoprotein making it cytotoxic. J Leukocyte Biol 38;341, 1985
26. Chen J-K, Hoshi H, McKeehan WL: Transforming growth factor type β specifically stimulates synthesis of proteoglycan in human adult arterial smooth muscle cells. Proc Natl Acad Sci USA 84:5287, 1987
27. Clowes AW, Karnovsky MJ: Suppression by heparin of smooth muscle cell proliferation in injured arteries. Nature 265:625, 1977
28. Clowes AW, Schwartz SM: Significance of quiescent smooth muscle migration in the injured rat carotid artery. Circ Res 56:139, 1985
29. Collins T, Ginsburg D, Boss JM, Orkin SH, Pober JS: Cultured human endothelial cells express platelet-derived growth factor B chain: cDNA cloning and structural analysis. Nature 316:748, 1985
30. Collins T, Pober JS, Gimbrone MA Jr, Hammacher A, Betsholtz C, Westermark B, Heldin C-H: Cultured human endothelial cells express platelet-derived growth factor A chain. Am J Pathol 127:7, 1987
31. Cotran RS: The endothelium and inflammation: new insights. In Inflammation and infection, edited by Majno G, Cotran RS, p. 18. Baltimore, Williams & Wilkins, 1982
32. Daoud AS, Jarmolych J, Augustyn JM, Fritz KE: Sequential morphologic studies of regression of advanced atherosclerosis. Arch Pathol Lab Med 105:233, 1981
33. Davies PF: Vascular cell interactions with special reference to the pathogenesis of atherosclerosis. Lab Invest 55:5, 1986
34. Davies PF, Dewey CF Jr, Bussolari SR, Gordon EJ, Gimbrone MA Jr: Influence of hemodynamic forces on vascular endothelial function: *in vitro* studies of shear stress and pinocytosis in bovine aortic cells. J Clin Invest 73:1121, 1984.
35. Davies, PF, Reidy MA, Goode TB, Bowyer DG: Scanning electron microscopy in the evaluation of endothelial integrity of the fatty lesion in atherosclerosis. Atherosclerosis 25:125, 1976
36. Davies PF, Remuzzi A, Gordon EJ, Dewey CF Jr, Gimbrone MA Jr: Turbulent fluid shear stress induces vascular endothelial cell turnover *in vitro*. Proc Natl Acad Sci USA 83:2114, 1986
37. Denholm EM, Lewis JC: Moncocyte chemoattractants in pigeon aortic atherosclerosis. Am J Pathol 126:464, 1987
38. Deuel TF, Senior RM, Huang JS, Griffin GL: Chemotaxis of monocytes and neutrophils to platelet-derived growth factor. J Clin Invest 69:1046, 1982
39. DiCorleto PE, Bowen-Pope DF: Cultured endothelial cells produce a platelet-derived growth factor-like protein. Proc Natl Acad Sci USA 80;1919, 1983
40. Duff GL, McMillan GC: Pathology of atherosclerosis. Am J Med 11:92, 1951
41. Endemann G, Pronzcuk A, Friedman G, Lindsey S, Alderson L, Hayes KC: Monocyte adherence to endothelial cells *in vitro* is increased by β-VLDL. Am J Pathol 126:1, 1987
42. Fabricant CG: Atherosclerosis: The consequence of infection with a herpes virus. Adv Vet Sci Comp Med 30:39, 1985
43. Faggiotto A, Ross R: Studies of hypercholesterolemia in the

nonhuman primate: II. Fatty streak conversion to fibrous plaque. Arteriosclerosis 4:341, 1984
44. Faggiotto A, Ross R, Harker L: Studies of hypercholesterolemia in the nonhuman primate. I. Changes that lead to fatty streak formation. Arteriosclerosis 4:323, 1984
45. Fialkow PJ: The origin and development of human tumors studied with cell markers. N Engl J Med 291:26, 1974
46. Fisher-Dzoga K, Frazer R, Wissler RW: Stimulation of proliferation in stationary primary cultures of monkey and rabbit aortic smooth muscle cells. I. Effects of lipoprotein fractions of hyperlipidemic serum and lymph. Exp Mol Pathol 24:346, 1976
47. Florentin RA, Nam SC, Daoud AS, Jones R, Scott RF, Morrison ES, Kim DN, Lee KT, Thomas WA, Dodds WJ, Miller KD: Dietary-induced atherosclerosis in miniature swine, I-V. Exp Mol Pathol 8:263, 1968
48. Fogelman AM, Schechter I, Seager J, Hokom M, Child JS, Edwards PA: Malondialdehyde alteration of low density lipoproteins leads to cholesteryl ester accumulation in human monocyte-macrophages. Proc Natl Acad Sci USA 77:2214, 1980
49. Frater-Schroder M, Risau W, Hallmann R, Gautschi P, Bohlen P: Tumor necrosis factor type α, a potent inhibitor of endothelial cell growth *in vitro*, is angiogenic *in vivo*. Proc Natl Acad Sci USA 84:5277, 1987
50. Friedman RJ, Stemerman MB, Wenz B, Moore S, Gauldie J, Gent M, Giell ML, Spaet TH: The effect of thrombocytopenia on experimental arteriosclerotic lesion formation in rabbits: smooth muscle cell proliferation and reendothelialization. J Clin Invest 60:1191, 1977
51. Fritze LM, Reilly CF, Rosenberg RD: An antiproliferative heparan sulfate species produced by post-confluent smooth muscle. J Cell Biol 100;1041, 1985
52. Gerrity RG, Naito HK, Richardson M, Schwartz CJ; Dietary induced atherogenesis in swine: morphology of the intima in prelesion stages. Am J Pathol 95:775, 1979
53. Gerrity RG: The role of the monocyte in atherogenesis: I. Transition of blood-borne monocytes into foam cells in fatty lesions. Am J Pathol 103:181, 1981
54. Gerrity RG: The role of the monocyte in atherogenesis: II. Migration of foam cells from atherosclerotic lesions. Am J Pathol 103:191, 1981
55. Gerrity RG, Goss JA, Soby L: Control of monocyte recruitment by chemotactic factor(s) in lesion-prone areas of swine aorta. Arteriosclerosis 5:55, 1985
55a. Gerrity RG: Vesicular transport and intimal accumulation of macromolecules in atherosclerosis-susceptible areas is augmented by hyperlipidemia (abstr) circulation (suppl) 76:IV-295, 1987
56. Ghinea N, Leabu M, Hasu M, Muresan V, Colceag J, Simionescu N: Prelesional events in atherogenesis: Changes induced by hypercholesterolemia in the cell surface chemistry of arterial endothelium and blood monocytes, in rabbit. J Submicrosc Cytol 19:209, 1987
57. Gianturco SH, Bradley WH: β-VLDL receptor pathway of macrophages. In Atherosclerosis VII, edited by Fidge NH, Nestel PG, p. 495. Amsterdam, Excerpta Medica, 1986
58. Gimbrone MA Jr: Endothelial dysfunction and the pathogenesis of atherosclerosis. In Atherosclerosis-V, Proceedings of the Vth International Symposium on Atherosclerosis, edited by Gotto A, p. 415, New York, Springer-Verlag, 1980
59. Glagov S: Hemodynamic risk factors: Mechanical stress, mural architecture, medial nutrition, and the vulnerability of arteries to atherosclerosis. In The Pathogenesis of Atherosclerosis, edited by Wissler RW, Geer JC, p. 164. Baltimore, Williams & Wilkins, 1972
60. Glenn KC, Ross R: Human monocyte-derived growth factor(s) for mesenchymal cells: Activation of secretion by endotoxin and concanavalin A. Cell 25:603, 1981
61. Goldberg ID, Stemerman MB, Handin RI: Vascular permeation of platelet factor 4 after endothelial injury. Science, 209:611, 1980
62. Gordon D, Guyton JR, Karnovsky MJ: Intimal alterations in rat aorta induced by stressful stimuli. Lab Invest 45:14, 1981
63. Gown AM, Tsukada T, Ross R: Human atherosclerosis. II. Immunocytochemical analysis of the cellular composition of human atherosclerotic lesions. Am J Pathol 125:191, 1986
64. Grotendorst FR, Seppa HEJ, Martin GR: Attachment of smooth muscle cells to collagen and their migration toward platelet-derived growth factor. Proc Natl Acad Sci (USA) 78:3669, 1982
65. Hajjar KA, Hajjar DP, Silverstein RL, Nachman RL: Tumor necrosis factor-mediated release of platelet-derived growth factor from cultured endothelial cells. J Exp Med 166:235, 1987
66. Halfon S-T, Kark JD, Baras M, Friedlander Y, Eisenberg S: Smoking, lipids and lipoproteins in Jerusalem 17-year-olds. Israel J Med Sci 18:1150, 1982
67. Hannan R, Kourembanas S, Flanders K, Rogelj S, Roberts A, Faller D, Klagsburn M: Human endothelial cells synthesize fibro blast growth factor and transforming growth factor beta (abstr). J Mol Cell Cardiol 19 (Suppl IV):S.9, 1987
68. Harker LA, Harlan JM, Ross R: Effect of sulfinpyrazone on homocystein-induced endothelial injury and arteriosclerosis in baboons. Circ Res 53:731, 1983
69. Harlan JM: Leukocyte-endothelial interactions. Blood 65:513, 1985
70. Hartung H-P, Kladetzky RG, Hennerici M: Chemically modified low density lipoproteins as inducers of enzyme release from macrophages. FEBS Lett 186:211, 1985
71. Hartung H-P, Kladetzky RG, Melnik B, Hennerici M: Stimulation of the scavenger receptor on monocytes-macrophages evokes release of arachidonic acid metabolites and reduced oxygen species. Lab Invest 55:209, 1986
72. Hawkins RI: Smoking, platelets and thrombosis. Nature 236:450, 1972
73. Henriksen T, Evensen SA, Carlander B: Injury to human endothelial cells in culture induced by low density lipoproteins. Scand J Clin Lab Invest 39:361, 1979
74. Henriksen T, Mahoney EM, Steinberg D: Enhanced macrophage degradation of low-density lipoprotein previously incubated with cultured endothelial cells: Recognition by receptors for acetylated low-density lipoprotein. Proc Natl Acad Sci USA 78:6499, 1981
75. Hessler JR, Robertson AL Jr, Chisolm GM III: LDL-induced cytotoxicity and its inhibition by HDL in human vascular smooth muscle and endothelial cells in culture. Atherosclerosis 32:213, 1979
76. Jackson RL, Gotto AM Jr: Hypothesis concerning membrane structure, cholesterol, and atherosclerosis. In Atherosclerosis Reviews, Vol. 1, edited by Paoletti R, Gotto AM Jr, p 1. New York, Raven Press, 1976
77. Jaffe EA: Cell biology of endothelial cells. Human Pathol 18:234, 1987
78. Janoff A: Elastases and emphysema. Current assessment of the protease-antiprotease hypothesis. Am Rev Respir Dis 132:417, 1985
79. Jonasson L, Holm J, Skalli O, Bondjers G, Hansson GK: Regional accumulations of T cells, macrophages, and smooth muscle cells in the human atherosclerotic plaque. Arteriosclerosis 6:131, 1986
80. Jonasson L, Holm J, Skalli O, Gabbiani G, Hansson GK: Expression of class II transplantation antigen on vascular smooth muscle cells in human atherosclerosis. J Clin Invest 76:125, 1985
81. Joris I, Majno G: Atherosclerosis and inflammation. Adv Exp Med Biol 104:227, 1977
82. Joris I, Zand T, Nunnari JJ, Krolikowski FJ, Majno G: Studies on the pathogenesis of atherosclerosis. I. Adhesion and emigration of mononuclear cells in the aorta of hypercholesterolemic rats. Am J Pathol 113:341, 1983
83. Kita T, Nagaro Y, Yukode M, Ishii K, Kume N, Ooshima A, Yoshida H, Kawai C: Probucol prevents the progression of atherosclerosis in Watanable heritable hyperlipidemic rabbit, an animal model for familial hypercholesterolemia. Proc Natl Acad Sci USA 84:5928, 1987
84. Klotz O, Manning MF: Fatty streaks in the intima of arteries. J Pathol Bacteriol 16:211, 1911
85. Kramsch DM, Franzblau C, Hollander W: The protein and lipid composition of arterial elastin and its relationship to lipid accumulation in the atherosclerotic plaque. J Clin Invest 50:1666, 1971
86. Ku DN, Giddens DP, Zarins CK, Glagov S: Pulsatile flow and atherosclerosis in the human carotid bifurcation. Positive correlation between plaque location and low and oscillating shear stress. Arteriosclerosis 5:293, 1985
87. Leibovich SJ, Ross R: A macrophage-dependent factor that stimulates the proliferation of fibroblasts *in vitro*. Am J Pathol 84:501, 1976
87a. Leibovich SJ, Polverini PJ, Shepard HM, Wiseman DM, Shively V, Nuseir N: Macrophage-induced angiogenesis is mediated by tumor necrosis factor-α. Nature 329:630, 1987
88. Lewis JC, Taylor RG, Jones ND, St. Clair RW, Cornhill JF: Endothelial surface characteristics in pigeon coronary artery ath-

erosclerosis. I. Cellular alterations during the initial stages of dietary cholesterol challenge. Lab Invest 46:123, 1982

89. Lipid Research Clinics Program: The Lipid Research Clinics coronary primary prevention trial results. J Am Med Assoc 251:365, 1984
90. Loft B, Olsen F: Delayed hypersensitivity and arteriosclerosis in man. Acta Pathol Microbiol Scand [B] 81:779, 1973
90a. Luger TA, Charon JA, Colot M, Micksche M, Oppenheim JJ: Chemotactic properties of partially purified human epidermal cell-derived thymocyte-activating factor for polymorphonuclear and mononuclear cells. J Immunol 131:816, 1983
91. Madtes DK, Raines EW, Sakariassent, Assoian RK, Sporn MB, Bell GI, Ross R: Induction of EGF and TGF α gene transcription and secretion of EGF competitive activity in activated human alveolar macrophages (abstr). J Cell Biochem II (Suppl): 33, 1987
91a. Majesky MW, Reidy MA, Benditt EP, Juchau MR: Focal smooth muscle proliferation in the aortic intima produced by an initiation-promotion sequence. Proc Natl Acad Sci USA 82:3450, 1985
92. Malinow MR: Atherosclerosis: Progression, regression, and resolution. Am Heart J 108:1523, 1984
93. Martin BM, Gimbrone MA Jr, Unanue ER, Cotran RS: Stimulation of nonlymphoid mesenchymal cell proliferation by a macrophage-derived growth factor. J Immunol 126:1510, 1981
94. Mathur SN, Field FJ, Spector AA, Armstrong ML: Increased production of lipoxygenase products by cholesterol-rich mouse macrophages. Biochim Biophys Acta 837:13, 1985
95. Mazzone T, Jensen M, Chait A: Human arterial wall cells secrete factors that are chemotactic for monocytes. Proc Natl Acad Sci USA 80:5094, 1983
96. McGill HC Jr, Arias-Stella J, Carbonell LM, Correa P, de Veyra EA Jr, Donoso S, Eggen Da, Galindo L, Guzmán MA, Lichtenberger E, Løken AC, McGarry PA, McMahan CA, Montenegro MR, Moossy J, Perez-Tamayo R, Restrepo C, Robertson WB, Salas J, Solberg LA, Strong JP, Tejada C, Wainwright J: General findings of the International Atherosclerosis Project. Lab Invest 18:498, 1968
97. McGill HC Jr: Fatty streaks in the coronary arteries and aorta. Lab Invest 18:560, 1968
98. McGill HC Jr: Persistent problems in the pathogenesis of atherosclerosis. Arteriosclerosis 4:443, 1984
99. Montenegro MR, Eggen DA: Topography of atherosclerosis in the coronary arteries. Lab Invest 18:586, 1968
100. Moyer CF, Reinisch CL: The role of vascular smooth muscle cells in experimental autoimmune vasculitis. I. The initiation of delayed type hypersensitivity agiitis. Am J Pathol 117:380, 1984
101. Munro JM, van der Walt JD, Munro CS, Chalmers JAC, Cox EL: An immunohistochemical analysis of human aortic fatty streaks. Human Pathol 18:375, 1987
102. Murata K, Motayama T, Kotake C: Collagen types in various layers of the human aorta and their changes with the atherosclerotic process. Atherosclerosis 60:251, 1986
103. Nakao J, Ooyama T, Chang W-C, Murota S, Orimo H: Platelets stimulate aortic smooth muscle cell migration *in vitro*. Atherosclerosis 43:143, 1982
104. Nathan CF: Secretory products of macrophages. J Clin Invest 79:319, 1987
105. Parthasarathy S, Printz DJ, Boyd D, Joy L, Steinberg D: Macrophage oxidation of low density lipoprotein generates a modified form recognized by the scavenger receptor. Arteriosclerosis 6:505, 1986
106. Penn A, Garte SJ, Warren L, Nesta D, Mindich B: Transforming gene in human atherosclerotic plaque DNA. Proc Natl Acad Sci USA 83:7951, 1986
107. Pober JS, Bevilacqua MP, Mendrick DL, Lapierre LA, Fiers W, Gimbrone MA Jr: Two distinct monokines, IL-1 and TNF, each independently induce biosynthesis and transient expression of the same antigen on the surface of cultured vascular endothelial cells. J Immunol 136:1680, 1986
108. Polverini P, Cotran RS, Gimbrone MA Jr, Unanue ER: Activated macrophages induce vascular proliferation. Nature, 269:804, 1977
109. Pooling Project Research Group: Relationship of blood pressure, serum cholesterol, smoking habit, relative weight and ECG abnormalities to incidence of major coronary events: Final report of pooling project. J Chron Dis 31:201, 1978
110. Quinn MT, Parthasarathy S, Steinberg D: Endothelial cell-derived chemotactic activity for mouse peritoneal macrophages and the effect of modified forms of low-density lipoprotein. Proc Natl Acad Sci USA 82:5949, 1985
111. Quinn MT, Parthasarathy S, Fong LG, Steinberg D: Oxidatively modified low density lipoproteins: A potential role in recruitment and retention of monocyte/macrophages during atherogenesis. Proc Natl Acad Sci USA 84:2995, 1987
112. Rayer P: Memoire sur l'ossification morbide, consideree comme une terminaison des phlegmasies. Arch Gen de Med (Paris) 1:313, 1823
113. Reidy MA, Schwartz SM: Recent advances in molecular pathology: Arterial endothelium assessment of *in vivo* injury. Exp Mol Pathol 41:419, 1984
113a. Reidy MA: A reassessment of endothelial injury and arterial lesion formation. Lab Invest 53:513, 1985
114. Rogers KA, Hoover RL, Castellot JJ Jr, Robinson JM, Karnovsky MJ: Dietary cholesterol-induced changes in macrophage characteristics: Relation to athersclerosis. Am J Pathol 125:284, 1986
115. Rosenberg RD, Reilly C, Fritze L: Atherogenic regulation by heparin-like molecules. Ann NY Acad Sci 454:270, 1985
116. Ross R, Glomset J, Kariya B, Harker L: A platelet-dependent serum factor that stimulates the proliferation of arterial smooth muscle cells *in vitro*. Proc Natl Acad Sci USA 71:1207, 1974
117. Ross R, Glomset JA: I. The pathogenesis of atherosclerosis. N Engl J Med 295:369, 1976
118. Ross R, Glomset JA: II. The pathogenesis of atherosclerosis. N Engl J Med 295:420, 1976
119. Ross R: The pathogenesis of atherosclerosis: An update. N Engl J Med 314:488, 1986
120. Ross R, Raines EW, Bowen-Pope DF: The biology of platelet-derived growth factor. Cell 46:155, 1986
121. St. Clair RW: Atherosclerosis regression in animal models: current concepts of cellular and biochemical mechanisms. Prog Cardiovasc Dis 26:109, 1983
122. Salisbury BGJ, Falcone DJ, Minick CR: Insoluble low-density lipoprotein-proteoglycan complexes enhance cholesteryl ester accumulation in macrophages. Am J Pathol 120:6, 1985
123. Sanchez-Madrid F, Nagy JA, Robbins E, Simon P, Springer TA: A human leukocyte differentiation antigen family with distinct alpha-subunits and a common beta-subunit. J Exp Med 158:1785, 1983
124. Saphir O, Gore I: Evidence for an inflammatory basis of coronary arteriosclerosis in the young. Arch Pathol 49:418, 1950
125. Schwartz CJ, Mitchell JRA: Cellular infiltration of human arterial adventitia associated with atheromatous plaques. Circulation 26:73, 1962
126. Schwartz SM, Reidy MA: Common mechanisms of proliferation of smooth muscle in atherosclerosis and hypertension. Human Pathol 18:240, 1987
127. Seifert RA, Schwartz SM, Bowen-Pope DF: Developmentally regulated production of platelet-derived growth factor-like molecules. Nature 311:669, 1984
128. Shimokado K, Raines EW, Madtes DK, Barrett TB, Benditt EP, Ross R: A significant part of macrophage-derived growth factor consists of at least two forms of PDGF. Cell 43:277, 1985
129. Sieffert GF, Keown K, Moore SW: Pathologic effect of tobacco smoke inhalation on arterial intima. Surg Forum 32:333, 1981
130. Sinzinger H, Bergmann H, Kaliman J, Angelberger P: Imaging of human atherosclerotic lesions using ^{123}I-low-density lipoprotein. Eur J Nucl Med 12:291, 1986
131. Smith EB: The relationship between plasma and tissue lipids in human atherosclerosis. Adv Lipid Res 12:1, 1974
132. Sporn MB, Roberts AB: Peptide growth factors and inflammation, tissue repair, and cancer. J Clin Invest 78:329, 1986
133. Stary HC: Atheroma arises in eccentric intimal thickening from concurrent fatty streak lesions (abstr). Fed Proc 46;418, 1987
134. Steinberg D: Current theories of the pathogenesis of atherosclerosis. In Hypercholesterolemia and Atherosclerosis. Pathogenesis and Prevention, edited by Steinberg D, Olefsky JM, p 5. New York, Churchill/Livingstone, 1987
135. Still WJS, O'Neal RM: Electron microscopic study of experimental atherosclerosis in the rat. Am J Pathol 40:21, 1962.
136. Still WJS, Marriott PR: Comparative morphology of the early atherosclerotic lesion in man and cholesterol-atherosclerosis in the rabbit. An electronmicroscopic study. J Atheroscler Res 4:373, 1964
137. Stratford N, Britten K, Gallagher P: Inflammatory infiltrates in

human coronary atherosclerosis. Atherosclerosis 59:271, 1986
138. Strong JP, Richards ML: Cigarette smoking and atherosclerosis in autopsied men. Atherosclerosis 23:451, 1976
139. Territo M, Berliner JA, Fogelman AM: Effect of monocyte migration on low density lipoprotein transport across aortic endothelial cell monolayers. J Clin Invest 74:2279, 1984
140. Thomas WA, Reiner JM, Florentin RA, Scott RF: Population dynamics of arterial cells during atherogenesis: VIII. Separation of the roles of injury and growth stimulation in early aortic atherogenesis in swine originating in pre-existing intimal smooth muscle cell masses. Exp Mol Pathol 31:124–144, 1979
141. Thomas WA, Kim DN: Atherosclerosis as a hyperplastic and/or neoplastic process. Lab Invest 48:245, 1983
142. Valente AJ, Fowler SR, Sprague EA, Kelley JL, Suenram CA, Schwartz CJ: Initial characterization of a peripheral blood mononuclear cell chemoattractant derived from cultured arterial smooth muscle cells. Am J Pathol 117:409, 1984
143. Vedeler CA, Nyland H, Matre R: *In situ* characterization of the foam cells in early human atherosclerotic lesions. Acta Pathol Microbiol Immunol Scand [C] 92:133, 1984
144. Vijayagopal P, Srinivasan SR, Radhakrishnamurthy B, Berenson GS: Hemostatic properties and serum lipoprotein binding of a heparan sulfate proteoglycan from bovine aorta. Biochim Biophys Acta 758:70, 1983
145. Virchow R: Der atheromatose prozess der arterien. Wien Med Wochenschr 6:825, 1856
146. Wahl SM, Hunt DA, Wakefield LM, McCartney-Francis N, Wahl LM, Roberts AB, Sporn MB: Transforming growth factor type β induces monocyte chemotaxis and growth factor production. Proc Natl Acad Sci USA 84:5788, 1987
147. Walker LN, Bowen-Pope DF, Ross R, Reidy MA: Intimal vascular smooth muscle cells secrete PDGF-like activity (abstr). Fed Proc 44:737, 1985
148. Wallis WJ, Harlan JM: Effector functions of endothelium in inflammatory and immunologic reactions. Pathol Immunopathol Res 5:73, 1986
149. Wang JM, Bersani L, Mantovani A: Tumor necrosis factor is chemotactic for monocytes and polymorphonuclear leukocytes. J Immunol 138:1469, 1987.
150. Wang JM, Collela S, Allavena P, Mantovani A: Chemotactic activity of human recombinant granulocyte-macrophage colony-stimulating factor. Immunology 60:439, 1987
151. Watanabe T, Hirata M, Yoshikawa Y, Nagafuchi Y, Toyoshima H, Watanabe T: Role of macrophages in atherosclerosis. Lab Invest 53:80, 1985
152. Webster WS, Bishop SP, Geer JC: Experimental aortic intimal thickening. I. Morphology and source of intimal cells. Am J Pathol 76:245, 1974
153. Werb Z, Banda MJ, Jones PA: Degradation of connective tissue matrices by macrophages. J Exp Med 152:1340, 1980
154. Yla-Herttuala S, Sumuvuori H, Karkola K, Mottonen M, Nikkari T: Glycosaminoglycans in normal and atherosclerotic human coronary arteries. Lab Invest 54:402, 1986

Section III

Tumor Biology

Biology of Disease

The Role of Extracellular Proteases in Cell Proliferation and Differentiation

WILLIAM SCHER

Chemotherapy Foundation Laboratory, Division of Medical Oncology, Department of Medicine, Mount Sinai School of Medicine, New York, New York

INTRODUCTION

Proteases play critical roles in a vast number of reactions that are important in regulating anabolic as well as catabolic cellular metabolism and, in addition, many extra- and intracellular physiologic functions (158, 165, 288). Although regulation of specific and general protein levels by catabolism was not as emphasized in early studies as that of the regulation of protein synthesis, this is now recognized as an error (4, 200). The importance of proteases in "molding" a final protein product by converting a zymogen, a pro-hormone, or a pro-growth factor to an active moiety, or by removing a signal peptide to have the protein "delivered" to the proper location, is clear (see Refs. 295, 338, 397). Specific examples include the activation of epidermal growth factor (EGF) by the proteolytic EGF-binding protein (123, 384) or the autoproteolytic processing of pro-β nerve growth factor (NGF) to NGF by its own γ-subunit (142, 389). The importance of studying protease induction of cell proliferation and DNA synthesis is now recognized (see Refs. 265, 266 for earlier reviews) and it has also been suggested that proteases may act as growth factors for malignant cells (41, 254) or in wound healing (see Ref. 30). Proteases appear to be able to act as true growth factors and not simply in a process directed toward supplying nutrient amino acids, as carefully defined by Gospodarowicz and Moran (140), although the latter case has not been ruled out as an augmenting process.

More recently, extracellular proteases such as trypsin or Clostridial collagenase have been shown to directly initiate another fundamental cellular physiologic process in addition to mitosis, *i.e.*, differentiation of several hemopoietic cell types (343).

Extracellular proteases can stimulate the secretion of other proteases. For example, trypsin induces plasminogen activator secretion and a number of proteases can stimulate the secretion of collagenase in rabbit synovial fibroblasts (424). It appears, therefore, that extracellular proteases may indirectly stimulate cell multiplication or differentiation through the induction of other proteases in a multipath cascade of proteolytic events. For example, trypsin can cleave procollagenase to collagenase, as well as induce plasminogen activator. Plasminogen activator can then activate plasmin from plasminogen and the resulting plasmin can then also activate collagenase.

Extracellular proteases may activate an intracellular protease(s). Traktman and Baltimore (393) found that trypsin, chymotrypsin or thermolysin could abrogate the temperature-sensitivity of NIH/3T3 mouse cells that were infected with temperature-sensitive Moloney murine leukemia virus, by affecting the cleavage and normal intracellular muturation of the viral precursor proteins, $Pr65^{gag}$ and $Pr180^{gag\text{-}pol}$. It was considered unlikely that these proteases, of approximately 25 kilodaltons (kd) entered the cell but rather that they activated an intracellular protease thereby substituting for the putative defective viral protease.

Many intracellular proteases involved in the regulation of cell multiplication, or differentiation and development, will not be discussed (*e.g.*, 80, 96, 184, 250, 290, 350) except for the case of nuclear proteases, nor will the role of extracellular proteases in reproduction (293, 347, 406) be discussed.

PROTEASE INDUCTION OF MITOGENESIS

Early History

Trypsin was used in all of the early reports of protease-induced mitosis, although additional proteases were later found to also be effective (Table 1). In 1937, Simms and Stillman (366) reported that proteases stimulate cell multiplication *in vitro*. Treatment with trypsin for 2.5 to 24 hours resulted in an increase in multiplication of several cell types assayed after 2 to 5 days in media without trypsin. Division of chick adult thoracic and abdominal aortic fibroblasts, adult liver fibroblasts and epithelial cells, adult thyroid and muscle fibroblasts, Rous sarcoma tissue cells, Walker rat sarcoma cells, dog muscle granulation tissue cells, and human brain meningioma and glioma cells are displayed increased proliferation. Papain was also noted to be a mitogen.

A quarter of a century later, Ershoff and Bajwa (107) reported that chymotrypsin, trypsin, papain, and protease P6, but not pepsin, induced hypertrophy with a 2-fold or more increase in the dry weight of the submaxillary glands of rats that were fed these proteases for 12 days *ad libitum*. The mechanism of proteases in this process was not understood, since it was not anticipated that a protease could be absorbed from either the intestinal tract or the buccal cavity. In this case, the proteases may not have been acting as growth factors, but possibly by allowing an increase in nutrient supply. On the other hand, protease-fed rats did not undergo an increase in weight when compared with untreated rats, which would have been expected if the mechanism were related to nutrient supply. Considering the studies of thrombin-induced mitogenesis (see below), it is possible that this effect was due to actions of these proteases at the surface of the submaxillary gland. However, as noted by the authors, further study will be necessary to locate the specific site of protease action in this process.

Two years later the trypsin stimulation of Walker tumor cells was confirmed, independently, and the trypsin stimulation of embryonic chick neural retinal cells *in vitro* was also reported (280).

Mazzei *et al.* (243, 244) were the first to report that proteases could stimulate mitogenesis of hematopoietic cells or of cells in suspension cultures. They found that treatment with either chymotrypsin, trypsin, or papain for 4 days was mitogenic for human peripheral blood lymphocytes *in vitro*, and suggested that this might be due to nonspecific damage of the cell surface rather than a specific mechanism related to an antigen function.

Rubin (324, 325) reported that a growth factor may be a protease, and based on this and work from his own laboratory (44, see also Ref. 267), Burger (43) reported that mouse 3T3 fibroblast mitogenesis was stimulated by trypsin, pronase (a mixture of proteases from *Streptomyces griseus*, or ficin. Soon after, Sefton and Rubin (357) reported that trypsin, pronase and ficin stimulated DNA synthesis in chick embryo cells. Burger's laboratory demonstrated commitment to mitosis by showing that mitosis occurred 2 to 4 days after a 45-minute exposure to a protease. Burger (46) suggested that the protease probably acted on the cell surface for these reasons: (a) medium pretreated with a protease did not simulate the effect, (b) a protein protease inhibitor (ovomucoid trypsin inhibitor, OTI) that presumably could not enter the cell, inhibited the effect, and (c) "particulate trypsin" (not described further), that also presumably could not be taken up by the cell, was also effective. Further, it was suggested that intracellular mediators, such as cAMP, might be activated or released intracellularly by these proteases acting at the cell surface. They demonstrated not only increases in mitosis and cell number after protease treatment of fibroblasts, but a rapid (3 hours) increase in DNA synthesis which was maximal within about 6 hours. The peak in mitosis occurred about 5 hours after the peak in DNA synthesis. They also reported that trypsin-treated medium did not mimic the effect of trypsin if the trypsin was eliminated before adding the mixture to the cells with a protein protease inhibitor (soybean trypsin inhibitor, SBTI). SBTI did not inhibit the induction of mitosis by pronase, a protease against which SBTI is ineffective, therefore SBTI only acted in conjunction with trypsin and not by a direct toxic effect.

Vaheri, Ruoslahti, and Hovi (401) confirmed the finding that trypsin was mitogenic for chick embryo fibroblasts and found that papain was also a mitogen. Frank, Ristow, and Veser (122) added embryonic rat fibroblasts to the growing list of cell types responsive to trypsin mitogenesis. Although some other types of human cells were finally shown to respond mitogenically to proteases (412, see below), human fibroblasts were not shown to be sensitive to proteases until 1977 (292). This was thought to be related to the finding that calf (the most

TABLE 1. CELL TYPES MITOGENICALLY STIMULATED BY PROTEASES

Cell type	Protease	Reference
Human		
Brain meningioma and glioma cells	Trypsin, papain	366
Lymphocytes	Chymotrypsin, papain, pronase, trypsin, elastase, human PMN cathepsin G	185, 243, 244, 370, 412, 413
Leukemia lymphoblasts	Thrombin	40
Cervical carcinoma (HeLa) cells, placental fibroblasts, tonsillar lymphocytes	Trypsin, pronase	412
Embryo fibroblasts	Thrombin, trypsin, plasmin	292
Neonatal diploid foreskin cells	Thrombin, trypsin	58
Fibrosarcoma cells	Thrombin	366
Canine		
Muscle granulation tissue cells	Trypsin	366
Rodent		
Rat Walker sarcoma cells	Trypsin, papain	366
Rat submaxillary glands	Chymotrypsin, trypsin, papain, protease P6	107
Rat embryo fibroblasts	Trypsin	122
Mouse 3T3 fibroblasts	Trypsin, pronase, ficin	43
Mouse embryo cells	Thrombin, trypsin	58, 444
Mouse macrophage	Thrombin	15
Mouse lymphocytes	Trypsin, pronase, thrombin, elastase, human PMN cathepsin G, chymotrypsin	67, 185, 410, 412, 413
Rabbit lymphocytes	Trypsin, pronase	136
Rabbit lens epithelial cells	Thrombin	305
Rabbit corneal fibroblasts	Thrombin	41
Hamster kidney cells	Trypsin, plasmin, pronase	36
CHL (CCL39 and V79) fibroblasts	Thrombin	283, 366
Chinese hamster ovary and embryo cells	Thrombin	see 257
Syrian hamster embryo (NIL) cells	Thrombin	60
Chicken		
Aortic, liver and breast muscle fibroblasts	Trypsin, papain	366
Thyroid, liver epithelial, Rous sarcoma, embryo and neural retinal cells	Trypsin	280, 366
CEF	Trypsin, pronase, elastase, 2 mouse submaxillary enteropeptidases and γ-subunit of NGF, human thrombin and urine plasminogen activator, bromelin, ficin, papain	42, 65, 143, 281, 357, 401

PMN, polymorphonuclear neutrophilic granulocyte; CHL, Chinese hamster lung.

frequently used), horse, and rabbit serum inhibited the effect, while chick, dog, and monkey serum supported protease induction. Greene, Shooter, and Varon (143) demonstrated that three of the major esteropeptidases of the mouse submaxillary gland could stimulate cell division in chick embryo body wall fibroblasts. One of these esteropeptidases was the γ-subunit of NGF, so NGF has both a subunit that is a protease and a growth-stimulator and another subunit(s) that induces nerve cell differentiation with cessation of cell proliferation.

PROTEASE INHIBITORS

Schnebli and Burger (348, 349) found that five protease inhibitors, OTI (with and without coupling to Sepharose beads, noted in 344), tosyl-arginine methyl ester (TAME), tosyl-phenylalanylchloromethylketone (TPCK), tosyl-lysyl-chloromethylketone (TLCK), and Trayslol, inhibited the protease-induced growth of three transformed mouse fibroblast cell lines and a polyoma virus-transformed baby hamster kidney cell line, but were less effective in inhibiting nontransformed cell lines. As with many experiments involving the use of inhibitors, the targets of these inhibitors are unknown and not necessarily the proteases themselves. One cannot rule out the possibility that moietes such as nonproteolytic esterases could have been the targets. Again, it was assumed that the site of action of these inhibitors was at the cell surface. Although this is apparently the case for the high molecular weight OTI and Trasylol, no such constraint necessitates that assumption for the low molecular weight protease inhibitors, TAME, TPCK, and TLCK, that can and probably did enter the cell. Furthermore, inhibition of growth by Sepharose-bound OTI may have been due to the Sepharose itself since Sepharose or contaminants on it have been noted to be cytotoxic (E. A. Slosberg, B. M. Scher, W. Scher, and S. Waxman: Induction of differentiation in mouse erythroleukemia cells by the action of papain at the cell surface, submitted for publication). Since Schnebli and Burger (349) found that SBTI by itself was not effective as a growth inhibitor of these cell lines, it is possible that the low molecular weight protease inhibitors may have been acting intracellularly (see below). If so, the targets of the low molecular weight protease inhibitors would not have been extracellular proteases. Therefore, the experiments with these inhibitors cannot be clearly interpreted, as discussed by Burger (47) or Vischer (411), and demonstrated by Noonan and Noonan (268). However, since large molecular weight protease inhibitors were effective, a cell-surface proteolytic activity may be involved in regulating cell growth. Evidence was presented that trypsin not only bound to the surface of HeLa and CBM17 baby mouse kidney cells but also entered the cells (162). More trypsin-like proteolytic activity was observed in lysates prepared from trypsin-treated cells than from nontreated cells so that the possibility that trypsin may act intracellularly was also suggested. Kast (186, 187) reported that SBTI and lima bean trypsin inhibitor inhibited the phytohemagglutinin (PHA)-induced mitogenesis of lymphocytes. However, other workers reported that neither SBTI nor OTI inhibited the PHA stimulation of human lymphocyte DNA or RNA synthesis, whereas the low molecular weight protease inhibitors, TPCK, TLCK, *M*-benzoyl-L-tyrosine ethyl ester, *N*-benzoyl-L-arginine amide or TAME did (93). Saito *et al.* (330) found that another low molecular weight protease inhibitor, leupeptin, inhibited PHA-induced lymphocyte (guinea pig) transformation. Goetz, Weinstein, and Roberts (134) noted that beef pancreas trypsin inhibitor, SBTI, and TLCK also depressed proliferation of golden hamster fibrosarcoma cells, whereas OTI did not. Similar to the findings of Schnebli and Burger (349), these workers also found that beef pancreas trypsin inhibitor did not inhibit mitosis in nontumorous cells, *i.e.*, hamster embryo cells.

Darzynkiewicz and Arnason (93) reported that preparations of chymotrypsin, pronase, or trypsin, when linked to Sepharose beads, had no effect on RNA synthesis after 3 hours of exposure to lymphocytes. However, the level of protease activity was not given, so these results cannot be adequately compared with those of other investigators. Presumably the lack of a stimulation in these experiments was due to the addition of insufficient active protease, insufficient incubation time, toxic contaminants "trapped" or bound to the Sepharose (as noted above), protease inhibitors in the culture medium, or to some combination of these factors.

Brown and Kiehn (36), however, found only "insignificant" inhibition of trypsin stimulation of baby hamster kidney cell proliferation by beef pancreas trypsin inhibitor and SBTI and, therefore, suggested that trypsin may act by a nonproteolytic mechanism, as has been shown for some effects of thrombin (see below). They also found that pronase and plasmin were mitogenic for these cells. Pronase was more effective than either trypsin or plasmin, probably due to the potent mitogenic action of a protease present in pronase, which was later purified by Ueki *et al.* (398, 399) (see below).

Cunningham and Ho (88) confirmed the report of Sefton and Rubin (357) that continuous treatment of chicken embryo fibroblasts (CEF) with trypsin (or pronase) stimulated mitogenesis, and that the stimulation was obviated by SBTI. However, they found that 4 to 8 hours of continuous trypsin treatment was required in order to detect an increase in cell number at 24 hours, a longer period of treatment than had been previously reported (43, 47).

Lymphocyte Mitogenesis

Five years after Mazzei, Novi, and Bazzi (243, 244) reported protease induction of mitogenesis, further studies on similar lymphocyte systems appeared. Goodall et al. (136) reported that trypsin or pronase induced DNA synthesis in rabbit lymphocytes. The data in this report also suggested that these proteases not only acted individually, but could also act synergistically with PHA in inducing mitogenesis. Synergism of several agents with proteases has also been seen in differentiating systems (see below). Shortly thereafter Steffan (370) reported that pronase stimulated mitosis in human peripheral blood lymphocytes, and the data presented indicate that pronase acted synergistically with PHA in this system also.

Vischer (410) demonstrated that BALB/c mouse B, but not T lymphocyte mitosis was stimulated by trypsin. At the earliest time tested, 6 hours, commitment to DNA synthesis was noted, when SBTI was used to block subsequent trypsin action. A 24-hour treatment with trypsin was required to reach the maximum increase in DNA synthesis when scored after 3 days. However, data demonstrating commitment to mitosis at 3 days, after only 30 minutes of trypsin treatment, was noted in several, but not all, experiments of this type when the trypsin activity was removed by washing the cells, instead of by SBTI addition. Therefore, the possibilities that either SBTI may have had additional inhibitory effects, or that the trypsin was not completely removed, still exist. Proteolytic action was required for the trypsin effect, since SBTI was shown to inhibit the trypsin induction of mitosis, but not the induction of B or T cell mitosis by lipopolysaccharide or PHA, respectively.

Kaplan and Bona (185) also reported that proteases induced lymphocyte mitogenesis. Both trypsin and pronase were effective in inducing AKR mouse and human lymphocyte mitogenesis. A 30-minute preincubation of mouse cells with trypsin was generally sufficient to commit a culture to approximately the same level of DNA synthesis, when tested 3 days later, as that of cultures treated continuously with the protease. Differences noted in the kinetics, and differences seen in the optimal concentration of trypsin required for induction in these experiments when compared with those of Vischer (40), were attributed to the different strains of mice utilized. However, since no measurements of the level of trypsin activity actually added to the incubations or to the preincubations were made, the differences could have been due to different specific activities of the trypsin preparations used and to different levels of trypsin activity "carried" over from the preincubations to the long-term incubations.

Grayzel and colleagues (141) identified at least four proteases in human peripheral blood lymphocytes. None of these were specifically noted to be involved in PHA-induced mitogenesis, and a neutral protease, bound to the lymphocyte surface, was specifically ruled out due to its resistance to TLCK, a normally effective inhibitor of the PHA effect.

However, a possibly different surface protease has been implicated in lymphocyte mitogenesis, since Moreau, Dornand, and Kaplan (253) found that "free" SBTI or SBTI covalently linked to Sepharose beads inhibited human peripheral blood lymphocyte mitogenesis in the mixed lymphocyte reaction or when induced by concanavalin A (Con A). They suggested that different proteases were independently sufficient, since both TLCK and TPCK, which differ in their mode of action, also inhibited the process (98). Some of these findings were summarized by Ranney (304).

Vischer and colleagues further extended the list of cell types and proteases that could take part in this process (412). They found that a human cervical carcinoma (HeLa) cell line and primary human placental fibroblasts or tonsillar lymphocytes could be induced to divide by proteases, and that another protein protease inhibitor, aprotinin, could inhibit these processes. These workers also found that elastase and a chymotrypsin-like cathepsin G from human polymorphonuclear leukocytes induced mitogenesis in human peripheral blood and mouse spleen lymphocytes. Therefore, it was proposed that proteases released during inflammatory reactions might induce mitogenesis of several cell types (413). Further work demonstrated that the protein protease inhibitors, SBTI and aprotinin inhibited mouse spleen lymphocyte induction by all mitogens tested (PHA, Con A, lipopolysaccharide, and dextran sulfate) whereas other protein protease inhibitors, α-1 trypsin inhibitor and α-2 macroglobulin, as well as the low molecular weight protease inhibitors, antipain and leupeptin, had little or no effect (411). These findings are consistent with the previous hypothesis that a specific protease(s) was involved in this process and that it acted on the cell surface. Vischer also found that the marked inhibitory effect of TLCK on protease-induced mitogenesis could be ameliorated by reduced glutathione. Since, in this case the effect could have been on the intracellular level of glutathione, it appears again that, in this in vivo experiment, the effect of a protease inhibitor may not have been on a protease. However, since no determination of the stability of TLCK was made, it is also possible that glutathione mediated the metabolism of TLCK so that it could no longer act as an effective protease inhibitor.

Mitogenic Action of Thrombin

Induction of Mitosis. In 1974, Chen and Buchanan (65) demonstrated that human thrombin was mitogenic for serum-free grown CEF. Prothrombin was mitogenic only if it was converted to thrombin. This was the first of many reports that utilized thrombin to study the mechanism of protease-induced mitogenesis (66). Thrombin was also found to be mitogenic for mouse splenocytes which suggested to Chen, Teng, and Buchanan (67) that thrombin may play a role in wound healing not only by stimulating fibroblast, but also B lymphoblast, proliferation. It was thought that the lymphoblast proliferation would aid in defending the host against infection during wound healing. Subsequently, thrombin was found to stimulate DNA synthesis and/or cell proliferation of several (although not all, see Ref. 265) other cell types tested (Table 1). In some systems, thrombin alone was not mitogenic, but it enhanced the activity of three growth factors: epidermal, fibroblast, and platelet-derived growth factors (139, 442) and could therefore, be considered to act synergistically with them.

Thrombin is a trypsin-like serine protease glycoprotein (bovine: M_r, 35,404 excluding the carbohydrate moiety of approximately 1.06 kd; human: approximately 36.6 kd) with most notably, homology to chymotrypsin (23, 50, 95, 105, 232). It has 2 chains (see 112), the catalytic B chain of 259 residues and the 36-49-residue (depending on the species) A chain, which is possibly "regulatory" (262). The human α-thrombin B-chain migrates at 32 kd on sodium dodecyl sulfate-polyacrylamide gels. This is relevant to the study of thrombin-receptor complexes since reducing conditions remove the A chain. Although thrombin is known to cleave at least 22 proteins, sometimes at more than 1 site, as well as some synthetic substrates (10, 24, 42, 64, 112, 294, 427), it is still considered to be fairly specific, particularly when compared with chymotrypsin or trypsin (66, 112, 233). For example, trypsin, which cleaves C-terminally to almost any arginyl or lysyl residue, thrombin is able to cleave C-terminally to only certain arginyl and rare lysyl residues (233). The residues immediately adjacent to cleavable arginyl sites ($\geq$8 N-terminally, $\geq$9 C-terminally) may impart moderate additional specificity (discussed in 294). In addition, steric hinderance, due to the tertiary structure of the substrate (294), may alter specificity.

Surface Action and Receptors. The first experiments that localized the site of action of mitogenic proteases to the cell-surface membrane were performed with trypsin. Burger (43, 44, 46) noted that "trypsin in a large particulate form", which could not be taken up by the cell, was mitogenic for mouse 3T3 fibroblasts. A further experiment utilizing trypsin bound to ^{3}H-labeled beads was also briefly described (45). This preparation was mitogenic after incubating the cells with it and then washing it away. Although very few radiolabeled beads remained in the culture after washing, these experiments were not definitive since no measurements of the level of remaining trypsin activity, nor the effect of the beads alone were made, nor was the type of beads (some types can be endocytosed), the method of radiolabelling the beads, or the method of linking the beads to trypsin given.

Carney and Cunningham (54) demonstrated that trypsin immobilized on 926 nm diameter polystyrene (latex) beads, was mitogenic for CEF and that the small amount of protein that was released from the beads during the assay was not sufficient to account for the mitogenic activity. They then found the same result with polystyrene bead-immobilized human α-thrombin (55, 56). Subsequently, thrombin has been utilized in most studies of the mechanism of protease-induced mitosis.

Thrombin was found to bind to the cell-surface by both high- and low-affinity receptors. The high-affinity receptors for thrombin were found on cells that were inducible for mitogenesis by thrombin and their occupancy by thrombin was required for the effect, whereas occupancy of the low-affinity receptors was not (9, 57,

282). Thrombin, as well as other growth factors, may bind covalently to cell-surface receptors or to fragments of receptors (11, 222, 365). It is likely that the covalent binding of thrombin is essential for its induction of mitogenesis and/or for its subsequent breakdown necessary to halt the mitogenic signal. Cell-surface receptors for another protease, plasminogen activator, have also been found in several cell types (6, 371, and references therein). In addition, proteases themselves have been found bound to the surface of several cell types, *e.g.*, monocytes (87, 407), fibroblasts (89, 352), and neutrophils (296).

The continuous occupancy of the receptor by thrombin seems to be required for the optimal mitogenic response of fibroblasts (59, 404) although this idea is controversial (226). Continuous occupancy would be required if the half-life of putative second messenger molecules (such as phospholipids, see below) involved in agonist signal transmission are very short. There appears to be only a single major thrombin receptor type (≥148 to 153 kd on fibroblastoid cells such as Chinese hamster lung fibroblasts, (both strain V79 and line CCL39), and mouse embryo cells (52, 59, 258, 405). However, it is not known if this receptor mediates thrombin-induced mitogenesis. The requirement for thrombin surface receptors in the thrombin stimulation of fibroblast proliferation has similarities to the apparent requirement of a high-affinity thrombin receptor for the actions of thrombin on platelets. In this case the receptor is equivalent to glycoprotein Ib (GIb) and is composed of two unequal linked chains that together have a molecular weight of approximately 170 kd (391, and see Refs. 77, 154, 161, 289, 425, 430). It is noteworthy that this molecule also binds von Willebrand factor (factor VIII), albeit at a different site. The receptor on endothelial cells is termed thrombomodulin (68 kd) (108, 224, 225, and see 77). Activation of the thrombin receptor on neuroblastoma cells stimulates cGMP formation (369). Thrombin-mediated activities in macrophages depend upon a thrombin receptor, but do not seem to depend on the proteolytic action of thrombin (see below) (18).

Thrombin binds to cells by a site on its B chain, and the B chain not only contains the active esteratic site, which is not at the cell-binding locus (59, 61), but also thrombin's only carbohydrate moiety. In addition, the B chain appears to contain all of the sites by which thrombin binds to other substances that have been studied; either low molecular weight compounds such as benzamide, or proteins such as antithrombin III, fibrinogen, or fibrin (112).

Thrombin may cleave its own receptor on fibroblasts (52). It is not known whether or not this is a required step in thrombin-induced mitogenesis, although it appears to correlate with it. It was shown that the putative 43 kd thrombin receptor fragment on CEF, mouse embryo fibroblasts, or human foreskin fibroblasts (132), but not on Chinese hamster lung fibroblasts (257), was cleaved during thrombin- or trypsin-induced mitogenesis (132). It is possible that the cleavage is similar to the proteolysis of the insulin receptor (90, 190) or the chorionic gonadotropin receptor (191, 436). After binding of the glycopeptide hormone, proteolytic processing of the chorionic gonadotropin receptor in rat ovarian or granulosa cell membranes and possibly those of porcine granulosa or rat luteal cells (see 191 for references) appears to play an important role in this hormone's function (191, 426).

It was also shown that in cultures of CEF cells that were unresponsive to thrombin, neither thrombin nor trypsin treatment removed the 43-kd protein (257). In addition, after treating CEF with ^{125}I-thrombin, a major radiolabeled protein of approximately 79 kd was detected. This protein has the appropriate molecular weight for a complex of the 43 kd possible thrombin receptor fragment and of thrombin itself. A possible receptor for thrombin on platelets (in addition to GIb), glycoprotein V, is also cleaved by thrombin (see 425). Other cell surface proteins such as the fibronectin are also cleaved *in situ* by thrombin, but no absolute requirement for this cleavage has been linked to its mitogenic activity (25, 42, 386, 443). Therefore, although a proteolytic event at the cell-surface is required for protease-induced mitogenesis, neither the specific substrate(s) nor the precise mechanism has been unequivocally identified.

Although proteolytically active thrombin is required to induce mitogenesis in most systems, this does not always seem to be the case. The proteolytically inactive diisopropylfluorophosphate (DIP)-thrombin was found to stimulate DNA synthesis (14, 15, 18) and chemotaxis (18) in the mouse monocytic line, J774, human peripheral blood monocytes, or other macrophage-like cell lines (14, 15, 18). The growth factor-like and chemotactic activities were found to reside in a tetradecapeptide (or shorter) fragment of the human thrombin B chain (residues 367–380 by prothrombin nomenclature) (14, 18). As noted above, the B chain contains a cell-surface receptor-specific site(s). However, these two putative receptor sites on the thrombin B chain are located evidently at opposite ends of the molecule (K. C. Glenn, G. J. Herbosa, and D. H. Carney: Identification of domains in thrombin involved in high affinity thrombin receptor binding and initiation of cell proliferation, submitted for publication).

DIP-thrombin also has been reported to mediate one of thrombin's effects in human renal vascular endothelial cells where both α-thrombin and DIP-thrombin treatment increase the cellular levels of c-*sis* mRNA (91). The c-*sis* gene codes for chain 2 of platelet-derived growth factor (PDGF). The expression of this gene is stimulated after 2 hours or less of thrombin treatment and its level is maximal at 4 hours after treatment. There is also an increase in PDGF activity released into the medium as well as an increase in the levels of auto-phosphorylated PDGF receptor (180 kd). In human umbilical endothelial vein cells, a similar, although not identical system, only active α- (not DIP-) thrombin was able to stimulate the release of PDGF activity (153).

In still another system, the intact rat diaphragm, insulin's growth factor activity was also mimicked by proteolytically inactive protease-related proteins (311) (see below). In this report, both porcine pepsinogen and alkali-inactivated pepsin were found to stimulate both the uptake of 3-*O*-methylglucose and the synthesis of glycogen in rat diaphragm as did insulin. Further, Kuo *et al.* (208) demonstrated that pronase, which displays insulin-like effects on glucose metabolism of isolated rat epididymal fat cells, was still active when over 95% of its proteolytic activity was abolished. However, the remaining proteolytic activity in this case may have still contained a sufficient amount of the insulin-mimetic protease that can be purified from pronase (399), to be an active preparation (398, see below).

Based upon these findings, homology between the possible receptor-binding sites in porcine pepsin or pepsinogen and the human thrombin B chain was sought, even though these proteases have different active proteolytic sites: *i.e.*, the former is an aspartyl protease and latter a serine protease. Porcine pepsinsogen and human thrombin B chain were compared by the Microgenie Program (Beckman, Inc.) and no perfect homology of over 3 adjacent amino acids was found although 10 homologous tripeptides were found (DSG, GAS, ISD, KLK, LLG, PSV, PVA, QEL, SGG, SLL) as well as several regions of 5-10 amino acids with 50 to 70% homology (W. Scher, D. Bishop, unpublished data). Since no obvious possible receptor-binding site was recognized by this method, further studies will be necessary to make an identification of this receptor-binding site, if it exists. However, a receptor-binding site may consist of only three adjacent amino acids and one of the homologous tripeptides observed may fill this role.

Recently Ruoslahti and Pierschbacher (328) have reviewed the low affinity receptor-binding properties of the tripeptide Arg-Gly-Asp. This tripeptide has been noted to be present in at least a dozen proteins where it appears to play a receptor-binding site role (171, 216, 260, 270, 328, 375). Although this tripeptidyl residue is present at positions 517–519 (prothrombin numbering) in human thrombin and in the pepsin-related enzyme, calf chymosin, it is not present in porcine, rat, or human pepsinogen. The reverse sequence, Asp-Gly-Arg, may also play a role in agonist binding. It was suggested that it may inhibit binding by the Arg-Gly-Asp sequence or be a binding sequence itself (1, 328). This reverse sequence is also found in thrombomodulin (174) and in the protein-binding fibroblast growth factor (noted in K. C. Glenn, G. J. Herbosa and D. H. Carney: Identification of domains in thrombin involved in high affinity thrombin receptor binding and initiation of cell proliferation, submitted for publication).

Mechanism of Thrombin Signal Transmission. Thrombin binds to cells and may require an active proteolytic site to induce mitosis. However, in an elegant series of experiments it has been demonstrated that for thrombin-induced fibroblast mitogenesis, both a proteolytic event(s) and the occupancy of a thrombin receptor(s) are required (52). It was shown that neither the proteolytically inactivate DIP-thrombin nor the nonbinding γ-thrombin (produced from active α-thrombin by autoproteolysis or by trypsin cleavage (62, 197)) can, by themselves, induce mitogenesis. However, when both of these agents are added to fibroblasts, mitogenic stimulation nearly equivalent to that induced by α-thrombin alone occurs (59, 61). Monoclonal antibody to the thrombin fibroblast receptor (59, G. J. Herbosa, W. C. Thompson, and D. H. Carney: Monoclonal antibody to the thrombin receptor stimulates DNA synthesis in combination with γ-thrombin or phorbol myristate acetate, submitted for publication, 1987) can substitute for the action of DIP-thrombin in an apparently similar fashion to that of the insulin- or EGF-mediated events that can be mimicked by antibody to the insulin or EGF receptor, respectively (*e.g.*, 175, 351, 385), or possibly to the anti-Ig-mediated activation of rabbit B lymphocytes (198). The sites of DIP-thrombin binding to its high affinity cell receptor and for proteolytic activity both appear to reside within amino acid residues 508–530 (prothrombin numbering), but are distinct (K. C. Glenn, G. J. Herbosa, and D. H. Carney: Identification of domains in thrombin involved in high affinity thrombin receptor binding and initiation of cell proliferation, submitted for publication). The active site serine is at position 525 and the DIP-thrombin receptor binding site, consisting of the cell-binding sequence Arg-Gly-Asp, is at position 517–519.

The actual thrombin-induced transmembrane signal(s), leading to the stimulation of mitosis, is unknown, but may involve phosphoinositides (360, and see Refs. 82, 167, 234, 235, 360), other types of second messengers such as prostaglandins or cyclic nucleotides, and/or phosphoprotein metabolism. Thrombin has been known for some time to affect phospholipid metabolism (219, 256, and see Refs. 234, 361) and protein phosphorylation (230). Alterations in phospholipid metabolism have been implicated in thrombin-induced fibroblast mitogenesis (60, 300, and for review Ref. 52). The proteolytically active α- or γ-thrombins stimulated both phosphoinositide turnover and the release of inositol triphosphate, whereas DIP-thrombin had little effect (59, 60). Thrombin-induced inositol phosphate formation is rapid and one of the earliest known intracellular responses to this enzyme (31, 209, 231, 396). Therefore, the proteolytic action of thrombin seems to be required for the activation of a phospholipase C activity thereby stimulating phosphoinositide turnover (232, 276).

Protein kinase C is the cell receptor for the tumor-promoting phorbol ester, phorbol 12-myristate 13-acetate (PMA) (263). PMA can induce mitosis in some systems and has been shown to enhance the expression of the c-*sis* gene as well as the level of its secreted product, PDGF-immunoprecipitable protein, as can thrombin. For example, PMA has these effects while inducing monocyte/macrophage-like differentiation of HL-60 and U937 cell lines (273). In addition, since PMA (binds to and) activates protein kinase C (as does thrombin in platelets) (see Ref. 86, 361), the effect of PMA on thrombin-induced mitogenesis was tested. PMA was found to act synergistically with either DIP-thrombin or a monoclonal antibody to the thrombin fibroblast receptor in stimulating mitogenesis (59, 137), which, again, suggests that at least two signals are required in thrombin-induced mitogenesis. Studies with inhibitors of proteases (leupeptin) and of arachidonate metabolism (indomethacin) also suggest that a combination of signals are involved in the sequence of steps after thrombin treatment (326). PMA in some systems, increases arachidonate release with subsequent increases in synthesis of leukotrienes, prostaglandins, prostacyclin, and thromboxanes. These, in turn, may act as second mesengers and have growth-promoting or inhibitory effects (245). In addition, since pretreatment of resting CCL39 cells with PMA inhibited the thrombin-induced inositol phosphate formation by up to 70%, it was suggested that protein kinase C activity was involved in a feedback regulation of thrombin induction (209).

PMA is thought to activate protein kinase C by posing as the natural lipid substrate, diacyclgylcerol, which is normally released from cell membrane phospholipids by the indirect action of some hormones and growth factors, resulting in the activation of protein kinase C (263). This process occurs in platelets (22 and see Ref. 211) and can be triggered by thrombin or trypsin. After the activation of protein kinase C, the phosphorylation of several proteins is increased, particularly an approximately 40-kd protein (327). Thrombin treatment has also been shown to stimulate the phosphorylation of two (other?) proteins of about this molecular weight (*i.e.*, 41 and 43 kd) as well as other proteins in CCL39 fibroblasts (199). In human umbilical vein endothelial cells, thrombin stimulates the phosphorylation of vimentin, an intermediate filament cytoskeletal protein, as well as other proteins (28). Thrombin or trypsin treatment of platelets inhibits the pertussis toxin induction of ADP-ribosylation of a protein of similar size (41 kd) (210).

A portion of the thrombin-mediated mitogenic signal may be mediated by cAMP and cGMP since thrombin treatment elevates the levels of these nucleotides in fibrosarcoma, neuroblastoma, and fibroblast cell lines (19, 52, 138, 369). In those cells responsive to the thrombin mitogenic signal, thrombin induces a rapid, transient increase in cAMP levels (52, 138). In another system (rat thymocytes), treatment with an exogenous protease, trypsin, also increases cAMP levels (358). The thrombin effect was also found to be mediated by DIP-inactivated thrombin, and not by γ-thrombin. Therefore, it appears that one portion of the thrombin mitogenic signal is mediated by its proteolytic action leading to diacylglycerol release, protein kinase C activation, and phosphorylation of specific proteins, whereas another portion of the signal may be mediated through a receptor binding site on thrombin leading to increased cAMP levels, presumably important for phosphorylation of additional proteins (138).

However, thrombin action is not always associated with processes that lead to an increase in protein phosphorylation. Thrombin treatment of platelets inhibits adenylate cyclase activity, thereby decreasing cAMP-dependent kinase activity and presumably, therefore, a decrease in the phosphorylation of at least some proteins (2, 176 and references therein). Of course, in platelets, thrombin action is not mitogenic so that these findings do not conflict.

Stimulation of DNA Synthesis in Isolated Nuclei by Proteases

Although there is no convincing evidence that exogenous mitogenic proteases can act in this process after being internalized, partially intact thrombin can be internalized by CEF (42, 444) and therefore could initiate a mitogenic signal from an intracellular site. However, in other cells (mouse embryo cells) that are responsive to the thrombin mitogenic signal, thrombin was not found to be internalized (21, 53). Other growth factors, including insulin, whose activity may be mediated by protease action, and NGF, cannot only be internalized, but can be bound by nuclear components where they would be at a suitable site to stimulate DNA synthesis (49, 181, 301, 302, 368). In addition, a growth factor may bind to its cell-surface receptor and the complex may then be internalized and "home" to the nucleus. It has been suggested that this process is critical in insulin's stimulation of growth and that the insulin receptor itself carries the growth signal to the nucleus (*e.g.*, see Refs. 49 and 291). This could occur even though insulin itself need not be the agent that activates the insulin receptor (299, 318, 385). This sequence of events could also require protease action. Therefore, a brief account of the effects of proteases on DNA synthesis in isolated nuclei is included.

Brown and Stubblefield (38) noted that trypsin or α-chymotrypsin, but not pronase, enhanced DNA synthesis in lysates of the Don strain of Chinese hamster fibroblasts. The effect appeared to be on the nucleus and not the cytosol. It was suggested that the reported trypsin stimulation of DNA methylation in isolated nuclei might be associated with its stimulation of DNA synthesis. Trypsin was found to stimulate DNA synthesis in Chinese hamster fibroblast nuclei from cells in G1, but not S, phase and, therefore, appeared to accelerate the G1 to S phase transition (37).

Recently, evidence that a physiologic protease is involved in the interleukin 2 stimulation of lymphocyte DNA synthesis has been presented (81). These workers found that cytoplasmic extracts from interleukin 2-treated human peripheral blood lymphocytes contain a proteins(s) (ADR) that activates DNA replication in isolated nuclei from untreated lymphocytes (147, 148). Aprotinin, leupeptin, *p*-amino-benzamidine, and TLCK (although not SBTI) were found to inhibit ADR activity, so that ADR activity appears to require a serine protease. A heat-stable, pH 5-stable, approximately 50-kd protein that can inhibit ADR action was found to appear in cytoplasmic extracts from lymphocytes that were cultured *in vitro* for 2 to 6 hours (149, 429). This inhibitor might be a physiologic protein protease inhibitor.

As noted in the discussion of several reports above as well as others (74, 150, 155, 330, 348), several protease inhibitors, that are capable of entering the cell, have been shown to inhibit DNA synthesis. This type of experiment also points to the possible involvement of intracellular protease activity in the control of cell proliferation. However, since the specificity and location of the protease inhibitor action was not ascertained, the effects could have been mediated by either a cell-surface component, or by toxic effects that did not involve a protease(s).

As noted earlier, extracellular trypsin treatment appears to activate an intracellular protease, *i.e.*, NIH/3T3 cells infected with certain temperature-sensitive Moloney leukemia virus mutants that produce virion precursor proteins, but are not able to proteolytically process them to mature active proteins, do so after treatment with exogenous trypsin (393).

Insulin-Like Activities of Proteases

Insulin is a required growth factor for many tissues and cultured cell lines (see Refs. 13 and 116). Insulin-like growth factors 1 and 2 have many structural and functional similarities to insulin (see Ref. 264 for references). These growth factors, as well as EGF and PDGF, appear to effect their growth-promoting activities by similar pathways. Although protease activity is required for processing several of these growth factors from precursor forms (*e.g.*, insulin, insulin-like growth factor 1, insulin-like growth factor 2, EGF, and NGF) to active forms, the involvement of a protease(s) itself in the generation of intracellular signals has so far only been suggested for insulin (213), prolactin (see Refs. 69, 212, and 388), or antigens binding to cell-surface antigen receptor immunoglobulins (and thereby activating rabbit B lymphocytes) (198). EGF-binding protein, which is a serine protease, also has growth promoting activities (217). In addition to extracellular proteases mimicking the action of insulin, an intracellular protease has been suggested as a mediator of insulin action (160).

Rieser and Rieser (312, 313) appear to be the first to observe that some proteases can have insulin-like effects (Table 2). Both chymotrypsin and trypsin were found to stimulate sugar and amino acid uptake in rat diaphragm. Surprisingly, Rieser (311) also found that proteolytically inactive proteases, *i.e.*, pepsinogen and alkali-denatured pepsin, were nearly as insulinomimetic in rat diaphragm as active pepsin, as noted above (311), and suggested a membrane-receptor mechanism of action for these agents. Kuo *et al.* (208) determined that pronase was insulinomimetic in rat adipose cells and that the insulin-like activity remained after 95% of the proteolytic activity was abolished by acid treatment. Therefore, the insulin-like activity may have been due to a protein without proteolytic activity, or to an active protease that accounted for only a small proportion of the bovine serum albumin-hydrolyzing activity present. The latter suggestion is consistent with the numerous reports of Ueki *et al.* (399) who purified a protease B-like enzyme from pronase that had powerful insulinomimetic effects on the mouse diaphragm. Hayashi *et al.* (156) then found that pronase induced hypoglycemia in fasted rabbits. Similarly, chymotrypsin was noted to induce hypoglycemia in rats (314). Trypsin also stimulated sugar accumulation in frog sartorius muscle (423). In addition to chymotrypsin, trypsin, and pronase, insulin-like action in rat adipocytes was also accorded to another bacterial protease, as well as to papain and ficin (195, 203, 206, 207, 208). Pepsin was found not to mimic insulin's effects on glucose metabolism in rat epididymal adipose cells (207), but the concentrations used were lower than those used by Rieser (311). Cherqui *et al.* (70, 71) found that endoproteinase Arg-C (which cleaves post-arginyl residues) effectively mimicked insulin action in rat adipocytes and liver plasma membranes, whereas endoproteinase Lys-C (which cleaves post-lysinyl residues) did not. This finding demonstrates a clear specificity for this process.

Table 2. Insulinomimetic Proteases

Protease	System studied	Reference
Chymotrypsin, trypsin	Rat diaphragm	312, 313
Pepsin	Rat diaphragm	312, 313
Pronase	Rat adipocyte	207, 208
Protease B-like pronase protease	Mouse diaphragm	399
Pronase	Rabbit	156
Chymotrypsin	Rat	314
Trypsin	Frog sartorius	423
Subtilopeptidase A, papain, ficin	Rat adipocyte	195, 202, 206, 207, 208
Endoproteinase Arg-C	Rat liver membranes, diaphragm	70, 71

Rieser and Rieser (310, 312) found that insulin itself had proteolytic activity on myoglobin, urea-denatured hemoglobin, and some rabbit muscle proteins and noted that others had found that insulin could also hydrolyze *p*-nitrophenyl acetate. This activity also demonstrated some specificity as it did not hydrolyze elastin, casein, ribonuclease, or muscle actin. The activity did not appear to be due to a contamination of pancreatic proteases since there was no cleavage of the trypsin-specific substrate, TAME, and the chymotrypsin-specific substrates, benzoyl-L-tyrosine ethyl ester and acetyl-L-tyrosine ethyl ester (312). Insulin was found to hydrolyze not only myoglobin and hemoglobin, but fibrinogen and possibly cell-surface receptors for insulin, glucagon, wheat germ agglutinin, and Con A as well (169, 173). However, in these reports the proteolytic activity of insulin was considered to be weak and possibly not physiologically significant. It was suggested that in artificial systems, proteolysis of the insulin receptor might mimic insulin action. Incubation of insulin with ^{125}I-labeled liver plasma membranes for 30 minutes was found to release trichloroacetic acid-soluble radioactive material (17). This was considered to be due to the activation of a serine protease (due to findings with specific protease inhibitors), but could have, been partially due to proteolytic action of insulin itself.

Possible Protease Involvement in the Action of Insulin

Ever since the finding that insulin when covalently bound to Sepharose beads, acted similarly to exogenous soluble insulin on the metabolism of rat adipocytes and the existence of a cell-surface insulin receptor was hypothesized (84), a search for the mechanism of transducing the insulin signal(s) across the cellular plasma membrane has been continuing. One of the early hypotheses for this transduction suggested that the cellular levels of specific, relatively small molecules (second messengers) that mediate insulin's activities may be increased following the binding of insulin to its cell-surface receptor (215, 416). These workers found that treatment of intact rat hemidiaphragms with insulin resulted in an increase in glycogen synthase I activity, and concomitant decreases in cAMP-dependent protein kinase and [^{3}H]cAMP binding activities. Although some cell-free systems that are responsive to insulin had been previously reported (*e.g.*, 408 and see Ref. 336), it was about this time that extensive use of Jarett's insulin-responsive cell-free system began (356). It was shown that an isolated rat adipocyte plasma membrane-mitochondrion (both required) preparation responded to insulin by the activation of mitochondrial pyruvate dehydrogenase. Within 30 seconds, a decrease in incorporation of radioactive phosphorus from γ-^{32}P-ATP into the 42-kd α-subunit of the enzyme occurred. Insulinomimetic agents such as Con A or antibody to the insulin receptor (see 299, 318, 385 for references), were also effective. Whatever the insulin-generated intracellular signals are, at least one of them is very short-lived ($t_{1/2}$ − 18 minutes) and is reminiscent of the rate at which insulin dissociates from its receptor (307).

Larner *et al.* (214) then found that after insulin treatment of rats, material extracted from hindleg skeletal muscle also inhibited rat skeletal muscle cAMP-dependent protein kinase and stimulated glycogen synthase phosphoprotein phosphatase activities, in a similar fashion to its action in rat diaphragm. The insulin-mediating active principle in the extract appeared to have a molecular weight of 1 to 1.5 kd. In an adjoining report, Jarett and Seals (178, 355) found that this muscle extract contained an insulin-mediating factor(s) that also affected the pyruvate dehydrogenase in the mitochondrion cell-free system as insulin had previously been shown to do. Of the four different insulinomimetic agents tested, trypsin had the most insulin-like effect in rat adipocytes, and it was found to also increase the levels of the putative insulin mediator (195).

Using a more sophisticated system, also containing isolated plasma membranes and mitochondria, evidence was then presented that insulin might act by activating a trypsin-like enzyme in the membrane that was crucial to the release of the putative insulin second messenger (353). First, it was noted that after adding insulin to a plasma membrane fraction, the supernatant fluid alone stimulated pyruvate dehydrogenase activity when added to a mitochondrial preparation. Then it was shown that trypsin treatment of the plasma membrane preparation mimicked insulin action and that protease inhibitors (SBTI, ovomucoid) blocked it. The "insulin-mediator" appeared to have a peptide component since treatment of the "mediator-containing" supernatant fluid with trypsin, chymotrypsin, or papain abolished its activity. Subsequently, it was observed that this mediator had a molecular weight of approximately 2 kd (354), which was in good agreement with the previously reported M_r. Evidence for an insulin second messenger was then forthcoming in other systems, *i.e.*, human lymphocytes (177) and rat liver plasma membranes (336), as well as a putative messenger for another hormone, prolactin (388). The putative insulin mediator was partially purified from rat and rabbit hindleg skeletal muscle. These preparations were capable of inhibiting purified rabbit muscle cAMP-dependent protein kinase in an insulin-like fashion (390). The active material appeared to consist of a 1 to 3 kd peptide of 13–14 amino acids or a derivatized peptide. However, since this mediator did not activate mitochondrial pyruvate dehydrogenase (390), more than one type of mediator appeared to be involved in insulin action (213). Saltiel *et al.* (336) had noted earlier that there appeared to be two insulin-activated agents in rat liver: one that stimulated pyruvate dehydrogenase activity and one that inhibited the insulin activation of both pyruvate dehydrogenase and adenyl cyclase. The same agents were able to either stimulate or inhibit the activity of insulin-regulated liver acetyl CoA carboxylase, respectively (334). However, there are conflicting reports concerning the inhibitory/stimulatory nature of the mediator (335). In relationship to the findings with adenyl cyclase, an earlier report found that trypsin treatment activated adenylate cyclase in another system, a rat kidney fibroblast line (417).

The insulin receptor is made up of four subunits linked by disulfide bonds: two 125 to 135 kd α-subunits (to which insulin binds) and two 90 to 95 kd β-subunits (103, and see Refs. 97 and 135). Kasuga *et al.* (188, 189) demonstrated that insulin stimulates the incorporation of ^{32}P into the β-subunits of its own receptor in human lymphocytes and rat hepatoma cells. This was found to be a general receptor phenomenon (see 441 for references) although possibly not required for all insulin-stimulated effects (255). Insulin was observed to activate a protein kinase that specifically phosphorylated tyrosine residues similar to other growth-regulating protein agents (287). It was then found that the insulin receptor itself was an insulin-sensitive tyrosine-specific protein kinase which was capable of not only autophosphorylation, but the phosphorylation of other protein and peptide substrates (441 and references therein).

Trypsin was shown to affect the insulin receptor. Relatively low levels of trypsin increased insulin binding (76, 202) whereas high levels of trypsin decreased the binding of insulin to its receptor in rat adipocytes (85, 201, 202, 203). It appears, therefore, that if trypsin acts directly on the receptor, the cleavage of a small and/or particularly sensitive portion of the receptor enhances insulin binding, and that the cleavage of a large or relatively protease-resistant segment(s) of the receptor destroys binding. It has been demonstrated that the binding of insulin to its receptor in rat liver membranes led to both an increase in the affinity of the receptor for insulin and an 11% reduction in the molecular weight of the α-subunit of the receptor and, in addition, that inhibition by serine protease inhibitors blocked the α-subunit cleavage, but not the affinity change (223). Therefore, the change in affinity of insulin for its receptor appears to depend on insulin binding and not on serine proteolytic activity. Regardless of whether or not the direct proteolysis of the insulin receptor by trypsin was required for the insulin-like effects previously reported, it was subsequently demonstrated that a concentration of trypsin that was insulinomimetic in rat adipocytes, and that cleaved the insulin receptor, also stimulated the insulin receptor protein kinase to autophosphorylate on a tyrosine residue and to phosphorylate an exogenous protein (382). Taking into account the caveats entailed in studies with inhibitors, this laboratory also showed that arginine-analog protease inhibitors or substrates (BAEE, TAME) inhibited the insulin stimulation of the phosphorylation of its own receptor in purified preparations from rat adipocytes and human placenta (383). There is additional indirect evidence that trypsin's insulin-like activity may be due to cleavage of the insulin receptor, *i.e.*, in Madin-Darby canine kidney cells which lack insulin receptors, trypsin does not have insulin effects, but other insulinomimetic agents, such as Con A and wheat germ agglutinin do (163). Furthermore, Rutter (329) has noted that the removal of much of the extramembrane portion of the insulin receptor has a similar effect as insulin's binding to its receptor.

The peptide nature of the putative insulin mediators has recently been questioned since apparently at least two similar, but distinct, mediators from liver plasma membranes have been partially characterized (236, 240, 333, 335). These mediators stimulated adipocyte cAMP-dependent phosphodiesterase in an insulin-like manner. However, these mediators, although similar in size (approximately 1.4 kd) and having some of the properties attributed to the apparently peptide-containing mediators suggested in earlier reports (212), were glycolipids that contained inositol, glucosamine, phosphate, and other monosaccharides. These glycolipid mediators appeared to be identical to the mediators from rat liver that affected pyruvate dehydrogenase and adenyl cyclase activities, even though one agent appeared to be an inhibitor of these very enzyme activities (332, 334, 336). Another putative insulin second messenger glycophospholipid that does not contain *myo*-inositol has also been described (240). The activity of at least eight different enzymes that are regulated by insulin appear to be affected by low molecular weight mediators (see 334, 376 for references). It is not known if any of these mediators contain a protease-sensitive peptide portion, but some might. The model of the anchoring structure for several cell surface proteins has many similarities to the hypothesized glycolipid mediators and there is a protease-sensitive region just distal to the glycolipid "anchoring" portion (83, 111, 227). This would suggest that the putative glycolipid mediator might be located on the external side of the plasma membrane, but in this location this "mediator" would not, however, fit easily into the currently suggested models.

A preliminary model has been proposed to link the phosphorylation of the insulin receptor to the release of insulin mediators (168). The mechanism of action of insulinomimetic proteases or the identity of possible substrates of the insulin receptor protein kinase (other than itself) are not known. Other than the regulation of several insulin-sensitive enzymes by phosphorylation-dephosphorylation reactions, no phosphoproteins are known to be definitely involved in protease- and insulin-mediated physiologic events. However, several phosphoproteins are candidates for involvement in hormone-regulated cell-growth or other functions (97), *e.g.*, the 32 kd ribosomal protein, S6 (78, 79, 157, 284, 285), a dexamethasone-enhanced, insulin-stimulated 120 kd liver protein (306), and the major protein-tyrosine kinase substrates of approximately 36 kd that were first observed to be retroviral $pp60^{src}$ substrates. Recently, the 36 kd substrates of $pp60^{src}$ have been found to be homologous to membrane proteins lipocortin I and II and part of calpactin I (39, 192, 205).

PROTEASE INDUCTION OF HEMOPOIETIC DIFFERENTIATION

Lymphoid Differentiation

Proteases can induce the expansion of primarily the B (and possibly a portion of the T) lymphocyte pool in cultures of mixed lymphocytes. This induction of cell proliferation may also be considered to be part of the induction of differentiation since the blastic transformation of resting lymphocytes into actively dividing cells is accompanied by the expression of specific differentiated functions (445). However, B cell proliferation can be stimulated independently of differentiation (121, 445). Reports of *in vivo* lymphocyte DNA synthesis and cell proliferation, but not differentiation, show that other factors, in addition to the cell proliferation, signal(s), are required for lymphocyte differentiation (445). Therefore, it is possible that exogenous proteases induce only lymphocyte proliferation and not differentiation. Additional evidence, obtained using serine-protease inhibitors, implicated membrane protease activity in the activation of lymphoid (B cells (20, 198) and cytotoxic T cells (277, 400)) as well as other non-erythroid hematopoietic cells such as neutrophils (102, 395), macrophages (259), and platelets (5). None of these activation processes appeared to involve DNA synthesis or cell proliferation, so that they may be considered examples of differentiation. However, irreversible commitment to differentiation was not shown, that is experiments in which a short exposure of an inducer followed by inducer withdrawal resulted in both the production of a differentiation product and the cessation of cell proliferation were not reported.

Erythroid Differentiation

Mouse Erythroleukemia (MEL) Cells and Other In Vitro Systems. In the early experiments testing the effect of proteases on erythroid differentiation, Rowley *et al.* (322) found that brief treatment (10 to 20 minutes) with trypsin, pronase, and chymotrypsin (as well as a nonproteolytic enzyme, phospholipase D) of suspensions of human adult marrow and fetal liver cells increased both the number and the size of erythroid bursts and/or colonies (322). In these seminal experiments, as with those reported earlier with lymphocyte systems as discussed above, the relationship between the stimulation of the multiplication of cells committed to a particular differentiation program as opposed to the stimulation of a differentiation program within individual cells, is not clear.

Nineteen different protease preparations (343) and carboxypeptidase A (344) were shown to stimulate hemoglobin synthesis, a marker for erythrodifferentiation, in rapidly proliferating Friend leukemia virus-infected MEL cells. These proteases were also shown to increase cell yield, but not the initial rate of cell proliferation (339). The characteristics of this stimulation depended upon the protease used, the time of exposure of the protease, the concentration of the protease, and the particular cell line (342). Treatment with various proteases yielded anywhere from 3% hemoglobin-containing (benzidine-stained, B^+) cells, as with plasmin or thrombin, to over 70% B^+ cells with chymotrypsin, whereas untreated cultures contained 0 to 1% B^+ cells. The protease-induced increase in the cell yield was shown to be due to a different mechanism than the protease stimulation of hemoglobin synthesis, since there were differences in several characteristics of these two processes.

The addition of dimethylsulfoxide (DMSO) (124), a known inducer of MEL cell differentiation as assayed by hemoglobin accumulation, at a concentration (0.25% v/v) that induced only about 2.5% of the culture to become B^+, acted synergistically in stimulating hemoglobin synthesis with all of the proteases tested. Several other low molecular weight inducers also acted synergistically with proteases in stimulating hemoglobin synthesis (Table 3) (344). These low molecular weight agents did not, however, act synergistically with proteases to increase cell yields. Butyrate, a member of a different class of inducers than DMSO (320, 346), did not act synergistically with proteases in stimulating hemoglobin synthesis. This finding is consistent with earlier reports that more than one mechanism is involved in the induction of MEL cell maturation (*e.g.*, 320).

Both erythroid as well as nonerythroid cells have now been found to be inducible by proteases, and the level of induction is also synergistically increased by the addition of suboptimal concentrations of some low molecular weight inducers. Seven of the proteases that were inducers of MEL cell hemoglobin synthesis were also tested on a human multilineage leukemia cell line, K562. All of these proteases induced K562 hemoglobin synthesis, and all but protease K stimulated its cell yield (341). Trypsin, papain, protease K, and protease V8 were the most effective. When added individually, they yielded between 25 and 44% B^+ cells over those present in untreated cultures. Hemin, a known potent low molecular weight inducer of hemoglobin synthesis in K562 cells at a relatively high concentration (60 μM), when added at a suboptimal inducing concentration (10 μM), acted synergistically with all of the proteases tested in augmenting hemoglobin synthesis, but as in MEL cells, not in augmenting cell yield. However, differences were found in the effects of other low molecular weight inducers, *i.e.*, although thymidine acted synergistically with protease V8 in inducing hemoglobin production in K562 cells, it did not do so with either trypsin or chymotrypsin. Cytosine arabinoside was found not to act synergistically with protease V8, the only protease with which it was tested. These results again suggest different modes of action for different inducers. However, it is of interest that the protease stimulation of hemoglobin synthesis did share some common features with the protease stimulation of cell yield.

K562 cells have not been shown to increase commitment to terminal differentiation after hemin treatment (94, 106, 321) above the low level of commitment that occurs spontaneously (3, 114). However, other low molecular weight inducers do commit K562 cells to terminal cell division (269, 321). With respect to the inability of hemin to induce commitment to terminal differentiation, K562 cells react similarly to MEL cells (146). The addition of trypsin during hemin treatment also did not induce commitment to terminal differentiation in K562 cell cultures (341). With the present data, it can be noted that proteases act differently than hemin in the production of hemoglobin in MEL cells since they act synergistically. However, in K562 cells, trypsin, at least, is similar to hemin in that it stimulates hemoglobin synthesis and does not commit the cells to terminal erythroid differentiation. This is in contradistinction to the finding that the one protease tested, chymotrypsin, was capable of committing MEL cells to terminal erythroid differentiation in the presence of a suboptimal inducing concentration of DMSO (0.25%) (noted in 343).

TABLE 3. SYNERGY IN INDUCTION OF DIFFERENTIATION BY A PROTEASE AND A LOW MOLECULAR WEIGHT INDUCER[a]

Low molecular weight inducer	Cell line		
	HL-60	K562	MEL
Actinomycin D	ND[b]	ND	+
AMS[c]	ND	ND	+
5-Azacytidine	ND	ND	+
Butyrate	+	+[d]	−
DMSO	+	−	+
Hemin	ND	+	+
HMBA	+	ND	+
Hypoxanthine	ND	ND	+
Retinoate	+	ND	ND

[a] Cells were grown with a protease with and without the addition of a low molecular weight inducer. The level of differentiation and synergy in its induction by the inducers added was determined (115, 341, 344).

[b] ND, not done.

[c] AMS, aminonucleoside of puromycin, *i.e*, 6-dimethylamino-9-(3′-amino-3′-deoxyribosyl) purine.

[d] K562 cells were grown with and without trypsin (0.3 mg/ml, Millipore Corporation, Bedford, Massachusetts) and/or butyrate (0.1 mM). After 5 days, untreated, trypsin-, butyrate-, and trypsin + butyrate-treated cultures contained 13, 33, 14, and 59% B^+ cells, respectively. The combination of trypsin plus butyrate yielded 12% more B^+ cells than expected, *i.e.*, the percentage of B^+ cells in the trypsin-treated cultures plus the percentage in the butyrate-treated cultures.

In addition to the induction of differentiation in some erythroid cells, exogenous proteases can also stimulate the mobilization of erythroid precursors (burst-forming units-erythroid) as well as pluripotent stem cells (colony-forming units-stem) or granulocyte/macrophage progenitors (colony-forming units-granulocyte/macrophage) from haemopoietic tissues into the peripheral blood (252, 415). In mice, intravenous administration of either trypsin or a crystalline bacterial protease was found to increase the concentration of these hemopoietic progenitor cells in the peripheral blood. Since the effect was observed rapidly (10 to 30 minutes), it was considered not to be due to differentiation, but to release of previously partially differentiated cells. These mobilized cells were committed since they then went on to fully differentiate in their new environment in the absence of specific added inducers.

Protease Site of Action. Proteases induce MEL cell differentiation and increase cell yield via their proteolytic action, since (a) a noncytotoxic protease inhibitor, aprotinin, inhibited the induction of both processes, and (b) heat-treated, heat-sensitive proteases failed to induce either process. Heat-treatment did not generate an inhibitor in the growth medium, since heat-treatment (in medium) of a heat-resistant protease, protease V8, did not inhibit its inducing capability. Other nonproteolytic proteins, such as albumin and erythropoietin, are not inducers and neither are the protease-related, but proteolytically inactive zymogens, α-chymotrypsinogen A and plasma plasminogen (343). Therefore, enzymatically active protease was required for induction. Induction of MEL cell differentiation by proteases appears to require cleavage of a cell-surface component(s) for several reasons. Protease induction takes place in serum-free medium (339). This medium did contain two potential protease substrates, albumin and insulin. However, protease treatment of serum-containing medium, which contains both albumin and insulin, followed by inactivation of the protease with either a non-toxic protease inhibitor (aprotinin) or by heat-treatment, did not activate an inducer. Therefore, it is not likely that either albumin or insulin served as precursors of an inducer by being a substrate for an added protease. Similar protease treatment of cell-conditioned medium (*i.e.*, medium in which untreated cells had grown for 3 days) also did not produce an inducer. However, in these experiments it was difficult to inactivate the proteolytic activity of the protease used since it was substantially protected by the serum present in the medium. The final amino acid products of protease degradation, (either individually or in mixtures), were shown not to be able to reproduce the protease induction, although a few amino acids were found to be weak inducers (339). Finally, it was shown that papain, when covalently linked to Sepharose beads, was capable of inducing erythrodifferentiation and that no significant amount of active papain was released from the beads during the induction period (367, E. A. Slosberg, B. M. Scher, W. Scher, and S. Waxman: Induction of differentiation in mouse erythroleukemia cells by the action of papain at the cell surface, submitted for publication). This methodology allowed a more clear-cut result than the pioneering studies of the induction of mitosis with immobilized trypsin and thrombin since in those experiments the latex (polystyrene) beads that were used as the immobilizing vehicle were small enough (926 nm diameter) to be endocytosed. Therefore, in those studies additional control experiments were performed in order to be certain that the proteases were acting on the cell surface and not intracellularly (see Ref. 52 for review). In summary, proteases do not induce differentiation by acting on a component of the medium to form an inducer and, therefore, must act on the cell or on a cell product. If the proteases act upon a cell product to form an inducer, the product must be bound to the outer surface of the cell where it is accessible, or it must be a labile product (or the inducer formed must be labile) since protease treatment of cell-conditioned media did not form a detectable inducer.

The initial mechanisms of action of physiologic erythroid inducers are not known other than that the inducers, burst-forming-unit erythroid (interleukin 3) and erythropoietin, presumably first bind to plasma membrane receptors, and that in MEL and K562 cells proteases act initially on the external surface of the plasma membrane. Erythropoietin is known to also increase cAMP and cGMP levels in rabbit bone marrow cell suspensions (27, 72, 317) apparently in a similar fashion to that in which hormones act on cell-surface receptors in other systems. In addition, the recently described homodimeric protein, erythroid differentiating factor (EDF), appears to act via a cell-surface receptor (W. Vale, personal communication, 1987) as suggested by Eto *et al.* (109). EDF is identical to both follicle-stimulating hormone-releasing protein (402) and to homoactivin (221), which can induce MEL cell erythrodifferentiation. Heteroactivin, a heterodimer, which is over 50% homologous to homoactivin (220), does not seem to have been tested for EDF activity yet. It is likely that heteroactivin could act as an EDF, since, like EDF, it possesses follicle-stimulating hormone-releasing protein activity (220).

Historically, it is of interest that EDF may also have been present in the human placental extract preparations that were previously shown to stimulate MEL cell differentiation (172, 378) or mouse erythropoiesis (179, see also 26). Not only has placenta been shown to contain inhibin, a heterodimer with one subunit identical with that of homoactivin (12, 241, 246), but EDF may also have been present in the preparations of prolactin that were shown to stimulate erythropoiesis (180) since inhibin, like prolactin, is present in the pituitary (303, 394, 402). Actually EDF may be responsible for at least a portion of the uncharacterized extrarenal erythropoietin activity (118, 126, 363, 446).

It is thought-provoking that MEL cells respond to EDF, but in general, appear to respond only weakly to erythropoietin (297, 298, 364), even though they possess specific erythropoietin receptors (242, 337). This may be because MEL cells produce their own erythropoietin, which might act as an autocrine factor to promote MEL cell replication in the absence of other differentiation inducers (73, 151, 381). Erythropoietin may be able only to potentiate differentiation in the presence of an inducer. However, erythroid cells "freshly" infected with Friend leukemia virus and therefore of low oncogenic potential, do respond well to erythropoietin, although they are generally altered in the presence of serum which could provide other factors (*e.g.*, see 196, 337, 364). K562 cells are not known to secrete erythropoietin, but evidentally can also respond weakly, in a possible synergistic fashion, to a combination of erythropoietin plus butyrate (126, 164).

Both K562 and HEL cells (also a human "erythroid" line), in addition to displaying erythroid characteristics, have characteristics typical of other hematopoietic lineages such as megakaryocytes. Both of these lines also appear to secrete a possible autocrine factor, PDGF (183, 275, 422). PDGF has erythropoietin-like activity (see 248) and like erythropoietin, is not known to have proteolytic activity. However, all of these protein factors and their cell-surface receptors are, presumably, protease-sensitive, and, therefore, could be regulated by proteases.

K-562 cells secrete at least two other protein growth factors which are probably protease-sensitive. One of these (the 20-kd leukemia-derived growth factor-I) is an autocrine factor (249). This growth factor contains ubiquitin (8.6 kd) which may "mark" it for rapid proteolytic degradation (see 418 for references). If such a growth factor bound to the surface of the cell were altered by an exogenous protease the cells might be directed away from a growth mode and toward a differentiation program.

It was also shown that transforming growth factor β-1, which has 36% amino acid homology to EDF (119, 238), does not stimulate MEL cell differentiation as EDF does (109). It is, however, capable of homoactivin (EDF)-like follicle-stimulating hormone-releasing activity (437). Therefore, it appears that transforming growth factor-β-1 acts on the same receptors as EDF does in the pituitary, but either not at all or on different receptors in MEL cells, as suggested by Eto *et al.* (109).

None of the protein erythroid inducers is known to have protease activity or to have sequence similarity with a protease although this has not been ruled out except for the case of erythropoietin (251). There are some apparent similarities in the mechanisms of action of these protein differentiation inducers and those of thrombin in inducing mitogenesis, as discussed above. Of the known inducers (approximately 300) of MEL cell differentiation (421), no specific initial step(s) in their mechanism of action has yet been identified. However, as discussed for the thrombin induction of mitogenesis, DMSO and some other known low molecular weight inducers also affect early alterations in the metabolism of possible second messengers such as phospholipids (110, 152, 315, 372, 447) and cAMP (*e.g.*, 63, 129, 323, 362).

Various inducers have different effects on the differentiation of MEL cells. Three major classes of inducers have been described: DMSO-like-acting, butyrate-like-acting, and hemin (320). One of the characteristics that varies upon induction is the ratio of hemoglobin major to hemoglobin minor with DMSO-like-acting agents inducing a high ratio, butyrate-like-acting agents a nearly equivalent amount of the two hemoglobins, and hemin inducing a low ratio. In this respect, all of the three proteases tested, chymotrypsin, trypsin, and protease V8, induced in a hemin-like fashion (342). This result is one of several that has complicated the simple classification of MEL cell inducers, since, hemin appears to have different inducing characteristics than the proteases, as shown by its ability to induce differentiation synergistically with them (344), while at the same time it induces a ratio of hemoglobin types similar to that induced by these proteases (342). Furthermore, it is possible that even different proteases induce by somewhat different mechanisms.

In addition to there being different capabilities in the level of differentiation by different proteases (343), different agents vary in their ability to inhibit differentiation induced by different proteases (346). This, again, indicates different mechanisms of induction. Dexamethasone (345 and see 346 for references) and PMA (see Refs. 127, 346, 431) are probably the two most highly studied inhibitors of induction of MEL cell differentiation. Dexamethasone substantially inhibited induction of MEL cell differentiation by chymotrypsin, but not by protease V8, whereas PMA inhibited protease V8 induction of differentiation more potently than that induced by chymotrypsin (346).

Other Proteases. Protease activities in differentiating erythroid cells have not been widely studied. One MEL cell line's (745) soluble acid-protease activity, that appears to be lysosomal, was shown to increase during the first 2 days of growth in fresh medium and to decrease late in butyrate-, DMSO-, or hexamethylene bisacetamide (HMBA)-induced differentiation (193). This activity did not change during DMSO treatment of a non-inducible line 745 variant, so that the change in activity appears to be correlated with the differentiation process.

A particle-associated ATP-dependent protease activity was shown to increase 2-fold in MEL cells after 4 days of treatment with 0.2 M (1.3%) DMSO, but not after induction of K562 cell differentiation with hemin (309). One of the ATP-dependent proteases identified in reticulocytes has some characteristics in common with this enzyme, but also differs in other aspects (309). Both proteases require a divalent cation and are inhibited by hemin or vanadate, but the reticulocyte enzyme is soluble. Therefore, the lack of increase in activity observed during hemin induction of K562 cell differentiation may have been due to direct inhibition of the protease activity by the exogenously supplied hemin.

A soluble ATP-dependent protease has also been identified in MEL cells, but the effect of differentiation on the activity of the enzyme has not been reported (419). This high molecular weight enzyme (approximately 600 kd) also appears to be inhibited by hemin. One of the ATP-dependent proteases in reticulocytes requires ubiquitin for activity (418). In contrast, MEL cells contain ubiquitin and can conjugate it to proteins, but ubiquitin was found not to be required for the MEL cell ATP-dependent proteolysis.

Another activity that may be associated with proteolysis has been reported in MEL cells. Several apparently related fluoride-inhibitable, fatty acid ester, neutral-acting esterases that are present both in lysosomal-like granules and in the cytoplasm (possibly due to release from lysosomes during staining), have been reported to increase during the induction of differentiation in certain, but not all, MEL sublines (117, 340). It is not known if these esterases are proteolytic, but they do cleave several types of esters, including both fatty acid esters and naphthol AS-D chloracetate (340). These two activities reside within the same isozyme molecules in mouse erythrocytes, giving these enzymes broader specificities than those of the analogous enzymes in human erythrocytes that preferentially cleave only one or the other of these two types of substrates (see 340 for references). Several other proteases have been detected in undifferentiated MEL cells, but changes in their activities during differentiation have not been reported (420). In addition, several proteases detected in mature non-nucleated erythroid cells have not been studied in nucleated erythroid cells (247).

The activity of one protease, plasminogen activator, is known to be affected in MEL cells by an inhibitor of differentiation, PMA (432). PMA, as noted above, is a tumor promoter. At concentrations that are not markedly cytotoxic, PMA inhibits the induction of MEL cell differentiation by DMSO and several other (346) inducers tested (see Ref. 431 for review). It should, therefore, reverse the reduction in the oncogenic potential of the cells due to DMSO treatment, *i.e.*, PMA treatment should make DMSO-treated cells more oncogenic since DMSO treatment reduces MEL cell oncogenic potential (124). However, this possibility does not seem to have been tested. PMA treatment increased plasminogen activator activity extracellulary within 6 hour in cultures of PMA-sensitive MEL cell clones, but not in cultures of PMA-resistant clones (also see Ref. 114). It is not known if this activity is altered during simultaneous treatment with both an inducer such as DMSO and an inhibitor such as PMA. However, since DMSO not only induces MEL cell differentiation, but also reduces the malignant potential of these cells (124) as well as that of other tumor cells (*e.g.*, 271), and reduces both cell-associated and released urokinase type plasminogen activator activity within 6 hours in a non-erythroid cell line, human carcinoma HEp-3 cells (271), there appears to be no simple relationship between plasminogen activator levels and differentiation.

PMA has other effects on MEL cells that appear to involve a protease activity. It increases the adhesiveness of the cells to the surface of the culture dish (adherence) and to each other (agglutination) (114). The increase in adhesiveness was detected after only 30 minutes of treatment. Two inhibitors of trypsin-like proteases, pentamidine isethionate and TPCK, inhibited both PMA-induced adherence and agglutination. PMA treatment rapidly increased a cellular protease activity that acted at alkaline pH. Pentamide isethionate inhibited this proteolytic activity. HMBA induction of erythroid differentiation decreased both PMA-induced cell adhesion and the proteolytic activity. Therefore, it appears that this serine-like alkaline proteolytic activity may be associated with the regulation of MEL cell differentiation (114).

Some of the effects that PMA has on MEL cells appear to resemble its effects on other cell lines. In human erythroleukemia cells, PMA induces adherence of the cells to the culture dish and inhibition of maturation along the erythroid path, but also induces macrophage-like morphology and function (99, 125, 274). With K562 cells, PMA induces cell adherence to plastic in some (374), but not all (99, and see Ref. 100), sublines and inhibits erythroid differentiation (120, 274, 409), while at the same time it induces granulocyte-monocyte characteristics and some megakaryocyte characteristics (130, 377, 387). In HL-60 cells, PMA also induces cell adherence and an increase in plasminogen activator activity as it induces monocyte/macrophage-like maturation (194). However, the effect of PMA on either plasminogen activator activity or other proteases in the "erythroleukemic" cell lines does not seem to have been studied.

GRANULOCYTE AND MONOCYTIC/ MACROPHAGE DIFFERENTIATION

HL-60 Cells. HL-60 cells (a human myeloid multilineage leukemia cell line, 392) are induced to undergo granulocytic differentiation by trypsin (115) as well as low molecular weight inducers such as DMSO. Chymotrypsin, elastase, and collagenase (but not plasmin, pepsin, papain, streptokinase, or urokinase) also induced granulocytic differentiation in this line (115). By changing the medium and adding fresh protease inducer, macrophage differentiation was seen after 10 to 14 days. A summary of the types of proteases that have been found to induce differentiation in hematopoietic cell lines is presented in Table 4. Several of the characteristics of protease HL-60 cell induction are similar to those of protease-induced erythrodifferentiation, such as synergism in induction by proteases and low molecular weight inducers (Table 3), increased "late" cell yield, requirement for continuous protease activity for maximal induction of differentiation, lack of (or reduced) requirement for serum in the medium for protease induction, and inhibition of protease induction by a protease inhibitor (in the HL-60 studies, SBTI). Other myelocytic and monocytic cell lines as well as cells from patients with acute myeloid leukemia were also inducible by trypsin (115).

Chemotaxis. Thrombin, which is both a mitogen for several cell lines and a weak differentiation inducer in MEL cells (343), has not, evidently, been tested for its effect on differentiation in HL-60 cells. However, it has been found to induce chemotaxis in these cells after they have undergone 1,25-dihydroxy-vitamin D_3-induced monocytic/macrophage-like differentiation (16), as it did in peripheral blood monocyte and J774 cells (see 18). Also, this effect in HL-60 cells apparently did not require the proteolytic activity of thrombin, but only a fragment of thrombin that was proteolytically inactive.

Plasminogen Activator. In contrast to its inhibition of induced MEL, human erythroleukemia, and K562 cell erythrodifferentiation, PMA induces monocytic/macrophage-like differentiation of HL-60 cells, as it does in other human leukemia cell lines. This type of differentiation is characterized by adherence of the cells to the substratum. PMA induced both cell-associated and released plasminogen activator activity in HL-60 cells (194). The prevention of PMA-induced cell adherence (*e.g.*, by continuous shaking) also prevented the increase in plasminogen activator activity, and therefore, the increase in proteolytic activity was considered to be a consequence of the adherence and related to the differentiation process. PMA-stimulates an increase in plasminogen activator activity in many cell types (8, 29, 113, 331) including MEL cells. The level of plasminogen activator activity is increased in many tumors and malignant cell lines and may correlate with tissue invasiveness and the capacity to metastasize (review 75, 92, 182,

TABLE 4. PROTEASE INDUCTION OF DIFFERENTIATION[a]

Cell type	Differentiation	Protease type			
		Acid	Metallo	Serine	Thiol
HL-60, human	Granulocytic	–[b]	±[c]	+	–[d]
HL-60, human	Macrophage	–[b]	±[c]	+	–[d]
K562, human	Erythroid	ND[e]	+	+	+
MEL, mouse	Erythroid	ND	+	+	+

[a] Cells were grown with and without a protease for 5 days (or more for macrophage differentiation) and the level of differentiation determined (115, 341, 343).
[b] Only pepsin tested.
[c] Only collagenase (clostridiopeptidase A) tested.
[d] Papain and streptokinase tested.
[e] ND, not done.

316, 331). However, since PMA can either induce or inhibit differentiation (thereby generally decreasing or increasing malignant potential, respectively) in the same cell lines that it induces plasminogen activator activity, there does not appear to be a strict correlation between the induction of this activity and either malignant potential or cell differentiation. Furthermore, two potent inducers of HL-60 cell granulocytic differentiation have the opposite effects on the amount of plasminogen activator activity released from the cells, i.e., retinoate (RA) stimulates, and DMSO inhibits, the amount released (131).

Other Proteases. Nonerythroid myeloid cells contain several proteases that may be associated with the differentiated state (see 159, 237, 296, 380, 428). Specific relationships to differentiation are most easily studied in differentiation-inducible cell lines. PMA has not only been shown to induce monocyte/macrophage-like characteristics and plasminogen activator activity in HL-60 cells, but, in addition, the activity of two other proteases: procoagulent activity (PCA, tissue factor, thromboplastin, factor III) (204) and cathespin B (48). PCA is also induced in monocytic cells that do not have granulocytic characteristics. PCA was first shown to be induced by PMA in white blood cells (human granulocytes and myeloblasts) (229) where it is considered to be a characteristic of monocyte-macrophage differentiation (see 228 for references). PCA was also shown to be present in HL-60 cells (439) where it is rapidly (within 8 hours) and markedly increased during PMA induction along the monocyte/macrophage path, whereas DMSO induction along the granulocytic path resulted in only a slight and delayed increase (204). The increase in PCA is one of the earliest known changes in HL-60 cells after PMA induction although more rapid effects are known such as the increase in neopterin and biopterin levels (359). In an apparently similar fashion (although a time course has not been reported) PMA, but not DMSO, treatment increased both the synthesis and activity of cathespin B in HL-60 cells (48). It is of interest that dexamethasone reduced the PMA-induced production of cathepsin B in this system, whereas in the MEL cell system, PMA and dexamethasone have generally similar phenotypic effects.

HL-60 cells, as MEL cells, contain fluoride-inhibitable nonspecific fatty acid ester esterase isozymes. It is not known whether or not these isozymes have proteolytic activity, but their esterase activity is markedly increased during monocyte/macrophage-like differentiation during growth in the presence of PMA (319, 440). At least some of these nonspecific esterases may actually be proteases, but even if they are not, they appear to be activated by a protease(s). In the study by Yourno *et al.* (440) evidence was presented that although PMA treatment increased the activities of these esterases, it did not increase the synthesis of their zymogens. Therefore, it was postulated that the PMA-dependent event that increased the activities of these esterases was the activation of their zymogens. If true, this presumably would occur due to protease action on the zymogens (440).

One extracellular serine esterase that appears to physiologically alter the cellular function of neutrophils is leukocyte migration inhibition factor (316). Leukocyte migration inhibition factor (approximately 68 kd) is produced by antigen-stimulated lymphocytes and may be a protease since it acts on esters that are trypsin substrates. Leukocyte migration inhibition factor halts the random migratory activity of polymorphonuclear leukocytes, presumably at a site of inflammation, where the neutrophils can undertake anti-inflammatory action. This could be considered to be a late step in neutrophil maturation. It is not known if macrophage inhibition factor (MIF) is an esterase. MIF, which has been found to consist of at least two moieties of approximately 25 and 55 kd, is also produced by lymphocytes, but it decreases macrophage, rather than PMN, migration. In testing MIF for esterase activity, it was found that serine protease inhibitors enhanced MIF activity. This was thought to be due to the inhibition of macrophage surface protease activity which otherwise would degrade MIF.

One protease that HL-60 cells do not seem to elaborate is collagenase (17). However, these cells do produce a collagenase inhibitor in response to monocyte/macrophage-like induction by either PMA or 1,25-dihydroxyvitamin D_3 (17). The relationship of the collagenase inhibitor to the regulation of differentiation is not known, but it has sequence similarity to the human tissue inhibitor of metalloproteinase and to human erythroid potentiating activity (see 373 and 128 for references), as well as to portions of avian, bovine, mouse, and human retroviral *gag* proteins, human granulocyte-macrophage colony stimulating factor (278), the mouse fibroblast growth-responsive gene, 16C8, and the 3′-end of mouse β-interferon (104). Since this factor potentiates erythroid precursor cell proliferation, it may play a role in white cell-mediated or infection-induced anemia. That is, it may block protease-induced erythrodifferentiation until a substantial number of erythroid precursor cells are available for subsequent maturation processes, which may then in turn be stimulated by proteases. On the other hand, it may play a role in ameliorating this type of anemia as a human erythroid potentiating activity. Human erythroid potentiating activity could act on a membrane protease, as has been shown for some activities of Bowman-Birk protease inhibitors on mouse C3H/$10_{T1/2}$ fibroblasts (433, 434).

Protease Site of Action. The site of action of proteases in their induction of HL-60 and myeloid cell maturation is unknown. A plasma membrane site appears to be most likely just as it does in MEL cells (367, E. A. Slosberg, B. M. Scher, W. Scher, and S. Waxman: Induction of differentiation in mouse erythroleukemia cells by the action of papain at the cell surface, submitted for publication). It has been reported that RA acts at the plasma membrane of HL-60 cells because RA, putatively covalently linked through its carbonyl moiety to glass beads or polystyrene by a carbodiimide reaction, induced cell differentiation without being released or internalized (436). This report, however, has been considered controversial. As pointed out by Breitman (T. R. Breitman, personal communication, 1986), polystyrene does not have amino groups so that carboxyl groups cannot be linked to it via the well-described carbodiimide reaction stipulated. In addition, the carboxyl group of RA appears to be essential for maximum inducer activity, since inducers lacking this group, *e.g.*, retinal and retinol, are not as potent (32, 33, 34, 166, 435 for other references). It is possible that free RA was left in the culture dishes after the coupling reaction when washed with phosphate-buffered saline (which is not a solvent of RA) and then 50% ethanol (which may not be a sufficiently powerful solvent of RA). A more appropriate wash solution would be methanol, or serum containing-medium.

Several of the same cell-associated moieties that have been implicated in the regulation of the transmembrane signals produced during the induction of MEL cell differentiation or the thrombin induction of mitogenesis (as well as the thrombin activation of platelets) have also been suggested as mediators of the induced differentiation of HL-60 and other myeloid cells. These include cAMP (33), phospholipids (51), protein kinase C (399) as activated by PMA (see 51), and prostaglandins and other arachidonate metabolites (133). Trypsin also induces an increase in cAMP in rat thymocytes (358). It appears that similar agents are involved in these various processes, but that they have different or even opposite effects in different systems. These differences may be due to the production of different intracellular second messenger molecules (332) and/or different levels or ratios of these putative messengers in the various systems. If the internalization of a membrane receptor or a receptor fragment (291) plays a role in the intracellular signal, then it may interact with some of the other proposed second messenger moieties.

HL-60 and similar cells secrete protein factors that are known to act in an autocrine fashion (7, 35, 248, 273, 279, 286, 438), which has not been shown in MEL and K562 cells. These factors are not known to have protease activity, but they are possible protease substrates. Therefore, the modification of an autocrine factor by a protease inducer could play a role in induction, e.g., by "steering" the cell away from cell replication.

Other protein inducers of HL-60 cell differentiation are known, but their relationship to proteases, if any, is not yet characterized (101, 144, 145, 170, 218).

SUMMARY

Proteases have been shown to be capable of inducing two of the most fundamental biologic processes: mitogenesis and cellular differentiation. Their proteolytic activity has been the most widely studied enzymatic activity implicated in inducing these processes. Protease induction of mitogenesis is a major system for studying the control of this process and studies of possible transmembrane signals have been initiated. Proteases have only recently begun to be used as tools for probing the induction of differentiation, but at least three cell line systems have been studied.

Extracellular proteases such as thrombin may play physiologic roles in inducing mitogenesis in vivo as suggested by several laboratories. Although the amount of data bearing on the similar possibility of the induction of differentiation by extracellular proteases is negligible, it remains a possibility. For example, macrophages not only have surface-bound proteases (6), but also release proteases (261, 308) as well as cytokines. Any of these agents, individually or in combination, may play a role in inducing erythroid differentiation *in vivo* and may provide a raison d'etre for the "blood islands" consisting of erythroblasts surrounding a "nurse" macrophage which are so frequently seen in bone marrow.

ADDENDUM

Hematopoietic cell lines, other than MEL cells, that are induced to differentiate by proteases also produce other autocrine factors for growth (K562 cells) (249) and differentiation (HL-60 cells) (97a). The growth factor for K-562 cells is a protein (249) and it and/or its hypothetical receptor could be subject to control by proteolytic degradation. The factors produced by HL-60 cells have not been characterized yet. However, the synthesis and the secretion of a protease, cathespin D, have recently been reported to occur in HL-60 cells and to be increased during induction of differentiation (370a). This protease might act in an autocrine fashion on growth and/or differentiation. The molecular weight of its mature form, 31 kd, is perhaps coincidentally, similar to those of some other growth factors that act on, and/or are released by, hematopoietic elements (see Refs. 35, 272, 279).

Specific receptors for a protease, human urokinase, which have been demonstrated on monocytic cells and A431 epidermal carcinoma cells as discussed (6, 87, 371, 407), have now been shown by Del Rosso et al. (96a) to be present on MEL cells. In addition, urokinase was observed to increase the induction of differentiation due to HMBA, and to shorten the period of time required for HMBA to induce commitment to terminal differentiation (96a). An earlier report found urokinase to be ineffective in stimulating MEL cell differentiation (343). Del Rosso *et al.* (96a) were able to demonstrate these effects of urokinase apparently by reducing both the plasminogen present in the serum supplement of the cell growth medium and the serum concentration.

A protein inducer of MEL cell differentiation, EDF, has been found to rapidly increase cytosolic calcium, cellular diacylglycerol, and phosphoinositide turnover (363a) in an apparently similar fashion to thrombin action (60, 219, 225, 232, 276, 300, 396). These effects were rapid (occurring in seconds to minutes) and the increase in calcium was transient so these findings do not necessarily conflict with the earlier reported DMSO-induced decreases in calcium levels (110a) and phosphoinositide turnover which were observed after a few hours (110, 152).

Acknowledgments: I would like to thank Dr. Samuel Waxman for his encouragement during the preparation of this article, Drs. Waxman, George Coppola, and Barbara M. Scher for critical reading of the manuscript, and Joreatha Jones-Martin for typing the manuscript.

This work was supported in part by the Chemotherapy Foundation and a grant from the National Cancer Institute.

REFERENCES

1. Akiyama SK, Yamada KM: Synthetic peptides competitively inhibit both direct binding to fibroblasts and functional biological assays for the purified cell-binding domain of fibronectin. J Biol

Chem 260:10402, 1985

2. Aktories K, Jakobs KH: N_i-mediated inhibition of human platelet adenylate cyclase by thrombin. Eur J Biochem 145:333, 1984
3. Alder S, Ciampi A, McCulloch EA: A kinetic and clonal analysis of heterogeneity in K562 cells. J Cell Physiol 118:186, 1984
4. Amenta JS, Brocher SC: Mechanisms of protein turnover in cultured cells. Life Sci 28:1195, 1981
5. Aoki N, Naito K, Yoshida N: Inhibition of platelet aggregation by protease inhibitors: possible involvement of proteases in platelet aggregation. Blood 52:1, 1978
6. Appella E, Robinson EA, Ullrich SJ, Stoppelli MP, Corti A, Cassani G, Blasi F: The receptor-binding sequence of urokinase. A biological function for the growth-factor module of proteases. J Biol Chem 262:4437, 1987
7. Ascensao JL, Mickman JK: Differentiation of human leukemic cell lines (HL60, U937) toward macrophages is accompanied by production of colony-stimulating activity (CSA). Exp Hematol 12:177, 1984
8. Ashino-Fuse H, Opdenakker G, Fuse A, Billiau A: Mechanism of the stimulatory effect of phorbol 12-myristate 13-acetate on cellular production of plasminogen activator. Proc Soc Exp Biol Med 176:109, 1984
9. Awbrey BJ, Hoak JC, Owen WG: Binding of human thrombin to cultured human endothelial cells. J Biol Chem 254:4092, 1979
10. Baenziger NL, Brodie GN, Majerus PW: A thrombin-sensitive protein of human platelet membranes. Proc Natl Acad Sci USA 68:240, 1971
11. Baker JB, Simmer RL, Glenn KC, Cunningham DD: Thrombin and epidermal growth factor become linked to cell surface receptors during mitogenic stimulation. Nature 278:473, 1979
12. Bandivdekar AH, Vijayalakshimi S, Jaswaney VL, Sheth AR: Inhibin in human placenta. Indian J Exp Biol 19:744, 1981
13. Barnes D, Sato G: Serum-free cell culture: a unifying approach. Cell 22:649, 1980
14. Bar-Shavit R, Kahn AJ, Mann KG, Wilner GD: Identification of a thrombin sequence with growth factor activity on macrophages. Proc Natl Acad Sci USA 83:976, 1986
15. Bar-Shavit R, Kahn AJ, Mann KG, Wilner GD: Growth-promoting effects of esterolytically inactive thrombin on macrophages. J Cell Biochem 32:261, 1986
16. Bar-Shavit R, Kahn AJ, Wilner GD: Chemotactic response to thrombin in HL-60 cells: Correlation with increased cytoskeletal actin. J Cell Biol 99:No. 4, Pt 2, No. 1027, p 279a, 1984
17. Bar-Shavit R, Teitelbaum SL, Stricklin GP, Eisen AZ, Kahn AJ, Welgus HG: Differentiation of a human leukemia cell line and expression of collagenase inhibitor. Proc Natl Acad Sci USA 82:5380, 1985
18. Bar-Shavit R, Wilner GD: Biologic activities of nonenzymatic thrombin: elucidation of a macrophage interactive domain. Semin Thromb Hemost 12:244, 1986
19. Becherer PR, Mertz LF, Baenziger NI: Regulation of prostaglandin synthesis mediated by thrombin and B2 bradykinin receptors in a fibrosarcoma cell line. Cell 30:243, 1982
20. Becker EL, Unanue ER: The requirement for esterase activity in the antimmunoglobulin-triggered movement of B lymphocytes. J Immunol 117:27, 1976
21. Bergmann JS, Carney DH: Receptor-bound thrombin is not internalized through coated pits in mouse embryo cells. J Cell Biochem 20:247, 1982
22. Berridge MJ: Inositol triphosphate and diacylglycerol as second messengers. Biochem J 220:345, 1984
23. Bing D, Laura R: A computer-generated three-dimensional model of the B chain of bovine alpha-thrombin. Ann NY Acad Sci 370:496, 1981
24. Blomback B, Hessel B, Hogg D, Claesson G: Substrate specificity of thrombin on proteins and synthetic substrates. In Chemistry and Biology of Thrombin, edited by Lundblad RL, Fenton JW II, Mann KG, p 275. Ann Arbor, Michigan, Ann Arbor Science Publishers Inc, 1977
25. Blumberg PM, Robbins PW: Effect of proteases on activation of resting chick embryo fibroblasts and on cell surface proteins. Cell 6:137, 1975
26. Boime I, Boguslawski S, Caine J: The translation of a human placental lactogen mRNA fraction in heterologous cell-free systems: the synthesis of a possible precursor. Biochem Biophys Res Commun 62:103, 1975
27. Bonanou-Tzedaki SA, Setchenska MS, Arnstein HRV: Stimulation of the adenylate cyclase activity of rabbit bone marrow immature erythroblasts by erythropoietin and haemin. Eur J Biochem 155:363, 1986
28. Bormann B-J, Huang C-K, Lam GF, Jaffe EA: Thrombin-induced vimentin phosphorylation in cultured human umbilical vein endothelial cells. J Biol Chem 261:10471, 1986
29. Bosman F, Opdenakker G, Van Damme J, Billiau A: Phorbol ester stimulates the synthesis and phosphorylation of a 48 kDa-intracellular protein in plasminogen activator secreting melanoma cells. Biochem Biophys Res Commun 137:263, 1986
30. Boyle MDP, Young M: Nerve growth factor: activation of the classical complement pathway by specific substitution for component CI. Proc Natl Acad Sci USA 79:2519, 1982
31. Brass LF, Laposata M, Banga HS, Rittenhouse SE: Regulation of the phosphoinositide hydrolysis pathology in thrombin-stimulated platelets by a pertussis toxin-sensitive guanine nucleotide-binding protein: evaluation of its contribution to platelet activation and comparison with the adenylate cyclase inhibitory protein G_i. J Biol Chem 261:16838, 1986
32. Breitman TR: Induction of terminal differentiation of HL-60 and fresh leukemic cells by retinoic acid. In Expression of Differentiated Functions in Cancer Cells, edited by Revoltella RP, Pontieri GM, Basilico C, Rovera G, Gallo RC, Subak-Sharpe JH, p 257. New York, Raven Press, 1982
33. Breitman TR, Keene BR, Hemmi H: Retinoic acid-induced differentiation of fresh human leukemia cells and the human myelomonocytic leukemia cell lines, HL-60, U-937, and THP-1, Cancer Surv 2:263, 1983
34. Breitman TR, Selonick SE, Collins SJ: Induction of differentiation of the human promyelocytic leukemia cell line (HL-60) by retinoic acid. Proc Natl Acad Sci USA 77:2936, 1980
35. Brennan JK, Abboud CN, DiPersio JF, Barlow GH, Lichtman MA: Autostimulation of growth by human myelogenous leukemia cells (HL-60). Blood 58:803, 1981
36. Brown M, Kiehn D: Protease effects on specific growth properties of normal and transformed baby hamster kidney cells. Proc Natl Acad Sci USA 74:2874, 1977
37. Brown RL, Clark RW, Chiu J-K, Stubblefield E: Protease activation of G1 nuclei isolated from Chinese hamster fibroblasts. Exp Cell Res 104:207, 1977
38. Brown RL, Stubblefield E: Enhancement of DNA synthesis in a mammalian cell-free system by trypsin treatment. Proc Natl Acad Sci USA 71:2432, 1974
39. Brugge JS: The p35/p36 substrates of protein-tyrosine kinases as inhibitors of phospholipase A_2. Cell 46:149, 1986
40. Bruhn HD: On the biochemistry of tumor cell thrombosis: thrombin acts as growth hormone. Behring Inst Mitt 79:31, 1986
41. Buchanan JM, Chen LB, Zetter BR: Reaction of thrombin with fibroblasts and mouse splenocytes. In Chemistry and Biology of Thrombin, edited by Lundblad RL, Fenton JW II, Mann KG, p 519. Ann Arbor, Michigan, Ann Arbor Science Publishers Inc., 1977
42. Buchanan JM, Chen LB, Zetter BR: Are high-molecular weight glycoproteins regulators of cellular growth? Ann NY Acad Sci 312:293, 1978
43. Burger MM: Proteolytic enzymes initiating cell division and escape from contact inhibition of growth. Nature 227:170, 1970
44. Burger MM: Changes in the chemical architecture of transformed cell surfaces: In Permeability and Function of Biological Membranes, edited by Katchalsky A, Keynes RD, Loewenstein WR, Pethica BA, p 107. Amsterdam, North-Holland Publishing Co Inc, 1970
45. Burger MM: Surface changes detected by lectins and implications for growth regulation in normal and in transformed cells. In Biomembranes, Vol 2, edited by Manson LA, p 247, New York, Plenum Press, 1971
46. Burger MM: The significance of surface structure changes for growth control under crowded conditions. In Growth Control in Cell Cultures, Ciba FDN Symposium, edited by Wolstenholme GEW, Knight J, p 45. Edinburgh, Churchill Livingstone, 1971
47. Burger MM: Surface changes in transformed cells detected by lectins. Fed Proc 32:91, 1973
48. Burnett D, Crocker J, Vaughan ATM: Synthesis of cathepsin B by cells derived from the HL60 promyelocytic leukaemia cell line. J Cell Physiol 115:249, 1983

49. Burwen SJ, Jones AL: The association of polypeptide hormones and growth factors with the nuclei of target cells. Trends Biochem Sci 4:159, 1987
50. Butkowski RJ, Elion J, Downing MR, Mann KG: Primary structure of human prethrombin 2 and α-thrombin. J Biol Chem 252:4942, 1977
51. Cabot MC, Welsh CJ, Callaham MF, Huberman E: Alterations in lipid metabolism induced by 12-O-tetradecanoylphorbol-13-acetate in differentiating human myeloid leukemia cells. Cancer Res 40:3674, 1980
52. Carney DH: Characterization of the thrombin receptor and its involvement in initiation of cell proliferation. In Control of Animal Cell Proliferation, Vol 2, edited by Boynton AL, Leffert HL, p 265. New York, Academic Press, Inc, 1987
53. Carney DH, Bergmann JS: ^{125}I-Thrombin binds to clustered receptors on noncoated regions of mouse embryo cell surfaces. J Cell Biol 95:697, 1982
54. Carney DH, Cunningham DD: Initiation of chick cell division by trypsin action at the cell surface. Nature 268:602, 1977
55. Carney DH, Cunningham DD: Transmembrane action of thrombin initiates chick cell division. J Supramol Struct 9:337, 1978
56. Carney DH, Cunningham DD: Cell surface action of thrombin is sufficient to initiate division of chick cells. Cell 14:811, 1978
57. Carney DH, Cunningham DD: Role of specific cell surface receptors in thrombin-stimulated cell division. Cell 15:1341, 1978
58. Carney DH, Glenn KC, Cunningham DD: Conditions which affect initiation of animal cell division by trypsin and thrombin. J Cell Physiol 95:13, 1978
59. Carney DH, Herbosa GJ, Stiernberg J, Bergmann JS, Gordon EA, Scott D, Fenton JW II: Double-signal hypothesis for thrombin initiation of cell proliferation. Semin Thromb Hemost 12:231, 1986
60. Carney DH, Scott DL, Gordon EA, Labelle EF: Phosphoinositides in mitogenesis: neomycin inhibits thrombin-stimulated phosphoinositide turnover and initiation of cell proliferation. Cell 42:479, 1985
61. Carney DH, Stiernberg J, Fenton JW II: Initiation of proliferative events by human α-thrombin requires both receptor binding and enzymic activity. J Cell Biochem 26:181, 1984
62. Chang J-Y: The structures and proteolytic specificities of autolysed human thrombin. Biochem J 240:797, 1986
63. Chapman LF: Changes in cyclic nucleotide levels during erythroid differentiation in Friend leukemia cells. Exp Cell Res 135:415, 1981
64. Chen K, Simpson I, Lorand L: Specificity of thrombin-like enzymes. In Chemistry and Biology of Thrombin, edited by Lundblad RL, Fenton II JW, Mann KG, p 297. Ann Arbor, Michigan, Ann Arbor Science Publishers Inc., 1977
65. Chen LB, Buchanan JM: Mitogenic activity of blood components. I. Thrombin and prothrombin. Proc Natl Acad Sci USA 72:131, 1975
66. Chen LB, Teng NNH, Buchanan JM: The mitogenic activity and related effects of thrombin on chick embryo fibroblasts. In Proteases and Biological Control, Cold Spring Harbor Conference on Cell Proliferation, Vol 2, edited by Reich E, Rifkin DB, Shaw E, p 957. Cold Spring Harbor, New York, Cold Spring Harbor Laboratory, 1975
67. Chen LB, Teng NNH, Buchanan JM: Mitogenicity of thrombin and surface alterations on mouse splenocytes. Exp Cell Res 101:41, 1976
68. Deleted in proof.
69. Cheng K, Larner J: Intracellular mediators of insulin action. Annu Rev Physiol 47:405, 1985
70. Cherqui G, Caron M, Capeau J, Lascols O, Wicek D, Picard J: Insulin activation of a membrane proteolytic step at the postreceptor level. In Regulatory Peptides in Digestive, Nervous and Endocrine Systems, INSERM Symp No. 25, edited by Lewin MJM, Bonfils S, p 205. Amsterdam, Elsevier North-Holland Biomedical Press, 1985
71. Cherqui G, Caron M, Capeau J, Picard J: Further evidence for the involvement of a membrane proteolytic step in insulin action. Biochem J 227:137, 1985
72. Chiuini F, Della Torre G, Fano G, Viti A: Early increase of cyclic adenosine monophosphate level induced by erythropoietin on rabbit bone marrow cell suspensions. Acta Haematol (Basel) 61:251, 1979
73. Choppin J, Egrié J, Casadevall N, Lacombe C, Muller O, Varet B: Biochemical analyses of murine erythropoietin from plasma and from cloned erythroleukemia cells. Exp Hematol 15:171, 1987
74. Chou I-N, Black PH, Roblin R: Effects of protease inhibitors on growth of 3T3 and SV3T3 cells. In Cold Spring Harbor Symposium on Control of Proliferation in Animal Cells, edited by Clarkson B, Baserga R., p 339. Cold Spring Harbor, New York, Cold Spring Harbor Laboratory, 1974
75. Christman JK, Silverstein SC, Acs G: Plasminogen activators. In Proteases in Mammalian Cells and Tissues, edited by Barrett AJ, p 91. Amsterdam, Elsevier/North-Holland Biomedical Press, 1977
76. Clark S, Larkins RG, De Luise M, Melick RA: The effects of trypsin and phospholipase C on insulin binding and action in the isolated adipocyte. Biochem J 186:535, 1980
77. Clouse LH, Comp PC: The regulation of hemostasis: the protein C system. N Engl J Med 314:1298, 1986
78. Cobb MH: An insulin-stimulated ribosomal protein S6 kinase in 3T3-L1 cells. J Biol Chem 261:12994, 1986
79. Cobb MH, Borr JG, Linder ME, Gray TB, Gregory JS: A similar ribosomal protein S6 kinase activity is found in insulin-treated 3T3-L1 cells and chick embryo fibroblasts transformed by Rous sarcoma virus. Biochem Biophys Res Commun 137:702, 1986
80. Cockle SM, Dean RJ: Derangement of regulation of protein degradation in transforming fibroblasts. Biosci Rep 2:102, 1982
81. Cohen S, Wong R, Gutowski J, Goldfarb RH: The cytoplasmic protein (ADR) that triggers DNA synthesis in interleukin 2-stimulated lymphocytes appears to be a protease. 6th Internatl Cong Immunol 2.65.41, 236, 1986
82. Connolly TM, Bansal VS, Bross TE, Irvine RF, Majerus PW: The metabolism of tris- and tetraphosphates of inositol by 5-phosphomonoesterase and 3-kinase enzymes. J Biol Chem 262:2146, 1987
83. Cross GAM: Eukaryotic protein modification and membrane attachment via phosphatidylinositol. Cell 48:179, 1987
84. Cuatrecasas P: Interaction of insulin with the cell membrane: the primary action of insulin. Proc Natl Acad Sci USA 63:450, 1969
85. Cuatrecasas P: Perturbation of the insulin receptor of isolated fat cells with proteolytic enzymes: direct measurement of insulin-receptor interactions. J Biol Chem 246:6522, 1971
86. Cuatrecasas P: Hormone receptors, membrane phospholipids, and protein kinases. Harvey Lect 80:89, 1986
87. Cubellis MV, Nolli ML, Cassani G, Blasi F: Binding of single-chain prourokinase to the urokinase receptor of U937 cells. J Biol Chem 261:15819, 1986
88. Cunningham DD, Ho T-S: Effects of added proteases on concanavalin A-specific agglutinability and proliferation of quiescent fibroblasts. In Proteases and Biological Control, Cold Spring Harbor Conference on Cell Proliferation, edited by Reich E, Rifkin DB, Shaw E, Vol 2, p 795. Cold Spring Harbor, New York, Cold Spring Harbor Laboratory, 1975
89. Cunningham DD, Van Nostrand WE, Farrell DH, Campbell CH: Interactions of serine proteases with cultured fibroblasts. J Cell Biochem 32:281, 1986
90. Czech MP: The nature and regulation of the insulin receptor: structure and function. Annu Rev Physiol 47:357, 1985
91. Daniel TO, Gibbs VC, Milfay DF, Garovoy MR, Williams LT: Thrombin stimulates c-*sis* gene expression in microvascular endothelial cells. J Biol Chem 261:9579, 1986
92. Danø K, Andreason A, Grøndahi-Hansen J, Kristensen P, Nielsen LS: Plasminogen activators, tissue degradation, and cancer. Adv Cancer Res 44:139, 1985
93. Darzynkiewicz Z, Arnason BGW: Suppression of RNA synthesis in lymphocytes by inhibitors of proteolytic enzymes. Exp Cell Res 85:95, 1974
94. Dean A, Erard F, Schneider AB, Schechter AN: Induction of hemoglobin accumulation in human K562 cells by hemin is reversible. Science 212:459, 1981
95. Degan SJF, MacGilvary RTA, Davie EW: Characterization of the complementary deoxynucleic acid and gene coding for human prothrombin. Biochemistry 22:2087, 1983
96. DeLotto R, Spierer P: A gene required for the specification of dorsal-ventral pattern in *Drosophilla* appears to encode a serine protease. Nature 323:688, 1986
96a. Del Rosso M, Pucci M, Fibbi G, Dini G: Interaction of urokinase with specific receptors abolishes the time of commitment to terminal differentiation of murine erythroleukemia (Friend) cells.

Brit J Haematol 66:289, 1987

97. Denton RM: Early events in insulin actions. Adv Cyclic Nucleotide Protein Phosphorylation Res 20:293, 1986

97a. Djulbegovic B, Christmas SE, Moore M: Differentiated HL-60 promyelocytic leukaemia cells produce a factor inducing differentiation. Leuk Res 11:259, 1987

98. Dornand J, Moreau P, Kaplan JG: The effect of prolonged ouabain treatment and of protease inhibitors on the mixed lymphocyte reaction (MLR). In Leukocyte Membrane Determinants Regulating Immune Reactivity, Proceedings of the 10th Leukocyte Culture Conference edited by Eijsvoogel VP, Roos D, Zeijlemaker WP, p 491. New York, Academic Press Inc, 1976

99. Drexler HG, Gaedicke G, Minowada J: Erythroleukemia cell lines HEL and K562: changes in isozyme profiles and morphology during induction of differentiation. Hematol Oncol 4:163, 1986

100. Drexler HG, Klein M, Komiyama A, Bhoopalam N, Minowada J: Induction of hemoglobin synthesis in the human leukemia cell line SP1-802 (abstr). Blood 64 (Suppl):140a, 1984

101. Drexler HG, Otsuka K, Gaedicke G, Minowada J: Modulation of isoenzymes in myeloid cell lines induced by T-cell derived differentiation inducing factor (DIF) and by 12-*O*-tetradecanoylphorbol 13-acetate (TPA) (abstr). Proc Am Assoc Cancer Res 25:38, 1984

102. Duque RE, Phan SH, Sulavik MC, Ward PA: Inhibition by tosyl-L-phenylalanyl chloromethyl ketone of membrane potential changes in rat neutrophils: correlation with the inhibition of biological activity. J Biol Chem 258:8123, 1983

103. Ebina Y, Ellis L, Jarnagin K, Edery M, Graf L, Clauser E, Ou J, Masiarz F, Kan YW, Goldfine ID, Roth RA, Rutter WJ: The human insulin receptor cDNA: the structual basis for hormone-activated transmembrane signalling. Cell 40:747, 1985

104. Edwards DR, Waterhouse P, Holman ML, Denhardt DT: A growth-responsive gene (16C8) in normal mouse fibroblasts homologous to a human collagenase inhibitor with erythroid-potentiating activity: evidence for inducible and constitutive transcripts. Nucleic Acids Res 14:8863, 1986

105. Elion J, Downing MR, Butkowski RJ, Mann KG: Structure of human thrombin: comparison with other serine proteases. In Chemistry and Biology of Thrombin, edited by Lundblad RL, Fenton JW II, Mann KG, p 97. Ann Arbor, Michigan, Ann Arbor Science Publishers, 1977

106. Erard F, Dean A, Schechter AN: Inhibitors of cell division reversibly modify hemoglobin concentration in human erythroleukemia K 562 cells. Blood 58:1236, 1981

107. Ershoff BA, Bajwa GS: Submaxillary gland hypertrophy in rats fed proteolytic enzymes. Proc Soc Exp Biol Med 113:879, 1963

108. Esmon NL, Owen WG, Esmon CT: Isolation of membrane-bound cofactor for thrombin-catalyzed activation of protein C. J Biol Chem 257:859, 1982

109. Eto Y, Tsuji T, Takezawa M, Takano S, Yokogawa Y, Shibai H: Purification and characterization of differentiation factor (EDF) isolated from human leukemia cell line THP-1. Biochem Biophys Res Commun 142:1095, 1987

110. Faletto DL, Arrow AS, Macara IG: An early decrease in phosphatidylinositol turnover occurs on induction of Friend cell differentiation and precedes the decrease in c-*myc* expression. Cell 43:315, 1985

110a. Faletto DL, Macara IG: The role of Ca^{2+} in dimethyl sulfoxide-induced differentiation of Friend erythroleukemia cells. J Biol Chem 260:4884, 1985

111. Fatemi SH, Haas R, Jentoft N, Rosenberry TL, Tartakoff AM: The glycolipid anchor of Thy-1: biosynthetic labeling experiments with wild-type and class E Thy-1 negative lymphomas. J Biol Chem 262:4728, 1987

112. Fenton JW II: Thrombin specificity. Ann NY Acad Sci 370:468, 1981

113. Ferraiuolo R, Stoppelli MP, Verde P, Bullock S, Lazzaro P, Blasi F, Peitropaolo TC: Transcriptional induction of urokinase in cultured human kidney carcinoma cells by tetradecanoyl-phorbol-acetate. J Cell Physiol 121:368, 1984

114. Fibach E, Kidron M, Nachshon I, Mayer M: Phorbol ester-induced adhesion of murine erythroleukemia cells: possible involvement of cellular proteases. Carcinogenesis 4:1395, 1983

115. Fibach E, Treves A, Kidron M, Mayer M: Induction of differentiation in human myeloid leukemic cells by proteolytic enzymes. J Cell Physiol 123:228, 1985

116. Filer JS, Usher P, Moses AC: Monoclonal antibody to the type I insulin-like growth factor (IGF-I) receptor blocks IGF-I receptor-mediated DNA synthesis: clarification of the mitogenic mechanisms of IGF-I and insulin in human skin fibroblasts. Proc Natl Acad Sci USA 83:664, 1986

117. Fioritoni G, Bertolini L, Toriontano G, Revoltella R: Cytochemical characteristics of leukopoietic differentiation in murine erythroleukemic (Friend) cells. Cancer Res 40:866, 1980

118. Fisher JW: Control of erythropoietin production. Proc Soc Exp Biol Med 173:289, 1983

119. Forage RG, Ring JM, Brown RW, McInerney BV, Cobon GS, Gregson RP, Robertson DM, Morgan FJ, Hearn MTW, Findlay JK, Wettenhall REH, Burger HG, De Kretser DM: Cloning and sequence analysis of cDNA species coding for the two subunits of inhibin from bovine follicular fluid. Proc Natl Acad Sci USA 83:3091, 1986

120. Forsbeck K, Nilsson K, Jemsson A, Skoglund G, Ingelman-Sundberg M: Phorbol ester-induced alteration of differentiation and proliferation in human hematopoietic/tumor cell lines: relationship to the presence and subcellular distribution of protein kinase C. Cancer Res 45:6194, 1985

121. Fothergill JJ, Wistar R, Woods JN, Parker DC: A mitogen for human B cells: anti Ig coupled to polyacrylamide beads activates blood mononuclear cells independently of T cells. J Immunol 128:1945, 1984

122. Frank W, Ristow H-J, Veser J: Stimulation of embryonic rat cells in culture by calf serum. Z Naturforsch [C] 29:169, 1974

123. Frey P, Forand R, Maciag T, Shooter EM: The biosynthetic precursor of epidermal growth factor and the mechanism of its processing. Proc Natl Acad Sci USA 76:6294, 1979

124. Friend C, Scher W, Holland JG, Sato T: Hemoglobin synthesis in murine virus-induced leukemic cells in vitro: stimulation of erythroid differentiation by dimethyl sulfoxide. Proc Natl Acad Sci USA 68:378, 1971

125. Fukuda M: Tumor-promoting phorbol diester-induced specific changes in cell surface glycoprotein profile of K562 human leukemic cells. Cancer Res 41:4621, 1981

126. Fyhrquist F, Rosenlöf K, Grönhagen-Riska C, Hortling L, Tikkanen I: Is renin substrate an erythropoietin precursor? (abstr). Nature 308:649, 1984

127. Gambari R, Fibach E, Rifkind RA, Marks PA: Inhibition of induced murine erythroleukemia cell differentiation by tumor promoters: relation to the cell cycle. Biochem Biophys Res Commun 94:867, 1980

128. Gasson JC, Golde DW: Physiological relevance of erythroid-potentiating activity or TIMP—reply. Nature 321:628, 1985

129. Gazitt Y, Reuben RC, Deitch AD, Marks PA, Rifkind RA: Changes in cyclic adenosine 3′:5′-monophosphate levels during induction of differentiation in murine erythroleukemia cells. Cancer Res 38:3779, 1978

130. Gewirtz AM, Burger D, Rado TA, Benz EJ Jr., Hoffman R: Constitutive expression of platelet glycoproteins by the human leukemia cell line K562. Blood 60:785, 1982

131. Ghezzo F, Pegoraro L: Effects of retinoic acid on the fibrinolytic activity of HL-60 human promyelocytic leukemia cells. Experentia 37:425, 1981

132. Glenn KC, Cunningham DD: Thrombin-stimulated cell division involves proteolysis of its cell surface receptor. Nature 278:711, 1979

133. Goerig M, Habenicht AJR, Heitz R, Zeh W, Katus H, Kommerell B, Ziegler R, Glomset JA: *sn*-1,2-Diacylglycerols and phorbol diesters stimulate thromboxane synthesis by *de novo* synthesis of prostaglandin H synthase in human promyelocytic leukemia cells. J Clin Invest 79:903, 1987

134. Goetz IE, Weinstein C, Roberts E: Effects of protease inhibitors on growth of hamster tumor cells in culture. Cancer Res 32:2469, 1972

135. Goldstein JL, Brown MS, Anderson RGW, Russell DW, Schneider WJ: Receptor-mediated endocytosis: concepts emerging from the LDL receptor system. Annu Rev Cell Biol 1:1, 1985

136. Goodall DM, Pardoe GI, Gregory JK: Lymphocyte surface components. Clin Exp Immunol 9:655, 1971

137. Gordon EA, Carney DH: Thrombin receptor occupancy initiates cell proliferation in the presence of phorbol myristate acetate. Biochem Biophys Res Commun 141:650, 1986

138. Gordon EA, Fenton JW II, Carney DH: Thrombin receptor occupancy initiates a transient increase in cAMP levels in mitogenically responsive hamster (NIL) fibroblasts. Ann NY Acad Sci, in press 1986
139. Gospodarowicz D, Brown KD, Birdwell CR, Zetter BR: Control of proliferation of human vascular endothelial cells. Characterization of the response of human umbilical vein endothelial cells to fibroblast growth factor, epidermal growth factor and thrombin. J Cell Biol 77:774, 1978
140. Gospodarowicz D, Moran JS: Growth factors in mammalian cell culture. Annu Rev Biochem 45:531, 1976
141. Grayzel AI, Hatcher VB, Lazarus GS: Protease activity of normal and PHA stimulated human lymphocytes. Cell Immunol 18:210, 1975
142. Greene LA, Shooter EM, Varon S: Enzymatic activities of mouse nerve growth factor and its subunits. Proc Natl Acad Sci USA 60:1383, 1968
143. Greene LA, Tomita JT, Varon S: Growth-stimulating activities of mouse submaxillary esteropeptidases on chick embryo fibroblasts in vitro. Exp Cell Res 64:387, 1971
144. Gullberg U, Nilsson E, Olsson I: Properties of a T-lymphocyte derived differentiation inducting factor (DIF) for the myeloid leukemic cell line HL-60. In Experimental Hematology Today-1985, edited by Baum SJ, Pluznik DH, Rozenszajn LA, p 72. New York, Springer-Verlag, 1986
145. Gullberg U, Nilsson E, Sarngadharan MG, Olsson I: T lymphocyte-derived differentiation-inducing factor inhibits proliferation of leukemic and normal hemopoietic cells. Blood 68:1333, 1986
146. Gusella JF, Weil SC, Tsiftsoglou AS, Volloch V, Neumann JR, Keys C, Housman DE: Hemin does not cause commitment of murine erythroleukemia (MEL) cells to terminal differentiation. Blood 56:481, 1980
147. Gutowski JK, Innes JB, Weksler ME, Cohen S: Impaired nuclear responsiveness to cytoplasmic signals in lymphocytes from elderly humans with depressed proliferative responses. J Clin Invest 78:40, 1986
148. Gutowski JK, Mukherji B, Cohen S: The role of cytoplasmic intermediates in IL 2-induced T cell growth. J Immunol 133:3068, 1984
149. Gutowski JK, West A, Cohen S: The regulation of DNA synthesis in quiescient lymphocytes by cytoplasmic inhibitors. Proc Natl Acad Sci USA 82:5160, 1985
150. Hagiwara T, Aoyagi T, Nagi Y: Leupeptin, a protease inhibitor, inhibits the PHA-stimulated DNA synthesis in guinea pig blood lymphocytes. Jpn J Exp Med 42:509, 1972
151. Hankins WD, Schooley J, Eastment C: Erythropoietin, an autocrine regulator? Serum-free production of erythropoietin by cloned erythroid cell lines. Blood 68:263, 1986
152. Harel L, Lacour F, Friend C, Durbin P, Semmel M: Early inhibition of phospholipid synthesis in dimethyl sulfoxide (DMSO) treated Friend erythroleukemia (FL) cells. J Cell Physiol 101:25, 1979
153. Harlan JM, Thompson PJ, Ross RR, Bowen-Pope DF: α-Thrombin induces release of platelet-derived growth factor-like molecule(s) by cultured human endothelial cells. J Cell Biol 103:1129, 1986
154. Harmon JT, Jamieson GA: Activation of platelets by α-thrombin is a receptor-mediated event: D-phenylalanyl-L-prolyl-L-arginine chloromethyl ketone-thrombin, but not N^{α}-tosyl-L-lysine chloromethyl ketone-thrombin, binds to the high affinity thrombin receptor. J Biol Chem 261:15928, 1986
155. Hart DA, Streilein JS: Effect of protease inhibitors on mitogen stimulation of hamster lymphoid cells. Exp Cell Res 102:253, 1976
156. Hayashi S, Ueki H, Hamamura K, Tsukada M: On the hypoglycemic activity of protease preparation of *Streptomyces griseus*, pronase P. Chem Pharm Bull 12:1393, 1964
157. Hecht LB, Straus DS: Insulin-sensitive protein kinase activity that phosphorylates ribosomal protein S6 in cultured fibroblast-melanoma hybrid cells. Endocrinology 119:470, 1986
158. Heinrich PC: Proteolytic processing of polypeptides during the biosynthesis of subcellular structures. Rev Physiol Biochem Pharmacol 93:115, 1982
159. Helin H: Macrophage procoagulant factors —mediators of inflammatory and neoplastic tissue lesions. Med Biol 64:107, 1986
160. Helm BA, Gunn JM: The effect of insulinomimetic agents on protein degradation in H35 hepatoma cells. Mol Cell Biochem 71:159, 1986
161. Henriksen RA, Brotherton AFA: Evidence that activation of platelets and endothelium by thrombin involves distinct sites of interaction: studies with the dysthrombin, Thrombin Quick I. J Biol Chem 258:13717, 1983
162. Hodges GM, Livingston DC, Franks LM: The localization of trypsin in cultured mammalian cells. J Cell Sci 12:887, 1973
163. Hoffmann C, Crettaz M, Bruns P, Hessel P, Hadawi G: Cellular responses elicited by insulin mimickers in cells lacking detectable plasma membrane insulin receptors. J Cell Biochem 27:401, 1985
164. Hoffman R, Murnane MJ, Benz Jr EJ, Prohaska R, Floyd V, Dainiak N, Forget BG, Furthmayr H: Induction of erythropoietic colonies in a human chronic myelogenous leukemia cell line. Blood 54:1182, 1979
165. Holzer H, Heinrich PC: Control of proteolysis. Annu Rev Biochem 49:63, 1980
166. Honma Y, Takenaga K, Kasukabe T, Hozumi M: Induction of differentiation of cultured human promyelocytic leukemia cells by retinoids. Biochem Biophys Res Commun 95:507, 1980
167. Houslay MD: Egg activation unscrambles a potential role for IP_4. Trends Biochem Sci 12:1, 1987
168. Houslay MD, Wakelam MJO, Pyne NJ: The mediator is the message: is it part of the answer of insulin's action? Trends Biochem Sci 11:393, 1986
169. Huang D, Cuatrecasas P: Insulin-induced reduction of membrane receptor concentrations in isolated fat cells and lymphocytes: independence from receptor occupation and possible relation to proteolytic activity of insulin. J Biol Chem 250:8251, 1975
170. Hunter RF, Mold NG, Mitchell RB, Huang AT: Differentiation of normal marrow and HL60 cells induced by antithymocyte globulin. Proc Natl Acad Sci USA 82:4823, 1985
171. Hynes RO: Integrins: a family of cell surface receptors. Cell 48:549, 1987
172. Ikawa Y, Aida M: Hemoglobin production in cultured Friend leukemia cells induced by a human placental extract preparation. Gann 66:583, 1975
173. Illiano G, Cuatrecasas P: Glucose transport in fat cell membranes. J Biol Chem 246:2472, 1971
174. Jackman RW, Beeler DL, Van De Water L, Rosenberg RD: Characterization of a thrombomodulin cDNA reveals structural similarity to the low density lipoprotein receptor. Proc Natl Acad Sci USA 83:8834, 1986
175. Jacobs S, Chang K-J, Cuatrecasas P: Antibodies to purified insulin receptor have insulin-like activity. Science 200:1283, 1978
176. Jakobs KH, Bauer S, Watanabe Y: Modulation of adenylate cyclase of human platelets by phorbol ester. Eur J Biochem 151:425, 1985
177. Jarett L, Kiechle FL, Popp DA, Kotagal N, Gavin JR III: Differences in the effect of insulin on the generation by adipocytes and IM-9 lymphocytes of a chemical mediator which simulates the action of insulin on pyruvate dehydrogenase. Biochem Biophys Res Commun 96:735, 1980
178. Jarett L, Seals JR: Pyruvate dehydrogenase activation in adipocyte mitochondria by an insulin-generated mediator from muscle. Science 206:1407, 1979
179. Jepson JH, Friesen HG: The mechanism of action of human placental lactogen on erythropoiesis. Br J Haematol 15:465, 1968
180. Jepson JH, Lowenstein L: Effect of prolactin on erythropoiesis in the mouse. Blood 24:726, 1964
181. Jochen A, Berhanu P: Effects of metalloendoprotease inhibitors on insulin binding, internalization and processing in adipocytes. Biochem Biophys Res Commun 142:205, 1987
182. Kadouri A, Bohak Z: Production of plasminogen activator by cells in culture. Adv Biotechnol Process 5:275, 1985
183. Kalmaz GD: Differentiation of multipotential human leukemia cell line (K-562) in diffusion chambers (abstr). In Vitro Cell Dev Biol 23:16A, 1987
184. Kaneko A, Enomoto K, Oyamada M, Sawada N, Demp K, Mori M: Induction of a novel Ca^{2+}-dependent chymotrypsin-like serine protease by tumor promoters in rat livers. JNCI 77:121, 1986
185. Kaplan JG, Bona C: Proteases as mitogens. Exp Cell Res 88:388, 1974
186. Kast RE: Inhibition of the lymphocyte blast transformation response to PHA by trypsin inhibitors from lima bean and soya bean. Scand J Immunol 2:449, 1973

187. Kast RE: A theory of lymphocyte blast transformation (LBT) and malignant change based on proteolytic cleavage of a trigger peptide: the detendomer. Oncology 29:249, 1974
188. Kasuga M, Karlsson FA, Kahn CR: Insulin stimulates the phosphorylation of the 95,000-dalton subunit of its own receptor. Science 215:185, 1982
189. Kasuga M, Zick Y, Blith DL, Karlsson FA, Häring HU, Kahn CR: Insulin stimulation of phosphorylation of the β subunit of the insulin receptor. J Biol Chem 257:9891, 1982
190. Kathuria S, Hartman S, Grunfeld C, Ramachandran J, Fujita-Yamaguchi Y: Differential sensitivity of two functions of the insulin receptor to the associated proteolysis: kinase action and hormone binding. Proc Natl Acad Sci USA 83:8570, 1986
191. Kellokumpu S, Rajaniemi H: Involvement of plasma membrane enzymes in the proteolytic cleavage of luteinizing hormone receptor. Endocrinology 116:707, 1985
192. Khanna NC, Tokuda M, Waisman DM: Phosphorylation of lipocortins *in vitro* by protein kinase C. Biochem Biophys Res Commun 141:547, 1986
193. Kidron M, Fibach E, Klemes Y, Mayer M: Changes in acid proteolytic activity during differentiation of murine erythroleukemic cells. Cell Differ 10:309, 1981
194. Kidron M, Nachshon I, Mayer M, Fibach E: Plasminogen activator activity in differentiating leukemia cells. FEBS Lett 177:66, 1984
195. Kikuchi K, Schwartz C, Creasy S, Larner J: Independent control of insulin-sensitive cell membrane and intracellular functions—the linkage of cell membrane and intracellular events controlled by insulin. Mol Cell Biochem 37:125, 1981
196. Kimura N, Mak TW: Isolation and characterization of an erythroid cell line highly inducible to form erythroid burst-like colonies. J Cell Physiol 128:41, 1986
197. Kingdon HS, Noyes CM, Lundblad RL: Some aspects of the primary structure of bovine alpha, beta, and gamma thrombins. In Chemistry and Biology of Thrombin, edited by Lundblad RL, Fenton II JW, Mann KG, p 91. Ann Arbor, Michigan, Ann Arbor Science Publishers Inc, 1977
198. Kishimoto T, Kikutani H, Nishizawa Y, Sakaguchi N, Yamamura Y: Involvement of anti-Ig-activated serine protease in the generation of cytoplasmic factor(s) that are responsible for the transmission of Ig-receptor-mediated signals. J Immunol 123:1504, 1979
199. Kohno M, Pouysségur J: α-thrombin-induced tyrosine phosphorylation of 43000- and 41000-M_r proteins is independent of cytoplasmic alkalinization in quiescent fibroblasts. Biochem J 238:451, 1986
200. Kolata GB: Protein degradation: putting the research together. Science 198:596, 1977
201. Kono T: Destruction of insulin effector system of adipose tissue cells by proteolytic enzymes. J Biol Chem 244:1772, 1969
202. Kono T, Barham FW: Insulin-like effects of trypsin on fat cells: localization of the metabolic steps and the cellular site affected by the enzyme. J Biol Chem 246:6204, 1971
203. Kono T, Barham FW: The relationship between the insulin-binding capacity of fat cells and the cellular response to insulin: studies with intact and trypsin-treated fat cells. J Biol Chem 246:6210, 1971
204. Kornberg A, Treves A, Rachmilewitz EA, Fibach E: Generation of procoagulent activity (PCA) by phorbol-esters-induced macrophages derived from a leukemia promyelocytic cell line (HL-60). Blood 59:1061, 1982
205. Kristensen T, Saris CJM, Hunter T, Hicks LJ, Nonnan DJ, Glenney JR Jr, Tack BF: Primary structure of bovine calpactin I heavy chain (p 36), a major cellular substrate for retroviral protein-tyrosine kinases: homology with the human phospholipase A_2 inhibitor lipocortin. Biochemistry 25:4497, 1986
206. Kuo JF, Dill IK, Holmlund CE: Comparisons of the effects of *Bacillus subtilis* protease, type VIII (subtilopeptidase A), and insulin on isolated adipose cells. I. Glucose and palmitic acid metabolism. J Biol Chem 242:3659, 1967
207. Kuo JF, Holmlund CE, Dill IK: The effect of proteolytic enzymes on isolated adipose cells. Life Sci 5:2257, 1966
208. Kuo JF, Holmlund CE, Dill IK, Bohonos N: Insulin-like activity of a microbial protease on isolated fat cells. Arch Biochem Biophys 117:269, 1966
209. L'Allemain G, Paris S, Magnaldo I, Pouysségur J: alpha-Thrombin-induced inositol phosphate formation in Go-arrested and cycling hamster lung fibroblasts: evidence for a protein kinase C-mediated desensitization response. J Cell Physiol 129:167, 1986
210. Lapetina EG, Reep B, Chang K-J: Treatment of human platelets with trypsin, thrombin, or collagen inhibits the pertussis toxin-induced ADP-ribosylation of a 41-kDa protein. Proc Natl Acad Sci USA 83:5880, 1986
211. Lapetina EG, Reep B, Ganong BR, Bell RM: Exogenous *sn*-1,2, diacylglycerols containing saturated fatty acids function as bioregulators of protein kinase C in human platelets. J Biol Chem 260:1358, 1985
212. Larner J: Insulin mediator—fact or fancy? J Cyclic Nucleotide Res 8:289, 1982
213. Larner J: Biochemical mechanism of insulin action-1986. Resident Staff Physician Jan:63, 1986
214. Larner J, Galasko G, Cheng K, DePaoli-Roach AA, Huang L, Daggy P, Kellogg J: Generation by insulin of a chemical mediator that controls protein phosphorylation and dephosphorylation. Science 206:1408, 1979
215. Larner J, Huang LC, Brooker G, Murad F, Miller TB: Inhibitor of protein kinase formed in insulin-treated muscle. Fed Proc 33:261, 1974
216. Lawler J, Hynes RO: The structure of human thrombospondin, an adhesive glycoprotein with multiple calcium-binding sites and homologies with several different proteins. J Cell Biol 103:1635, 1986
217. Lembach KJ: Induction of human fibroblast proliferation by epidermal growth factor (EGF): enchancement by an EGF-binding arginine esterase and by ascorbate. Proc Natl Acad Sci USA 73:183, 1976
218. Leung K, Chiao JW: Human leukemia cell maturation induced by a T-cell lymphokine isolated from medium conditioned by normal lymphocytes. Proc Natl Acad Sci USA 82:1209, 1985
219. Lewis N, Majerus PW: Lipid metabolism in human platelets II. *De novo* phospholipid synthesis and the effect of thrombin on the pattern of synthesis. J Clin Invest 48:2114, 1969
220. Ling N, Ying S-Y, Ueno N, Shimasaki S, Esch F, Hotta M, Guillemin R: Pituitary FSH is released by a heterodimer of the beta-subunits from the two forms of inhibin. Nature 321:779, 1986
221. Ling N, Ying S-Y, Ueno N, Shimasaki S, Esch F, Hotta M, Guillemin R: A homodimer of the β-subunits of inhibin A stimulates the secretion of pituitary follicle stimulating hormone. Biochem Biophys Res Commun 138:1129, 1986
222. Linsley PS, Blifeld C, Wrann M, Fox CF: Direct linkage of epidermal growth factor to its receptor. Nature 278:745, 1979
223. Lipson KE, Yamada K, Kolhatkar AA, Donner DB: Relationship between the affinity and proteolysis of the insulin receptor: evidence that higher affinity receptors are preferentially degraded. J Biol Chem 261:10833, 1986
224. Lollar P, Hoak JC, Owen WG: Binding of thrombin to cultured human endothelial cells: nonequilibrium aspects. J Biol Chem 255:10279, 1980
225. Lollar P, Owen WG: Evidence that the effects of thrombin on arachidonate metabolism in cultured human endothelial cells are not mediated by a high affinity receptor. J Biol Chem 255:8031, 1980
226. Low DA, Wiley HS, Cunningham DD: Role of cell-surface thrombin-binding sites in mitogenesis. In Cancer Cells, Growth Factors and Transformation, edited by Feramisco J, Ozanne B, Stiles C, Vol 3, p 401. Cold Spring Harbor, New York, Cold Spring Harbor Laboratory, 1985
227. Low MG, Ferguson MAJ, Futerman AH, Silman I: Covalently attached phosphatidylinositol as a hydrophobic anchor for membrane proteins. Trend Biochem Sci 11:212, 1986
228. Lyberg T, Nilsson K, Prydz H: Synthesis of thromboplastin by U-937 cells. Br J Haematol 51:631, 1982
229. Lyberg T, Prydz H: Phorbol esters induce synthesis of thromboplastin activity in human monocytes. Biochem J 194:699, 1981
230. Lyons RM, Stanford N, Majerus PW: Thrombin-induced protein phosphorylation in human platelets. J Clin Invest 56:924, 1975
231. Magnaldo I, L'Allemain G, Chambard JC, Moenner M, Barritault D, Pouysségur J: The mitogenic signaling pathway of fibroblast growth factor is not mediated through phosphoinositide hydrolysis and protein kinase C activation in hamster fibroblasts. J Biol

Chem 261:16916, 1986

232. Magnaldo I, Talwar H, Anderson WB, Pouysségur J: Evidence for a GTP-binding protein coupling thrombin receptor to PIP-phospholipase C in membranes of hamster fibroblasts. FEBS Lett 210:6, 1987
233. Magnusson S, Petersen TE, Sottryp-Jensen L, Claeys H: Complete primary structure of prothrombin: isolation, structure and reactivity of ten carboxylated glutamic acid residues and regulation of prothrombin activation of thrombin. In Proteases and Biologic Control. Cold Spring Harbor Conference on Cell Proliferation, Vol 2, edited by Reich E, Rifkin DB, Shaw E, p 123. Cold Spring Harbor, New York, Cold Spring Harbor Laboratory, 1975
234. Majerus PW: The production of phosphoinositide-derived messenger molecules. Harvey Lect 82, in press, 1987
235. Majerus PW, Connolly TM, Deckmyn H, Ross TS, Bross TE, Ishii H, Bansal VS, Wilson DB: The metabolism of phosphoinositide-derived messenger molecules. Science 234:1519, 1986
236. Malchoff CD, Huang L, Gillespie N, Villar Palasi C, Schwartz CFW, Cheng K, Hewlett EL, Larner J: A putative mediator of insulin action which inhibits adenylate cyclase and adenosine 3′,5′-monophosphate-dependent protein kinase: partial purification from rat liver: site and kinetic mechanism of action. Endocrinology 120:1327, 1987
237. Marossy K, Hauck M, Elödi P: Purification and characterization of the chymotrypsin-like enzyme of the bovine granulocyte. Biochim Biophys Acta 662:36, 1981
238. Mason AJ, Hayflick JS, Ling N, Esch F, Ueno N, Ying S-Y, Guillemin R, Niall H, Seeburg PH: Complementary DNA sequences of ovarian follicular fluid inhibin show precursor structure and homology with transforming growth factor-beta. Nature 318:659, 1985
239. Deleted in proof
240. Mato JM, Kelly KL, Abler A, Jarett L: Identification of a novel insulin-sensitive glycophospholipid from H35 hepatoma cells. J Biol Chem 262:2131, 1987
241. Mayeux P, Billat C, Jacquot R: Murine erythroleukemia (Friend Cells) possess high-affinity binding sites for erythropoietin. FEBS Lett 211:229, 1987
242. Mayo KE, Cerelli GM, Spiess J, Rivier J, Rosenfeld MG, Evans RM, Vale W: Inhibin A-subunit cDNAs from porcine ovary and human placenta. Proc Natl Acad Sci USA 83:5849, 1986
243. Mazzei D, Novi C, Bazzi C: Mitogenic action of trypsin and chymotrypsin. Lancet 2:232, 1966
244. Mazzei D, Novi C, Bazzi C: Mitogenic action of papain. Lancet 2:802, 1966
245. McColl SR, Hurst NP, Cleland LG: Modulation by phorbol myristate acetate of arachidonic acid release and leukotriene synthesis by human polymorphonuclear leukocytes stimulated with A23187. Biochem Biophys Res Commun 141:399, 1986
246. McLachlan RI, Healy DL, Robertson DM, Burger HG, de Kretser, DM: The human placenta: a novel source of inhibin. Biochem Biophys Res Commun 140:485, 1986
247. Melloni E, Salamino F, Sparatore B, Michetti M, Morelli A, Benatti U, De Flora A, Pontremoli S: Decay of proteinase and peptidase activities of human and rabbit erythrocytes during cellular aging. Biochim Biophys Acta 675:110, 1981
248. Michalevicz R, Katz F, Stroobant P, Janossy G, Tindle RW, Hoffbrand AV: Platelet-derived growth factor stimulates growth of highly enriched multipotent haemopoietic progenitors. Br J Haematol 63:591, 1986
249. Mihara A, Fujiwara K, Sato S, Okabe T, Fujiyoshi N: N-Terminal amino acid sequence of leukemia derived growth factor (LGF) from human erythroleukemia cell culture. In Vitro Cell Dev Biol 23:317, 1987
250. Min HY, Spiegelman BM: Adipsin, the adipocyte serine protease: gene structure and control of expression by tumor necrosis factor. Nucleic Acids Res 74:8879, 1986
251. Mok M, Spivak JL: Protease activity in human urine erythropoietin preparations. Exp Hematol 10:300, 1982
252. Molendijk WJ, van Oudenaren A, van Dijk H, Daha MR, Benner R: Complement split product C5a mediates the lipopolysaccharide-induced mobilization of CFU-s and haemopoietic progenitor cells, but not the mobilization induced by proteolytic enzymes. Cell Tissue Kinet 19:407, 1986
253. Moreau P, Dornand J, Kaplan JG: Inhibition of lymphocyte transformation: effect of soy bean trypsin inhibitor and synthetic anti-proteases. Can J Biochem 53:1337, 1975
254. Morisset M, Capony F, Rochefort H: The 52-kDa estrogen-induced protein secreted by MCF_7 cells is a lysosomal acidic protease. Biochem Biophys Res Commun 138:102, 1986
255. Morrison BD, Pessin JE: Insulin stimulation of the insulin receptor kinase can occur in the complete absence of β subunit autophosphorylation. J Biol Chem 262:2861, 1987
256. Moscat J, Moreno F, Iglesias S, Garcia-Barreno P, Municio AM: Ionophore A23187 induces a refractory state in thrombin-activated release of inositol phosphates. Biochem J 238:709, 1986
257. Moss M, Cunningham DD: Cleavage of cell surface proteins by thrombin. J Supramol Struct Cell Biochem 15:49, 1981
258. Moss M, Wiley HS, Fenton JW II, Cunningham DD: Photoaffinity labeling of specific α thrombin binding sites on Chinese hamster lung cells. J Biol Chem 258:3996, 1983
259. Nagai K, Nakamura T, Koyama J: Characterization of macrophage proteases involved in the ingestion of antigen-antibody complexes by the use of protease inhibitors. FEBS Lett 92:299, 1978
260. Naidet C, Sémériva M, Yamada KM, Thiery JP: Peptides containing the cell-attachment recognition signal Arg-Gly-Asp prevent gastrolation in *Drosophila* embryos. Nature 325:348, 1987
261. Nathan CF: Secretory products of macrophages. J Clin Invest 79:319, 1987
262. Neurath H: Proteolytic enzymes, past and present. Fed Proc 44:2907, 1985
263. Nishizuka Y: Studies and perspective of protein kinase C. Science 233:305, 1986
264. Nissley SP, Haskell JF, Sasaki N, De Vroede MA, Rechler MM: Insulin-like growth factor receptors. J Cell Sci 3 (Suppl):39, 1985
265. Noonan KD: Proteolytic modification of cell surface macromolecules: mode of action in stimulating cell growth. Curr Top Membr Transp 11:397, 1978
266. Noonan KD: Lectins as probes of the transformed cell surface. In Virus Transformed Cell Membranes, edited by Nicolau C, p 281. New York, Academic Press Inc, 1978
267. Noonan KD, Burger MM: Induction of 3T3 cell division at the monolayer stage. Exp Cell Res 80:405, 1973
268. Noonan NE, Noonan KD: The effect of TLCK on transcription and its role in modifying cell growth. J Cell Physiol 92:137, 1977
269. Ohlsson-Wilhelm BM, Farley BA, Rudolph HS, Rowley PT: Erythroid induction of K562 human leukemia cell lines: enhancement by purines. Arch Biochem Biophys 239:567, 1985
270. Oldberg A, Franzén A, Heinegård D: Cloning and sequence analysis of rat bone sialoprotein (osteopontin) cDNA reveals an Arg-Gly-Asp cell-binding sequence. Proc Natl Acad Sci USA 83:8819, 1986
271. Ossowski L, Belin D: Effect of dimethyl sulfoxide on human carcinoma cells. Inhibition of plasminogen activator synthesis, change in cell morphology, and alteration of response to cholera toxin. Mol Cell Biol 5:3552, 1985
272. Pantazis P, Lanfrancone L, Pelicci PG, Dalla-Favera R, Antoniades HN: Human leukemia cells synthesize and secrete proteins related to platelet-derived growth factor. Proc Natl Acad Sci USA 83:5526, 1986
273. Pantazis P, Sariban E, Kufe D, Antoniades HN: Induction of c-*sis* gene expression and synthesis of platelet-derived growth factor in human myeloid leukemia cells during monocytic differentiation. Proc Natl Acad Sci USA 83:6455, 1986
274. Papayannopoulou T, Nakamoto B, Yokochio T, Chait A, Kannagi R: Human erythroleukemia cell line (HEL) undergoes a drastic macrophage-like shift with TPA. Blood 62:832, 1983
275. Papayannopoulou T, Raines E, Collins S, Nakamoto B, Tweeddale M, Ross R: Constitutive and inducible secretion of platelet-derived growth factor analogs by human leukemic cell lines coexpressing erythroid and megakaryocytic markers. J Clin Invest 79:859, 1987
276. Paris S, Chambard J-C, Pouysségur J: Coupling between phosphoinositide breakdown and early mitogenic events in fibroblasts: studies with fluoroaluminate, vanadate and pertussis toxin. J Biol Chem 262:1977, 1987
277. Pasternak MS, Eisen HN: A novel serine esterase expressed by cytotoxic T lymphocytes. Nature 314:743, 1985

278. Patarca R, Haseltine W: A major retroviral core protein related to EPA and TIMP. Nature 318:390, 1985
279. Paukovits JB, Paukovits WR, Laerum OD: Identification of a regulatory peptide distinct from normal granulocyte-derived hemoregulatory peptide produced by human promyelocytic HL-60 leukemia cells after differentiation induction with retinoic acid. Cancer Res 46:4444, 1986
280. Peck D, Byvoet P: The growth-promoting effect of crystalline trypsin on embryonic chick and Walker tumor cells in vitro. Anat Rec 151:398, 1965
281. Perdue JF, Kivity E, Lubenskyi W: Characterization of thrombin binding to cultured avian and mouse fibroblasts and mouse epithelial cells. J Cell Biol 83:255a, 1979
282. Perdue JF, Lubenskyi W, Kivity E, Sonder SA, Fenton JW II: Protease mitogenic response of chick embryo fibroblasts and receptor binding/processing of human α-thrombin. J Biol Chem 256:2767, 1981
283. Pæerez-Rodriguez R, Franchi A, Pouysségur J: Growth factor requirements of Chinese hamster lung fibroblasts in serum-free media: high mitogenic action of thrombin. Cell Biol Int Rep 5:347, 1981
284. Perisic O, Traugh JA: Protease-activated kinase II as the potential mediator of insulin-stimulated phosphorylation of protein S6. J Biol Chem 258:9589, 1983
285. Perisic O, Traugh JA: Protease-activated kinase II as the mediator of epidermal growth factor-stimulated phosphorylation of ribosomal protein S6. FEBS Lett 183:215, 1985
286. Perkins SL, Andreotii PE, Sinha SK, Wu M-C, Yunis AA: Human myeloid leukemic cell (HL-60) autostimulator: relationship to colony-stimulating factor. Cancer Res 44:5169, 1984
287. Petruzzelli LM, Ganguly S, Smith CJ, Cobb MH, Rubin CS, Rosen OM: Insulin activates a tyrosine-specific protein kinase in extracts of 3T3-L1 adipocytes and human placenta. Proc Natl Acad Sci USA 79:6792, 1982
288. Phadke K: Fibroblast growth factor enhances the interleukin-1-mediated chondrocytic protease release. Biochem Biophys Res Commun 142:448, 1987
289. Philips DR, Agin PP: Platelet plasma membrane glycoproteins: evidence for the presence of nonequivalent disulfide bonds using nonreduced-reduced two-dimensional gel electrophoresis. J Biol Chem 252:2121, 1977
290. Phillips M, Djian P, Green H: The nucleotide sequence of three genes participating in the adipose differentiation of 3T3 cells. J Biol Chem 261:10821, 1986
291. Podlecki DA, Smith RM, Kao M, Tsai P, Huecksteadt T, Brandenburg D, Lasher RS, Jarett L, Olefsky JM: Nuclear translocation of the insulin receptor. J Biol Chem 262:3362, 1987
292. Pohjanpelto P: Proteases stimulate proliferation of human fibroblasts. J Cell Physiol 91:387, 1977
293. Polakoski KL, Zanveld LJD: Proacrosin. In Methods in Enzymology, Proteolytic Enzymes, Vol 45, Part B, edited by Lorand L, p 325. New York, Academic Press Inc, 1976
294. Ponstingl H, Krauhs E, Little M, Kemp T, Hofer-Warbinek R: Approaches to the sequence of tubulin. In Methods in Peptide and Protein Sequence Analysis, edited by Birr C, p 225. Amsterdam, Elsevier/North Holland Press, 1980
295. Pontremoli S, Melloni E: Extralysosomal protein degradation. Annu Rev Biochem 55:455, 1986
296. Pontremoli S, Melloni E, Michetti M, Sacca O, Sparatore B, Salamino F, Damiani G, Horecker BL: Neutrophils: role for a membrane-bound neutral proteinase. Proc Natl Acad Sci USA 83:1685, 1986
297. Preisler HD, Giladi M: Erythropoietin responsiveness of differentiating Friend leukemia cells. Nature 251:645, 1974
298. Preisler HD, Zanjani ED: Erythropoietin-induced stimulation of heme synthesis by dimethylsulfoxide-treated Friend leukemic cells in vitro. J Lab Clin Med 84:667, 1974
299. Purrello F, Burnham DB, Goldfine ID: Insulin receptor antiserum and plant lectins mimic the direct effects of insulin on nucleur envelope phosphorylation. Science 221:462, 1983
300. Raben DM, Cunningham DD: Effects of EGF and thrombin on inositol-containing phospholipids of cultured fibroblasts: stimulation of phosphotidylinositol synthesis by thrombin but not EGF. J Cell Physiol 125:582, 1985
301. Rakowicz-Szulczynska EM, Koprowski H: Identification of NGF receptor in chromatin of melanoma cells using monoclonal antibody to cell surface NGF receptor. Biochem Biophys Res Commun 140:174, 1986
302. Rakowicz-Szulczynska EM, Rodeck U, Herlyn M, Koprowski H: Chromatin binding of epidermal growth factor, nerve growth factor, and platelet-derived growth factor in cells bearing the appropriate surface receptors. Proc Natl Acad Sci USA 83:3718, 1986
303. Ramasharma K, Li CH: Human seminal alpha-inhibins: detection in human pituitary, hypothalamus, and serum by immunoreactivity. Proc Natl Acad Sci USA 83:3484, 1986
304. Ranney DF: An integrative approach to activation and sequential metabolic regulation of the immune response. In Regulatory Mechanisms in Lymphocyte Activation, Proceedings of the 11th Leukocyte Conference, edited by Lucas DO, p 3. New York, Academic Press, Inc, 1977
305. Reddan JR, Dziedzid DC, McGee SJ: Thrombin induces cell division in rabbit lens cultured in a completely defined serum-free medium. Invest Ophthalmol Visual Sci 22:486, 1982
306. Rees-Jones RW, Taylor SI: An endogenous substrate for the insulin receptor-associated tyrosine kinase. J Biol Chem 260:4461, 1985
307. Reid TW, Reid WA: The labile nature of the insulin signal(s) for the stimulation of DNA synthesis in mouse lens epithelial and 3T3 cells. Proc Natl Acad Sci USA 262:229, 1987
308. Reiko T, Werb Z: Secretory products of macrophages and their physiological functions. Am J Physiol 246:1, 1984
309. Rieder RF, Ibrahim A, Etlinger JD: A particle-associated ATP-dependent proteolytic activity in erythroleukemia cells. J Biol Chem 260:2015, 1985
310. Rieser P: The catalytic nature of insulin. Am J Med 40:759, 1966
311. Rieser P: The insulin-like action of pepsin and pepsinogen. Acta Endocrinol 54:375, 1967
312. Rieser P, Rieser CH: Insulin-catalyzed proteolysis. Biochem Biophys Res Commun 17:373, 1964
313. Rieser P, Rieser CH: Anabolic responses of diaphragm muscle to insulin and to other pancreatic proteins. Proc Soc Exp Biol Med 116:669, 1964
314. Rieser P, Rieser CH: Enzymatic hypoglycemia in alloxan-diabetic rats. Proc Soc Exp Biol Med 119:532, 1965
315. Rittmann LS, Jelsema CL, Schwartz EL, Tsiftsoglou AS, Sartorelli AC: Lipid composition of Friend leukemia cells following induction of erythroid differentiation by dimethyl sulfoxide. J Cell Physiol 110:50, 1982
316. Rocklin RE, Bendtzen K, Greineder D: Mediators of immunity: lymphokines and monokines. Adv Immunol 29:55, 1980
317. Rodgers GM, Fisher JW, George WJ: Elevated cyclic GMP concentrations in rabbit bone marrow culture and mouse spleen following erythropoietic stimulation. Biochem Biophys Res Commun 70:287, 1976
318. Roth RA, Cassell DJ, Wong KY, Maddux BA, Goldfine IO: Monoclonal antibodies to the human insulin receptor block insulin binding and inhibit insulin action. Proc Natl Acad Sci USA 79:7312, 1982
319. Rovera G, Santoli D, Damsky C: Human promyelocytic leukemia cells in culture differentiate into macrophage-like cells when treated with a phorbol diester. Proc Natl Acad Sci USA 76:2779, 1979
320. Rovera G, Surrey S: Use of resistant or hypersensitive variant clones of Friend cells in analysis of mode of action of inducers. Cancer Res 38:3737, 1978
321. Rowley PT, Ohlsson-Wilhelm BM, Farley BA: K562 human erythroleukemia cells demonstrate commitment. Blood 65:862, 1985
322. Rowley PT, Ohlsson-Wilhelm B, Farley B, Kosciolek B: Trypsin enhances erythropoiesis in vitro. J Lab Clin Med 96:433, 1980
323. Rubin CS: Effects of cyclic AMP on the growth of differentiating and undifferentiated Friend erythroleukemia cells. J Cell Physiol 94:57, 1978
324. Rubin H: Growth-regulating interactions among cultured animal cells. In Permeability and Function of Biological Membranes, edited by Katchalsky A, Keynes RD, Loewenstein WR, Pethica BA, p 103. Amsterdam, North-Holland Publishing Co., Inc, 1970
325. Rubin H: Overgrowth stimulating factor released from Rous sarcoma cells. Science 167:1271, 1970
326. Ruggiero M, Lapetina EG: Protease and cyclooxygenase inhibitors synergistically prevent activation of human platelets. Proc Natl

Acad Sci USA 83:3456, 1986

327. Ruggiero M, Lapetina EG: Thrombin and trypsin activate phospholipase C in human platelets via a proteolytic-mediated pathway. Semin Thromb Hemost 12:241, 1986
328. Ruoslahti E, Pierschbacher MD: Arg-Gly-Asp: a versatile cell recognition signal. Cell 44:517, 1986
329. Rutter W: In Chimeric receptors give clues to oncogene action. Science 233:160, 1986
330. Saito M, Yoshizawa T, Aoyagi T, Nagai Y: Involvement of proteolytic activity in early events in lymphocyte transformation by phytohemagglutinin. Biochem Biophys Res Commun 52:569, 1973
331. Saksela O: Plasminogen activation and regulation of pericellular proteolysis. Biochim Biophys Acta 823:35, 1985
332. Saltiel AR: Insulin generates an enzyme modulator from hepatic plasma membranes: regulation of adenosine 3′,5′-monophosphate phosphodiesterase, pyruvate dehydrogenase, and adenylate cyclase. Endocrinology 120:967, 1987
333. Saltiel AR, Cuatrecasas P: Insulin stimulates the generation from hepatic plasma membranes of modulators derived from an inositol glycolipid. Proc Natl Acad Sci USA 83:5793, 1986
334. Saltiel AR, Doble A, Jacobs S, Cuatrecasas P: Putative mediators of insulin action regulate hepatic acetyl CoA carboxylase activity. Biochem Biophys Res Commun 110:789, 1983
335. Saltiel AR, Fox JH, Sherline P, Cuatrecasas P: Insulin-stimulated hydrolysis of a novel glycolipid generates modulators of cAMP phosphodiesterase. Science 233:967, 1986
336. Saltiel AR, Siegel MI, Jacobs S, Cuatrecasas P: Putative mediators of insulin action: regulation of pyruvate dehydrogenase and adenylate cyclase activities. Proc Natl Acad Sci USA 79:3513, 1982
337. Sawyer ST, Krantz SB, Goldwasser E: Binding and receptor-mediated endocytosis of erythropoietin in Friend virus-infected erythroid cells. J Biol Chem 262:5554, 1987
338. Schekman R: Protein transport—it's what's up front that counts. Trends Biochem Sci 5:177, 1985
339. Scher BM, Scher W, Waxman S: Lack of evidence for activation of a serum factor in protease-induced differentiation of mouse erythroleukemia cells. In Vitro Cell Devel Biol 21:260, 1985
340. Scher W, Ansley H, Gilbert H, Ornstein L: Monocyte-like esterase in Friend leukemia cells and mouse erythrocytes. In Prevention and Detection, Part II. Detection, Vol 2, Cancer Detection in Specific Sites, edited by Nieburgs HE, p 2339. New York, Marcel Dekker, Inc, 1980
341. Scher W, Hellinger N, Waxman S: Protease induction of hemoglobin synthesis but not terminal cell division in K562 cells. Exp Hematol 13:36, 1985
342. Scher W, Scher BM, Hellinger N, Waxman S: The proportions of hemoglobin types induced in mouse erythroleukemia cells vary with the inducer or combination of inducers, the inducer concentration and the time of induction. Hemoglobin 9:577, 1985
343. Scher W, Scher BM, Waxman S: Proteases stimulate mouse erythroleukemia cell differentiation and multiplication. Biochem Biophys Res Commun 109:348, 1982
344. Scher W, Scher BM, Waxman S: Proteases act synergistically with low molecular weight inducers to stimulate mouse erythroleukemia cell differentiation. Exp Hematol 11:490, 1983
345. Scher W, Tsuei D, Sassa S, Price P, Gabelman N, Friend C: Inhibition of dimethyl sulfoxide-stimulated Friend cell erythrodifferentiation by hydrocortisone and other steroids. Proc Natl Acad Sci USA 75:3851, 1978
346. Scher W, Waxman S: Effects of dexamethasone and phorbol myristate acetate on the induction of differentiation in mouse erythroleukemic cells by dimethyl sulfoxide, proteases, and other compounds. Ann NY Acad Sci 411:180, 1983
347. Schleuning W-D, Fritz H: Sperm acrosin. In Methods in Enzymology, Proteolytic Enzymes, Part B, Vol 45, edited by Lorand L, p 330. New York, Academic Press, Inc, 1976
348. Schnebli HP: Growth inhibition of tumor cells by protease inhibitors: consideration of the mechanisms involved. In Cold Spring Harbor Symp, Control of Proliferation in Animal cells, edited by Clarkson B, Baserga R, p 327. Cold Spring Harbor, Cold Spring Harbor Laboratory, 1974
349. Schnebli HP, Burger MM: Selective inhibition of growth of transformed cells by protease inhibitors. Proc Natl Acad Sci USA 69:3825, 1972
350. Schollmeyer JE: Possible role of calpain I and calpain II in differentiating muscle. Exp Cell Res 163:413, 1986
351. Schreiber AB, Lax I, Yarden Y, Eshhar Z, Schlessinger J: Monoclonal antibodies against receptor for epidermal growth factor induce early and delayed effects of epidermal growth factor. Proc Natl Acad Sci USA 78:7535, 1981
352. Scott GK, Seow HF: Further evidence for a cell surface proteinase essential to the growth of cultured fibroblasts. Exp Cell Res 158:43, 1985
353. Seals JR, Czech MP: Evidence that insulin activates an intrinsic plasma membrane protease in generating a secondary chemical mediator. J Biol Chem 255:6529, 1980
354. Seals JR, Czech MP: Production by plasma membranes of a chemical mediator of insulin action. Fed Proc 41:2730, 1982
355. Seals JR, Jarett L: Activation of pyruvate dehydrogenase by direct addition of insulin to an isolated plasma membrane/mitochondria mixture: evidence for generation of insulin's second messenger in a subcellular system. Proc Natl Acad Sci USA 77:77, 1980
356. Seals JR, McDonald JM, Jarett L: Direct effect of insulin on the labeling of isolated plasma membranes by [γ^{32}P]ATP. Biochem Biophys Res Commun 83:1365, 1978
357. Sefton BM, Rubin H: Release from density dependent growth inhibition by proteolytic enzymes. Nature 227:843, 1970
358. Segal J: Trypsin-induced increase in cyclic AMP concentration in rat thymocytes: an effect independent of calcium and calmodulin. Biochem J 239:603, 1986
359. Seidl J, Borchert M, Ziegler I: Phorbol ester causes short term and transient accumulation of pteridines in T cells and in cell lines. Biochem Biophys Res Commun 141:494, 1986
360. Sekar MC, Dixon JF, Hokin LE: The formation of inositol 1,2-cyclic 4,5-trisphosphate and inositol 1,2-cyclic 4-bisphosphate on stimulation of mouse pancreatic minilobules with carbamylcholine. J Biol Chem 262:340, 1987
361. Sekar MC, Hokin LE: The role of phosphoinositides in signal transduction. J Memb Biol 89:193, 1986
362. Sherman ML, Shafman TD, Kufe DW: Inhibitory effects of theophylline and dibutyryl cAMP on murine erythroleukemia cell differentiation. Biochem Biophys Res Commun 134:845, 1986
363. Sherwood JB: The chemistry and physiology of erythropoietin. In Vitamins and Hormones Advances in Research and Applications, edited by Aurbach GD, McCormic DB, Vol 41, p 161, New York, Academic Press, Inc, 1984
363a. Shibata H, Ogata E, Etoh Y, Shibai H, Kojima I: Erythroid differentiation factor stimulates hydrolysis of polyphosphoinositide in Friend erythroleukemia cells. Biochem Biophys Res Commun 146:187, 1987
364. Shibuya T, Mak TW: Induction of erythroid tumorigenic colonies by Friend helper virus F-MuLV alone and isolation of a new class of Friend erythroleukemic cells. J Cell Physiol 1 (Suppl):185, 1982
365. Simmer RL, Baker JB, Cunningham DD: Direct linkage of thrombin to its cell surface receptors in different cell types. J Supramolec Struct 12:245, 1979
366. Simms HS, Stillman NP: Substances affecting adult tissue in vitro I. The stimulating action of trypsin on fresh adult tissue. J Gen Physiol 20:603, 1937
367. Slosberg EA, Scher BM, Scher W, Josephson S, Waxman S: Localization of the site of action of protease inducers of erythroid differentiation of mouse erythroleukemia (MEL) cells to the cell surface. Exp Hematol 14:442, 1986
368. Smith RM, Jarett L: Ultrastructural evidence for the accumulation of insulin in nuclei of intact 3T3-L1 adipocytes by an insulin-receptor-mediated process. Proc Natl Acad Sci USA 84:459, 1987
369. Snider RM, McKinney M, Richelson E: Thrombin binding and stimulation of cyclic guanosine monophosphate formation in neuroblastoma cells. Semin Thromb Hemostas 12:253, 1986
370. Steffan JA: Changes of *in vitro* proliferation patterns of human lymphocytes following pronase pretreatment. In Lymphocyte Recognition and Effector Mechanisms, Proceedings of the 8th Leukocyte Culture Conference, edited by Lindagl-Kiessling K, Osoba D, p 565. New York, Academic Press, Inc, 1974
370a. Stein M, Braulke T, Von Figura K, Hasilik A: Effects of differentiation-inducing agents on synthesis, maturation and secretion of cathepsin D in U937 and HL-60 cells. Biol Chem Hoppe-Seyler 368:413, 1987
371. Stoppelli MP, Tacchetti C, Cubellis MV, Corti A, Hearing VJ, Cassani G, Appella E, Blasi F: Autocrine saturation of pro-

urokinase receptors on human A431 cells. Cell 45:675, 1986

372. Storm G, Bosman GJCGM, Boer P, Roelofsen B, Op den Kamp JAF, van Deenen LLM: Studies on phospholipid turnover in Friend erythroleukaemic cells. Biochem Intern 5:169, 1982
373. Stricklin GP, Welgus HG: Physiologic relevance of erythroid-potentiating activity or TIMP. Nature 321:628, 1986
374. Sutherland JA, Turner AR, Mannoni P, McGann LE, Turc J-M: Differentiation of K562 leukemia cells/along erythroid, macrophage, and megakaryocyte lineages. J Biol Response Mod 5:250, 1986
375. Suzuki S, Argraves WSA, Pytela R, Arai H, Krusius T, Pierschbacher MD, Ruoslahti E: cDNA and amino acid sequences of the cell adhesion protein receptor recognizing vitronectin reveal a transmembrane domain and homologies with other adhesion protein receptors. Proc Natl Acad Sci USA 83:8614, 1986
376. Suzuki S, Toyota T, Tamura S, Kikuchi K, Tsuiki S, Huang L, Villar-Palasi C, Larner J, Goto Y: ATP-Mn^{2+} stimulates the generation of a putative mediator of insulin action. J Biol Chem 262:3199, 1987
377. Tabilio A, Pelicci PG, Vinci G, Mannoni P, Civin CI, Vainchenker W, Testa U, Lipinski M, Rochant H, Breton-Gorius J: Myeloid and megakaryocytic properties of K-562 cell lines. Cancer Res 43:4569, 1983
378. Takahashi E, Nagasawa T, Sato S, Matsushima T, Sugimura T, Ohashi A: Induction of delta-aminolevulinic acid synthetase in cultured Friend leukemia cells by dimethyl sulfoxide and human placental extract. Gann 65:261, 1974
379. Takamatsu J, Horne III, MK, Gralnick HR: Identification of the thrombin receptor on human platelets by chemical crosslinking. J Clin Invest 77:362, 1986
380. Takemura R, Werb Z: Secretory products of macrophages and their physiological functions. Am J Physiol 246:1, 1984
381. Tambourin P, Casadevall N, Choppin J, Lacombe C, Heard JM, Fichelson S, Wendling F, Varet B: Production of erythropoietin-like activity by a murine erythroleukemia cell line. Proc Natl Acad Sci USA 50:6269, 1983
382. Tamura S, Fujita-Yamaguchi Y, Larner J: Insulin-like effect of trypsin on the phosphorylation of rat adipocyte insulin receptor. J Biol Chem 258:14749, 1983
383. Tamura S, Schwartz CFW, Whipple JH, Dubler RE, Fujita-Yamaguchi Y, Larner J: Selective inhibition of the insulin-stimulated phosphorylation of the 95,000 dalton subunit of the insulin receptor by TAME or BAEE. Biochem Biophys Res Commun 119:465, 1984
384. Taylor JM, Mitchell WM, Cohen S: Characterization of the binding protein for epidermal growth factor. J Biol Chem 249:2188, 1974
385. Taylor R, Soos MA, Wells A, Argyraki M, Siddle K: Insulin-like and insulin-inhibitory effects of monoclonal antibodies for different epitopes on the human insulin receptor. Biochem J 242:123, 1987
386. Teng NNH, Chen LB: Thrombin-sensitive surface protein of cultured chick embryo cells. Nature 259:578, 1976
387. Tetteroo PAT, Massaro F, Mulder A, Schreuder-van-Gelder R, von dem Borne AEG KR: Megakaryoblastic differentiation of proerythroblastic K562 cell-line cells. Leuk Res 8:197, 1984
388. Teyssot B, Djiane J, Kelly PA, Houdebine L-M: Identification of the putative prolactin second messenger activating beta-casein gene transcription. Biol Cell 43:51, 1982
389. Thomas KA, Baglan NC, and Bradshaw RA: The amino acid sequence of the γ-subunit of mouse submaxillary gland 7 S nerve growth factor. J Biol Chem 256:9156, 1981
390. Thompson MP, Larner J, Kilpatrick DL: Purification and partial characterization of a putative mediator of insulin action on cyclic AMP-dependent protein kinase. Mol Cell Biochem 62:67, 1984
391. Tollefsen DM, Feagler JR, Majerus PW: The binding of thrombin to the surface of human platelets. J Biol Chem 249:2646, 1974
392. Tomonaga M, Gasson JC, Quan SG, Golde DW: Establishment of eosinophilic sublines from human promyelocytic leukemia (HL-60) cells: demonstration of multipotentiality and single-lineage commitment of HL-60 stem cells. Blood 67:1433, 1986
393. Traktman P, Baltimore D: Protease bypass of temperature-sensitive murine leukemia virus maturation mutants. J Virol 44:1039, 1982
394. Tsonis CG, Sharpe RM: Dual gonadal control of follicle-stimulating hormone. Nature 321:724, 1986
395. Tsung P-K, Kegeles SW, Becker EL: The evidence for the existence of chymotrypsin-like esterase activity in the plasma membranes of rabbit neutrophils and the specific chemotactic peptide binding activity of the subcellular fractions. Biochim Biophys Acta 541:150, 1978
396. Tysnes O-B, Verhoeven AJM, Holmsen H: Phosphate turnover of phosphatidylinositol in resting and thrombin-stimulated platelets. Biochim Biophys Acta 889:183, 1986
397. Uchida M, Watanabe Y, Fujimoto Y: Is phospholipid a required cofactor for the activity of mammalian signal peptidase? FEBS Lett 200:343, 1986
398. Ueki H, Araki M, Nagayoshi A, Funakoshi T, Shoji S, Kubota Y: Insulin-like activity of proteases. VI. Chem Pharm Bull (Tokyo) 30:4144, 1982
399. Ueki H, Furuta K, Funakoshi T, Matsunami Y, Kubota Y: Insulin-like activity of proteases. V. Chem Pharm Bull (Tokyo) 30:1054, 1982
400. Utsunomiya N, Nakanishi M: A serine protease triggers the initial step of transmembrane signalling in cytotoxic T cells. J Biol Chem 261:16514, 1986
401. Vaheri A, Ruoslahti E, Hovi T: Cell Surface and growth control of chick embryo fibroblasts in culture. In Control of Proliferation in Animal Cells, edited by Clarkson B, Baserga R, p 305. Cold Spring Harbor, Cold Spring Harbor Laboratory, 1974
402. Vale W, Rivier J, Vaughan J, McClintock R, Corrigan A, Woo W, Karr D, Spiess J: Purification and characterization of an FSH releasing protein from porcine ovarian follicular fluid. Nature 321:776, 1986
403. Vandenbark GR, Kuhn LJ, Niedel JE: Possible mechanism of phorbol diester-induced maturation of human promyelocytic leukemia cells: activation of protein kinase C. J Clin Invest 73:448, 1984
404. Van Obberghen-Schilling E, Chambard JC, Paris S, L'Allemain G, Pouysségur J: Alpha-thrombin-induced early mitogenic signalling events and Go to S-phase transition of fibroblasts require continual external stimulation. EMBO J 4:2927, 1985
405. Van Obberghen-Schilling E, Pouysségur J: Affinity labeling of high-affinity α-thrombin binding sites on the surface of hamster fibroblasts. Biochim Biophys Acta 847:335, 1985
406. Van Winkle LJ: Chymotrypsin stimulated development of delayed implantation mouse blastocysts. Biochem Biophys Res Commun 98:562, 1981
407. Vassalli, J-D, Baccino D, Belin D: A cellular binding site for the M_r 55,000 form of the human plasminogen activator, urokinase. J Cell Biol 100:86, 1985
408. Vester JW, Reino ML: Hepatic glucokinase: a direct effect of insulin. Science 142:590, 1963
409. Villeval JL, Pelicci PG, Tabilio A, Titeux M, Henri A, Houesche F, Thomopoulous P, Vainchenker W, Garbaz M, Rochant H, Breton-Gorius J, Edwards PHW, Testa U: Erythroid properties of K562 cells: effect of hemin, butyrate and TPA induction. Exp Cell Res 146:428, 1983
410. Vischer TL: Stimulation of mouse B lymphocytes by trypsin. J Immunol 113:58, 1974
411. Vischer TL: Protease inhibitors reduce mitogen induced lymphocyte stimulation. Immunology 36:811, 1979
412. Vischer TL, Bertand L: Stimulating effect of neutral proteases on cells in vitro. Agents Actions 6:180, 1976
413. Vischer TL, Bretz U, Baggiolini M: In vitro stimulation of lymphocytes by neutral proteinases from human polymorphonuclear leukocyte granules. J Exp Med 144:863, 1976
414. von Melchener H, Hoffken K: Changes in self-renewal potential of human leukemic cells (K562): A bidirectional stochastic process. J Cell Physiol 123:249, 1985
415. Vos O, Burman WA, Ploemacher RE: Mobilization of haemopoietic stem cells (CFU) into the peripheral blood of the mouse; effects of endotoxin and other compounds. Cell Tissue Kinet 5:467, 1972
416. Walkenbach RJ, Hazen R, Larner J: Reversible inhibition of cyclic AMP-dependent protein kinase by insulin. Mol Cell Biochem 19:31, 1978
417. Wallach D, Anderson W, Pastan I: Activation of adenylate cyclase in cultured fibroblasts by trypsin. J Biol Chem 253:24, 1978
418. Waxman L, Fagan JM, Goldberg AL: Demonstration of two

distinct high molecular weight proteases in rabbit reticulocytes, one of which degrades ubiquitin conjugates. J Biol Chem 262:2451, 1987

419. Waxman L, Fagan JM, Tanaka K, Goldberg AL: A soluble ATP-dependent system for protein degradation from murine erythroleukemia cells: evidence for a protease which requires ATP hydrolysis but not ubiquitin. J Biol Chem 260:11994, 1985
420. Waxman L, Tanaka K: The cytoplasmic proteases in undifferentiated murine erythroleukemia cells. J Cell Biol 97:118, 1983
421. Waxman S, Scher W, Scher BM: Basic principles for utilizing combination differentiation agents. Cancer Detect Prev 9:395, 1986
422. Weich HA, Herbst D, Schairer HU, Hoppe J: Platelet-derived growth factor. Phorbol ester induces the expression of the B-chain but not of the A-chain in HEL cells. FEBS Lett 213:89, 1987
423. Weis LS, Narahara HT: Regulation of cell membrane permeability in skeletal muscle. I. Action of insulin and trypsin on the transport system for sugar. J Biol Chem 244:3084, 1969
424. Werb Z, Aggler J: Proteases induce secretion of collagenase and plasminogen activator by fibroblasts. Proc Natl Acad Sci USA 75:1839, 1978
425. Wicki AN, Clemetson KJ: Structure and function of platelet membrane glycoproteins Ib and V. Eur J Biochem 153:1, 1985
426. Wilks JW, Hui OJ: Aprotinin antagonizes the binding of human chorionic gonadotropin to its receptor. Endocrinology 120:946, 1987
427. Williams WJ: Biochemistry of plasma coagulation factors. In Hematology, Edited by Williams WJ, Beutler E, Erslev AJ, Rundles RW, p 1057. New York, McGraw-Hill Book Co., 1972
428. Wilson EL, Jacobs P, Dowdle EB: The secretion of plasminogen activators by human myeloid leukemic cells in vitro. Blood 6:568, 1983
429. Wong RL, Gutowski JK, Katz M, Goldfarb RH, Cohn S: Induction of DNA synthesis in isolated nuclei by cytoplasmic factors: inhibition by protease inhibitors. Proc Natl Acad Sci USA 84:241, 1987
430. Yamamato K, Tamamoto N, Kitagawa H, Tanoue K, Kosaki G, Yamazaki H: Localization of a thrombin-binding site on human platelet membrane glycoprotein Ib determined by a monoclonal antibody. Thromb Hemost 55:162, 1985
431. Yamasaki H, Drevon C, Martel N: *In vitro* studies on the mechanism of tumor promoter-mediated inhibition of cell differentiation. Carcinogenesis 7:359, 1982
432. Yamasaki H, Fibach E, Weinstein IB, Nudel U, Rifkind RA, Marks PA: Inhibition of Friend leukemia cell differentiation by tumor promoters. In Oncogenic Viruses and Host Cell Genes, edited by Ikawa Y, Odaka T, p 365. New York, Academic Press, Inc, 1979
433. Yavelow J, Caggana M, Beck KA: Proteases occurring in the cell membrane: a possible cell receptor for the Bowman-Birk type of protease inhibitors. Cancer Res 47:1598, 1987
434. Yavelow J, Scott CB, Mayer TC: Fluorescent visualization of binding and internalization of the anticarcinogenic Bowman-Birk type protease inhibitors in transformed fibroblasts. Cancer Res 47:1602, 1987
435. Yen A, Powers V, Fishbaugh J: Retinoic acid induced HL-60 myeloid differentiation: dependence of early and late events on isomeric structure. Leuk Res 10:619, 1986
436. Yen A, Reece SL, Albright KL: Membrane origin for a signal eliciting a program of cell differentiation. Exp Cell Res 152:493, 1984
437. Ying S-Y, Becker A, Baird A, Ling N, Ueno N, Esch F, Guillemin R: Type beta transforming growth factor (TGF-β) is a potent stimulator of the basal secretion of follicle stimulating hormone (FSH) in a pituitary monolayer system. Biochem Biophys Res Commun 135:950, 1986
438. Young DC, Griffin JD: Autocrine secretion of GM-CSF in acute myeloblastic leukemia. Blood 68:1178, 1986
439. Young TH, Niemetz J, Ohnuma T: Procoagulent activity in HL-60, ML-2, and KG-1 human myelogenous leukemia cell lines. Blood 58, No. 55, 1 (Suppl):81, 1981
440. Yourno J, Walsh J, Kornatowski G, O'Conner D, Kumar SA: Nonspecific esterases of leukemia cell lines: evidence for activation of myeloid-associated zymogens in HL-60 by phorbol esters. Blood 63:238, 1984
441. Yu K-T, Czech MP: Tyrosine phosphorylation of the insulin receptor β subunit activates the receptor-associated tyrosine kinase activity. J Biol Chem 259:5277, 1984
442. Zetter BR, Antoniades MN: Stimulation of human vascular endothelial cell growth by a platelet-derived growth factor and thrombin. J Supramolec Struct 11:361, 1979
443. Zetter BR, Chen LB, Buchanan JM: Effects of protease treatment on growth, morphology, adhesion, and cell surface proteins of secondary chick embryo fibroblasts. Cell 7:407, 1976
444. Zetter BR, Chen LB, Buchanan JM: Binding and internalization of thrombin by normal and transformed chick cells. Proc Natl Acad Sci USA 74:596, 1977
445. Zola H: Differentiation and maturation of human B lymphocytes: a review. Pathology 17:365, 1985
446. Zuckerman GB, Naughton BA, Gaito A, Preti RA, Gordon AS: The effect of methylcellulose on extrarenal erythropoietin production. Proc Soc Exp Biol Med 176:197, 1984
447. Zwingelstein G, Tapiero H, Portoukalian J, Fourcade A: The effect of dimethylsulfoxide on the lipid composition of inducible and noninducible Friend leukemia cells. Biochem Biophys Res Commun 108:437, 1982

Biology of Disease

Dietary and Nutritional Influences on Cancer: A Review of Epidemiologic and Experimental Data

ADRIANNE E. ROGERS AND MATTHEW P. LONGNECKER

Department of Pathology, Boston University School of Medicine and Mallory Institute of Pathology; and Harvard School of Public Health, Boston, Massachusetts

INTRODUCTION

Investigation of dietary and nutritional influences on induction and development of cancer has produced a vast amount of data. This information has furthered understanding of basic mechanisms of carcinogenesis and explained certain aspects of cancer epidemiology. As is true in many areas, some relationships that were initially recognized and appeared simple have proved to be complex and to require major modification or qualification. Because the literature on diet and cancer is extensive we have limited our review of epidemiologic results to the more intensively studied nutrients and foods and to the cancers that occur most frequently in Western societies. The nutrients and foods examined in relation to cancer risk are: total calories, fat, cholesterol, fiber, alcohol, carotenoids, vitamin A, vitamin E, vitamin C, selenium, coffee, cruciferous vegetables, and protein. The sites considered are lung, breast, large bowel, prostate, ovary and pancreas. The experimental results discussed include many of the same subjects with the addition of nutrients and target organs that form a significant segment of the experimental literature. Additional nutrients discussed are: zinc, choline and methionine. Additional target organs are: liver, esophagus, urinary bladder. The review is concerned primarily with nutritional influences on cancer and carcinogenesis and not with the effects of dietary additives or contaminants. The emphasis is on recent studies, questions and research directions.

The 1982 evaluation of the evidence on dietary and nutritional influences on cancer (184) served as a starting point for parts of the review, although in several cases older publications were used. The 1982 evaluation concluded in part that:

1. Epidemiologic and experimental data support an association between high dietary fat and carcinoma of breast, large bowel and prostate, although not all data are consistent with the association.

2. Reduction in total diet intake reduces tumor incidence in laboratory animals, possibly because of reduced caloric intake, but reduction of other diet components may be responsible; epidemiologic studies have not confirmed a relationship between caloric intake and cancer.

3. There are data suggesting an association of high dietary protein and cancer, but clear separation of effects of fat and protein cannot be made.

4. Laboratory studies show that vitamin A inhibits chemical carcinogenesis at several sites; epidemiologic studies indicate that ingestion of foods containing vitamin A or beta-carotene reduces cancer risk in lung, larynx and bladder.

5. Epidemiologic and experimental data suggest that selenium may reduce cancer risk, but the results are not conclusive.

6. Limited epidemiologic evidence suggests an association of ingestion of foods containing vitamin C and decreased risk for esophageal and gastric cancer; laboratory studies show that vitamin C can reduce formation of carcinogenic nitrosamines.

7. Results of studies of carbohydrate, fiber, vitamin E and the B vitamins are inconclusive.

8. Alcohol acts synergistically with tobacco smoking to increase risk for cancers of the upper gastrointestinal and respiratory tracts. There is inconsistent evidence of an association of colorectal, particularly rectal, cancer with excessive beer consumption, limited evidence that excessive alcohol intake contributes to hepatic injury and cirrhosis and, in turn, to hepatoma.

Since the 1982 National Academy of Sciences review, many noteworthy studies of diet and cancer have been reported. Understanding of relationships suggested by epidemiologic studies and supported by experimental data, such as the association of breast cancer with diets relatively high in fat, is being modified by more detailed examination of caloric balance and use of newer analytical and experimental approaches. Major inconsistencies in epidemiologic and experimental data have been revealed in investigations of the possible association between colon cancer and diets relatively high in fat. Inconsistent results in studies of the influence of dietary vitamin A have stimulated the development of new chemical, epidemiologic and experimental methods. Recent studies on alcohol consumption in relation to breast cancer have found, fairly consistently, a modest direct association which suggests that sites not directly involved in absorption and metabolism of alcohol may be affected by it. In mechanistic studies of the effect of diet on carcinogenesis, the lipotrope-deficient rat has provided the first clear evidence of carcinogenesis by a dietary deficiency per se. The importance of physical activity and relative body weight, which are related to total caloric intake and balance, is now becoming recognized in evaluating dietary intake.

The data reviewed were critically evaluated according to specific considerations. Epidemiologic considerations and data precede the parallel experimental sections; in the concluding section data from both sources are synthesized.

EPIDEMIOLOGIC STUDIES OF DIETARY AND NUTRITIONAL INFLUENCES IN CANCER RISK

Method of Evaluation of Data from Epidemiologic Studies

General Epidemiologic Considerations. The epidemiologic data on each diet-cancer relation were assessed according to the considerations outlined below. Epidemiologic study designs can be classified according to the method of obtaining data: simple observation (nonexperimental studies) or observation after some type of intervention (experimental studies). Study designs can be classified further according to the basic unit of analysis: a population (*e.g.*, geographic correlation studies) or individuals (*e.g.*, follow-up and case-control studies). Epidemiologic study designs vary with respect to the types of bias most likely to occur and the likelihood that bias may materially affect the result.

In epidemiology, experimental studies (clinical trials) are in theory the best method by which to assess diet-cancer relations. Data so obtained are the most powerful available for making causal inference and are least likely to be biased. Unfortunately, clinical trials are frequently infeasible for practical, financial or ethical reasons.

Follow-up and case-control studies are the two nonexperimental study designs most commonly used in nutritional epidemiology. In a follow-up study comparison is made of the occurrence of disease among exposed and unexposed individuals. In case-control studies, the prior exposure experience of diseased individuals is contrasted with exposure in nondiseased (control) individuals, sampled from the population that gave rise to the cases.

Data obtained with geographic correlation studies, including migration studies, are less powerful than other nonexperimental studies, and their usefulness is a subject of debate. There are two problems with geographic correlation studies: first, it is not known if the individuals exposed are the ones affected by the disease, and, second, there is often no way to separate the influence of potentially confounding factors from the influence of the exposure under study. Geographic correlation studies are useful for hypothesis generation and support of hypotheses when better data are unavailable, but they are not reliable sources of information for causal inference.

In general, the goal of an epidemiologic study is to estimate accurately the direction and magnitude of association, if any, between the exposure and disease of interest in the population studied. Bias in the measured association can arise for several reasons, *e.g.*, when compared groups differ with respect to unmeasured risk factors, or because of poor data on disease or exposure status. Further discussion of bias in epidemiologic research can be found elsewhere (123, 249).

Nutritional Epidemiology. The fundamental principles of diet assessment and analysis of diet in relation to disease are reflected more fully in recent epidemiologic studies than they were in older studies. More frequent employment of diet assessment techniques that allow measurement of total caloric intake is one manifestation of progress. For individuals in caloric balance (*e.g.*, not experiencing weight gain or loss) with a consistent level of physical activity, total caloric intake is a relatively constant. However, the proportion of total calories coming from fats, carbohydrates, and protein (macronutrients) may vary and is amenable to manipulation for experimental, therapeutic or preventive reasons. For meaningful analyses with public health implications, the proportion of total calories coming from each macronutrient, or a functionally similar quantity known as the calorie adjusted residual, should be examined in relation to disease risk (326). Causal interpretation of data on macronutrient intake in relation to disease risk must take account of the fact that, at a fixed caloric intake, an increase in calories from fat means a decrease in calories from carbohydrate and protein (or alcohol). If consumption of a high proportion of calories from fat is associated with an increased risk of disease, the reciprocal interpretation is equally valid, *i.e.*, the reduced consumption of calories from carbohydrate and protein could be the key association. In other words it is the effect of diet as a whole, as opposed to the effect of a single nutrient, that can be examined.

Measurement of diet is inherently error prone. Errors in classifying individuals' long-term intake of a given diet, food, or nutrient make diet-cancer associations difficult to detect. Individuals do not remember what they have eaten with perfect accuracy; their diet may have varied substantially over time. Therefore, it is possible that an association exists but is not detectable with current methods.

The survey instruments in dietary epidemiology are used to gather information on the consumption of foods, not individual nutrients directly. Data on the frequency of consumption of foods and on portion size can be used to calculate nutrient intakes. The accuracy of the translation depends, in part, upon the quality of information in the food composition data used. Nutrient content of foods can vary due to environmental, seasonal, and processing effects (5).

When the interest is in associations between consumption of certain foods and cancer risk, then data collected on food intake (regardless of nutrient content) can be examined in relation to disease directly. However, when associations between consumption of certain nutrients and cancer risk are the focus, data on food or food-group intake should be presented also in terms of nutrient content. For this review in discussing studies in which only food or food-group data were presented, the intake of foods that account for the greatest variance in intake of the nutrient of interest was used as a surrogate measure of nutrient intake when appropriate. For example, in studies reviewed for the section on fat and cancer, many investigators presented only an analysis of meat intake in relation to cancer risk. Since meat accounts for a large amount of the variance in fat intake in the United States (26), meat intake was used as a surrogate for fat intake. Likewise, in many studies the relation between fiber intake and cancer risk was inferred from data relating intake of foods from certain groups (vegetables, fruits and cereals) to cancer risk. The surrogate exposure method was used in evaluating cancer risks associated with intakes of protein (meat and milk), carotenoids (fruits and vegetables), and cholesterol (meat, eggs, and milk).

Use of surrogate measures poses two difficulties. First, if there truly is an association between the disease and nutrient, the magnitude of the association is underestimated. If a high fat intake actually causes colon cancer, and if the intake of meat is used as surrogate measure of fat intake, the association between meat intake and risk of colon cancer will be smaller than the true but unmeasured association between fat intake and colon cancer. This underestimate is a consequence of having imperfect data on exposure. Second, certain foods are important sources of more than one nutrient of interest. For example, foods that account for the greatest proportion of variation in protein intake (hamburgers, whole milk and steak in the United States) also are important sources of cholesterol and fat (26). The correlation between protein intake and fat intake, unadjusted for total caloric intake, is about 0.4 to 0.5, and between protein intake and cholesterol intake is 0.5 to 0.6 (322). Thus, an association between intake of protein-containing foods and cancer may be due to an effect of fat or cholesterol in those foods. For these reasons, findings from studies in which only surrogate measures of nutrient intake were available were given less weight than data from studies in which associations between nutrient intake and cancer risk could be directly assessed.

Biochemical markers are useful to characterize intake of several micronutrients. Serum concentrations of β-carotene, vitamin E, and selenium (Se) and toenail Se content reflect dietary intake (183, 290, 330). However, the relation between intake and blood levels of micronutrients is often complex. For example, smokers have lower serum concentrations of Se and carotene than nonsmokers when both groups report the same intakes (102, 282). Serum retinol (vitamin A) is buffered by tissue stores and reflects nutritional status only at extremes of depletion or excess (329).

Despite the inaccuracies in diet measurement, nutritional epidemiologic studies can provide useful information, as reviewed below. As diet assessment methods improve and analytical techniques advance, it is likely that currently unrecognized subtle, relationships will be found.

Method of Summarizing Epidemiologic Data. Investigators analyze their data in a multitude of ways. Some authors compare disease risk between groups in upper and lower nutrient intake quintiles; others dichotomize intakes and compare risks, and others compare mean intakes of diseased and nondiseased groups. These inconsistencies make assessment of dose-response (other than within a single study) difficult, and in most cases, permit only qualitative evaluation of associations.

When relative risks are weak it is particularly difficult to know if the association observed is attributable to the food or nutrient studied or to a confounding factor, such as another food, which also influences the risk of disease and is associated with the food of interest.

The importance placed on the data from a particular epidemiologic study was determined by the size of the study, the quality of the dietary assessment method, the appropriateness of the analysis and the degree of potential bias suspected. Every epidemiologic study reviewed was evaluated on each of these criteria according to a scoring system described in the "Appendix."

FAT

Although data in geographic correlation studies support high diet fat content as a risk factor in breast cancer, in case-control and follow-up studies breast cancer risk appears to be only weakly related or not related to intake of fat or fat-containing foods (Table 1). In two of the studies in which the largest direct association was found (94, 153) the findings may reflect the effect of factors other than fat. In Hirayama's data (94), the analysis of meat intake, as surrogate for fat intake, in relation to breast cancer risk may be confounded by reproductive determinants of breast cancer and degree of "Westernization." In the study of Lubin *et al.* (153), cases and controls were interviewed by somewhat different procedures, and the information obtained may, therefore, not be entirely comparable. Breast cancer risk in relation to fat intake appears not to vary according to menopausal status (Table 1) or to the type of fat eaten (115, 327).

Two hypotheses have been advanced to explain why the evidence for a relationship is weaker in case control and follow-up studies than in the international comparisons. First, it has been proposed that, because of the homogeneous fat intakes within the populations studied, the contrasts are not great enough to demonstrate an effect (335). Second, it has been proposed that an adverse effect of high fat intake could occur early in a woman's life and that differences in early intake may not be detected by questioning of adult women. In any case the current epidemiologic evidence, gathered in Western populations, does not indicate that a moderate reduction in fat intake by adult women will have a detectable influence on their breast cancer risk.

TABLE 1. A SUMMARY OF EPIDEMIOLOGIC STUDIES IN WHICH TOTAL FAT INTAKE WAS EXAMINED AS A RISK FACTOR FOR BREAST CANCER

References	Study design	Number of		Intake categories compared	RR			Notes[a]
		Cases	Non-cases		pre	post	Combined	
Most informative								
Katsouyanni *et al.* (119)	cc	120	120	High:low deciles	—	—	1.4	
Willett *et al.* (327)	fu	601	89,538	High:low quintiles	0.9	0.8	0.8	
Jones *et al.* (115)	fu	99	5,386	High:low quartiles	—	—	0.7	
Hirohata *et al.* (97)	cc	344	688	High:low quartiles	—	—	"1.2"	
Hirohata *et al.* (98)	cc	212	424	High:low quartiles	—	1.0	1.0	
Miller *et al.* (174)	cc	400	400	High:low quartiles	1.6	1.8	"1.7"	
Others								
Lubin *et al.* (154)	cc	818	1,556	High:low quartiles	"1.1"	"1.4"	"1.3"	
Talamini *et al.* (286)	cc	368	373	High:low frequency	—	—	1.3	1
Kolonel *et al.* (129)	cc	268	591	Adjusted means	—	">1.0"	—	2
Phillips *et al.* (214)	fu	186	21,295	High:low frequency	—	—	1.2	1
Graham *et al.* (68)	cc	2024	1,463	Not given	—	—	"1.0"	3
Lubin *et al.* (153)	cc	577	826	High:low quartiles	—	—	1.8	4,5
Hirayama (94)	fu	139	142,857	Daily *vs.* < daily	1.3	2.4	"1.8"	1
Phillips *et al.* (213)	cc	77	166	Not given	—	—	"1.0"	6

Abbreviations and legend, cc, case-control study; fu, follow-up study; pre- and post- refer to menopausal status; —, data not given; ip, in press, RR, relative risk. Quotation marks indicate values that best summarize original data although the value was not presented by the authors.

[a] Notes:

1. Meat consumption was used as a surrogate for total fat intake.
2. Japanese cases had a greater mean fat intake than Japanese controls. Young Caucasians cases ate less fat than Caucasian controls; in older Caucasians the reverse was true.
3. The authors state there were no differences by menopausal status.
4. Animal fat as opposed total fat was compared.
5. In an analysis of risk associated with high beef or pork intake, postmenopausal women with frequent intakes were at greater risk than premenopausal women.
6. The frequency of meat, fish, and poultry consumption was examined.

A remarkable feature of the many studies of colorectal cancer in relation to intake of fat and fat-containing foods is the inconsistency of the results (Table 2). Even the findings from the two most informative follow-up studies are divergent (274, 275). There is a tendency to find a small direct association between fat intake and colon cancer risk. In several studies, fat intake was more directly associated with rectal cancer than colon cancer (Table 2) (66, 111, 222, 275, 285). In all studies in which risk of large bowel cancer was examined in relation to intake of both saturated and polyunsaturated fats (111, 274, 275), it was found that polyunsaturated or polyunsaturated plus monounsaturated fat intake was not associated with increased colorectal cancer risk. Jain *et al.* (111) and Stampfer *et al.* (274) found intake of saturated fat to be associated with increased risk of large bowel cancer; Stemmerman *et al.* (275) found that ingestion of calories from saturated fat was a direct risk factor for rectal cancer but was inversely related to risk of colon cancer. Several authors have presented data on fat intake

TABLE 2. A SUMMARY OF EPIDEMIOLOGIC STUDIES IN WHICH FAT INTAKE WAS EXAMINED AS A RISK FACTOR FOR COLORECTAL CANCER[a]

References	Study design	Number of		Intake categories compared	Colon	Rectum	RR[b]	Comments[c]
		Cases	Non-cases					
Most informative								
Jain *et al.* (111)	cc	542	1,077	High:low tertiles	"2.6"	"3.4"	"2.9"	Saturated fat
Maquart-Moulin *et al.* (159)	cc	399	399	High:low quartiles			0.7	Total fat
Potter *et al.* (222)	cc	419	732	High:low quintiles	"1.6"	"2.0"	"1.7"	Saturated fat
Stemmerman *et al.* (275)	fu	106	7,074	High:low quintiles	0.4	2.3	"1.0"	Saturated fat
Stampfer *et al.* (274)	fu	103	89,534	High:low quintiles	1.7			Total fat
Garland *et al.* (61)	fu	49	1,954	Means		"1.0"		Total fat
Kune *et al.* (134)	cc	715	727	High:low			1.5	Total fat
Others								
Bjelke (17)	cc	380	1,394	Means			"1.0"	Meat intake
Bjelke (18)	cc	651	3,051	Means			"1.0"	Meat intake
Dales *et al.* (44)	cc	99	280	High:low		1.6	1.6	Foods >=5% Saturated fat
Graham *et al.* (66)	cc	586	1,411	High:low categories	0.7	0.9	"0.8"	Beef
Haenzel *et al.* (77)	cc	588	1,176	High:low		0.8	0.8	Beef, veal, lamb
Haenzel *et al.* (76)	cc	179	357	High:low			"2.2"	Beef
Higginson (89)	cc	340	1020	Daily:<daily			"0.8"	Beef
Hirayama (96)	fu	725	265,118	Daily:<daily			0.4	Meat
Manousos *et al.* (162)	cc	100	100	High:low quartiles			2.6	Meat
Martinez *et al.* (165)	cc	461	461	High:low categories			3.8	Fat
Modan *et al.* (179)	cc	275	550	Means			"1.0"	High fat foods
Phillips *et al.* (215)	fu	172	21,295	High:low categories	1.1	0.8	0.9	Meat or poultry
Pickle *et al.* (216)	cc	86	176	High:low	1.7	1.1	"1.5"	Meat
Tajima *et al.* (285)	cc	93	93	High:low	1.8	2.2	"1.9"	Beef
Wynder *et al.* (338)	cc	791	409	Not given			"1.0"	Meat
Wynder *et al.* (337)	cc	157	307	Not given			"1.0"	Meat
Phillips *et al.* (213)	cc	41	123	High:low tertiles		3.1		Beef

[a] See comments in Table 1.

[b] When the original authors presented data separately for colon and rectum, a RR for presentation in this table was calculated by weighting the colon RR by 0.67 and the rectum by 0.33 and combining the results to get a RR near that which would have been seen had these two sites been combined.

[c] Comments refer to the nutrient or food intake that was compared.

in relation to large bowel cancer risk stratified by gender (17, 111, 215, 222) and found no strong evidence that gender influences the association with fat.

In all four studies reviewed in which fat intake was examined in relation to risk of lung cancer, there was a small direct association (25, 136, 262). However, Hunter *et al.* (D. J. Hunter, W. C. Willett, M. J. Stampfer, and G. C. Colditz, unpublished data) have found a significant direct relation between calorie adjusted fat intake and smoking, suggesting that the apparent fat-lung cancer association may be entirely due to residual confounding by smoking (see section on carotenoids for a discussion of residual confounding).

In the handful of studies on pancreatic cancer risk and intake of fat or fat-containing foods, a moderate direct association has more frequently been found than not (51, 64, 93, 160, 201). However, in only one of these studies was fat intake per se examined as the exposure measure (51); in other studies, in which surrogates were used, the apparent associations could be due to effects of protein, cholesterol or other constituents of fat-containing foods.

In dietary studies of prostatic cancer risk, a small to moderate positive association with intake of fat or fat-containing foods has been found consistently (67, 129, 245, 247, 257, 270), but the studies are not sufficiently informative to be considered definitive.

In three studies of ovarian cancer risk in relation to diet there was a small to moderate direct association with intake of fat (27, 43) or fat-containing foods (138).

Cholesterol

McMichael *et al.* (171) exhaustively reviewed the evidence regarding the relations between dietary and endogenous cholesterol and human cancer in 1984. They concluded: "With respect to dietary cholesterol, there is moderately consistent evidence, both descriptive and analytic, of a small to medium increase in risk of cancer of the colon and female breast in association with increased dietary cholesterol. However, the close correlation of cholesterol with other foods and nutrients precludes causal inference," and "Observational studies on blood cholesterol and cancer thus afford substantial evidence that preclinical cancer causes a lowering of blood cholesterol and limited, but biologically plausible, evidence that males with naturally low blood cholesterol levels are at increased risk of colon cancer." Several years have passed since that review; data presented since 1984 have been scrutinized to see if any amendments to the conclusions of McMichael *et al.* (171) are merited.

In the two most informative studies of dietary cholesterol in relation to breast cancer risk, an inverse association was found (115, 327). In two additional case-control studies the findings regarding dietary cholesterol and breast cancer were equivocal (97, 119). The recent data do not support a direct association between dietary cholesterol and breast cancer risk.

Three groups (175, 222, 275) have presented data on dietary cholesterol in relation to risk of colorectal cancer since the 1984 review. In all three, an association between colorectal cancer risk and dietary cholesterol was observed, but examination of the data suggests that if the authors had adjusted for total caloric intake the association would no longer be present. In two follow-up studies of blood cholesterol and risk of colorectal cancer no association was found (265, 276).

In a recent review of diet and lung cancer, Colditz *et al.* (42), examined the role of cholesterol and concluded: "The data from the serum and dietary intake studies are thus inconclusive and do not support an association between cholesterol intake and lung cancer risk." In the one paper on lung cancer and diet published since the review by Colditz *et al.* (42), the authors found no association between dietary cholesterol and risk of lung cancer (25).

There are no published data on cholesterol intake in relation to pancreatic cancer, although data on intake of cholesterol-containing foods are available (64, 93, 201). An association between meat intake and risk of pancreatic cancer is present more often than not, but the data are inconclusive (64, 93, 201).

Similarly for prostatic cancer, the data do not permit separation of the effects of fat and cholesterol (67, 129, 245, 257, 270).

Cramer *et al.* (43) found no association between cholesterol intake and risk of ovarian cancer. La Vecchia *et al.* (138) found cases ate fewer eggs but significantly more meat than controls, an observation that does not support an association between cholesterol intake and risk of ovarian cancer.

Protein

Katsouyanni *et al.* (119) found protein intake, adjusted for total caloric intake, not to be a determinant of breast cancer. In other studies with no control for total caloric intake, there was a small positive association between both protein intake (97, 98, 153, 154) and meat intake (94, 214, 286) and risk of breast cancer. Even if total caloric intake is not a major risk factor for breast cancer (see section on total caloric intake), it is important to adjust for total calories in case-control studies because disease may have affected the cases' recall of total amount eaten.

Several authors examined protein intake in relation to colorectal cancer (61, 111, 134, 222, 275); overall the results are consistent with no association. Results from studies in which meat intake was measured and related to risk of colorectal cancer are variable but in aggregate suggest no association (18, 44, 66, 76, 77, 89, 96, 159, 162, 165, 215).

In the limited data available on the relation of protein intake to risk of lung cancer (25, 262) there is no association.

Durbec *et al.* (51) found protein intake, unadjusted for total caloric intake, was not an important factor for pancreatic cancer. In most (93, 160, 201) but not all (64) other investigations meat intake was directly related to risk of pancreatic cancer. The association could be due to confounding by fat, total calories or other factors.

Ross *et al.* (245) and Heshmat *et al.* (85) investigated protein intakes as a possible determinant of prostatic cancer and found no association (245) or a very small direct but not statistically significant association (85).

Byers *et al.* (27) found a very slight direct association between protein intake and risk of ovarian cancer.

β-Carotene and Vitamin A

In addition to studies of dietary β-carotene and vitamin A and cancer risk, studies were reviewed in which prediagnostic levels of serum β-carotene and retinol were examined in relation to cancer risk. Serum retinol levels are tightly regulated and do not reflect intake of vitamin A except at the extremes of intake; however the review included studies on serum retinol and cancer for completeness.

Potter and McMichael (222), Paganini-Hill *et al.* (207), and Kune *et al.* (134) assessed dietary β-carotene in relation to risk of large bowel cancer. The data of Kune *et al.* (134) suggest that β-carotene intake may be inversely related to risk of colorectal cancer, but in the other two studies this was not the case. There appears to be no association between dietary vitamin A and colorectal cancer risk (134, 159, 207, 222). In several studies intakes of foods containing β-carotene (carrots, spinach, and green leafy vegetables) were evaluated with respect to risk of colorectal cancer; an inverse association was found in some (77, 162, 215), but not all (17, 76). Attributing associations between fruit and vegetable intake and risk of cancer to their β-carotene content is risky since the association may be confounded by effects of other constituents of these foods. In two follow-up studies, risk of colorectal cancer was examined in relation to prediagnostic serum β-carotene and retinol levels (200, 273). In both studies cases had lower β-carotene levels than controls, but in neither was the difference statistically significant. Retinol differences were unremarkable. Overall, the data regarding vitamin A and β-carotene intake and colorectal cancer risk are inconclusive.

In three studies in which dietary vitamin A was evaluated with respect to risk of breast cancer, an inverse association was found (68, 119, 207). In two the statistical test for a trend in dose-response was significant (68, 119). Results from studies in which breast cancer risk and serum levels of β-carotene and retinol was evaluated are inconsistent, and in no case were any strong associations found (210, 306, 325). The results of the dietary and blood studies are not necessarily in conflict since intake of preformed vitamin A (within the normal range) would not be reflected by serum levels (329).

Graham *et al.* (67) reported a moderate direct association between dietary vitamin A and risk of prostatic cancer. Paganini-Hill *et al.* (207) found a moderate direct association between intake of vitamin supplements containing vitamin A and risk of prostatic cancer, but high intakes of vitamin A from sources other than supplements and of β-carotene were not associated with an increased risk of prostatic cancer. Others have found no association between risk of prostatic cancer and carotenoid or vitamin A intake (245, 262). In other studies, the intakes of carotene-containing foods were inversely associated with risk of prostate cancer in two (94, 257) and directly associated in one other (85). Serum levels of retinol (210, 325) or carotenoids (325) showed essentially no differences between prostatic cancer cases and controls in follow-up studies.

The relation between risk of lung cancer and dietary and serum β-carotene and vitamin A has recently been reviewed (42). There are persuasive data in support of an inverse association between β-carotene intake and risk of lung cancer. Evidence has emerged suggesting that smokers eat less β-carotene than nonsmokers (207) and have even lower blood levels of β-carotene than would be expected from reduced intake alone (282). This means that smoking is a potentially more important confounding factor for the β-carotene-lung cancer relation than has been previously recognized. Incomplete control of confounding by smoking could result in finding a greater inverse association between β-carotene and lung cancer risk than actually exists. In several of the studies on lung cancer and β-carotene, stratification levels for smoking were relatively few (69, 72, 92, 136). It would be of interest to see reanalyses of these data with more complete control of confounding by smoking.

The relations between risk of pancreatic cancer and intake of vegetables (93), fruits and vegetables (64, 160), and carrots (201), have been examined, and most (64, 160, 201), but not all (93) investigators reported inverse associations.

Byers *et al.* (27) evaluated the risk of ovarian cancer in individuals in the highest intake category of vitamin A relative to those in the lowest and found a very small direct association. La Vecchia *et al.* (138) found no association between risk of ovarian cancer and intake of vitamin A or β-carotene.

Vitamin E

In dietary studies, vitamin E (α-tocopherol) intake per se was not calculated, but intake of foods high in polyunsaturated fats, the main source of vitamin E in the diet, can be used to indicate vitamin E intake. In five studies of colorectal cancer (89, 111, 159, 274, 275), the results are consistent with a modest inverse association or no association. Wald *et al.* (308), Nomura *et al.* (200) and Stahelin *et al.* (273) found lower concentrations of α-tocopherol in the blood of colorectal cancer cases than in controls, but the differences were not statistically significant.

Dietary evidence does not support an association between intake of fats containing vitamin E and risk of breast cancer (97, 98, 115, 174, 327). Wald *et al.* (306) and Willett *et al.* (325) found breast cancer cases to have lower serum levels of α-tocopherol than controls, but only in the study by Wald *et al.* (306), was the difference statistically significant.

Shekelle *et al.* (262) and Byers *et al.* (25) found no association between indices of dietary vitamin E intake and risk of lung cancer. Results of studies of serum α-tocopherol levels in relation to risk of lung cancer have been inconsistent, although more investigators have found lower α-tocopherol levels in lung cancer cases (173, 252, 273, 308) than not (200, 325).

Dietary studies of relations between intake of vitamin E and risks of prostatic, pancreatic, or ovarian cancer have not been reported. Willett *et al.* (325) found no association between serum α-tocopherol level and risk of prostate cancer; the analysis is based on only a small number of cases.

The amount of α-tocopherol in serum is determined in part by serum lipid levels. As serum lipid concentrations increase, a greater amount of α-tocopherol is present in the lipophilic compartment of serum. Controlling for serum lipid levels in studies of serum α-tocopherol may increase ability to detect associations with cancer risk. The same point applies to β-carotene, but adjustment for serum lipids affects results less markedly than for α-tocopherol.

Vitamin C

Graham *et al.* (68) and Katsouyanni *et al.* (119) found no relation between intake of vitamin C and risk of breast cancer.

In studies in which vitamin C intake was examined in relation to risk of colorectal cancer, the findings suggest either no association or a very modest inverse association (17, 111, 134, 159, 222, 273, 334). In two studies in which an inverse association was found (17, 273), no adjustment was made for other, possibly confounding, dietary risk factors.

In studies of vitamin C intake and lung cancer risk, there was no evidence of an association (25, 28, 128, 136, 262). Stahelin *et al.* (273) investigated the relation between serum vitamin C levels and risk of lung cancer in a follow-up study and found cases had slightly lower levels than controls.

Norell *et al.* (201) found that frequent consumption of citrus juices was inversely associated with pancreatic cancer.

Graham *et al.* (67) found a high intake of vitamin C to be a risk factor for cancer of the prostate, but neither Heshmat *et al.* (85) or Kolonel *et al.* (128) found this association.

Byers *et al.* (27) found no association between vitamin C intake and risk of ovarian cancer.

Selenium

Food Se content varies widely, and intake cannot be accurately measured by questionnaire (102). Blood or nail Se levels do reflect intake (102). Since malignancy may be associated with decreased food intake, only studies in which the investigators evaluated prediagnostic Se status in relation to the occurrence of malignancy were reviewed (127, 173, 197, 211, 251, 252, 295, 324).

In all five studies in which risk of gastrointestinal malignancy was examined in relation to serum Se levels, the average Se level among cases was lower than among controls (197, 211, 251, 252, 324). This finding was remarkably consistent, but, since each study was based on a small number of cases, it is not clear whether the result represents an association for large bowel cancer, pancreatic cancer, stomach cancer, or more than one of these malignancies. Nomura *et al.* (197) found the inverse association with serum Se was present for large bowel cancer but not stomach cancer.

In studies in which risk of breast cancer was examined in relation to Se levels (211, 295, 324), case-control differences were not remarkable.

Low serum Se was found to be a risk factor for lung cancer in some (251, 252, 324), but not all (174, 197, 211) studies. Menkes *et al.* (173), found that high serum Se was associated with increased risk of lung cancer when α-tocopherol levels were low.

Smokers have lower levels of blood and nail Se than nonsmokers (102, 152). Statistical adjustment for smoking was made by the original authors in all analyses evaluated except in the study of breast cancer by Van Noord *et al.* (295) in which smoking apparently had no effect on Se levels.

Willett *et al.* (324) and Peleg *et al.* (211) examined prostate cancer risk in relation to serum Se levels; Willett *et al.* found an inverse association and Peleg *et al.* found a direct association, but in neither were the results statistically significant.

Willett *et al.* (324) found that individuals in the lowest category of both serum α-tocopherol and serum Se were at the greatest risk of cancer (all sites combined), a finding corroborated by Salonen *et al.* (252), but not by Nomura *et al.* (197). The Finnish population studied twice by Salonen *et al.* (251, 252) has a markedly lower Se intake than most Western populations, and showed the strongest inverse associations between serum Se and cancer risk. This suggests that an increase in Se intake up to the point of saturation of glutathione peroxidase (290) has a greater effect in decreasing cancer risk than increasing intake above that level.

Fiber

The physiologic effects of different fiber types may vary widely (271). Differentiating between their health effects in epidemiologic studies is difficult and may be unnecessary since dietary intake of different fiber types is highly correlated with total dietary fiber intake (C. J. Masters, J. Buring, C. Hennekens, and W. C. Willett, unpublished data). The term fiber is used in a generic sense in the following discussion.

Most epidemiologic studies of fiber or fiber-containing food intake in relation to risk of colorectal cancer are consistent with a very small inverse association or no association (17, 18, 44, 89, 96, 111, 134, 159, 162, 165, 179, 213, 216, 222, 274, 285, 337, 338). In all but one (222) of the studies in which a direct, rather than an inverse, association was found, there are possible reasons for the unusual findings (165, 213, 216, 285). In three studies (213, 216, 285) the small number of subjects may have resulted in disparate findings by chance. In one (165), the direct association may have been due to the fact that cases reported eating more of everything than controls. The direct association between fiber intake and colon cancer in females reported by Potter *et al.* (222), however, is not easily explained. There are not sufficient data to evaluate whether fiber intake affects risk of colon and rectal cancers differently or whether effects of fiber differ between males and females.

Associations between fiber intake and other cancers have not been extensively studied. Two studies of fiber intake and breast cancer risk have been reported (119, 154). In one (154), fiber appeared to be protective in premenopausal women but not in postmenopausal women. In the second (119), in Greek women, high fiber intake was associated with a moderate increase in breast cancer risk, but the number of observations was small and a test for a trend in dose-response was not significant.

In two case-control studies of the relation between fiber consumption and lung cancer risk (25, 28), a small inverse association was found which was apparently not attributable to a lower total caloric intake among cases. In other studies (92, 136, 344), lung cancer risk was inversely associated with vegetable and fruit intake, an association possibly due to the carotenoids and other constituents in the fiber-containing foods.

Heshmat *et al.* (85) found no association between fiber intake and risk of prostate cancer. Schuman *et al.* (257) and Hirayama (92) reported data suggesting that frequent vegetable intake may be inversely associated with risk of prostate cancer, but, again, it is not possible to attribute this association to fiber as opposed to carotenoids or other constituents.

None of the studies of pancreatic cancer and diet allow differentiation of associations with fiber from associations with other food constituents. In three studies, frequent consumption of raw vegetables was found to be inversely associated with risk of pancreatic cancer (64, 160, 201). However in the follow-up study by Hirayama there was no association between green and yellow vegetable use and risk of pancreatic cancer (93).

In the dietary study of ovarian cancer by Byers *et al.* (27), frequent consumption of fiber was slightly protective. La Vecchia *et al.* (138) found frequent consumption of green vegetables and whole grain bread or pasta to be inversely associated with ovarian cancer risk; the associations persisted after controlling for intake of vitamin A and beta-carotene.

Calcium

Several investigators have examined the relation between calcium intake and colorectal cancer risk. Macquart-Moulin *et al.* (159) found an inverse association between calcium intake and risk of colorectal cancer in an analysis adjusting for total caloric intake. Kune *et al.* (134) found an inverse association between calcium intake and risk of colorectal cancer in females but not males in an analysis not adjusted for fat or total caloric intake. Garland *et al.* (61) found both calcium and vitamin D intake to be inversely associated with colorectal cancer risk in an analysis adjusted for total calories and fat intake (61). Lipkin *et al.* (148) conducted a controlled clinical trial in individuals at high risk of colorectal cancer and found that supplementary dietary calcium reduced the elevated proliferation in colonic epithelium.

Cruciferous Vegetables

Vegetables that are a members of the brassicaceae family (brussel sprouts, cabbage, and broccoli) have been purported to enhance inactivation of dietary and other carcinogens because they contain indoles and other compounds that can induce microsomal oxidases in liver, small intestine, and possibly other tissues. Their potential effect on cancer risk has been evaluated in several studies. Katsouyanni *et al.* (118) found intakes of cauliflower and cooked or raw cabbage were inversely associated with risk of breast cancer; the association was statistically significant only for raw cabbage. Graham *et al.* (68) did not find that cruciferae intake was associated with risk of breast cancer.

In several investigations frequent intake of cruciferae or cabbage alone was inversely related to colorectal cancer risk (66, 134, 162, 175); in two smaller studies the results were equivocal (216, 285). In three of the studies (134, 162, 175), the association persisted after the authors controlled for the potentially confounding effects of other dietary factors.

Kvale *et al.* (136) demonstrated a small inverse association between intake of cabbage and cauliflower and risk of lung cancer in a follow-up study, but did not control for potential confounding by other dietary constituents.

Graham *et al.* (67) and Schuman *et al.* (257) investigated cruciferous vegetable intake in relation to risk of prostate cancer; taken together, the results of these two studies do not suggest an association.

Byers *et al.* (27) found intake of cruciferae to have a very small inverse association with risk of ovarian cancer. Data on the relation between cruciferae intake and risk of pancreatic cancer are not available.

Coffee

Data on coffee consumption in relation to risk of breast cancer consistently demonstrate no association (110, 118, 139, 140, 155, 243, 254, 269).

Snowdon and Phillips (269) found an increased risk of colon cancer among Seventh Day Adventists drinking two or more cups of coffee daily compared with those drinking less than one. Seventh Day Adventists who do not strictly obey the church's food rules may consume not only coffee but also meat and perhaps alcohol more frequently than strict Seventh Day Adventists. Thus the apparent coffee-colon cancer association could have been due to confounding by several factors. In other studies coffee consumption and risk of colorectal cancer show no association (17, 18, 44, 66, 76, 89, 110, 159, 198, 285).

In two studies of coffee consumption in relation to risk of lung cancer, a modest direct association was found (110, 198). However, the possibility that residual confounding by smoking explains the observed association suggests cautious interpretation of these findings.

The data available on coffee consumption in relation to risk of prostate cancer do not suggest an association (110, 198).

Six investigators have found no association between coffee consumption and risk of ovarian cancer (27, 80, 110, 176, 269, 294), and one found a positive association (43).

In contrast to the data consistently showing no relationship of coffee consumption to the occurrence of breast, colorectal, prostatic or ovarian cancer, the findings on pancreatic cancer are varied. MacMahon *et al.* (158) reported a positive association between coffee consumption and risk of pancreatic cancer. In the numerous studies that followed, either no association or more modest associations than reported by MacMahon *et al.* (158) were found (64, 65, 86, 101, 110, 113, 120, 147, 160, 198, 201, 260, 269, 320, 336). The unequivocal absence of association in the large study by Wynder *et al.* (336) is notable, as are two large, well done, case-control studies in which a direct association was found (64, 160). Residual confounding by smoking is unlikely since smoking and pancreatic cancer are associated only to a moderate degree, and smoking and coffee consumption are weakly related ($r = 0.2$ (198)). An association between pancreatic cancer and coffee drinking cannot be excluded; the variability in the findings remains to be explained.

ALCOHOL

There are numerous large studies in which modest direct associations between alcohol consumption and certain of the major Western cancers are reported. Epidemiologic evidence regarding the relationship of alcohol consumption with risk of breast cancer is remarkably consistent (Table 3). In a high proportion of both follow-up (3 of 3) and case-control studies (8 of 11), a positive association has been reported. The association appears not be confounded by established breast cancer risk factors or altered by adjustment for dietary factors (141, 255, 286, 328). The increased risk is found at surprisingly low intakes; risk of breast cancer increased with amount of alcoholic beverage consumed in most studies in which dose-response was evaluated. In general, the magnitude of the increased risk is about 30% for women consuming on average one-half drink of an alcoholic beverage daily (relative risk (RR) = 1.3), and about 60% for women consuming 1.5 drinks or more daily (RR = 1.6). Harvey *et al.* (82) found that moderate alcohol consumption at age <30 years was more strongly related to breast cancer risk than consumption at later ages. The consistency of these findings, despite the different study settings and the variety of designs employed, is notable.

In aggregate, results of studies of breast cancer risk in relation to alcoholic beverage consumption support a moderate positive association. If the findings from the Nurses' Health Study (328) in which subjects are under 65 years of age apply also to older women, then 13%, or approximately 16,900 cases annually in the United States, of all cases of breast cancer might be attributable to alcohol consumption (123). Expressed as an etiologic fraction, of all cases of breast cancer in women consuming on average one-half drink or more of alcohol daily, 29% may be attributable to alcohol (246). Therefore alcohol, which is currently used by about 57% of American women (9), appears to be a potentially important risk factor for one of the most common cancers in females. The association between alcohol consumption and breast cancer risk makes more plausible the possibility that alcohol is associated with cancers at other sites remote from sites directly exposed and that small to moderate alcohol intake may have an effect.

Many investigators have looked for associations between colorectal cancer risk and alcohol consumption, (17, 44, 46, 66, 89, 96, 112, 116, 122, 135, 159, 162, 175, 216, 220, 222, 285, 321, 334, 337, 338). Collectively, the data suggest that alcohol may be directly associated to a moderate degree with risk of large bowel cancer, particularly rectal cancer. For rectal cancer the association is stronger in males than females; it appears that alcohol drunk in the form of beer is more strongly related to risk than an equal amount of alcohol in the form of wine or spirits. For colon cancer, evidence for gender and beverage specificity is not strong.

The magnitude of the association between beer consumption and rectal cancer risk is of the same order as was found for breast cancer. One to two beers daily increases risk in males by a factor of 1.5 to 2.0 (122, 220,

TABLE 3. A SUMMARY OF EPIDEMIOLOGIC STUDIES IN WHICH ALCOHOL CONSUMPTION WAS EXAMINED AS A RISK FACTOR FOR BREAST CANCER

References	Study design (1)	Number of Cases	Number of Non-cases	gm/day (2,3)	RR (4,5)	Comments[a]
Most informative						
Willett *et al.* (328)	fu	590	89,538	3	1.0	
				10	1.3	
				>15	1.6	
Schatzkin *et al.* (255)	fu	121	7,188	1	1.4	
				3	1.6	
				>5	2.0	
Hiatt *et al.* (88)	fu	838	88,477	52	1.4	
				>78	1.2	
Harvey *et al.* (82)	cc	1524	1,896	8	1.1	
				20	1.3	
				>26	1.7	
Others						
O'Connell *et al.* (202)	cc	276	1,519	>2	1.5	
Katsouyanni *et al.* (118)	cc	120	120	(12)	0.5	(6, 12)
La Vecchia *et al.* (137)	cc	437	437	26	1.3	
				>39	2.1	
Le *et al.* (141)	cc	500	945	6	1.0	
				17	1.4	
				29	1.5	
				>34	1.2	
Talamini *et al.* (286)	cc	368	373	32	2.4	(13)
				>65	16.7	
Webster *et al.* (312)	cc	1226	1,279	14	0.9	(7)
				25	1.1	
				32	1.1	
				40	1.0	
Paganini-Hill *et al.* (208)	cc	239	239	7	1.0	(8, 11)
				>26	1.0	
Bett *et al.* (7)	cc	572	449	7	0.9	(8)
				>13	1.4	
Byers *et al.* (24)	cc	1314	770	1	1.1	(8)
				3	1.0	
				7	1.1	
				>11	1.1	
Rosenberg *et al.* (244)	cc	1152	519 2,702			(9)
Williams *et al.* (321)	cc	1118	2,070			(10)

[a] Comments.
1. fu, follow-up study; cc, case control study; cs, cross-sectional study.
2. One beer, glass of wine, or drink of liquor was estimated to contain 13 grams of ethanol (Harvey *et al.* (82)).
3. Quantities listed are category medians (unless ">" is used to indicate an open-ended upper category).
4. RR, relative risk.
5. Reference category is nondrinkers.
6. Controls were all admitted for trauma or orthopedic conditions and may have consumed more alcohol than a more representative sample of the population.
7. It is unclear if matching on age was adequately controlled for in the analysis.
8. Letter to the editor only.
9. Ever/never alcohol consumption dichotomy was used. RR was 1.4 or 1.9 for imbibers, depending on control group.
10. The study showed a positive association: nondrinkers were compared with those with <5 "ounce-years" of ethanol consumption (RR, 1.3), and to those with >5 "ounce-years" of ethanol consumption (RR, = 1.6).
11. It is unclear how useful data on prevalent breast cancer cases is.
12. High and low intake quartiles were compared.
13. Wine only consumption data were presented.

334, 337). The strongest data in favor of such an association were reported by Pollack *et al.* (220), Klatsky *et al.* (122), and Wu *et al.* (334). All presented findings from well designed, carefully analyzed follow-up studies. Individuals that drink alcohol consume a slightly smaller proportion of their total calories as fat (90, 114, 322) and eat slightly less fiber and slightly more calories (53, 90, 114, 322) than abstainers. Therefore, the apparent association of small to moderate alcohol consumption with increased risk of colorectal cancer is unlikely to be due to confounding by fat intake. It might be slightly diminished once statistical control for intake of total calories and fiber is considered.

The strong association of smoking with both lung cancer and alcohol consumption makes it difficult to disentangle the effects of these two factors on lung cancer risk. In an analysis of alcohol consumption and lung cancer risk, statistical adjustment is made for smoking, and within categories of smoking, abstainers from alcohol are compared with imbibers. However, if within categories of smoking, individuals that drink smoke more heavily than abstainers, residual confounding has occurred. In some studies reporting a positive association between alcohol consumption and lung cancer risk (121, 220, 281), the confounding effect of smoking may not have been controlled to the extent that residual confounding is no longer a concern. However, Kvale *et al.* (136) carefully controlled for the effect of smoking and still found a modest association between alcohol consumption and risk of lung cancer. Williams and Horn (321) found no effect of alcohol after adjusting for smoking. As an alternative, attention can be focused entirely on individuals known never to have smoked. Hirayama (93) reported that nonsmokers who drink had twice the risk of lung cancer of nonsmokers who do not drink. Among smokers, consumption of alcohol was not associated with a greater risk of lung cancer (93). It may be that in smokers the additional effect of drinking is minimal, but in nonsmokers there is a significant effect.

Data on the relation between alcohol consumption and ovarian cancer risk are presented in six studies (27, 43, 75, 138, 319, 321). Most results are consistent with a very small inverse association (27, 43, 75, 321), although in one study (138), a direct association was found.

Pollack *et al.* (220) found an increased risk of prostate cancer among heavy drinkers; however, Ross *et al.* (245) found no association between alcohol consumption and risk of prostatic cancer. In a recent review of data on the relation between pancreatic cancer and alcohol consumption, it was concluded that there was insufficient evidence for a causal relationship (296).

Cancers associated with heavy alcohol intake arise largely in a different group of target organs: mouth, pharynx, larynx, esophagus and liver. These associations have recently been reviewed elsewhere (234).

Total Caloric Intake

In both follow-up studies of colorectal cancer in which data on total caloric intake were presented (61, 275), the average caloric intake among cases was less than for controls. Of the four case-control studies of colorectal cancer in which total caloric intake was measured, cases had a greater caloric intake than controls in two (111, 222), and the results were equivocal in two others (134, 159). More data are needed to determine the relation between total caloric intake and colorectal cancer.

In four dietary studies of breast cancer, data on total caloric intake were presented (115, 119, 174, 327). In the large follow-up study by Willett *et al.* (327), no association between caloric intakes and breast cancer risk was found. In the case-control study by Miller *et al.* (174), premenopausal cases reported total caloric intakes slightly greater than controls; in postmenopausal women there was essentially no difference. In the case-control study by Katsouyanni *et al.* (119) and the follow-up study by Jones *et al.* (115), caloric intake among cases was somewhat lower than for controls. Together, these studies do not support an association between breast cancer risk and total caloric intake.

Data on the effect of total caloric intake are not available for ovarian cancer and prostatic cancer. In the study of pancreatic cancer by Durbec *et al.* (51), greater energy intake appeared to be strongly protective, a result possibly related to the greater prevalence of smoking among cases or to the effect of disease on recall of amount of food eaten.

Shekelle *et al.* (262) presented data from a follow-up study showing that lung cancer cases had a lower mean caloric intake than controls, but no adjustment was made for an effect of smoking on total caloric intake. In the case-control study of Byers *et al.* (25), there was an inverse association between total caloric intake and lung cancer risk, even after controlling for smoking. The true relation between total caloric intake and lung or other smoking-related cancer risks may be obscured by the U-shaped relation between total caloric intake and smoking (D. J. Hunter, W. C. Willett, M. J. Stampfer, and G. C. Colditz, unpublished data). That is to say, nonsmokers and heavy smokers tend to have greater total caloric intake than smokers of 1 to 2 packs/day. An additional dimension of complexity in this, as in other sites, is that the effect of intake of calories or specific nutrients on cancer risk may vary with the cancer cell type.

The paucity of data on the relation between total caloric intake and cancer risk reflects the nascent state of nutritional epidemiology. Recently more epidemiologists have begun using diet assessment methods detailed enough to allow estimates of total caloric intake and to study effects of determinants of caloric intake.

Determinants of caloric Intake. Physical activity, body size, caloric balance, and metabolic efficiency determine the caloric needs of an individual (326). Physical activity is a major determinant of energy expenditure and caloric intake. Body size influences caloric needs but accounts for only a small proportion of variation between individuals. Caloric imbalance, an unequal flux of caloric intake and energy expenditure, results in alterations in body weight. Long-term caloric balance can be assessed by relative weight. Metabolic efficiency encompasses a variety of factors including efficiency of nutrient absorption from the gut, basal metabolic rate, and other factors. Studies of diet and cancer risk in which data on physical activity, body size, and energy balance are gathered in conjunction with data on total caloric intake would be extremely interesting but are not yet available. Factors determining caloric intake may also have independent effects on cancer risk so that data on caloric intake per se are not directly interpretable.

Physical Activity. Vena *et al.* (297) used occupation to classify individuals' physical activity and found an inverse relation between activity and breast cancer. Since education and socioeconomic status also were inversely related to occupational physical activity, the apparent relation between occupational physical activity and breast cancer may be confounded by the breast cancer risk factors that vary with socioeconomic status. Frisch *et al.* (55) reported that former college athletes, who were more likely to continue exercising than nonathletes, had a reduced risk of breast cancer. However, Paffenbarger *et al.* (206) found no association between college sports play and risk of breast cancer. In both studies the number of breast cancer cases was small. In aggregate, the data are inconclusive.

In studies of colorectal cancer risk in relation to physical activity in which occupation was used as a surrogate for physical activity, an inverse association has been found consistently (60, 63, 298) and appears not to be due to differences in social class (60, 63). Albanes (3) reported that occupational physical activity was inversely related to relative weight and suggested that confounding by relative weight explained the association between occupational activity and risk of colorectal cancer. Wu *et al.* (334) found that leisure time physical activity was inversely related to risk of colorectal cancer in a multivariate analysis adjusted for relative weight. Paffenbarger *et al.* (206) found an inverse relation between college sports play and colorectal cancer. In contrast, in 2 studies, physical activity appeared to be directly associated with colorectal cancer among college alumni and among longshoremen (206). The numbers of cases in both studies was relatively small. Most of the evidence favors an inverse association between physical activity and colorectal cancer but investigations considering the potentially confounding effects of dietary fat and relative weight are needed.

In three studies of physical activity in relation to risk of prostatic cancer an inverse relation was reported (206, 297), and in another, college sports play was directly related to risk of prostatic cancer (206). There are similar discrepancies between studies of pancreatic cancer risk and physical activity.

Because smoking is closely related to both lung cancer (directly) and physical activity (inversely), the relation between physical activity and lung cancer is unclear from available data (206).

In summary, studies of cancer risk in relation to physical activity suggest that an inverse relation exists for cancer of the large bowel and possibly breast. Further studies are needed to confirm these findings and to define the associations, if any, between physical activity and cancers at other sites.

Relative Body Weight

Obesity indicates caloric intake in excess of caloric expenditure. In epidemiologic studies relative weight (weight divided by the square of height, Quetelet's Index) is often used as an index of obesity. It correlates well ($r = 0.6 - 0.8$) with body fat measured by densitometry (322).

This review was generally restricted to follow-up studies in which the relation of relative body weight to cancer in specific sites was examined and in which cancer incidence (not mortality) was the outcome measure. In mortality studies, the potential effect of relative weight on cancer incidence cannot be separated from an effect on the case fatality rate. For pancreatic and lung cancers, data from mortality studies were included because the case fatality rates are so high that incidence and mortality are essentially tantamount. Data from case-control studies in which hospitalized controls were used were not considered because relative body weight may be related to hospitalization (323). For a recent review of all available data on relative body weight and risk of cancer, the reader is referred to Albanes (2).

In prospective studies of relative body weight and risk of breast cancer, relative weight was not a determinant of postmenopausal breast cancer (47, 323). Willett *et al.* (323) found leanness to be a risk factor for breast cancer in premenopausal women; the increased risk was not due to weight loss caused by preclinical disease.

Nomura *et al.* (199) found high relative weight and weight gain since age 25 to be associated with increased risk of colon but not rectal cancer. Wu *et al.* (334) reported that relative body weight was directly related to risk of colorectal cancer.

Lew and Garfinkel (146) examined body weight relative to "ideal weight" (a measure of relative weight highly correlated with Quetelet's Index) in relation to site-specific cancer mortality and found a reverse J-shaped relation with risk of lung cancer. Possible explanations for a relation of lean body habitus with increased risk of lung cancer are weight loss due to preclinical disease and cigarette smoking, which is associated with lean body habitus. Nomura *et al.* (199) found relative weight was inversely related to risk of lung cancer; the association was not due to confounding by smoking or an effect of preclinical disease on weight.

Lew and Garfinkel (146) found for males that relative body weight had a J-shaped relation with risk of pancreatic cancer; lean women and women just over ideal body weight also had an increased risk of pancreatic cancer compared with women at ideal weight.

Nomura *et al.* (199) found risk of prostatic cancer to have a weak direct relation with high relative body weight.

Follow-up data on the relationship between relative body weight and ovarian cancer risk are nonexistent.

In summary, most questions on the relation between relative body weight and cancer risk remain unanswered, but there is some evidence that greater relative body weight is a risk factor for cancer of the colon and possibly for cancer of the prostate, pancreas, and ovary. Lower relative weight also may be risk factor for cancers of the breast occurring before menopause, and lung. The association between lower relative weight and lung cancer is almost certainly due to an effect of smoking.

EXPERIMENTAL STUDIES OF DIETARY AND NUTRITIONAL INFLUENCES ON CARCINOGENESIS IN LABORATORY ANIMALS

Methodologic Considerations

There are two nonspecific nutritional or dietary effects on carcinogenesis that are important in design and interpretation of experiments in laboratory animals. The first is the positive correlation between intake of calories and tumor occurrence observed in most tumor models (131, 132). The second is the frequent, but not universal, observation that ingestion of diets composed of purified ingredients is associated with greater tumor induction than ingestion of diets composed of natural (relatively unrefined) ingredients, even if both diets are nutritionally complete by standard criteria (32, 71, 105, 231).

When testing for specific dietary or nutrient effects on carcinogenesis, caloric intake must be comparable in test groups, and the diets must differ only in the nutrient(s) of interest. If food intake and weight gain are altered by an experimental regimen in the same direction as alterations observed in carcinogenesis, one cannot attribute the alteration of carcinogenesis to the regimen tested. This conclusion applies to dietary regimens high in fat that increase body weight gain and to regimens deficient in protein, vitamins, or other nutrients or high in fiber that decrease weight gain. The sensitivity of tumor response to feed intake and weight gain may be surprisingly great. Ip (103) found that dietary intake restriction resulting in a 10% decrease in body weight over 24 weeks compared with *ad libitum* fed controls reduced 7,12-dimethylbenz(a)anthracene (DMBA) mammary tumorigenesis by 20%. Recent studies from three laboratories have reported significant positive correlations of mammary or colon carcinogenesis with feed intakes varying within relatively narrow ranges in rats fed *ad libitum* (10, 36, 37, 185, 187). High fat diets must be designed to maintain protein and micronutrient: total calorie ratios; high fiber diets must be designed to permit adequate caloric and nutrient ingestion (14–16, 186, 187, 191, 194, 231). Pair-feeding and other methods of compensating for different intakes of diet, and calculation of caloric intake and utilization have been discussed in recent publications (48, 49, 145, 196, 209).

Evaluation of nutritional status is another important consideration. Feeding a diet designed to induce nutritional alterations does not guarantee the expected result; tissue content or activity of nutrients should be measured, and body weight and histologic changes documented as manifestations of nutrient deficiency or excess. Interpretation of nutrient effects on carcinogenesis requires knowledge of tissue content, biologic activity, and form of the nutrient ingested. These considerations have been discussed extensively with respect to vitamin A (205), Se (103, 104, 177), and the lipotropes, choline, methionine, folate and vitamin B12 (52).

Diets are potentially variable in nutrient and contaminant content. Diets composed of natural ingredients (cereals, legumes, fish meal, and milk products) present greater potential for nutrient variability and contamination than diets composed of purified ingredients. Rao and Knapka (1987, 223) assayed batches of the NIH-07 open formula, natural ingredient diet and found that essential nutrient content met the published requirements for rodents, but varied considerably, particularly in vitamin A (up to 6-fold) and carotene (up to 20-fold), reflecting variations in the natural products used and in vitamin A added to allow for degradation between manufacture and use. There were low but detectable levels of carcinogenic nitrosamines, lead, cadmium, ethylene dibromide, other toxic or potentially carcinogenic substances, and of antioxidants and other compounds that can influence carcinogenesis. The results demonstrate the inadequacy of natural ingredient diets for use in studies of nutrient effects on carcinogenesis in which nutrient content must be consistent and subtle effects must be detectable.

The dietary studies reviewed are primarily in rat models in which tumors are induced by a chemical carcinogen. The models are reasonably predictable but vary sufficiently to require use of concurrent controls (237). The firmest end points for measurement of dietary effects on carcinogenesis are the cumulative incidence and mean latency period of malignant tumors. Number and size of tumors (tumor burden) and incidence and number of benign tumors are useful additional expressions of data, but alterations by diet probably represent a less powerful effect than alterations of incidence and latency. Early histologic changes, characteristically described as presumptive or potential preneoplastic lesions, are useful in screening for potential dietary effects or in mechanistic evaluations of demonstrated dietary effects on carcinogenesis. The relationship of the lesions to carcinoma is, at best, only roughly quantitative and far removed in time.

Nutrient Effects on Experimental Carcinogenesis

Dietary Fat and Experimental Mammary Gland Tumorigenesis. The effect of dietary fat content on mammary tumorigenesis is one of the most readily and consistently demonstrated dietary effects on experimental carcinogenesis (29, 105, 106, 237). ω-6 polyunsaturated fatty acid (PUFA)-containing vegetable oils, such as corn oil or sunflower oil, fed at levels of 20 to 30% by weight in the diet to rats given DMBA or *N*-methyl, *N*-nitrosourea (MNU), increase significantly the incidence and number of tumors induced and decrease tumor latency compared with results in rats fed 5% fat in the diet. Certain, but not all, other fats are effective in the same models. Current investigation of the phenomenon is focusing on differentiating a specific effect of fat from a nonspecific effect of the calories provided by fat.

In this review, fat content of diets is given as percentage weight, followed, in some cases, by percentages of calories supplied. For purified diets of the composition used most frequently in the rat models, percentage of energy can be calculated approximately by multiplying the percentage weight of fat by 2; exact calculations require knowledge of full diet composition and application of appropriate conversion factors (49).

The effect of high dietary fat in mammary tumor models has been demonstrated primarily by decreased tumor latency; increased tumor incidence and number are found if termination of experiments is relatively early (Tables 4 and 5). The fat content has generally been 3 to 5% for control diets and 20 to 25% for high fat diets. Diets that contain 3% fat or less may not support growth fully, may be deficient in essential fatty acids (EFA), may not permit the hormone synthesis and secretion needed for growth and differentiation of the mammary gland, and are not suitable controls for high fat diets (125, 313, 342). Diets that contain 5% fat support growth

TABLE 4. COMPARISON OF EFFECT ON MAMMARY TUMORIGENESIS IN RATS OF FEEDING HIGH LEVELS OF DIFFERENT TYPES OF FAT IN NUTRITIONALLY BALANCED DIETS[a]

Fat	Fat in diet	Carcinogen	Rat strain	Mammary tumors		References
				Incidence	Latency	
	%			%	wks	
Corn oil	5	MNU, 50 mg/kg	F344[b]	33	11	Chan *et al.*
	33			85	8	(33)
Lard	33[c]			63	9	
Beef tallow	33[c]			50	10	
Coconut oil	33[c]			43	13	
Lard	5[c]	DMBA, 2.5 mg	SD[b]	52	16	Rogers *et*
	24[c]			80	12	*al.*
	24[c,d]			70	13	(233)
Beef tallow	5[c]	DMBA, 2.5 mg	SD[b]	83	22	Lee and
	20[c]			80	19	Rogers (143)
Rapeseed oil	5[c]			71	16	
	20[c]			66	17	
Corn oil	5[e]	MNU, 50 mg/kg	F344[b]	66	17	Cohen *et*
	23[e]			87	11	*al.* (39)
Safflower oil	5[e]			63	17	
	23[e]			87	12	
Olive oil	23[e]			63	21	
Coconut oil	3[c]	DMBA, 5 mg	SD[b]	53	—	Kritch-
	18[c]			53	—	evsky *et al.* (133)
Corn oil	5	DMBA, 7.5 mg	SD[b]	47	12	Sylvester
	20[f]			56	10	*et al.*
Lard	20[f]			78	10	(284)
Corn oil	3	DMBA, 5 mg	SD	45	12	Braden
	10			45	11	and
	20			55	11	Carroll (20)
Menhaden	3			35	13	
oil	10			20	14	
	20			30	15	

—, data not given.

[a] Diets fed throughout experiment unless otherwise noted.

[b] Body weight not significantly different between groups and not correlated with tumor end points.

[c] Included 1% corn oil.

[d] Diet fed only before carcinogen exposure; 5% fat after exposure.

[e] Diets fed after carcinogen exposure; natural ingredient diet fed earlier.

[f] Diet fed before and 1 week after carcinogen exposure; 5% corn oil fed thereafter.

and mammary gland DNA synthesis at levels comparable to results with 20 to 25% fat diets in mice (313) and rats (142).

The effectiveness of a fat or mixture of fats in enhancing DMBA-induced mammary tumorigenesis in Sprague-Dawley (S-D) rats is correlated with its linoleic acid content; fats with little or no effect may become effective if supplemented with linoleic acid in amounts 4 to 5 times the nutritional requirement (105). This result was suggested by inconsistent observations in different laboratories on the influence of fat type on tumorigenesis enhancement. While virtually all laboratories showed enhancement by diet containing 20- to 25% PUFA oils, not all found enhancement by diets containing 20 to 25% saturated fats supplemented with vegetable oils to supply the EFA requirement (reviewed in reference 235). In contrast to the results of the study by Ip (105), a consistent pattern of response to linoleate was not found in the MNU-induced model in Fischer 344 (F344) rats, possibly because of the use of 10% rather than 5% total fat as the control diet (23).

Feeding diets that contain a single fat source induces metabolic patterns that may differ from patterns in animals fed mixed fat sources and may not be ideal models for human diets. The ω-6 PUFA, found in corn and other seed oils, inhibit the metabolism of the ω-3 PUFA found in fish and certain plant oils; the ω-3 acids similarly inhibit metabolism of the ω-6 acids, and monounsaturated fats compete with the metabolism of ω-3 and ω-6 PUFA (99). Mixed fats, of composition based on average Western or other diets, may give more realistic results (10, 11, 29, 99).

Examples of reports of the effects of dietary fat on mammary tumorigenesis, shown in Tables 4 and 5. Both end points used to quantitate tumorigenesis, final incidence and latency, show the effect of dietary fat, but in many cases one is more sensitive than the other. Conclusions that are apparent from the studies tabulated and others are: (a) Dietary fats that increase mammary gland tumorigenesis in rats are effective in both strains most often used, S-D and F-344, and influence tumorigenesis by either DMBA or MNU. (b) Body weight gain and caloric intake do not account entirely for the effect of high fat diets on tumorigenesis, but restriction of caloric intake can overcome the effect. (c) Corn and safflower oils and lard consistently enhance tumorigenesis when fed at high levels; coconut oil and fats high in ω-3 fatty acids do not, and beef tallow and olive oil are variably effective. (d) Often there is not a linear dose response of mammary tumorigenesis to fat content in the diet. Most experiments that have used 3 to 5% dietary fat as control and 20 to 25% as high fat have given clear evidence of increased tumorigenesis. Studies in which intermediate levels of fat, 10 to 15%, were fed have yielded inconsistent responses.

Effects on tumorigenesis of the timing and duration of feeding high fat diets have been studied using corn oil or lard (Tables 4 and 5). Both fats enhance tumorigenesis by DMBA even if they are fed only for the 4- to 5-week period between weaning and administration of DMBA (35, 233) or for that period plus 1 week (284). Diets high in corn oil are effective if fed only after carcinogen exposure (20, 36, 317); results with lard are variable (232,

TABLE 5. DOSE-RESPONSE OF MAMMARY TUMORIGENESIS IN RATS TO CORN OIL OR MIXED FAT CONTENT IN NUTRITIONALLY BALANCED, COMPLETE DIETS AND RESPONSE TO RESTRICTED FEEDING OF TUMORIGENESIS

%Corn oil in diet		Carcinogen[a]	Strain	Restriction[b]	Mammary tumors		References
Before Carcinogen	After				Incidence	Latency[a]	
					%	*wks*	
5	5	DMBA, (3 mg)	SD[c]	0	38	[27]	Clinton *et al.* (36)
10	10			0	36	[19]	
25	25			0	65	[17]	
5	10	DMBA, (3 mg)	SD[c]	0	55	[20]	Clinton *et al.* (35)
10	10			0	65	[18]	
25	10			0	76	[16]	
5	5	DMBA, 7.5 mg	SD[c]	0	47	12	Sylvester *et al.* (284)
20	5				56	10	
5	5	DMBA, 5 mg	SD[c]	0	76	11	Thompson *et al.* (293)
5	25			0	79	9	
14	14	DMBA, —	SD	0	80	—	Kritchevsky and Klurfeld (131)
14	14			40	20	—	
5	5	DMBA, 6.5 mg/100 gm	F344	10[d]	74[e]	—	
5	17.5			10	69	—	
5	30			10	82	—	
5	5	MNU, —	F344	0	30	—	Cohen (38)
5	10			0	56	—	
5	20			0	67	—	
5	10			25	8	—	
5	20			25	3	—	
Natural Product Diet	10[f]	MNU, 25 mg/kg	SD	0	67	18	Beth *et al.* (10)
	16			0	77	17	
	22			0	77	14	
	10			30	50	24	
	16			30	63	21	
	22			30	57	20	

—, data not given.

[a] Average carcinogen dose and tumor latency calculated from published data if not explicitly stated; calculated values in brackets.

[b] After carcinogen exposure.

[c] Effect of fat on tumorigenesis significant and not correlated with effect on caloric intake or body weight; tumor incidence correlated with caloric intake across diet groups.

[d] For 5 weeks, then ad libitum intake.

[e] Tumor incidence paralleled caloric intake irrespective of dietary fat content.

Mixed fat representative of West German diet.

233). There is a direct correlation of tumorigenesis with duration of feeding either high fat diet, irrespective of the relationship to time of exposure to carcinogen (45, 233). When diets are changed from high to control or control to high fat to permit evaluation of the effect of timing of feeding on tumorigenesis, results may be inconsistent with results of experiments in which the same diet is fed throughout (232). It is likely that metabolic adaptations and transient alterations of intake in response to the changed diet are responsible. Similar problems of adaptation were encountered in paired-feeding experiments in which rats fed reduced amounts of a high-fat diet to match amounts eaten by controls did not consume even the reduced amount of food (19).

Rats fed a high lard diet and given DMBA had a significantly increased fraction of tumors that were malignant and an approximately 4 times increase in number of malignant tumors compared with control rats (232). Clinton *et al.* (35, 36) reported a higher incidence of malignant tumors in DMBA-treated rats fed a high corn oil diet than in control rats. It may be necessary to use a relatively small dose of DMBA (2.5 to 3 mg) to demonstrate the effect of high fat diets on tumor histology, since it was not reported in earlier studies. The amount of fat in the diet does not influence tumor growth rate (10, 232).

In studies using transplanted mammary tumors, growth, and in some cases metastases, of transplants were inhibited by dietary levels of 12.5 to 20% ω-3 fatty acids compared with results in rats fed the same amounts of ω-6 fatty acids. The ω-3 fatty acid diets did not reduce tumor growth and metastasis below the level in rats fed control (5%) fat diets (1, 117, 130).

The effect of high fat diets can be reduced by supplementation of the diet with Se, by treatment with indomethacin, by endocrine manipulations and by reduction of total caloric intake. The experimental evidence suggests that fat influences mammary tumorigenesis by more than one mechanism and at more than one point in tumor development. Mechanisms may include more efficient utilization of calories from fat than from carbohydrate or protein, oxidative damage by metabolites of the PUFA, endocrine alterations, membrane alterations or altered metabolism of carcinogens and promoters (314, 315). Numerous studies investigating effects of dietary fat on serum prolactin, estrogen, progesterone and on mammary gland DNA synthesis have yielded negative results (142, 314, 315, 316, 318). Estrogen tumorigenesis has not been found to be responsive to dietary fat (30). High fat diets have no effect on absorption, clearance or tissue binding of labeled DMBA (59, 144).

Arguments against caloric excess as the sole basis for the effect of fat on mammary tumorigenesis are: (a) There is wide variation in the effectiveness of different types of fat despite their equivalent caloric contributions. (b) Paired feeding studies have shown an effect of a high fat diet although caloric intake was limited to match the intake of rats fed the control fat diet (233).

In studies of the relative role and importance of fat and of calories in carcinogenesis, experimental designs have been of two major types. In one, diets that provide different amounts and types of fat are fed *ad libitum* with measurement of daily intake; in the second diets are fed in amounts that restrict total calorie intake. In rats subjected to restricted intake, tumorigenesis is reduced compared with rats fed *ad libitum*, regardless of the fraction of calories supplied by fat (Table 5; 19, 124, 131–133). When caloric intake is not restricted, increasing the fraction of calories supplied by fat increases mammary tumor incidence and number and decreases tumor latency (Table 5) and may increase induction of other types of tumors as well (10, 11, 13, 15, 16, 132, 237, 314).

Clinton *et al.* (1986; 35) analyzed separately effects of caloric intake and fat intake on DMBA tumorigenesis in rats fed diets that contained 5, 10 or 25% corn oil (12, 24 or 48% calories as fat) before DMBA exposure and 10% corn oil for the remainder of the experiment. Body weight and caloric intake were the same in the 3 dietary fat groups up to the time of DMBA exposure; increasing dietary fat was associated with significant increases in tumor incidence and number and decreases in latency. Tumor incidence across the different groups correlated strongly with caloric intake after DMBA exposure (when all rats were eating the same diet).

Feeding a mixed fat, designed to reproduce the fatty acid profile of an average West German diet, at 10% (25% of calories) or 22% (45% of calories), Beth *et al.* (10) found a small enhancement of MNU-induced mammary tumorigenesis and weight gain by 22% dietary fat. Subsequently, they also tested an intermediate level, 16% (35% of calories) of the mixed fat. Indices of tumorigenesis tended to increase, but not at a statistically significant level, with an increase in fat from 10% to 16%; no further increase occurred at 22% fat; tumorigenesis was proportional to caloric intake. If caloric intake was restricted to 70% of *ad libitum* intake, there was comparable reduction in tumorigenesis at all levels of fat fed (10, 11).

Investigations of exercise, caloric balance, and mammary carcinogenesis have been reported in recent abstracts. Thompson *et al.* (293) reported that daily, standardized, treadmill exercise increased the enhancement by a high fat diet of mammary gland DMBA tumorigenesis in S-D rats that were fed *ad libitum* and maintained normal weight gain. Yedinak *et al.* (341) reported similar results. In contrast, Cohen (38) reported that voluntary wheel exercise by F-344 rats decreased mammary gland tumorigenesis in response to MNU, despite increased feed intake and body weight compared with nonexercising rats fed the same high corn oil diet.

Fat and Experimental Colon Cancer. Despite a large body of experimental data, the strength, or even the existence, of an effect of fat on colon carcinogenesis is controversial. There are major differences in protocols between experiments with respect to rat strain and sex, diet design, feed intake and weight gain, duration of study and detection and diagnosis of tumors, and the results have been reviewed (188, 190, 241).

In attempts to evaluate the influence of protocol differences, Nauss *et al.* (185, 187–189) and Locniskar *et al.* (149) performed a well-controlled, large series of experiments. They found no effect of isocaloric diets high (24%) in beef tallow, corn oil or hydrogenated vegetable oils compared with diets containing 5% fat, composed of a mixture of the three fats, on colon tumorigenesis in rats by 1,2-dimethylhydrazine (DMH) or MNU. Subsequently, they compared isocaloric diets containing 5 or 20% fat as a mixture of corn oil and beef tallow in F-344 and S-D rats given DMH. The S-D, but not the F-344 rats, fed 20% fat had a significantly increased colon tumor incidence. However, the increase was associated with increased caloric intake and weight gain compared with rats fed 5% fat and appeared to be explained by those factors. F344 rats did not show a consistent relationship between caloric intake, weight gain, and tumor incidence.

The results emphasize the need for careful measurements of feed intake, which requires individual housing of animals, in such experiments. In addition, the dependence of tumorigenesis on EFA content of the diet in the two models in which it has been most carefully studied, mammary gland neoplasia and pancreatic acinar preneoplasia (see below), strongly indicates the importance of an adequate dietary supply of EFA.

The questions that remain in this area are basic ones that should be answered before more elaborate mechanistic studies are performed. The early positive studies stimulated interest in the field, but their results may have been due more to nutrient imbalances induced by dilution of nutrients with fat or to excessive caloric intake than to fat *per se*. Defects in study design have been discussed by Clinton and Visek (37) and Nauss *et al.* (187).

Feeding a marine oil containing ω-3 fatty acids inhibited growth and pulmonary colonization of a transplanted colon tumor in mice compared with results in mice fed safflower oil (21).

Fat and Pancreatic Tumors. Two animal models of pancreatic neoplasia have been used: the rat given l-azaserine (l-aza) and the hamster given *N*-nitrobis(2-oxopropyl)amine (BOP) or other derivatives of *N*-nitroso-di-*n*-propylamine (151, 253). The two models differ in the histogenesis and histology of tumors induced but respond similarly to dietary fat content. In the rat given l-aza, pancreatic neoplasia was increased by concurrent feeding of a diet that contained 20% corn or sunflower oil compared with rats fed diets that contained 5% corn oil or 20% coconut oil. The increase was primarily in multiplicity rather than incidence of tumors. Subsequent experiments localized the effect of fat to the postcarcinogen treatment period and extended the results to the appearance of the putative preneoplastic lesions in the model, the atypical acinar cell nodules or foci (AACN). DNA synthesis, evaluated by labeling by [^{3}H]thymidine, of cells in the AACN but not in the surrounding pancreas was increased by the high corn oil diet. In rats fed mixtures of corn and coconut oils, the size and number of AACN increased with increasing concentrations above 4% of linoleic acid, the major PUFA in corn oil. Caloric intake and weight gain did not correlate with and were, therefore, judged not responsible for the influence of dietary fat on pancreatic tumorigenesis (227–230).

In contrast to results with corn oil, menhaden oil (ω-3 fatty acids) did not increase the number of AACN induced by 1-aza. (203).

The relationship of pancreatic neoplasia to dietary fat is similar to the relationship of mammary neoplasia in the following respects: (a) Tumor development is enhanced by diets high in ω-6 PUFA. (b) Enhancement occurs when fat composes about 20% of the diet by weight if the linoleic acid content is at least 3 to 5%; in addition, a dose response to linoleic acid above 3% can be demonstrated. (c) ω-3 fatty acid-containing fats do not increase tumor development when fed at high levels.

The mechanism by which fat acts in the pancreas is not known. In normal pancreas (107), as in mammary gland (142), high fat diets do not stimulate DNA synthesis. Cholecystokinin, a trophic hormone for pancreas, is not elevated in the blood of rats fed high fat diets (229).

In the hamster model, a high corn oil diet increased pancreatic tumor incidence and number, but the hamsters in the high fat groups had increased food intake and weight gain, and the result could not be clearly attributed to the dietary fat content (16). In a subsequent study, hamsters were fed the high fat diet *ad libitum* or in an amount restricted to the caloric intake of hamsters fed control diet; pancreatic carcinomas were increased equally in both groups fed the high fat diet, demonstrating a specific effect of fat (13).

Protein and Experimental Carcinogenesis. Effects of dietary protein content on carcinogenesis have been studied primarily in the mammary gland and liver. Dietary protein content has surprisingly little effect on tumorigenesis except at extremes of feeding (302); at both extremes reduction of mammary gland tumorigenesis occurs, probably as a result of reduced feed intake and growth. There may be an added protective effect of induction of hepatic mixed function oxidases (MFO) by high protein diets. (302).

In an exception to the general findings that dietary protein is not a major determinant of cancer in experimental models, Hawrylewicz *et al.* (81) reported an effect of dietary protein on mammary tumorigenesis in a two-generation model. They found that a high protein diet (31% casein) fed to dams from before mating through lactation and then fed to female offspring, accelerated sexual maturation and increased the incidence of DMBA-induced mammary tumors compared with results in offspring of rats fed control diet containing 19.5% casein. Protein deficiency (8% casein) retarded maturation and growth and inhibited mammary gland tumorigenesis. In a second study of MNU-induced mammary tumors (81), latency and incidence were not affected by the 33% casein diet, but tumor number and weight were greater than in controls fed 19% casein.

In the liver tumor model induced by aflatoxin B_1 (AFB_1) in male, F-344 rats, there was reduction of carcinogenesis in rats fed a severely protein restricted diet that markedly reduced growth (161). Studies examining the dose-response relationships between diet protein content and AFB_1 carcinogenesis, using gammaglutamyltranspeptidase foci as an index of carcinogenesis, showed that casein insufficient to support growth also did not support development of foci, that maximum development of foci occurred in rats fed 12% casein and that higher levels had no additional effect (50).

Vitamin A, β-Carotene, and Experimental Carcinogenesis. Recent reviews are available of effects of vitamin A and other retinoids on tumorigenesis in many models (180) and of molecular mechanisms by which retinoids may act (205, 225). Retinoids are thought to act by controlling cell differentiation (225) and by their function as antioxidants, reacting with peroxyl and other free radicals (157, 163). Vitamin A and other retinoids are unquestionably anticarcinogenic in several organs, including skin, mammary gland, and urinary bladder. They may also enhance carcinogenesis in lung, skin, liver and other tissues under some experimental conditions (12, 150, 169, 204, 267, 268, 280). In evaluation of retinoid and carotenoid effects, distinctions should be made between effects of deficiency and excess of vitamin A or vitamin A-like activity, between physiologic and pharmacologic vitamin A activity and between vitamin A and nonvitamin A activity of synthetic retinoids and carotenoids (205). Nonspecific reduction of tumorigenesis due to anorexia and weight loss resulting from toxicity of the compounds must also be considered.

Deficiency of vitamin A in rats, maintained over the long periods needed for carcinogenesis, increased urinary bladder tumorigenesis by *N*-[4-(5-nitro-2-furyl)-2-thiazolyl] formamide (40) and increased somewhat the incidence of colon tumors induced by DMH or AFB_1 (195, 236). Unrecognized deficiency may have been responsible for inconsistent results with vitamin A in the hamster lung tumor model, (discussed in references 267, 268). Maintenance of deficient animals is difficult, and the majority of studies have looked at effects of excessive, rather than deficient, vitamin A intake.

Feeding of excess vitamin A protected rats against bladder tumorigenesis by *N*-butyl-*N*-(4-hydroxybutyl) nitrosamine (72) and against mammary tumor induction by DMBA, MNU, or procarbazine (70, 71, 180). Protection against MNU was not found in a second laboratory using lower dietary levels of vitamin A (11). Dietary supplementation of vitamin A at levels 50 to 200 times the requirement reduced DMBA skin tumorigenesis in mice; both supplements reduced food intake; the higher supplement reduced body weight also (62). In mice fed vitamin A at approximately 150 times the requirement, survival and growth were reduced, and spontaneous tumor incidence was slightly, but not significantly, greater than in controls (277). High dietary vitamin A did not protect against colon or liver tumorigenesis in rats given DMH or AFB_1 (195, 236), or against bladder tumorigenesis in rats given *N*-[4-(5-nitro-2-furyl)-2-thiazolyl] formamide (40), despite the effects of deficiency in the same models.

Since the amounts of vitamin A fed are many times greater than the nutritional requirement and induce variable degrees of toxicity, the studies are only marginally relevant to a discussion of nutritional influences on cancer.

Research on β-carotene effects on tumorigenesis in laboratory animals has been hampered because absorption of the whole molecule into the blood is much lower in rodents than in humans; serum and tissue levels are, therefore, low and not easily increased (8, 73). Female S-D rats fed β-carotene at levels 4 to 400 times the dietary requirement showed variable tissue accumulation of β-carotene with apparent saturation after 2 to 10 weeks. Accumulation in lung and skin, tissues of major interest, was minimal. Depletion from lung was rapid; levels had dropped 50% by 1 week after feeding was stopped (261). Earlier studies had shown somewhat greater tissue accumulation of β-carotene in mice (167, 166).

Experimental evaluation of a role of beta-carotene in cancer prevention began in the mouse skin tumor models, in which beta-carotene, and in some cases carotenoids without vitamin A activity, were reported to reduce tumorigenesis by ultraviolet light or polycyclic aromatic hydrocarbons (8, 166). Reduction of growth of transplanted or virally induced mammary tumors (224, 256) and of DMH-induced colon tumorigenesis (289) in mice by β-carotene has been reported. In the DMH experiment, mice fed β-carotene, 22 mg/kg of natural product diet had significantly greater weight gain than controls fed 2 mg/kg; the colon tumor incidence was halved in mice with the greater carotene intake (289). Unexplained differences in weight gain between groups makes interpretation of the result difficult. In contrast, rats fed 1% β-carotene in the diet, about 1 gm/kg body weight/day, before, during, and after administration of a carcinogenic regimen of DMH, showed no evidence of protection against colon tumorigenesis (41).

S-D rats and caesarean-derived-1 mice fed β-carotene to supply 0.1 to 1 gm/kg/day for 2 years showed no alteration of spontaneous tumor incidence or type. Pigmentation of adipose tissue constituted evidence that β-carotene was absorbed and distributed to tissues, but measurement of tissue content was not reported (87).

Topical β-carotene markedly inhibited DMBA induction of squamous cell carcinoma in the hamster buccal pouch and was effective when applied with or after carcinogen application. In addition, there was a reduction in tumor size and histologic grade of malignancy (283). Suppressive activity of topical retinoids has been studied extensively in the DMBA-induced mouse skin tumor models (299, 301). Dietary administration of retinoids or vitamin A (retinyl palmitate) is less effective but can reduce tumor burden somewhat when fed at toxic or near-toxic levels (62, 300). Increased tumorigenesis also has been reported in similar models after topical or dietary exposure to retinoids. (169).

In vitro studies using chinese hamster ovary cells showed that accumulation of β-carotene, at levels comparable to levels found in human oral mucosal cells, inhibited genotoxic activity of methylmethanesulfonate and 4-nitroquinoline-1-oxide but not of H_2O_2 or several other agents. The effect appeared not to be due to conversion to retinol (278, 279).

Lipotropes and Carcinogenesis. Lipotropic nutrients have powerful effects on hepatic tumorigenesis. Deficiency of choline and methionine, *i.e.*, of methyl groups, is carcinogenic for the liver in the absence of known carcinogen exposure and is a powerful enhancer of hepatocarcinogenesis by a number of chemicals (190, 217, 218, 241, 263, 264). Hepatic DNA from deficient rats does not contain detectably increased alkyl or aromatic adducts, evidence against the hypothesis that deficient rats develop hepatocarcinomas in the absence of known carcinogen exposure because of heightened sensitivity to environmental carcinogens (74). Several possible mechanisms for the lipotrope effect in carcinogenesis have been demonstrated. They include accelerated hepatocyte turnover, altered xenobiotic metabolism, increased peroxidation and altered nucleic acid metabolism with hypomethylation of DNA, including oncogenes (218, 219, 241, 263, 264, 303, 304). The model is a provocative one, useful in examining mechanisms of carcinogenesis in the liver since the deficiency influences events during and after carcinogen administration (242). Deficient rats have been used to examine the altered morphology, molecular biology and biochemistry of preneoplastic and neoplastic liver cells. Carcinogens that are more effective in deficient rats include AFB_1, *N*-2-fluorenylacetamide, diethylnitrosamine and dibutylnitrosamine, ethionine and l-aza. Dimethylnitrosamine is the only hepatocarcinogen tested apparently not influenced by the deficiency (241).

Weanling, growing animals are highly susceptible to the deficiency, rapidly become severely deficient and may die with severe fatty liver and hemorrhagic renal necrosis within 10 to 14 days if not given small supplements of choline. Susceptibility declines with age and the fully expressed deficiency does not appear if feeding begins later than about 10 to 12 weeks of age. The deficiency need not be severe to enhance hepatocarcinogenesis in rats. In male mice, as in rats, induction of lipotrope deficiency depends on the age of the animal and type of fat fed. In deficient mice the response to AFB_1 and development of spontaneous liver tumors are increased. In older mice fed the deficient diet and in young mice fed the deficient diet containing beef tallow rather than cottonseed oil as the major fat source, deficiency was less severe, as measured by hepatocyte fat and hyperplasia, and there was no increase in spontaneous or induced liver lesions (190, 193).

The histologic and biochemical changes have been characterized more fully in rats than in mice, but when mice have been studied they have shown similar results. The deficient liver shows early and persistent increased turnover of hepatocytes and endothelial cells (238) and numerous biochemical abnormalities. One biochemical lesion induced by the deficiency that probably contributes to the increased development of hepatocarcinoma is altered capacity for methylation because of reduced hepatic *S*-adenosylmethionine (218, 242). Carcinogens including N-2-fluorenylacetamide, diethylnitrosamine, ethionine, and possibly others alter hepatic methyl metabolism by interfering with folate metabolism and by influencing metabolism of S-adenosylmethionine and t-RNA methylases (218, 303, 304). The reappearance in deficient mice of fetal RNA methyltransferases is inversely correlated with their spontaneous hepatic tumor incidence (303, 304) and is directly correlated with lipotrope deficiency. Other biochemical effects of the deficiency that may influence carcinogenesis include alteration of MFO and other enzyme systems that metabolize carcinogens, and alteration of cell membrane composition with changes in phospholipid ratios (see reference 242 for review).

Early reports of decreased lifespan (156) and increased mitosis and [^{3}H]thymidine labeling in hepatocytes of deficient rats and mice (238) and of deficient, carcinogen-treated rats (240, 241) have been expanded by recent studies (34). [^{3}H]Thymidine was administered by continuous infusion for 2 weeks to weanling, male F344 rats fed a complete, natural product diet, that were then fed a lipotrope-deficient or supplemented diet. Hepatic DNA labeling was measured at intervals from 1 to 16 weeks. Hepatocyte half-life was reduced from 112 weeks to 21 weeks in rats studied after 4 to 8 weeks of dietary deficiency, and from 416 weeks to 75 weeks after 8 to 16 weeks of deficiency. Rates of cell death and proliferation were significantly higher in deficient than control rats and correlated with rates of triglyceride accumulation, as previously reported (238). At 16 weeks, the label remaining in hepatic DNA or deficient rats was only approximately 7% of the initial level, whereas in controls it was approximately 90%. The authors discussed the problem of identifying mechanisms of the dietary effect in the face of the large numbers of degenerating and regenerating cells which may be reflected for example, in measurements of peroxidation, membrane composition changes and alterations of gene expression.

Glutathione (GSH) may have a role in the lipotropic effects on carcinogenesis. GSH is linked to methionine and choline through cysteine-methionine interconversions. Hepatic GSH is not reduced in lipotrope deficiency if the sulfur amino acid, cystine, is supplemented in adequate amount but is decreased in the absence of cystine supplementation (242). The effect of the combined deficiency was studied in rats given l-aza and fed deficient diet before and during l-aza administration, only after l-aza administration, or throughout the experiment. Hepatocarcinoma incidence was highest in rats fed deficient diet before and during carcinogen exposure (50%) or throughout the experiment (31%). It was low in control rats (12%), and there were no liver tumors in rats fed the deficient diet only after exposure. Hepatic glutathione-S-transferase activity was not altered by the deficiency or by l-aza; GSH increased in response to azaserine but remained significantly decreased in deficient compared with control rats (242).

Ascorbic Acid and Experimental Carcinogenesis. Ascorbic acid blocks nitrosation of amines to form carcinogenic nitrosamines in people and laboratory animals and can be, by that mechanism, anticarcinogenic (178). Evidence for a more general anticarcinogenic effect is lacking, and in some experiments ascorbic acid has enhanced chemical carcinogenesis. Colacchio and Memoli (41) reviewed earlier reports and presented results showing statistically significant inhibition of DMH-induced colon tumorigenesis in rats fed 7% ascorbic acid in a natural product diet. Weight gain was 7 to 10% less in ascorbic-acid fed rats than in DMH-treated or β-carotene fed controls, an indication of toxicity of the ascorbate or of dilution or destruction of other nutrients. Therefore, the decrease in tumorigenesis cannot be considered definitive for a specific effect of ascorbic acid. Similar reduction in weight gain was reported in Fischer rats fed 5% sodium ascorbate in the diet and found to have increased, not decreased, bladder tumorigenesis by N-butyl-N-(4-hydroxybutyl) nitrosamine. The increase in tumors was attributed to altered urinary pH and ion concentrations (56, 57, 182).

Minerals. Effects of minerals in experimental carcinogenesis include both reduction and enhancement by high levels in the diet and enhancement by dietary deficiency.

Deficiency of Zn induces hyperplasia of the esophageal epithelium in rats while reducing cell division and turnover in most other tissues. The deficiency is associated with increased susceptibility to methylbenzylnitrosamine carcinogenesis at that site (58).

Dietary Se content influences chemical carcinogenesis in several sites, generally reducing but sometimes enhancing tumor development (12). The rodent dietary requirement for Se is approximately 0.1 mg/kg. Ip (104) reviewed studies reporting Se inhibition of liver, mammary gland, and colon tumorigenesis in rats and of skin tumorigenesis in mice, and summarized the data in the DMBA-induced rat mammary tumor model. Reduction of mammary tumor incidence and number and lengthening of the latency period occurred in a dose-responsive manner in rats fed 1.5, 2.5, or 5.0 mg/kg but not in rats fed 0.5 mg/kg Se in diets that contained either 5 or 25% corn oil. There was a reduction of feed intake and weight gain in rats fed 5 mg/kg but not in rats fed the lower levels. The effect of Se on mammary tumorigenesis is exerted throughout the periods of tumor initiation and development, the reduction depending on duration of treatment and dose (104, 291, 292). Addition of vitamin E at approximately 20 times the requirement enhanced the tumor reduction due to Se; vitamin E alone had no effect. The protective effect of Se was nullified by addition of ascorbic acid (1.2%) to the diet (103, 104). In mice a dietary Se content of 2 mg/kg inhibited induction of mammary tumors by DMBA or murine mammary tumor virus and prevented development of tumors from transplanted precursor lesions. Growth of established tumors was not affected (172).

Se administered in drinking water at 4 mg/kg reduced the incidence of forestomach papillomas and carcinomas in male, S-D rats given N-methyl-N'-nitro-N-nitrosoguanidine to 14% compared with 49% in control rats (192). N-methyl-N'-nitro-N-nitrosoguanidine-induced carcinomas of the glandular stomach were reduced in Wistar rats fed Se 4 mg/kg diet, compared with rats fed 0.1 mg/kg (126).

In contrast to inhibitory effects of Se on tumorigenesis at several sites, hamsters fed Se, 2.5 mg/kg diet, showed increased BOP-induced pancreatic carcinogenesis if high fat (24%) diet was fed but not if control (6%) fat diet was fed (12).

The mechanism of action of Se is not known; in both the rat and the mouse models investigation of effects on tissue peroxidation and on glutathione peroxidase have shown no correlation with effects on tumorigenesis. (104, 172).

Se deficiency (dietary content 0.02 mg/kg) enhanced DMBA mammary tumorigenesis if a high (25%) corn oil diet was fed but not if control (5% corn oil) was fed (106). Deficiency of Se did not increase spontaneous tumors in male or female S-D rats observed for up to 2 years (164). Using the methylbenzylnitrosamine-induced esophageal cancer rat model that has been fruitful in demonstrating an influence of Zn deficiency on carcinogenesis, Nauss *et al.* (186) found no effect of Se deficiency; excess Se (4 mg/kg in diets) gave inconsistent results.

An enhancing effect of low Se (0.02 mg/kg) on AFB_1-induced, gammaglutamyltranspeptidase-positive hepatocyte foci was reported in rats fed a 20% corn oil diet; differences in body weight may have contributed to the effect (6).

Carcinogenesis in the glandular stomach of rats by *N*-methyl-*N′*-nitro-*N*-nitrosoguanidine was enhanced by simultaneous exposure to concentrated sodium chloride (192).

There is interest in calcium (Ca) as a potential protective agent against colon carcinogenesis. Reduction of toxicity of bile acids and other chemicals by Ca has been reported (22, 311). Definitive carcinogenesis studies using Ca supplementation have not been reported in full. Reduction of colorectal tumor number in azoxymethane (AOM)-treated rats given Ca drinking water was reported; tumor incidence and latency were not given (4). Reduction of colon tumor incidence was reported also in DMH-treated rats fed a 20% corn oil diet when dietary Ca was doubled; Ca had no effect in rats fed a 5% corn oil diet (212).

Dietary Fiber and Colon Carcinogenesis. Jacobs (108, 109) has summarized the data available on colon carcinogenesis and dietary fiber in laboratory animals. The majority of studies of wheat bran, fed at 15 to 40% of the diet, showed an inhibiting effect on colon tumor incidence or number when proximate carcinogens were used but not when MNU, a direct-acting carcinogen, was used. Jacobs pointed out the need for feeding a diet that provided at least 5% fat to support tumor development. He summarized his own studies showing that wheat bran could increase tumorigenesis if it was fed during carcinogen administration only, whereas it reduced carcinogenesis when fed after carcinogen exposure. Of the many other fiber types tested, only cellulose gave reasonably consistent evidence of reduction of tumorigenesis. Several fibers increased tumorigenesis in some experiments and reduced it or had no effect in others. The fibers that increased tumorigenesis in two or more experiments were corn bran, pectin, and undegraded carageenan in rats and agar in mice.

Jacobs (108) reviewed evidence that dietary fibers can stimulate or retard colon epithelial cell division and migration. He raised the possibility that fermentation of fiber components by intestinal flora, producing a decreased pH, may inhibit colon tumorigenesis. Bruce (22) in discussing several hypotheses about dietary influences on colon cancer, reviewed studies in animals of effects of colon pH and concluded that overall the studies "supported a protective effective of a slightly acidic pH." In a further review of fiber effects (187) cautions were raised about dilution of diet by fiber leading to reduced weight gain and nonspecific reduction of tumorigenesis. There is a possible contribution of short-chain fatty acids from fiber fermentation to energy supply of the colon mucosa.

In a study published since Jacob's review, psyllium husk and cellulose were tested in DMH-treated rats fed 20% fat diets designed to allow for increased diet intake in response to addition of fiber (226). The test groups were small (10/group), but they showed a significant decrease in colon tumor incidence, 40% in psyllium-fed and 60% in cellulose-fed rats compared with 100% in control rats. Rats fed the fiber-containing diets compensated by higher diet intake only partially (cellulose-fed) or not at all (psyllium-fed) so their weight gains were somewhat, but not significantly, smaller than gains of control rats, and their nutrient intakes were not entirely comparable. For these reasons the decrease in carcinogenesis cannot be attributed unequivocally to the dietary fiber. Fecal pH was reduced in psyllium-fed and increased in cellulose-fed rats; colonic pH or pH of fecal water were not measured.

Other Factors. There are reports of inhibition of colon (339) and mammary (288, 340) tumorigenesis in rats fed seaweed preparations. In some cases the inhibition may have result of reduced weight gain due to reduced intake from diet or to dilution of diet by the seaweed. The inhibition has not always correlated with reduced gain, and the subject deserves further study.

Lignans and phytoestrogens derived from plant foods have hormonal, principally estrogenic, and antioxidant properties. They are metabolized by intestinal flora, absorbed and excreted in the urine and have been associated with endocrine and other abnormalities in wild, domestic, and laboratory animals. They present an additional focus of research interest in the area of factors derived from plant food that could alter carcinogenesis (259).

Other components of plant-derived foods that have anticarcinogenic properties are the organic sulfides in products of the *Allium* genus. Diallyl sulfide, a thioether in garlic, prevents or reduces hepatic and colon epithelial necrosis induced by DMH in rats and mice, reduces colon tumorigenesis by DMH in mice (Table 6, 309), and reduces hepatic gammaglutamyltranspeptidase foci induced by DMH in rats (83). In both studies diallyl sulfide was given by gavage before administration of DMH and probably acted by altering DMH activation. Related compounds reduced benzo(a)pyrene induced gastric and pulmonary neoplasia in mice when administered 96 and 48 hours before benzo(a)pyrene; they induced glutathione-S-transferase in the target and other tissues (272).

The feeding of preparations of cruciferous vegetables to carcinogen-treated rats has reduced, or in some cases increased, tumor development, but diet design and poor dietary intake have raised questions of nutritional and caloric adequacy and comparability of the diets. In a large, well-designed study hamsters were given the pancreatic carcinogen BOP and fed approximately 10% dried cabbage with adjustment of all nutrients to compensate for the reduction of caloric density by cabbage (14). Pancreatic and gall bladder tumors and pancreatic ductal dysplasia were increased in hamsters fed cabbage beginning 4 weeks before BOP administration and continuing throughout the experiment (Table 6). The result is, therefore, contrary to expectation and further study is needed.

The protective effects of vegetable foods and preparations against carcinogenesis in some animal models may be the result of biochemical responses that alter carcinogen metabolism or metabolism of activated oxygen species that result from carcinogen exposure. Alteration of hepatic MFO, cytochromes P450, epoxide hydratase and of ability of tissue extracts to activate carcinogens was reported in mice fed vegetable or herb extracts (84). Induction of hepatic and intestinal diaphorase, an enzyme thought to protect against oxidative-cellular damage, and of intestinal MFO was reported in rats fed a diet containing 25% freeze-dried Brussels sprouts. Reduced feed intake and growth may have contributed to the effect (250). Since the studies were not performed in models in which an effect of the same extracts on carcinogenesis had been demonstrated, they are suggestive but not conclusive as to a mechanism of action for vegetable extracts.

Raw soybean flour contains a proteinaceous trypsin inhibitor that stimulates cholecystokinin release and induces pancreatic necrosis, hypertrophy, and hyperplasia followed by development of tumors in rats. When raw soybean flour is fed to 1-aza-treated rats, AACN are increased in number and size and tumor development is accelerated (181, 229). Other components of the flour, including its high content of PUFA may contribute to its effects (181).

Alcohol. Demonstration of a consistent effect of alcohol on carcinogenesis in laboratory animals has not been accomplished (for review see reference 234). There are studies suggesting that alcohol increases carcinogenesis by other agents. Alcohol ingestion was associated with increased nitrosamine hepatocarcinogenesis in a small number of lipotrope-deficient rats (221) and nitrosamine induction of hyperplastic hepatic nodules in hamsters (170). Increased respiratory tract and esophageal carcinogenesis by nitrosamines in alcohol-fed rats and hamsters have been reported (31, 58, 266). Spontaneous mammary tumors arose significantly earlier in alcohol-fed than in control mice (256). Investigation of alcohol and tumor induction in the colon gave evidence suggestive of an effect. Rats were fed 12% of calories as beer or 9% as ethanol and given AOM. Tumor incidence in the left colon was 42% (beer-fed) or 35% (ethanol-fed) compared with 15% in diet controls. Right colon tumor incidence was not affected, but higher alcohol intake (18 to 23% of calories) reduced right colon tumors and had no effect an left colon tumors (78). In a second study, tumorigenesis throughout the colon was decreased when ethanol was fed before and during AOM administration at 22 or 33% of calories but was not affected by ethanol at 11% of calories; ethanol fed after AOM exposure had no effect. AOM metabolism was reduced by the concurrent feeding of ethanol, presumably the mechanism of inhibition of tumorigenesis. There may have been a contribution also of lower body weight in rats fed the two higher amounts of ethanol. The rats were pair-fed by calories but, as is generally the case (234), weight gain was lower when the calories were provided in part by alcohol. In rats fed ethanol after AOM exposure, the reduction in weight gain was less marked and consistent than with the early feeding of ethanol (79).

Woutersen *et al.* (331) studied effects of ethanol on pancreatic neoplasia in 1-aza-treated rats. AACN were significantly increased in number and size if ethanol, 15% weight/volume, was supplied in place of drinking water. The increase occurred despite reduced weight gain and was much greater in rats fed 25% corn oil than rats fed 5% corn oil diets. In a subsequent study, in which pancreatic tumors rather than AACN were the end point, ethanol had no effect (K. A. Woutersen, unpublished data). Ethanol had no effect in the hamster BOP model (332).

SUMMARY

At this time, the epidemiologic data are inconclusive on specific relationships between diet or nutritional status and cancer risk. Certain relations have been found fairly consistently in multiple studies, *e.g.*, the inverse association between β-carotene intake and lung cancer risk. Another recent and fairly consistent finding is the direct association between alcohol consumption and breast cancer risk. At the other end of the spectrum is the consistent absence of association between coffee consumption and breast cancer risk. Epidemiologic methods of assessing the role of diet in cancer etiology are improving rapidly; their application in new studies is needed to detect and define associations with better precision.

TABLE 6. PLANT FOODS OR PRODUCTS AND CARCINOGENESIS

Plant food, product	Species	Carcinogen	Target organ	Change in tumors		References
				Malignant	Benign	
Cabbage in control fat diet	Hamster	BOP	Pancreas	0[a]	+170	Birt *et al.* (14)
Cabbage in high fat diet				+170[a]	0	
Cabbage in control diet	Mouse	DMBA	Skin	—	+117	Birt *et al.* (14)
Diallyl sulfide, gavage	Mouse	DMH	Colon		−380	Wargovich (309)

—, data not given.

[a] Gall bladder carcinoma increased 4-fold (from 3 to 12% incidence) irrespective of dietary fat.

In contrast research results in laboratory animals on three groups of nutrients, fat, vitamin A, and related compounds and lipotropes (choline, methionine, folate, and vitamin B_1) conclusively demonstrate significant effects at many target sites.

In case-control and follow-up epidemiologic studies of fat intake in relation to cancer of the breast and large bowel, the evidence is inconsistent; in neither case is the evidence in favor of a direct association strong. When an effect on large bowel cancer is found, it appears to be greater for saturated fats than for other types of fat. The small amount of epidemiologic evidence available on fat intake and cancer of the pancreas, prostate, and ovary is consistent with a small to moderate direct association. Studies are needed in populations with more heterogeneous fat intakes than are typically seen in the West to determine whether low fat diets confer a protective effect. Recent data suggest that dietary cholesterol is not associated with breast or lung cancer risk and that the small to medium association with large bowel cancer risk reported in the past may not be present when total caloric intake is considered.

Evaluation of the role of total caloric intake in the etiology of cancer is complex because intake and balance are related to physical activity, relative body weight, and other factors that may affect cancer risk independently. Findings on site-specific cancer risks and total caloric intake are inconclusive. Data on cancer risk in relation to physical activity suggest an inverse relation with risk of large bowel and possibly breast cancer. Leanness may be a risk factor for pre- but not postmenopausal breast cancer. Obesity may be a risk factor for cancer of the large bowel, ovaries, and prostate. Relations between lung or pancreatic cancer and relative body weight are difficult to interpret because of the influences of smoking. Collection of data on physical activity and relative body weight in dietary studies will allow assessment of the effect of total caloric intake after adjustment for its measurable determinants.

The enhancement of mammary gland tumorigenesis experimentally by diets high in certain fats is a consistent finding. Dietary fat influences carcinogenesis in rats at several sites; most extensively studies are mammary gland, colon, and pancreas. The evidence is strong that certain kinds of fat, fed in amounts three to five times greater than required for normal growth and reproduction, enhance mammary tumor development in rats and mice. The mechanism by which fat acts in the mammary tumor models is unknown; part of the effect can be attributed to caloric intake. The evidence that fat enhances colon tumor development in animal models is much less consistent, and the differences between laboratories are, at present, unresolved. Several mechanisms for the effect of fat have been proposed and investigated, but their relevance must remain in doubt until a clear effect of fat on colon tumorigenesis is demonstrated. The data on fat enhancement of pancreatic carcinogenesis in rats are more recent and less extensive than data in mammary gland and colon. The mechanism is unknown. Attempts to separate specific effects of fat from nonspecific caloric effects are in progress in several models and include studies of the effect of exercise. Mammary gland, colon and pancreatic tumorigenesis are directly related to caloric intake, irrespective of the percent of calories supplied by fat.

The most effective fats in the animal models are rich in ω-6 PUFA, but fats that or saturated can be largely monounsaturated are effective also, if supplemented with ω-6 PUFA. Oils composed largely of ω-3 PUFA are not effective. Enhancement of tumorigenesis by fat is related to timing and duration of feeding; reversibility of the effect of feeding a high fat diet early in life is not consistently demonstrated.

These results have stimulated expansion of research into examination of mechanisms and basic questions of the influence of caloric balance, exercise and body composition on carcinogenesis. The results should be applicable to other fat or calorie-modulated tumor models and to design of epidemiologic studies which at present, have not produced clear answers.

The apparent discrepancies between the epidemiologic and experimental data on an association of dietary fat and breast cancer risk may be the result of the different ranges of fat intake examined. In the animal studies 10 and 40% of calories from fat are generally compared, whereas in the Western populations, 30 and 40% of calories from fat are the extremes that can be compared. The geographic studies that were included in the National Academy of Sciences-National Research Council review (184) were not considered here for the reasons discussed in the section on epidemiologic methods.

In some epidemiologic studies of breast cancer risk in relation to protein intake, there is a small direct association. Data on protein intake and colorectal cancer risk do not suggest an association. Data on cancer of the lung, ovaries, and prostate are inconclusive.

Experimental studies for effects of protein on tumorigenesis support an enhancing effect of high dietary protein on mammary gland tumorigenesis in a two-generation model.

An inverse association between vitamin A intake and risk of breast cancer has been shown in several epidemiologic studies; serum β-carotene and retinol levels appear to be unrelated to risk. Vitamin A and β-carotene appear not to play on important role in determining risk of large bowel or prostate cancer. A moderate inverse association between risk of lung cancer and intake of foods high in β-carotene is consistently reported, but new data on the inverse relation between smoking and β-carotene intake and serum levels suggest the true magnitude of a protective effect may be slightly less that previously thought. Data on pancreatic and ovarian cancer in relation to intake of β-carotene and vitamin A are inconclusive.

In experimental studies, vitamin A and synthetic retinoids inhibit carcinogenesis in skin, mammary gland, and urinary bladder and have inconsistent effects in respiratory tract and other mucosae. The requirement of extremely large doses of vitamin A and the anticarcinogenic effect of synthetic retinoids that have variable vitamin A activity indicates that the effect is a nonnutritional or paranutritional one. Evaluation of β-carotene cannot be made since few studies are available; investigation is hampered by failure of rodents to absorb the whole molecule into the blood. Protection against carcinogenesis by large doses of vitamin A and related compounds in several target organs is a third generally consistent result in experimental studies; its applicability to epidemiologic questions again, is not clear because the amounts used are far greater than usual human intakes or requirements.

Deficiency of vitamin A increases somewhat susceptibility of urinary bladder, colon, and probably respiratory tract mucosae to chemical carcinogenesis in animal models. This suggests that the inverse association of β-carotene intake and smoking could be due to increased development of smoking-associated cancers if intake of preformed vitamin A also was low.

Results of epidemiologic studies of the relation between serum Se and cancer risk suggest a possible inverse association for gastrointestinal malignancy; for other sites the results are less consistent with an association. Several studies of risk of colorectal cancer in relation to calcium suggest a possible inverse association.

In animals, Se reduces development of mammary gland tumors in rats and mice and colon and liver tumors in rats. In mice Se deficiency increases the effect of high fat diets on mammary gland tumorigenesis. The experimental data, therefore, support the epidemiologic data on selenium and gastrointestinal cancer. Preliminary reports suggest that calcium may inhibit colon tumorigenesis under some experimental conditions. The experimental data, therefore, support the epidemiologic data on Ca and gastrointestinal cancer.

Epidemiologic data on fiber intake in relation to risk of large bowel cancer suggest a small inverse association or no association. Associations between fiber intake and other cancers have not been extensively studied; investigations suggesting an inverse relation between fiber intake and risk of lung cancer are provocative.

Dietary fiber has inconsistent effects on colon tumorigenesis in laboratory animals, as do preparations of whole vegetables.

In epidemiologic data, breast cancer risk and dietary vitamin E appear not to be associated, although an inverse association of serum α-tocopherol has been found in one small study. Data from studies of serum α-tocopherol in relation to risk of colorectal cancer suggest a modest inverse association; in dietary studies there appears to be an inverse association or no association. There are conflicting data on serum or dietary α-tocopherol and lung cancer; studies of vitamin E intake and risk of cancers of the prostate, pancreas, and ovaries have not been reported.

In rats, vitamin E increases the reduction by Se of mammary tumorigenesis but has no activity by itself.

Relatively little epidemiologic evidence was available to assess cancer-vitamin C relations. There appears to be no relation with breast cancer risk, either no association or a very small inverse association with large bowel cancer risk, and no association with prostatic or ovarian cancer risk.

Vitamin C reduces formation of carcinogenic nitrosamines in animals but no significant effect on carcinogenesis it self has been reported.

Studies of breast cancer risk in humans in relation to alcoholic beverage consumption support a moderate direct association. Data on the relation between colorectal cancer and alcohol consumption are less consistent, but suggest a modest association, possibly stronger for rectal than for colon cancer; beer is implicated more than other alcoholic beverages. The effect of alcohol consumption on risk of lung cancer cannot be evaluated from existing data. For cancers of the prostate, and pancreas, the evidence does not support a direct association. For ovarian cancer the evidence is consistent with a small inverse association.

Ethanol has only rarely increased chemical carcinogenesis in animal models. Feeding ethanol in significant amounts almost invariably reduces weight gain, a result that could negate any carcinogenic or cocarcinogenic effect it may have. Data suggestive of effects of alcohol on experimental carcinogenesis in colon and liver have been reported but are not consistent. An animal model for alcoholic cirrhosis, induced by deficiency of the lipotropic agents, choline and methionine, shows markedly enhanced susceptibility, hepatocarcinogenesis by many chemicals, and to development of spontaneous tumors. Deficiency of methylating capacity, abnormal activity of methylating and MFO enzyme systems and hyperplasia of hepatocytes all may contribute to the effect of the deficiency on carcinogenesis. The consistent effect of lipotrope deficiency on hepatocarcinogenesis is highly useful in examination of molecular mechanisms of carcinogenesis; its applicability to epidemiology of liver or other cancer is not clear.

In contrast to the epidemiologic data consistently showing no relation of coffee consumption to the occurrence of breast, colorectal, ovarian, or prostatic cancer, the findings on pancreatic cancer, although variable, are consistent with a modest direct association.

Experimental data have not shown consistent effects of coffee on mammary gland tumorgenesis.

Finally, addition of fiber, vitamin A, Se, or vegetable preparations to the diet has increased, rather than decreased, carcinogenesis under some experimental conditions.

These results indicate the need for further study of the relationships between diet and nutritional status and cancer risk. Improved design of epidemiologic and experimental studies should permit resolution of at least some of the inconsistencies discussed.

CONCLUSIONS

The recent epidemiologic data relating high dietary fat and breast or colon carcinoma are less consistent with a direct association than the data reviewed in the National Academy of Sciences-National Research Council report (184). The recent experimental data are consistent with an effect of certain fats on mammary and pancreatic tumorigenesis but are inconsistent in studies of colon tumor models. In both epidemiologic and experimental studies, consideration of the effect of total caloric intake has reduced somewhat the magnitude of the apparent specific effect of fat.

The recent experimental data directly relating caloric intake and mammary and colon carcinogenesis are consistent. The epidemiologic data on caloric intake are inconsistent but may become clearer as the independent effects of determinants of caloric intake on cancer risk are considered.

Epidemiologic data on the association of breast cancer risk with alcohol intake support the addition of breast to the cancer sites previously related to alcohol consumption.

Conclusions about the relations between other nutrients or foods and cancer risk discussed are not substantially changed from the 1982 publication (184).

The effects of nutrients and diet on cancer risk in people or laboratory animals are generally subtle. However, because of the great morbidity and mortality due to cancer, even small changes in incidence or latency due to dietary changes may be highly significant. Large international variations in cancer rates suggest that the effects of diet on cancer in humans may be more marked than in the data reviewed. Additional studies are warranted to: (a) refine current dietary guidelines; (b) support efforts in chemoprevention using foods, and related nutrient compounds; (c) identify other components of foods that may be anticarcinogenic; (d) examine interactions between nutrients that may influence carcinogenesis.

Acknowledgments: Grateful acknowledgment is made to three colleagues who read and criticized this review: Drs. Selwyn Broitman, Daniel Longnecker, and Walter Willett. While their comments were extremely helpful, the authors used them selectively and retain full responsibility for the interpretations and opinions expressed in the review.

This work was supported in part by grants from the American Institute for Cancer Research and the Alcoholic Beverage Medical Research Foundation.

Dr. Longnecker is a Medical Foundation Research Fellow supported by the Medical Foundation, Inc., Boston, Massachusetts.

REFERENCES

1. Adams LM, Cullinan CA, Karmali RA: Differential effect of dietary fish oil and a low fat diet on spontaneous and experimental metastasis of rat mammary tumor 13762 (abstr). Proc Am Assoc Cancer Res 28:159, 1987
2. Albanes D: Caloric intake, body weight, and cancer: a review. Nutr Cancer 9:199, 1987
3. Albanes D: Potential for confounding of physical activity risk assessment by body weight and fatness. Am J Epidemiol 125:745, 1987
4. Appleton GV, Davies PW, Bristol JB, Williamson RC: Inhibition of intestinal carcinogenesis by dietary supplementation with calcium. Br J Surg 74:523, 1987
5. Asenjo CF: Variations in the nutritive values of foods. Am J Clin Nutr 11:368, 1962
6. Baldwin S, Parker RS: Influence of Dietary fat and selenium and promotion of aflatoxin B_1-induced preneoplastic foci in rat liver. Carcinogenesis 8:101, 1987
7. Begg CB, Walker AM, Wessen B, Zelen M: Alcohol consumption and breast cancer. Lancet i:293, 1983
8. Bendich A, Shapiro SS: Effect of β-carotene and canthaxanthin on the immune responses of the rat. J Nutr 116:2254, 1986
9. Berkelman RL, Ralston M, Herndon J, Gwinn M, Bertolucci D, Dufour M: Patterns of alcohol consumption and alcohol-related morbidity and mortality. Center for Disease Control Surveillance Summaries 35:1SS, 1986
10. Beth M, Berger MR, Aksoy M, Schmahl D: Comparison between the effects of dietary fat level and of calorie intake on methylnitrosourea-induced mammary carcinogenesis in female SD rats. Int J Cancer 39:737, 1987
11. Beth M, Berger MR, Aksoy M, Schmahl D: Effects of vitamin A and E supplementation to diets containing two different fat levels on methylnitrosourea-induced mammary carcinogenesis in female SD-rats. Br J Cancer 56:445, 1987
12. Birt DF: Update on the effects of vitamins A, C, and E and selenium on carcinogenesis. Proc Soc Exp Biol Med 183:311, 1986
13. Birt DF, Julius AD, White LT, Pour PM: Enhancement of pancreatic carcinogenesis in hamsters fed a high fat diet at a restricted intake (abstr). Proc Am Assoc Cancer Res 28:153, 1987
14. Birt DF, Pelling JC, Pour PM, Tibbels MG, Schweickert L, Bresnick E: Enhanced pancreatic and skin tumorigenesis in cabbage-fed hamsters and mice. Carcinogenesis 8:913, 1987
15. Birt DF, Pour PM: Pancreatic cancer enhancement in the hamster model by diets high in fat and/or protein. In Experimental Pancreatic Carcinogenesis, edited by Scarpelli D, Reddy VK, Longnecker DS, p 175. Boca Raton, CRC Press Inc, 1987
16. Birt DF, Roebuck BD: Enhancement of pancreatic carcinogenesis by dietary fat in the hamster and rat models. In Dietary Fat and Cancer, edited by Ip C, Birt DF, Rogers AE, Mettlin C, p 331. New York, Alan R. Liss, Inc., 1986
17. Bjelke E: Case-control study of cancer of the stomach, colon, and rectum. In Oncology 1970: Proceedings of the Tenth International Congress, vol 5, p 320. Chicago: Yearbook Medical Publ, 1971
18. Bjelke E: Epidemiology of colorectal cancer with emphasis on diet. In Human Cancer: Its Characterization and Treatment. Proceedings of the Eight International Symposium on the Biological Characterization of Human Tumors, edited by Davis W, Harrap KR, Stathopoulos G, p 158. International Congress Series No. 484. Exerpta Medica, Amsterdam, Oxford, Princeton, 1980
19. Boissonneault GA, Elson CE, Pariza MW: Net energy effects of dietary fat on chemically induced mammary carcinogenesis in F344 rats. J Natl Cancer Inst 76:335, 1986
20. Braden LM, Carroll KK: Dietary polyunsatured fat in relation to mammary carcinogenesis in rats. Lipids 21:285, 1986
21. Broitman SA, Cannizzo F, Rogers A, Gottlieb LS: Comparison of dietary marine oil and safflower oil on growth and pulmonary colonization of Ct-26 implanted into bowel of mice (abstr). Fed Proc 46:437, 1987
22. Bruce WR: Recent hypotheses for the origin of colon cancer. Cancer Res 47:4237, 1987
23. Bunnik GSJ, Bosland MC, De Bie ATJ: Interactive effects of amount of fat and of linoleic acid in the diet on induction of mammary cancer by NMU in rats (abstr). Proc. AACR 28:158, 1987
24. Byers T, Funch DF: Alcohol and breast cancer. Lancet 1:799, 1982
25. Byers TE, Graham S, Haughey BP, Marshall JR, Swanson MK: Diet and lung cancer risk: findings from the western New York diet study. Am J Epidemiol 125:351, 1987
26. Byers T, Marshall J, Fiedler R, Zielezny M, Graham S: Assessing nutrient intake with an abbreviated dietary interview. Am J Epidemiol 122:41, 1985
27. Byers T, Marshall J, Graham S, Mettlin C, Swanson M: A case-control study of dietary and nondietary factors in ovarian cancer. JNCI 71:681, 1983
28. Byers T, Vena J, Miettlin C, Swanson M, Graham S: Dietary vitamin A and lung cancer risk: an analysis by histologic subtypes. Am J Epidemiol 120:769, 1984
29. Carroll KK, Braden LM, Bell JA, Kalamegham R: Fat and cancer. Cancer 58:1818, 1986
30. Carroll KK, Noble RL: Dietary fat in relation to hormonal induction of mammary and prostatic carcinoma in NB rats. Carcinogenesis 8:851, 1987
31. Castonguay A, Rivenson A, Trushin N: Effects of chronic ethanol consumption on the metabolism and carcinogenicity of N-nitrosonornicotine in F344 rats. Cancer Res 44:2285, 1984
32. Chan PC, Dao TL: Enhancement of mammary carcinogenesis by a high-fat diet in Fischer, Long-Evans, and Sprague-Dawley rats. Cancer Res 41:164, 1981
33. Chan PC, Ferguson KA, Dao TL: Effects of different dietary fats on mammary carcinogenesis. Cancer Res 43:1079, 1983
34. Chandar N, Amenta J, Kandala JC, Lombardi B: Liver cell turnover in rats fed a choline-devoid diet. Carcinogenesis 8:669,

1987
35. Clinton SK, Alster JM, Imrey PB, Nandkumar S, Truex CR, Visek WJ: Effects of dietary protein, fat and energy intake during an initiation phase study of 7, 12-dimethylbenz[a]anthracene-induced breast cancer in rats. J Nutr 116:2290, 1986
36. Clinton SK, Imrey PB, Alster JM, Simon J, Truex CR, Visek WJ: The combined effects of dietary protein and fat on 7,12-dimethylbenz[a]anthracene-induced breast cancer in rats. J Nutr 114:1213, 1984
37. Clinton SK, Visek WJ: The macronutrients in experimental carcinogenesis of the breast, colon, and pancreas. In Dietary Fat and Cancer, edited by Ip C, Birt DF, Rogers AE, Mettlin C, p 377. New York, Alan R. Liss, Inc., 1986
38. Cohen LA: The fat effect on n-nitrosomethylurea (NMU)-induced rat mammary carcinogenesis: inhibition by (A) voluntary energy expenditure and (B) caloric restriction (abstr). Proc Am Assoc Cancer Res 28:155, 1987
39. Cohen LA, Thompson DO, Maeura Y, Choi K, Blank ME, Rose DP: Dietary fat and mammary cancer. Promoting effects of different dietary fats on N-nitrosomethylurea-induced rat mammary tumorigenesis. JNCI 77:33, 1986
40. Cohen SM, Wittenberg JF, and Bryan GT: Effects of avitamin—osis A and hypervitaminosis A on urinary bladder carcinogenicity of N-[4-(5-nitro-z-furyl)-2-thiazolyl] formamide. Cancer Res 36:2334, 1976
41. Colacchio TA, Memoli VA: Chemoprevention of colorectal neoplasms. Arch Surg 121:1421, 1986
42. Colditz GA, Stampfer MJ, Willett WC: Diet and lung cancer: a review of the epidemiologic evidence in humans. Arch Intern Med 147:157, 1987
43. Cramer DW, Welch WR, Hutchison GB, Willett W, Scully RE: Dietary animal fat in relation to ovarian cancer risk. Obstet Gynecol 63:883, 1984
44. Dales LG, Friedman GD, Ury HK, Grossman S, Williams SR: A case-control study of relationships of diet and other traits to colorectal cancer in American blacks. Am J Epidemiol 109:132, 1979
45. Dao TL, Chan PC: Effect of duration of high fat intake on enhancement of mammary carcinogenesis in rats. JNCI 71:201, 1983
46. Dean G, MacLennan R, McLoughlin H, Shelley E: Causes of death of blue-collar workers at a Dublin brewery, 1954–73. Br J Cancer 40:581, 1979
47. De Waard F, Baander-van Halewijn EA: A prospective study in general practice on breast-cancer risk in postmenopausal women. Int J Cancer 14:153, 1974
48. Donato KA: Efficiency and utilization of various energy sources for growth. Am J Clin Nutr 45:164, 1987
49. Donato K, Hegsted DM: Efficiency of utilization of various sources of energy for growth. Proc Nat Acad Sci USA 82:4866, 1985
50. Dunaif GE, Campbell TC: Dietary protein level and Aflatoxin B_1-induced preneoplastic hepatic lesions in the rat. J Nutr 117:1298, 1987
51. Durbec JP, Chevillotte G, Bidart JM, Berthezene P, Sarles H: Diet, alcohol, tobacco and risk of cancer of the pancreas: a case-control study. Br J Cancer 47:463, 1983
52. Eto I, Krumdieck CL: Role of Vitamin B12 and Folate Deficiencies in Carcinogenesis. In Essential Nutrients in Carcinogenesis, edited by Poirier LA, Newberne PM, Pariza MW, p 313. New York, Plenum Press, 1986
53. Fisher M, Gordon T: The relation of drinking and smoking habits to diet: the lipid research clinics prevalence study. Am J Clin Nutr 41:623, 1985
54. Fong LYY, Sivak A and Newberne PM: Zinc deficiency and methy-benzylnitrosamine-induced esophageal cancer in rats. J Natl Cancer Inst 61:145, 1978
55. Frisch RE, Wyshak G, Albright NL, Albright TE, Schiff I, Jones KP, Witschi, Shiang E, Koff E, Marguglio M: Lower prevalence of breast cancer and cancers of the reproductive system among former college athletes compared to non-athletes. Br J Cancer 52:885, 1985
56. Fukushima SH, Imaida K, Sakata T, Okamura T, Shibata M, Ito N: Promoting effects of sodium L-ascorbate on two-stage urinary bladder carcinogenesis in rats. Cancer Res 43:4454, 1983
57. Fukushima S, Shibata MA, Shirai T, Kurata Y, Tamano S, Imaida K: Promotion by L-ascorbic acid of urinary bladder carcinogenesis in rats under conditions of increased urinary K ion concentration and pH. Cancer Res 47:4821, 1987
58. Gabrial GN, Schrager TF and Newberne PM: Zinc deficiency, alcohol, and a retinoid: association with esophageal cancer in rats. J Natl Cancer Inst 68:785, 1982
59. Gammal EB, Carroll KK and Plunkett ER: Effects of dietary fat on mammary carcinogenesis by 7,12-dimethylbenz(a)anthracene by rat mammary tissue. Cancer Res 28:384, 1968
60. Garabrant DH, Peters JM, Mack TM, Bernstein L: Job activity and colon cancer risk: Am J Epidemiol 119:1005, 1984
61. Garland C, Shekelle RB, Barrett-Connor E, Criqui MH, Rossof AH, Ogelsby P: Dietary vitamin D and calcium and risk of colorectal cancer: a 19-year prospective study in men. Lancet i:307, 1985
62. Gensler HI, Watson RR, Moriguchi S, Bowden GT: Effects of dietary retinyl palmitate or 13-cis-retinoic acid on the promotion of tumors in mouse skin. Cancer Res 47:967, 1987
63. Gerhardsson M, Norell SE, Kiviranta H, Pedersen NL, Ahlbom A: Sedentary jobs and colon cancer. Am J Epidemiol 123:775, 1986
64. Gold EB, Gordis L, Diener MD, Seltser R, Boitnott JK, Bynum TE, Hutcheon DF: Diet and other risk factors for cancer of the pancreas. Cancer 55:460, 1985
65. Goldstein HR: No association found between coffee and cancer of the pancreas. N Engl J Med 306:997, 1982
66. Graham S, Dayal H, Swanson M, Mittelman A, Wilkinson G: Diet in the epidemiology of cancer of the colon and rectum. JNCI 61:709, 1978
67. Graham S, Haughey B, Marshall J, Priore R, Byers T, Rzepka T, Mettlin C, Pontes JE: Diet in the epidemiology of carcinoma of the prostate gland. JNCI 70:687, 1983
68. Graham S, Marshall J, Mettlin C, Rzepka T, Nemoto T, Byers T: Diet in the epidemiology of breast cancer. Am J Epidemiol 116:68, 1982
69. Gregor A, Lee PN, Roe FJC, Wilson MJ, Melton A: Comparison of dietary histories in lung cancer cases and controls with special reference to vitamin A. Nutr Cancer 2:93, 1980
70. Grubbs CJ, Hill DL, Farnell DR: Effect of retinyl acetate in preventing mammary cancer induced by procarbazine a chemotherapeutic agent (abstr). Int Assn Vit Nutr Oncology P-1, 1985
71. Grubbs CJ, Juliana MM, Hill DL, Whitaker LM: Effect of laboratory diets on methylnitrosourea (MNU)-induced mammary cancers and on the efficacy of a chemopreventive agent (Retinyl Acetate) (abstr). Proc Am Assoc Cancer Res 28:160, 1987
72. Grubbs CJ, Moon RC, Squire RA, Farrow GM, Stinson SF, Goodman DG, Brown CC, Sporn MB: 13-cis-Retinoic acid: inhibition of bladder carcinogenesis induced by *N*-butyl-*N*-(4-hydroxybutyl)nitrosamine. Science 198:743, 1977
73. Grummer MA, Erdman JW: Effect of chronic alcohol consumption and moderate fat diet on vitamin A status in rats fed either Vitamin A or B-carotene. J Nutr 113:350, 1983
74. Gupta RC, Earley K, Locker J, Lombardi B: $^{32-}P^{-}$ Postlabeling analysis of liver DNA adducts in rats chronically fed a choline-devoid diet. Carcinogenesis 8:187, 1987
75. Gwinn ML, Webster LA, Lee NC, Layde PM, Rubin GL. The Cancer and Steroid Hormone Study Group: Alcohol consumption and ovarian cancer risk. Am J Epidemiol 123:759, 1986
76. Haenzel W, Berg JW, Segi M, Kurihara M, Locke FB: Large-bowel cancer in Hawaiian Japanese. JNCI 51:1765, 1973
77. Haenzel W, Locke FB, Segi M: A case-control study of large bowel cancer in Japan. JNCI 64:17, 1980
78. Hamilton SR, Hyland J, McAvinchey D, Chaudhry Y, Hartka I, Kim HT, Cichon P, Floyd J, Turjman N, Kessie G: Effects of chronic dietary beer and ethanol consumption on experimental colonic carcinogenesis by azoxymethane in rats. Cancer Res 47:1551, 1987
79. Hamilton SR, Sohn OS, Fiala ES: Effects of timing and quantity of chronic dietary ethanol consumption on azoxymethane-induced colonic carcinogenesis and azoxymethane metabolism in Fischer 344 rats. Cancer Res 47:4305, 1987
80. Hartge P, Lesher LP, McGowan L, Hoover R: Coffee and ovarian cancer. Int J Cancer 30:531, 1982
81. Hawrylewicz EJ: Fat-protein interaction, defined 2-generation

studies. In Dietary Fat and Cancer, edited by Ip C, Birt DF, Rogers AE, Mettlin C, p 403. New York, Alan R. Liss Inc., 1986
82. Harvey EB, Schairer MS, Brinton LA, Hoover RN, Fraumeni JF Jr: Alcohol consumption and breast cancer. JNCI 78:657, 1987
83. Hayes MA, Rushmore TH, Goldberg MT: Inhibition of hepatocarcinogenic responses to 1,2-dimethylhydrazine by diallylsulfide, a component of garlic oil. Carcinogenesis 8:1155, 1987
84. Hendrich S, Bjeldanes LF: Effects of dietary Schizandra Chinensis, Brussels sprouts and illicium verum extracts on carcinogen metabolism systems in mouse liver. Food Chem Toxicol 24:903, 1986
85. Heshmat MY, Kaul L, Kovi J, Jackson MA, Jackson AG, Jones GW, Edson M, Enterline JP, Worrell RG, Perry SL: Nutrition and prostate cancer: a case-control study. The Prostate 6:7, 1985
86. Heuch I, Kvale G, Jacobsen BK, Bjelke E: Use of alcohol, tobacco and coffee and risk of pancreatic cancer. Br J Cancer 48:637, 1983
87. Heywood R, Palmer AK, Gregson RL, Hummler H: The toxicity of beta carotene. Toxicology 36:91, 1985
88. Hiatt RA, Bawol RD: Alcoholic beverage consumption and breast cancer incidence. Am J Epidemiol 120:676, 1984
89. Higginson J: Etiologic factors in gastrointestinal cancer in man. JNCI 37:527, 1966
90. Hillers VN, Massey LK: Interrelationships of moderate and high alcohol consumption with diet and health status. Am J Clin Nutr 41:356, 1985
91. Hinds MW, Kolonel LN, Hankin JH, Lee J: Dietary vitamin A, carotene, vitamin C, and risk of lung cancer in Hawaii. Am J Epidemiol 119:227, 1984
92. Hirayama T: Diet and cancer. Nutr Cancer 1:67, 1979
93. Hirayama T: Prospective studies on cancer epidemiology based on census population in Japan. In Cancer Epidemiology: Environmental Factors, Proceedings of the Eleventh International Cancer Congress, Florence, vol 3, edited by Bucalossi P, Veronesi W, Cascinelle N, p 26. Amsterdam, Exerpta Medica, 1974
94. Hirayama T: Epidemiology of breast cancer with special reference to the role of diet. Prev Med 7:173, 1978
95. Hirayama T: Prospective studies on cancer epidemiology based on census population in Japan. In Prevention and Detection of Cancer, vol 1, Etiology, edited by Nieburgs HE, p 1139. New York, Marcel Dekker, 1978
96. Hirayama T: A large-scale cohort study on the relationship between diet and selected cancers of the digestive organs. In Banbury Report No. 7: Gastrointestinal Cancer: Endogenous factors, edited by Bruce WR, Correa P, Lipkin M, Tannenbaum SR, p 409. Cold Spring Harbor, N.Y.: Cold Spring Harbor Laboratory, 1981
97. Hirohata T, Nomura AMY, Hankin JH, Kolonel LK, Lee J: An epidemiologic study on the association between diet and breast cancer. JNCI 78:595, 1987
98. Hirohata T, Shigematsu T, Nomura AMY, Nomura Y, Horie A, Hirohata I: Occurrence of breast cancer in relation to diet and reproductive history: a case-control study in Fukuoka, Japan. Natl Cancer Inst Monogr 69:187, 1985
99. Holman RT: Nutritional and functional requirements for essential fatty acids. In Dietary Fat and Cancer, edited by Ip C, Birt DF, Rogers AE, Mettlin C, p 211. New York, Alan R. Liss, Inc., 1986
100. Howe GR, Miller AB, Jain M: Re: "Total energy intake: implications for epidemiologic analyses". Am J Epidemiol 124:157, 1986
101. Hsieh CC, MacMahon B, Yen S, Trichopoulos D, Warren K, Nardi G: Coffee and pancreatic cancer (chapter 2). N Engl J Med 315:587, 1986
102. Hunter DG, Chute CG, Kushner E, Colditz GA, Stampfer MJ, Speizer FE, Morris SJ, Willett WC: Predictors of selenium concentration in nail tissue. Am J Epidemiol 126:743, 1987
103. Ip C: Factors influencing the anticarcinogenic efficacy of selenium in dimethylbenz(a)anthracene induced mammary tumorigenesis in rats. Cancer Res 41:2683, 1981
104. Ip C: The chemopreventive role of selenium in carcinogenesis,In Essential Nutrients in Carcinogenesis, edited by Poirier LA, Newberne PM, Pariza MW, p 431. New York, Plenum Press, 1986
105. Ip C, Carter CA and Ip MM: Requirement of essential fatty acid for mammary tumorigenesis in the rat. Cancer Res 45:1997, 1985
106. Ip C, Sinha DK: Enhancement of mammary tumorigenesis by dietary selenium deficiency in rats with a high polyunsaturated fat intake. Cancer Res 41:31, 1981
107. Jacobs LR: Effect of short-term dietary fat on cell growth in rat gastrointestional mucosa and pancreas. Am J Clin Nutr 37:361, 1983
108. Jacobs LR: Modification of experimental colon carcinogenesis by dietary fibers. In Essential Nutrients in Carcinogenesis, edited by Poirier LA, Newberne PM, Pariza MW, p 105. New York, and London Plenum Press, 1986
109. Jacobs LR: Dietary fiber and cancer. J Nutr 117:1319, 1987
110. Jacobsen BK, Bjelke E, Kvale G, Heuch I: Coffee drinking, mortality, and cancer incidence: results from a Norwegian prospective study. JNCI 76:823, 1986
111. Jain M, Cook GM, Davis FG, Grace MG, Howe GR, Miller AB: A case-control study of diet and colo-rectal cancer. Int J Cancer 26:757, 1980
112. Jensen OM: Cancer morbidity and causes of death among Danish brewery workers. Int J Cancer 23:454, 1979
113. Jick H, Dinan BJ: Coffee and pancreatic cancer. Lancet ii:92, 1981
114. Jones BR, Barrett-Connor E, Criqui MH, Holdbrook MJ: A community study of calorie and nutrient intake in drinkers and non-drinkers of alcohol. Am J Clin Nutr 35:135, 1982
115. Jones DY, Schatzkin A, Green SB, Block G, Brinton LA, Ziegler RG, Hoover R, Taylor PR: Dietary fat and breast cancer in the national health and nutrition examination survey I epidemiologic follow-up study. JNCI 79:465, 1987
116. Kabat GC, Howson CP, Wynder EL: Beer consumption and rectal cancer. Int J Epidemiol 15:494, 1986
117. Karmali RA: Fatty acids: inhibition. Am J Clin Nutr 45:225, 1987
118. Katsouyanni K, Trichopoulos D, Boyle P, Xirouchaki E, Trichopoulou A, Lisseos B, Vasilaros S, MacMahon B: Diet and breast cancer: a case-control study in Greece. Int J Cancer 38:815, 1986
119. Katsouyanni K, Willett W, Trichopoulos D, Boyle P, Trichopoulou A, Vasilaros S, Papadiamantis J, MacMahon B: Risk of breast cancer among greek women in relation to nutrient intake. Cancer 61:181, 1988
120. Kinlen LJ, McPherson K: Pancreas cancer and coffee and tea consumption: a case-control study. Br J Cancer 49:93, 1984
121. Klatsky AL, Armstrong MA, Friedman GD: Alcohol comsumption and 17-year cancer mortality (abstract). Am J Epidemiol 126:770, 1987
122. Klatsky AL, Armstrong MA, Friedman GD, Hiatt RA: Alcoholic beverage use and colorectal cancer (abstr). Am J Epidemiol 126:770, 1987
123. Kleinbaum DG, Kupper LL, Morgenstern, H: Epidemiologic Research: Principles and Quantitative Methods. Belmont, California, Lifetime Learning Publications, 1982
124. Klurfeld DM, Weber MM, Kritchevsky D: Inhibition of chemically induced mammary and colon tumor promotion by caloric restriction in rats fed increased dietary fat. Cancer Res 47:2759, 1987
125. Knazak RA, Liu SC, Bodwin JS, Vonderhaar BK: Requirement of essential fatty acids in the diet for development of the mouse mammary gland. J Natl Cancer Inst 64:377, 1980
126. Kobayashi M, Kogata M, Yamamura M, Takada H, Hioki K, Yamamoto M: Inhibitory effect of dietary selenium on carcinogenesis in rat glandular stomach induced by N-methyl-N-nitronitrosoguanidine. Cancer Res 46:2266, 1986
127. Kok FJ, De Bruijn AM, Hofman A, Vermeeren R, Valkenburg HA: Is serum selenium a risk factor for cancer in men only? Am J Epidemiol 125:12, 1987
128. Kolonel LN, Hinds MW, Nomura AMY, Hankin JH, Lee J: Relationship of dietary vitamin A and ascorbic acid intake to the risk for cancers of the lung, bladder, and prostate in Hawaii. Natl Cancer Inst Monogr 69:137, 1985
129. Kolonel LN, Nomura AMY, Hinds MW, Hirohata T, Hankin JH, Lee J: Role of diet in cancer incidence in Hawaii. Cancer Res 43:2397s, 1983
130. Kort WJ, Weijma IM, Bijma AM, van Schalkwijk WP, Vergroesen AJ, Westbroek DL: Omega-3 fatty acids inhibiting the growth of a transplantable rat mammary adenocarcinoma. JNCI 79:593, 1987
131. Kirtchevsky D, Klurfeld DM: Influence of caloric intake on experimental carcinogenesis: a review. In Essential Nutrients in Carcinogenesis, edited by Poirier LA, Newberne PM, Pariza MW,

p 55. New York, and London, Plenum Press, 1986
132. Kritchevsky D, Klurfeld DM: Caloric effects in experimental mammary tumorigenesis. Am J Clin Nutr 45:236, 1987
133. Kritchevsky D, Weber MM, Klurfeld DM: Dietary fat versus caloric content in initiation and promotion of 7,12-dimethylbenz(a)anthracene-induced mammary tumorigenesis in rats. Cancer Res 44:3174, 1984
134. Kune S, Kune GA, Watson LF: Case-control study of dietary etiological factors: the Melbourne colorectal cancer study. Nutr Cancer 9:21, 1987
135. Kune S, Kune GA, Watson LF: Case-control study of alcoholic beverages as etiologic factors: the Melbourne colorectal cancer study. Nutr Cancer 9:43, 1987
136. Kvale G, Bjelke E, Gart JJ: Dietary habits and lung cancer risk. Int J Cancer 31:397, 1983
137. La Vecchia C, Decarli A, Francheschi S, Pampallona S, Tognoni G: Alcohol consumption and the risk of breast cancer in women. JNCI 75:61, 1985
138. La Vecchia C, Decarli A, Negri E, Parazzini F, Gentile A, Cecchetti G, Fasoli M, Franceschi S: Dietary factors and the risk of epithelial ovarian cancer. JNCI 79:663, 1987
139. La Vecchia C, Talamini R, Decarli A, Franceschi S, Parazzini F, Tognoni G: Coffee consumption and the risk of breast cancer. Surgery 100:477, 1986
140. Lawson DH, Jick H, Rothman KJ: Coffee and tea consumption and breast disease. Surgery 90:801, 1981
141. Le MG, Hill C, Kramar A, Flammat R: Alcoholic beverage consumption and breast cancer in a French case-control study. Am J Epidemiol 120:350, 1984
142. Lee SY, Ng SF, Busby WF, Rogers AE: Mammary gland DNA synthesis in rats fed high lard or control diets. J Nutr Growth and Cancer 4:167, 1988
143. Lee SY, Rogers AE: Dimethylbenzathracene mammary tumorigenesis in Sprague-Dawley rats fed diets differing in content of beef tallow or rapeseed oil. Nutrition Research 3:361, 1983
144. Lee SY, Walsh CT, Ng SF, Rogers AE: Toxicokinetics of 7,12-dimethylbenz(a)anthracene (DMBA) in rats fed high lard or control diets. J Nutr Growth and Cancer 3:167, 1986
145. Leveille GA, Cloutier PF: Isocaloric diets: effects of dietary changes. Am J Clin Nutr 45:158, 1987
146. Lew EA, Garfinkel L: Variations in mortality by weight among 750,000 men and women. J Chronic Dis 32:563, 1979
147. Lin RS, Kessler II: A multifactorial model for pancreatic cancer in man. JAMA 245:147, 1981
148. Lipkin M, Newmark H: Effect of added dietary calcium on colonic epithelial-cell proliferation in subjects at high risk for familial colonic cancer. N Engl J Med 313:1381, 1985
149. Locniskar M, Nauss KM, Kaufmann P, Newberne PM: Interaction of dietary fat and route of carcinogen administraton on 1,2-dimethylhydrazine-induced colon tumorigenesis in rats. Carcinogenesis 6:349, 1985
150. Longnecker DS, Kuhlmann ET and Curphey TC: Divergent effects of retinoids on pancreatic and liver carcinogenesis in azaserine treated rats. Cancer Res 43:3219, 1983
151. Longnecker DS: The Azaserine-induced model of pancreatic carcinogenesis in rats. In Experimental Pancreatic Carcinogenesis, edited by Scarpelli DG, Reddy JK, Longnecker DS, p 117. Boca Raton, FL, CRC Press, 1987
152. Longnecker MP, Taylor PR, Levander OA, Howe SM, Veillon C, McAdam PA, Patterson KY, Holden JM, Stampfer MJ, Morris SJ, Willett WC: Tissue selenium (Se) levels and indices of Se exposure in a seleniferous area (abstract). Fed Proc 46:587, 1987
153. Lubin JH, Burns PE, Blot WJ, Ziegler RG, Lees AW, Fraumeni JF Jr: Dietary factors and breast cancer risk. Int J Cancer 28:685, 1981
154. Lubin F, Wax Y, Modan B: Role of fat, animal protein, and dietary fiber in breast cancer etiology: a case-control study. JNCI 77:605, 1986
155. Lubin F, Ron E, Wax Y, Modan B: Coffee and methylxanthines and breast cancer: a case-control study. JNCI 74:569, 1985
156. MacDonald RA: Lifespan of liver cells. Autoradiographic study using tritiated thymidine in normal, cirrhotic, and partially hepatectomized rats. Arch Intern Med 107, 79, 1961
157. Machlin LJ, Bendich A: Free radical tissue damage: protective role of antioxidant nutrients. FASEB J 1:441, 1987
158. MacMahon B, Yen S, Trichopoulos D, Warren K, Nardi G: Coffee and cancer of the pancreas. N Engl J Med 304:630, 1981
159. Macquart-Moulin G, Riboli E, Cornee J, Charnay B, Berthezene P, Day N: Case-control study on colorectal cancer in diet in Marseilles. Int J Cancer 38:183, 1986
160. Mack TM, Yu MC, Hanisch R, Henderson BE: Pancreas cancer and smoking, beverage consumption, and past medical history. JNCI 76:49, 1986
161. Madhaven TV, Gopalan C: The effect of dietary protein on carcinogenesis of aflatoxin. Arch Pathol 85:133, 1968
162. Manousos O, Day NE, Trichopoulos D, Gerovassilis F, Tzonou A, Polychronopoulou A: Diet and colorectal cancer: case-control study in Greece. Int J Cancer 32:1, 1985
163. Marnett LJ: Peroxyl free radicals: potential initiators of tumor initiation and promotion. Carcinogenesis 8:1365, 1987
164. Marshall MV, Gleiser CA: 2-Acetylaminofluorene (AAF) carcinogenesis and dietary selenium (abstr). Proc. AACR 28:159, 1987
165. Martínez I, Torres R, Frías Z, Colón JR, Fernández N: Factors associated with adenocarcinomas of the large bowel in Puerto Rico. Adv Med Onc Res Educ 3:45, 1979
166. Matthews-Roth MM: Antitumor activity of B-carotene, canthaxanthin and phytoene. Oncology 39:33, 1982
167. Matthews-Roth MM, Crean C, Clancy M: The phytoene content of various organs of animals administered large doses of phytoene. Nutr Rep Int 17:581, 1978
168. Matthews-Roth MM, Hummel D, Crean C: The carotenoid content of various organs of animals administered large amounts of beta-carotene. Nutr Rep Int 16:419, 1977
169. McCormick DL, Bagg BJ, Hultin TA: Comparative activity of dietary or topical exposure to three retinoids in the promotion of skin tumor induction in mice. Cancer Res 47:5989, 1987
170. McCoy GD, Hecht SS and Furuya K: The effect of chronic ethanol consumption on the tumorigenecity of N-nitrosopyrrolidine in male Syrian golden hamsters. Cancer Lett 33:151, 1986
171. McMichael AJ, Jensen OM, Parkin DM, Zaridze DG: Dietary and endogenous cholesterol and human cancer. Epidemiol Rev 6:192, 1984
172. Medina D: Mechanisms of selenium inhibition of tumorigenesis. In Essential Nutrients in Carcinogenesis, edited by Poirier LA, Newberne PM, Pariza MW, p 466. New York, Plenum Press, 1986
173. Menkes MS, Comstock GW, Vuilleumier JP, Helsing KJ, Rider AA, Brookmeyer R: Serum beta-carotene, vitamins A and E, selenium, and the risk of lung cancer. N Engl J Med 315:1250, 1986
174. Miller AB, Kelly A, Choi NW, Matthews V, Morgan RW, Munan L, Burch JD, Feather J, Howe GR, Jain M: A study of diet and breast cancer. Am J Epidemiol 107:499, 1978
175. Miller AB, Howe GR, Jaon M, Craib KJP, Harrison L: Food items and food groups as risk factors in a case-control study of diet and colo-rectal cancer. Int J Cancer 32:155, 1983
176. Miller DR, Rosenberg L, Helmrich SP, Kaufman DW, Shapiro S: Ovarian cancer and coffee drinking in Banbury Report No. 17, Coffee and Health, edited by MacMahon B, Sugimura T, p 189. Cold Spring Harbor, New York, Cold Spring Harbor Laboratory, 1984
177. Milner JA. Inhibition of chemical carcinogenesis and tumorigenesis by selenium, In Essential Nutrients in Carcinogenesis, edited by Poirier LA, Newberne PM, Pariza MW, p. 449. New York, and London, Plenum Press, 1986
178. Mirvish SS: Formation of N-nitrose compounds, chemistry, kinetics and in vivo occurrence. Toxicol Appl Pharmacol 31:325, 1975
179. Modan B, Barell V, Lubin F, Modan M, Greenbery RA, Graham S: Low-fiber intake as an etiologic factor in cancer of the colon. JNCI 55:15, 1975
180. Moon RC, Mehta RG: Anticarcinogenic effects of retinoids in animals. In Essential Nutrients in Carcinogenesis, edited by Poirier LA, Newberne PM, Poirier LA, Newberne PM, Pariza MW, p 399. Plenum Press, New York, 1986
181. Morgan RGH: Raw soy flour and pancreatic cancer in experimental animals. In Experimental Pancreatic Carcinogenesis, edited by Scarpelli DG, Reddy JK, Longnecker DS, p 159. Chicago, CRC Press, 1987
182. Mori S, Kurata Y, Takeuchi Y, Toyama M, Makino S, Fukushima

S: Influences of strain and diet on the promoting effects of sodium L-ascorbate in two-state urinary bladder carcinogenesis in rats. Cancer Res 47:3492, 1987
183. Morris JS, Stampfer MJ, Willett W: Dietary selenium in humans: toenails as an indicator. Biological Trace Element Research 5:529, 1983
184. NAS-NRC: Diet, Nutrition, and Cancer. National Academy Press, 1982
185. Nauss KM, Bueche D, Newberne PM: Effect of beef fat on DMH-induced colon tumorigenesis: influence of rat strain and nutrient composition. J Nutr 117:739, 1987
186. Nauss KM, Bueche D, Soule N, Fu P, Yew K, Newberne PM: Effect of dietary selenium levels on methylbenzylnitrosamine induced esophageal cancer in rats. Cancer Lett 33:107, 1986
187. Nauss KM, Jacobs LR, Newberne PM: Dietary fat and fiber: relationship to caloric intake, body growth, and colon tumorigenesis. Am J Clin Nutr 45:243, 1987
188. Nauss KM, Locniskar M, Newberne PM: Effect of alterations in the quality and quantity of dietary fat on 1,2-dimethylhydrazine-induced colon tumorigenesis in rats. Cancer Res 43:4083, 1983
189. Nauss KM, Locniskar M, Sondergaard D, Newberne PM: Lack of effect of dietary fat on N-nitrosomethylurea (NMU)-induced colon tumorigenesis in rats. Carcinogenesis 5:255, 1984
190. Newberne PM: Lipotropic Factors and Oncogenesis. In Essential Nutrients in Carcinogenesis, edited by Poirier LA, Newberne PM, and Pariza MW, p 223. Plenum Press, New York and London, 1985
191. Newberne PM, Bieri JG, Briggs GM, Nesheim MC: Control of Diets in Laboratory Animal Experimentation. ILAR News 21:A3, 1978
192. Newberne PM, Charnley G, Adams K, Cantor M, Roth D, Supharkarn V: Gastric and oesophageal carcinogenesis: models for the identification of risk and protective factors. Food Chem Toxicol 24:1111, 1986
193. Newberne PM, De Camargo JV, Clark AJ: Choline deficiency, partial hepatectomy and liver tumors in rats and mice. Toxicol Pathol 2:95, 1982
194. Newberne PM, Nauss KM: Dietary fat and colon cancer: variable results in animal models. In Dietary Fat and Cancer, edited by Ip C, Birt DF, Rogers AE, Mettlin C, p 311. New York, Alan R. Liss Inc., 1966
195. Newberne PM, Rogers AE: Rat colon carcinomas associated with aflatoxin and marginal vitamin A J Natl Cancer Inst 50:439, 1973
196. Newmark HL: Nutrient density: an important and useful tool for laboratory animal studies. Carcinogenesis 8:871, 1987
197. Nomura A, Heilbrun LK, Morris JS, Stemmermann GN: Serum selenium and the risk of cancer, by specific sites: case-control analysis of prospective data. JNCI 79:103, 1987
198. Nomura A, Heilbrun LK, Stemmermann GN: Prospective study of coffee consumption and the risk of cancer. JNCI 76:587, 1986
199. Nomura A, Heilbrun LK, Stemmerman GN: Body mass index as a predictor of cancer in men. JNCI 74:319, 1985
200. Nomura AMY, Stemmermann GN, Heilbrun LK, Salkeld RM, Vuilleumier JP: Serum vitamin levels and the risk of cancer of specific sites in men of Japanese ancestry in Hawaii. Cancer Res 45:2369, 1985
201. Norell SE, Ahlbom A, Erwald R, Jacobson G, Lindberg-Navier I, Olin R, Tornberg B, Wiechel KL: Diet and pancreatic cancer: a case-control study. Am J Epidemiol 124:894, 1986
202. O'Connell DL, Hulka BS, Chambless LE, Wilkinson WE, Deubner DC. Cigarette smoking, alcohol consumption, and breast cancer risk: JNCI 78:229, 1987
203. O'Conner TP, Roebuck BD, Campbell TC: Dietary intervention during the post-dosing phase of L-azaserine-induced preneoplastic lesions. J Natl Cancer Inst 75:955, 1985
204. Ohshima M, Ward JM, Wenk ML: Preventive and enhancing effects of retinold on the development of naturally occurring tumors of skin, prostate gland, and endocrine pancreas in aged male ACI/segHapBR rats. JNCI 74:517, 1985
205. Olson JA: Some thoughts on the relationship between Vitamin A anc cancer. In Essential Nutrients in Carcinogenesis, edited by Poirier LA, Newberne PM, Pariza MW, p 379. Plenum Press, New York, 1986
206. Paffenbarger RS, Hyde RT, Wing AL: Physical activity and incidence of cancer in diverse populations: a preliminary report. Am J Clin Nutr 45:312, 1987
207. Paganini-Hill A, Chao A, Ross RK, Henderson BE: Vitamin A, B-carotene, and the risk of cancer: a prospective study. JNCI 79, 1987
208. Paganini-Hill A, Ross RK: Breast cancer and alcohol consumption. Lancet ii:826, 1983
209. Pariza MW: Fat, calories, and mammary carcinogenesis: net energy effects. Am J Clin Nutr 45:261, 1987
210. Peleg I, Heyden S, Knowles M, Hames CG: Serum retinol and risk of subsequent cancer: extension of the Evans County, Georgia, study. JNCI 73:1455, 1984
211. Peleg I, Morris S, Hames CG: Is serum selenium a risk factor for cancer? Med Oncol Tumor Pharmacother 2:157, 1985
212. Pence BC, Buddingh F: Inhibition of dietary fat promotion of colon carcinogenesis by supplemental calcium or vitamin D. Proc Am Assoc Cancer Res 28:154, 1987
213. Phillips RL: Role of life-style and dietary habits in risk of cancer among Seventh-Day Adventists. Cancer Res 35:3513, 1975
214. Phillips RL, Snowdon DA: Association of meat and coffee use with cancers of the large bowel, breast, and prostate among Seventh-Day Adventists: preliminary results. Cancer Res 43 (Suppl):2403, 1983
215. Phillips RL, Snowdon DA: Dietary relationships with fatal colorectal cancer among Seventh-Day Adventists. JNCI 74:307, 1985
216. Pickle LW, Greene MH, Ziegler RG, Toledo A, Hoover R, Lynch HT, Fraumeni JF Jr.: Colorectal cancer in rural Nebraska. Cancer Res 44:363, 1984
217. Poirier LA: Brief history of the role of nutrition in carcinogenesis. In Essential Nutrients in Carcinogenesis, edited by Poirier LA, Newberne PM, Pariza MW, p 5. New York and London, Plenum Press, 1986
218. Poirier LA: The role of methionine in carcinogenesis in vivo.In Essential Nutrients in Carcinogenesis, edited by Poirier LA, Newberne PM, Pariza MW, p 209. New York and London, Plenum Press, 1986
219. Poirier LA, Bhave MR: C-H-Ras and C-K-Ras gene hypomethylation and amplification in the livers and hepatomas of rats fed methyl-deficient, amino acid-defined diets (abstr). Proc Am Assoc Cancer Res 28:150, 1987
220. Pollack ES, Nomura AMY, Heilbrun LK, Stemmerman GN, Green SB: Prospective study of alcohol consumption and cancer. N Engl J Med 310:617, 1984
221. Porta EA, Markell N, Dorado RD: Chronic alcoholism enhances hepatocarcinogenecity of diethylnitrosamine in rats fed a marginally methyl-deficient diet. Hepatology, 5:1120, 1985
222. Potter RD, McMichael AJ: Diet and cancer of the colon and rectum: a case-control study. JNCI 76:557, 1986
223. Rao GN, Knapka JJ: Contaminant and nutrient concentrations of natural ingredient rat and mouse diet used in chemical toxicology studies. Fundam Appl Toxicol 9:329, 1987
224. Rettura G, Stratford F, Levenson SM, Seifter E: Prophylactic and therapeutic actions of supplemental B-carotene in mice inoculated with C3HBA adenocarcinoma cells: lack of therapeutic action of supplemental ascorbic acid. JNCI 69:73, 1982
225. Roberts AB, Sporn MB: Cellular biology and biochemistry of the retinoids. In The Retinoids, edited by Sporn MB, Roberts AB, Goodman DS, p 218. New York, Academic Press, 1986
226. Roberts-Andersen J, Mehta T, Wilson RB: Reduction of DMH-induced colon tumors in rats fed psyllium husk or cellulose. Nutr Cancer 10:129, 1987
227. Roebuck BD: Effects of high levels of dietary fats on the growth of azaserine-induced foci in the rat pancreas. Lipids 21:281, 1986
228. Roebuck BD: Enhancement of pancreatic carcinogenesis in the rat by dietary fats. In Experimental Pancreatic Carcinogenesis, edited by Scarpelli DG, Reddy JK, Longnecker DS, p 187. Boca Raton FL, CRC Press Inc., 1987
229. Roebuck BD, Kaplita PV, Edward BR, Praissman M: Effects of dietary fats and soybean protein on azaserine-induced pancreatic carcinogenesis and plasma cholecystokinin in the rat. Cancer Res 47:1333, 1987
230. Roebuck BD, Longnecker DS, Baumgartner KJ, Thron CD: Carcinogen-induced lesions in the rat pancreas: effects of varying levels of essential fatty acid. Cancer Res 45:5252, 1985
231. Rogers AE: Nutrition. In The Laboratory Rat, edited by Baker HJ, Lindsay JR, Weisbroth SJ, p 123. New York, Academic Press,

1979
232. Rogers AE, Conner B, Boulanger C, Lee S: Mammary tumorigenesis in rats fed diets high in lard. Lipids 21:275, 1986
233. Rogers AE, Conner BH: Boulanger CL, Lee SY, Carr FA, Dumouchel WH: Enhancement of 7,12-Dimethylbenz(a)anthracene mammary carcinogenesis by a high lard diet. In Dietary Fiber, edited by Vahouny GV, Kritchevsky D, p 449. Plenum Publishing Corp 1985
234. Rogers AE, Conner MW: Alcohol and Cancer. In Essential Nutrients in Carcinogenesis, edited by Poirier LA, Newberne PM, Pariza MW, p 473. New York and London, Plenum Press, 1985
235. Rogers AE, Fernstrom JD, Ge K, McConnell RG, Leavitt WW Wetsel WC, Yang SO, Camelio EA: Endocrine interactions in the nutritional modulation of mammary carcinogenesis in rats. In Molecular Interrelations of Nutrition and Cancer, edited by Arnott MS, Van Eys J, Wang YM, p 381. New York, Raven Press, 1982
236. Rogers AE, Herndon BJ, Newberne PM: Induction of dimethylhydrazine of intestinal carcinoma in normal rats and rats fed high or low levels of vitamin A. Cancer Res 33:1003, 1973
237. Rogers AE, Lee SY: Chemically-induced mammary gland tumors in rats: modulation by dietary fat. In Dietary Fat and Cancer, edited by Ip C, Birt DF, Rogers AE, Mettlin C, p 255. New York, Alan R. Liss Inc., 1966
238. Rogers AE, MacDonald RA: Hepatic vasculature and cell proliferation in experimental cirrhosis. Lab Invest 14:1710, 1965
239. Rogers AE, Nauss KM: Contributions of laboratory animal studies of colon carcinogenesis. In Studies of Large Bowel Cancer: Clinical and Basic Science Research edited by Mastromarino AJ, Brattain MG, p 1. New York, Prager, 1985
240. Rogers AE, Newberne PM: Aflatoxin B1 carcinogenesis in lipotrope-deficient rats. Cancer Res 29:1965, 1969
241. Rogers AE, Newberne PM: Lipotrope deficiency in experimental carcinogenesis. Nutr Cancer 2:104, 1981
242. Rogers AE, Nields HM, and Newberne PM: Nutritional and dietary influences on liver tumorigenesis in mice and rats. Arch Toxicol 10(Suppl):231, 1987
243. Rosenberg L, Miller DR, Helmrich SP, Kaufman DW, Schottenfeld D, Stolley PD, Shapiro S: Breast cancer and the consumption of coffee. Am J Epidemiol 122:391, 1985
244. Rosenberg L, Slone D, Shapiro S, Kaufman DW, Helmrich SP, Miettinen OS, Stolley PD, Levy M, Rosenshein NB, Schottenfeld D, Engle RL Jr: Breast cancer and alcoholic-beverage consumption. Lancet i:267, 1982
245. Ross RK, Shimizu H, Paganini-Hill A, Honda G, Henderson BE: Case-control studies of prostate cancer in blacks and whites in Southern California. JNCI 78:869, 1987
246. Rothman KJ: Modern Epidemiology. Boston, Little, Brown and Company, 1986
247. Rotkin ID: Studies in the epidemiology of prostate cancer: expanded sampling. Cancer Treat Rep 61:173, 1977
248. Russell-Briefel R, Bates MW, Kuller LH: The relationship of plasma carotenoids to health and biochemical factors in middle-aged men. Am J Epidemiol 122:741, 1985
249. Sackett DL: Bias in analytic research. J Chronic Dis 32:51, 1979
250. Salbe AD, Bjeldanes LF: Dietary influences on rat hepatic and intestinal DT-diaphorase activity. Food Chem Toxicol 24:851, 1986
251. Salonen JT, Alfthan G, Huttunen JK, Puska P: Association between serum selenium and the risk of cancer. Am J Epidemiol 120:342, 1984
252. Salonen JT, Salonen R, Lappetelainen R, Maenpaa PH, Alfthan G, Puska P: Risk of cancer in relation to serum concentrations of selenium and vitamins A and E: matched case-control analysis of prospective data. Br Med J 290:417, 1985
253. Scarpelli DG, Rao S: Experimental carcinogenesis of exocrine pancreas in the Syrian golden hamster (Mesocricetus Auratus). In Experimental Pancreatic Carcinogenesis, edited by Scarpelli DG, Reddy JK, Longnecker DS, p 45. Chicago, CRC Press, Inc., 1987
254. Schairer C, Brinton LA, Hoover RN: Methylxanthines and breast cancer. Int J Cancer 40:469, 1987
255. Schatzkin A, Jones DY, Hoover RN, Taylor PR, Brinton LA, Ziegler RG, Harvey EB, Carter CL, Licitra LM, Larson DB: Alcohol consumption and breast cancer in the epidemiologic follow-up study of The First National Health and Nutrition Examination Survey. N Engl J Med 316:1169, 1987
256. Schrauzer GN, McGinness JE, Ishamael D and Bell LJ: Alcoholism and Cancer I. Effects of long-term exposure to alcohol on spontaneous mammary adenocarcinoma and prolactin levels in C3H/St. Mice. Journal Stud Alcohol 40:240, 1979
257. Schuman LM, Mandel JS, Radke A, Seal U, Halberg F: Some selected features of the epidemiology of prostatic cancer: Minneapolis-St. Paul, Minnesota case-control study, 1976–1979. In Trends in Cancer Incidence: Causes and Practical Implications, edited by Magnus K, p 345. Washington DC, Hemisphere Press, 1982
258. Seifter E, Rettura G, Padawar J, Levenson SM: Moloney murine sarcoma virus tumors in CBA/J mice: chemopreventive and chemotherapeutic actions of supplemental B-carotene. JNCI 68:835, 1982
259. Setchell KDR, Adlerkreutz H: Mammalian lignans and phytoestrogens; recent studies on their formation, metabolism and biological role in health and disease. In The Role of Gut Microflora in Toxicity and Cancer, edited by Rowland I, p 420. Carshallton, BIBRA Press, 1987
260. Severson RK, Davis S, Pollisar L: Smoking, coffee, and cancer of the pancreas. Br Med J 285:214, 1982
261. Shapiro SS, Mott DJ, Machlin LJ: Kinetic characteristics of B-carotene uptake and depletion in rat tissue. J Nutr 114:1924, 1984
262. Shekelle RB, Lepper M, Liu S, Maliza C, Raynor WJ Jr, Rossof AH: Dietary vitamin A and risk of cancer in the western electric study. Lancet ii:1185, 1981
263. Shinozuka H, Katyal SL: Choline deficiency and chemical carcinogenesis. In Essential Nutrients in Carcinogenesis, edited by Poirier LA, Newberne PM, Pariza MW, p 253. New York and London, Plenum Press, 1986
264. Shinozuka H, Katyal SL, Perera MIR: Fat, lipotropes, hypolipidemic agents and liver cancer.In Dietary Fat and Cancer, edited by Ip C, Birt DF, Rogers AE, Mettlin C, p 461. New York, Alan R. Liss Inc., 1966
265. Sidney S, Friedman GD, Hiatt RA: Serum cholesterol and large bowel cancer: a case-control study. Am J Epidemiol 124:33, 1986
266. Siraj I, Mufi I, Sipes G: Promotion of MBN-induced esophageal carcinogenesis by dietary ethanol (abstr). Proc Am Assoc Cancer Res 28:170, 1987
267. Smith DM, Rogers AE, Herndon BJ, Newberne PM: Vitamin A (retinyl acetate) and benzo(a)pyrene-induced respiratory tract carcinogenesis in hamsters fed a commercial diet. Cancer Res 35:11, 1975
268. Smith DM, Rogers AE, Newberen PM: Vitamin A and benzo(a)pyrene carcinogenesis in the respiratory tract of hamsters fed a semisynthetic diet. Cancer Res 35:1485, 1975
269. Snowdon DA, Phillips RL: Coffee consumption and risk of fatal cancers. AJPH 74:820, 1984
270. Snowdon DA, Phillips RL, Choi W: Diet, obesity, and risk of fatal prostatic cancer. Am J Epidemiol 120:244, 1984
271. Southgate DAT: The relation between composition and properties of dietary fiber and physiologic effects. In Dietary Fiber: Basic and Clinical Aspects edited by Vahouny GV, Kritchevsky D, p 35. Plenum Press, 1986
272. Sparnins VL, Harany G, Wattenberg LW: Effects of allyl methyl disulfide (AMD) allyl methyl trisulfide (AMT), propyl methyl disulfide (PMD), and propyl methyl trisulfide (PMT) on glutathione S-transferase (GST) activity and benzo(a)pyrene (BP) carcinogenesis in mice (abstr). Proc Am Assoc Cancer Res 28:142, 1987
273. Stahelin HB, Rosel F, Buess E, Brubacher G: Cancer, vitamins, and plasma lipids: prospective Basel study. JNCI 73:1463, 1984
274. Stampfer MJ, Willett WC, Colditz GA, Rosner B, Hennekens C, Speizer FE: A prospective study of diet and colon cancer in a cohort of women (abstr). Fed Proc 46:883, 1987
275. Stemmerman GN, Nomura AMY, Heilbrun LK: Dietary fat and the risk of colorectal cancer. Cancer Res 44:4633, 1984
276. Stemmerman G, Nomura AMY, Heilbrun LK, Mower H, Hayashi T: Colorectal cancer in Hawaiian Japanese men: a progress report. Natl Cancer Inst Monogr 69:125, 1985
277. Stenback F, Mu B, Williams G: Retinyl acetate effects on the life span and the incidence of cryptogenic neoplasms in C3H mice. Nutr Cancer 10:119, 1987

278. Stich HF, Dunn BP: Relationship between cellular levels of beta-carotene and sensitivity to genotoxic agents. Int J Cancer 38:713, 1986
279. Stich HF, Hornby AP, Dunn BP: Beta-carotene levels in exfoliated mucosa cells of population groups at low and elevated risk for oral cancer. Int J Cancer 37:389, 1986
280. Stinson SF, Reznik G, and Donahoe R: Effect of three retinoids on tracheal carcinogenesis with N-methyl-N-nitrosources in hamsters. J Natl Cancer Inst 66:947, 1981
281. Stockwell HG, Matanoski GM: Re: "Association of alcohol consumption and cancer". N Engl J Med 311:256, 1984
282. Stryker WS, Stein EA, Kaplan L, Stampfer MJ, Sober A, Willett WC: Relations of diet and cigarette smoking with plasma beta-carotene levels (abstract). Am J Epidemiol 126:772, 1987
283. Suda D, Schwartz J, Shklar G: Inhibition of experimental oral carcinogenesis by topical beta carotene. Carcinogenesis 7:711, 1986
284. Sylvester PW, Russell M, Ip MM, Ip C: Comparative effects of different animal and vegetable fats fed before and during carcinogen administration on mammary tumorigenesis, sexual maturation, and endocrine function in rats. Cancer Res 46:757, 1986
285. Tajima K, Tominaga S: Dietary habits and gastrointestinal cancers: a comparative case-control study of stomach and large intestinal cancers in Nagoya, Japan. Jpn J Cancer Res 76:705, 1985
286. Talamini R, La Vecchia C, Decarli A, Franceschi S, Grattoni E, Grigoletto E, Liberati A, Tognoni G: Social factors, diet and breast cancer in a Northern Italian population. Br J Cancer 49:723, 1984
287. Tatematsu M, Takahaski M, Fukushimna S, Hananouchi M and Shirai T: Effects in rats of sodium chloride on experimental gastric cancer induced by MNNG or 4-nitroquinoline-1-oxide. JNCI 55:101, 1975
288. Teas J, Harbison ML and Gelman RS: Dietary seaweed (Laminaria) and mammary carcinogenesis in rats. Cancer Res 44:2758, 1984
289. Temple NJ, Basu TK: Protective effect of B-carotene against colon tumors in mice. JNCI 78:1211, 1987
290. Thompson CD, Ong LK, Robinson MF: Effects of supplementation with high selenium wheat bread on selenium, glutathione peroxidase and related enzymes in blood components of New Zealand residents. Am J Clin Nutr 41:1015, 1985
291. Thompson HJ, Meeker LD, Becci PJ, Kokoska S: Effect of short term feeding of sodium selenite on 7,12-dimethylbenz(a) anthracene induced mammary carcinogenesis in the rat. Cancer Res 42:4954, 1982
292. Thompson HJ, Meeker LD, and Kokoska S: Effect of an inorganic and organic form of dietary selenium on the promotional stage of mammary carcinogenesis in the rat. Cancer Res 44:2803, 1984
293. Thompson HJ, Ronan AM, Tagliaferro AR: Effect of exercise on the enhancement of mammary tumorigenesis by high dietary fat (abstr). Proc Am Assoc Cancer Res 28:157, 1987
294. Trichopoulos D, Tzonou, Polychronopoulou A, Day NE: A case-control investigation of a possible association between coffee consumption an ovarian cancer in Greece. In Banbury Report No. 17, Coffee and Health, edited by MacMahon B, Sugimura T, Cold Spring Harbor, New York, Cold Spring Harbor Laboratory, 1984
295. Van Noord PAH, Collette HJA, Maas MJ, De Waard F: Selenium levels in nails of premenopausal breast cancer patients assessed prediagnostically in a cohort-nested case-referent study among women screened in the DOM project. Int J Epidemiol 16(Suppl):318, 1987
296. Velema JP, Walker AM, Gold EB: Alcohol and pancreatic cancer: insufficient evidence for a causal relationship. Epidemiol Rev 8:28, 1986
297. Vena JE, Graham S, Zielezny M, Brasure BS, Swanson MK: Occupational exercise and risk of cancer. Am J Clin Nutr 45:318, 1987
298. Vena JE, Graham S, Zielezny M, Swanson MK, Barnes RE, Nolan J: Lifetime occupational exercise and colon cancer. Am J Epidemiol 122:357, 1985
299. Verma AK, Conrad EK, Boutwell RK: The differential effects of retinoic acid and 7,8-benzoflavone on the induction of mouse skin tumors by the complete carcinogenesis process and by the initiation-promotion regimen. Cancer Res 42:3519, 1982
300. Verma AK, Duvick L, Ali M: Modulation of mouse skin tumor promotion by dietary 13-cis-retinoic acid (RA) and o-difluoromethylornithine. Carcinogenesis 7:1019, 1986
301. Verma AK, Shapas BG, Rice HM, Boutwell RK: Correlation of the inhibition by retinoids of tumors promoter-induced mouse epidermal ornithine decarboxylase activity and of skin tumor promotion. Cancer Res 39:419, 1979
302. Visek WJ: Dietary protein and experimental carcinogenesis. In Essential Nutrients in Carcinogenesis, edited by Poirier LA, Newberne PM, Pariza MW, p 163. Plenum Press, New York, 1986
303. Wainfan E, Dizik M: Suppression by methionine and choline of onco-fetal patterns of liver tRNA methyltransferase activities in carcinogen-treated rats. Carcinogenesis 8:615, 1987
304. Wainfan E, Dizik M, Hluboky M, Balis ME: Altered tRNA methylation in rats and mice fed lipotrope-deficient diets. Carcinogenesis 7:473, 1986
305. Wald N, Boreham J, Bailey A: Serum retinol and subsequent risk of cancer. Br J Cancer 54:957, 1986
306. Wald NJ, Boreham J, Hayward JL, Bulbrook RD: Plasma retinol, B-carotene and vitamin E levels in relation to the future risk of breast cancer. Br J Cancer 49:321, 1984
307. Wald NV, Idle M, Boreham J: Low serum-vitamin-A and subsequent risk of cancer: preliminary results of a prospective study. Lancet ii:813, 1980
308. Wald NJ, Thompson SG, Densem JW, Boreham J, Bailey A: Serum vitamin E and subsequent risk of cancer. Br J Cancer 56:69, 1987
309. Wargovich MJ: Diallyl sulfide, a flavor component of garlic (Allium sativum), inhibits, dimethylhydrazine-induced colon cancer. Carcinogenesis 8:487, 1987
310. Wargovich MJ: Inhibition of colon carcinogenesis by the naturally occurring thioether diallyl sulfide (abstr). Proc Am Assoc Cancer Res 28:139, 1987
311. Wargovich MJ, Lointier PH: Calcium and vitamin D modulate mouse colon epithelial proliferation and growth characteristics of a human colon tumor cell line. Can J Physiol Pharmacol 65:472, 1987
312. Webster LA, Layde PM, Wingo PA, Ory HW, and the Cancer and Steroid Hormone Study Group: Alcohol consumption and risk of breast cancer. Lancet ii:724, 1983
313. Welsch CW, De Hoog JV, O'Connor DH, Sheffield LG: Influence of dietary fat levels on development and hormone responsiveness of the mouse mammary gland. Cancer Res 45:6147, 1985
314. Welsch CW: Enhancement of mammary tumorigenesis by dietary fat: review of potential mechanisms. Am J Clin Nutr 45:192, 1987
315. Welsch CW: Interrelationship between dietary fat and endocrine processes in mammary gland tumorigenesis. In Dietary Fat and Cancer, edited by Ip C, Birt DF, Rogers AE, Mettlin C, p 623. New York, Alan R. Liss Inc., 1986
316. Wetsel WC, Rogers AE: Hepatic prolactin binding in female Sprague-Dawley rats fed a diet high in corn oil. JNCI 75:531, 1984
317. Wetsel WC, Rogers AE, Newberne PM: Dietary fat and DMBA mammary carcinogenesis in rats. Cancer Detect Prev 4:535, 1981
318. Wetsel WC, Rutledge A, Rogers AE: Absence of an effect of dietary corn oil content on plasma prolactin, progesterone, and 17B-estradiol in female Sprague-Dawley rats. Cancer Res 44:1420, 1983
319. West RO: Epidemiologic study of malignancies of the ovaries. Cancer 19:1001, 1966
320. Whittemore AS, Paffenbarger RS, Anderson K, Halpern J: Early precursors of pancreatic cancer in college men. J Chronic Dis 36:251, 1983
321. Williams RR, Horm JW: Association of cancer sites with tobacco and alcohol consumption and socio-economic status of patients: interview study from The Third National Cancer Survey. JNCI 58:525, 1977
322. Willett WC (ed): Nutrition Epidemiology, New York, Oxford University Press, 1988
323. Willett WC, Browne ML, Bain C, Lipnick RJ, Stampfer MJ, Rosner B, Colditz GA, Hennekens CH, Speizer FE: Relative weight and risk of breast cancer among premenopausal women. Am J Epidemiol 122:731, 1985
324. Willett WC, Polk BF, Morris JS, Stampfer MJ, Pressel S, Rosner B, Taylor JO, Schneider K, Hames CG: Prediagnostic serum selenium and risk of cancer. Lancet ii:130, 1983
325. Willett WC, Polk BF, Underwood BA, Stampfer MJ, Pressel S,

Rosner B, Taylor JO, Schneider K, Hames CG: Relation of serum vitamins A and E to carotenoids to the risk of cancer. N Engl J Med 310:430, 1984
326. Willett WC, Stampfer MJ: Total energy intake: implications for epidemiologic analyses. Am J Epidemiol 124:17, 1986
327. Willett WC, Stampfer MJ, Colditz GA, Rosner BA, Hennekens CH, Speizer FE: Dietary fat and the risk of breast cancer. N Engl J Med 316:22, 1987
328. Willett WC, Stampfer MJ, Colditz GA, Rosner BA, Hennekens CH, Speizer FE: Moderate alcohol consumption and the risk of breast cancer. N Engl J Med 316:1174, 1987
329. Willett WC, Stampfer MJ, Underwood BA, Sampson LA, Hennekens CH, Wallingford JC, Cooper LC, Hsieh CC, Speizer FE: Vitamin A supplementation and plasma retinol levels: a randomized trial among women. JNCI 73:1445, 1984
330. Willett WC, Stampfer MJ, Underwood BA, Taylor JO, Hennekens CH: Vitamins A, E, and carotene: effects of supplementation on their plasma levels. Am J Clin Nutr 38:559, 1983
331. Woutersen KA, van Garderen-Hoetmer A, Bax J, Feringa AW, Scherer E: Modulation of putative preneoplastic foci in exocrine pancreas of rats and hamsters., I. Interaction of dietary fat and ethanol. Carcinogenesis 7:1587, 1986
332. Woutersen RA, van Garderen-Hoetmer A, Longnecker DS: Characterization of a 4-month protocol for the quantitation of BOP-induced lesions in hamster pancreas and its application in studying the effect of dietary fat. Carcinogenesis 8:833, 1987
333. Wu AH, Henderson BE, Pike MC, Yu MC: Smoking and other risk factors for lung cancer in women. JNCI 74:747, 1985
334. Wu AH, Paganini-Hill A, Ross RK, Henderson BE: Alcohol, physical activity and other risk factors for colorectal cancer: a prospective study. Br J Cancer 55:687, 1987
335. Wynder EL: Homogeneity in nutritional exposure: an impediment in cancer epidemiology. JNCI 79:605, 1987
336. Wynder EL, Hall NEL, Polansky M: Epidemiology of coffee and pancreatic cancer. 43:3900, 1983
337. Wynder EL, Kajitani T, Ishakawa S, Dodo J, Takano A: Environmental factors of cancer of the colon and rectum II: Japanese epidemiological data. Cancer 23:1210, 1969
338. Wynder EL, Shigematsu T: Environmental factors of cancer of the colon and rectum. Cancer 20:1520, 1967
339. Yamamoto I, Maruyama H: Effect of dietary seaweed preparations on 1,2-dimethylhydrazine induced intestinal carcinogenesis in rats. Cancer Lett 26:241, 1985
340. Yamamoto I, Maruyama H, Moriguchi M: The effect of dietary seaweeds on 7,12-Dimethyl-Benz(a)anthracene-induced mammary tumorigenesis in rats. Cancer Lett 35:109, 1987
341. Yedinak RA, Layman DK, Milner JA: Influences of dietary fat and exercise on DMBA-induced mammary tumors (abstr). Fed Proc 46:436, 1987
342. Zhang L, Bird RP, Bruce WR: Proliferative activity of murine mammary epithelium as affected by dietary fat and calcium. Cancer Res 47:4905, 1987
343. Ziegler Rg, Mason TJ, Stemhagen A, Hoover R, Schoenberg JB, Gridley G, Virgo PW, Altman R, Fraumeni JF Jr: Dietary carotene and vitamin A and risk of lung cancer among white men in New Jersey. JNCI 73:1429, 1984
344. Ziegler RG, Mason TJ, Stemhagen A, Hoover R, Schoenberg JB, Gridley G, Virgo PW, Fraumeni JF Jr: Carotenoid intake, vegetables, and the risk of lung cancer among white men in New Jersey. Am J Epidemiol 123:1080, 1986

APPENDIX

Scoring System for Evaluation of Epidemiologic Studies of Relations between Diet and Cancer

The weight given to the findings from a given study were a function of the study size and the total score. A total score of 9 points per study (3 points from each of the categories below) was possible, with lower scores being best (near-ideal studies got 3 points). Where a range of possible points is indicated, *e.g.*, > = 2 points the decision as to whether to give 2 or 3 points depended on the severity of the problem.

1. Evaluation of general design:
   a. Was the exposure period inquired about before disease onset? if not or if not specified, score > = 2 points.
   b. Was the control group appropriately chosen? if there was any doubt as to the appropriateness, score > = 2.
   c. Were the response rate among controls at least 70%? If not specified, score > = 2 (although if it was a hospital control group and the response rate was not specified, do not add any points).
   d. Were the cases and controls interviewed in a similar setting? If not (or not specified), score > = 2.
   e. if data on exposure could have been affected by disease status score > = 2.
   f. If two or more of the above problems are present, score > = 3.
2. Evaluation of diet assessment:
   a. Semiquantitative food frequency questionnaire (sqffq) and diet history methods, score > = 1.
   b. Partial sqffq or partial diet history or other focused, sensible approach, score > = 2.
   c. 24-Hour diet recall, score > = 2.
   d. Food frequency questionnaire, score > = 3.
3. Evaluation of analysis:
   a. Matched data with unmatched analysis, score > = 2.
   b. Case-control means but no relative risk presented, score > = 2.
   c. No adjustment for important confounders (*e.g.*, dietary), score > = 2.
   d. Had data on total caloric intake but did not adjust for it, score > = 2.
   e. More than one of the above present, score > = 3.
   f. No means or relative risks presented, score > = 3.

Section IV

Advances in Methodology

Biology of Disease

Advances in Flow Cytometry for Diagnostic Pathology

JOHN S. COON, ALAN L. LANDAY, AND RONALD S. WEINSTEIN

Departments of Pathology and Immunology/Microbiology, Rush Medical College and Rush-Presbyterian St. Luke's Medical Center, Chicago, Illinois

INTRODUCTION

Only 3 years have passed since Lovett *et al.* (147) first reviewed applications of flow cytometry (FCM) to diagnostic pathology in *Laboratory Investigation.* Progress in this field has been rapid, however, and the importance of having timely, practical knowledge of this technology has increased significantly for pathologists. Lovett's lucid explanation of the basic function of the instrument would still be difficult to improve upon. Therefore, this review is not intended to duplicate or replace the earlier substantial monograph. Rather, we will attempt to update the reader on what we regard to be important recent developments in the field. We will also consider some older work which seems in retrospect, to have been insufficiently covered in Lovett's review. Readers with little or no background in FCM may benefit from referring to the earlier review before starting this one, or else consulting other more comprehensive works, especially Shapiro's monograph (204). For the many pathologists who have been following the development of FCM, we hope this review will aid in bringing advances in the state-of-the-art into perspective.

This review, like its predecessor, focuses attention on those aspects of FCM which are relevant to diagnostic pathology. Basic research applications have been critically reviewed elsewhere (204).

TECHNICAL DEVELOPMENTS

INSTRUMENTS

A diagram of a modern clinical flow cytometer is shown in Figure 1. Flow cytometers have been impractical pieces of equipment for the vast majority of nonuniversity pathology laboratories, until recently. The high purchase price, in the range of $150,000, and service contract costs for an instrument to be used sporadically was an insurmountable barrier. The requirement to replace laser plasma tubes, costing $10,000 per tube, every 2 years added to the burden. Apart from the cost of the instrument itself, the expense of creating a suitable environment for these instruments has been an obstacle. The large lasers required three phase power and a copious, dependable supply of cooling water, which often required that special measures be taken to maintain pressure, especially on the upper floors of multistory laboratory buildings. Special provisions for control of dust, and ambient light and temperature were usually recommended. The instruments were large, required access from all sides, and thus consumed a significant amount of precious laboratory space.

The technical complexity of earlier generations of FCM instruments imposed significant drains on manpower resources of clinical laboratories. One has been

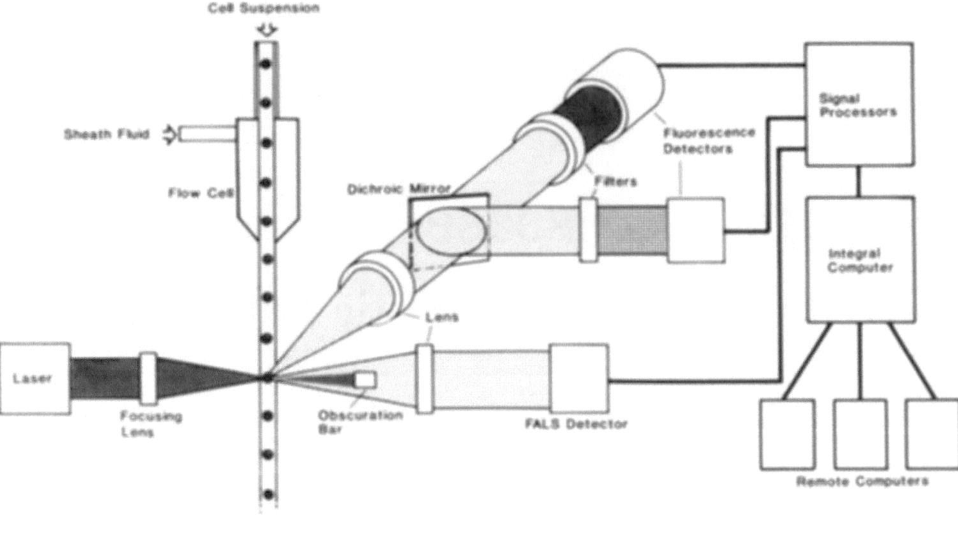

FIG. 1. Schematic representation of a modern flow cytometer suitable for clinical work. Stained cells enter the flow chamber where they pass into the center of a stream of sheath fluid in single file. They are then struck by a focused laser beam and emit scattered and fluorescent light, which is separated according to wavelength by appropriate mirrors and filters. An obscuration bar protects the forward angle light scatter (*FALS*) detector from exposure to the direct laser beam. Only two fluorescence detectors are shown, for sake of simplicity, but a typical instrument has three or four such detectors, one of which can be used to measure laser light scattered perpendicular to the laser beam by the cells. Signals from the detectors pass to amplifying processors and then to the integral (on-board) computer, which digitizes the signals, stores, and displays them. Detailed analysis of the data is often most efficiently done with stand alone computers.

the need for a highly trained technical specialist, not infrequently at the Ph.D. level, to be responsible for technical aspects of the FCM laboratory operations. Often such individuals have narrowly focused interests, and are unable to perform other duties in the clinical laboratory, making their relatively high salaries a substantial component of FCM test costs. Even where the funds to support such technical experts are available, pedigreed individuals are in short supply. Other, more subtle problems in implementation have been commonplace. The technical and esoteric nature of the instruments has tended to complicate the relationship of the FCM facility personnel with the technical staff of other clinical laboratories. Thus, the perceived need to "protect the instrument" from relatively unskilled or inexperienced personnel has hindered the integration of FCM tests into the regular clinical laboratory routine, where capable technicians gain competence with many of the important laboratory instruments. The technical complexity of flow cytometers has also posed a significant barrier to pathologists and other professional personnel, unless they possess a specialized background in FCM or allied areas of analytical cytology.

Compounding problems with optical and electronic components of flow cytometers have been serious limitations in data processing capabilities. Because of the large volumes of data generated by FCM (4 measurements on each of 50,000 cells is fairly typical) powerful, efficient, and convenient data analysis is highly desirable. Multiparameter analysis of samples containing few cells, *e.g.*, study of bladder barbotage specimens for detection of recurrent cancer, may require the capability to store all of the data for each cell in a list mode file for later analysis of selected subpopulations revealed by gating (electronic exclusion of data from irrelevant cells) (159). Analysis of list mode files, as well as extended analysis of processed data (histograms), should be done at a stand-alone computer, preferably at a separate site than the FCM laboratory itself. Otherwise, valuable instrument time is consumed for data analysis, and personnel who may be devoted specifically to data analysis without an understanding of the flow instrument *per se* must work in the flow laboratory. The flow laboratory is inherently a poor location for this data analysis because of the presence of biohazards, noise, often overcrowded conditions, and expensive, sensitive equipment. In this era of widespread use of inexpensive powerful microcomputers with "user-friendly" software, which can be run on machines from many manufacturers, the configuration of a satisfactory data analysis system seems clear. It is possible to transmit either list mode or processed data directly to an IBM compatible microcomputer. This data can then be analyzed at any convenient site with other microcomputers which may serve a variety of other functions. A few large academic departments of analytical cytology have in fact created systems like this (159), but nothing has been available commercially until very recently. Major FCM manufacturers have offered stand-alone computers for extended data analysis, but they have suffered from a number of drawbacks. The software has not been compatible with other common microcomputers, eliminating the convenience of low cost data analysis at multiple sites. The data from the flow cytometer's integral computer has generally been encrypted in such a way as to discourage its translation into a form that could be transferred to common microcomputers. The transfer of data from the flow cytometer to the FCM manufacturer's stand-alone computers, generally via the integral computer, has been slow and inconvenient, often requiring the use of inconvenient translation programs. Paradoxically the software used in some commercial stand-alones bears little resemblance to that used in their integral computer, forcing operators to learn two completely independent systems to accomplish similar tasks. The opportunity for the user to customize software for specialized tasks has been very limited. Ability to analyze list mode files with the stand-alones has been limited or nonexistent. Finally, the cost of pre-1987 systems seemed inflated considering their modest hardware. No doubt this cost reflects the considerable software development for a rather small market. However, the value of highly proprietary software designed to run only in a single type of specialized microcomputer is debatable, no matter how dazzling the graphics packages may be.

In light of this litany of problems, it is encouraging that the solution to many of them appears to be forthcoming. A new generation of instruments, such as the FACScan® and Profile® has been introduced which should be much more compatible with the clinical laboratory environment than earlier instruments with comparable analytical capability (42). These new multiparameter instruments (up to 3 fluorescence + 2 scatter measurements for each cell) are less expensive, smaller, and feature bench top installation. The lasers are air-cooled and have no special electrical requirements. A source of compressed gas is not required. Manual adjustments have been largely replaced by software control, much of it automatic, even extending to optical alignment and laser power. Optical filters for the photomultiplier tubes may be fixed, eliminating another potential source of human error. As operator safety features, the laser beam is completely enclosed, and further efforts have been made to contain biologically hazardous samples. Comprehensive service contracts are now offered by both major U.S. companies, a departure from the recent past. Clearly, an important goal of instrument manufacturers has been to make instruments which are both more "user friendly" and "user-proof." How well they have succeeded will be gauged by their future acceptance by the clinical laboratory community.

Apart from continuing technical progress in instrument design, a major factor in the introduction of the new generation of instruments has been an evolution in the maufacturer's concept of what the instruments are intended to do. Many past and current models have been designed for maximum versatility, including a preparative capability (*i.e.*, cell sorting) (145), fluorescence excitation at many different wavelengths, including ultraviolet (141), multibeam analysis (203), and pulse width measurements (204). Whereas there is a need for such multifunctional instruments in an academic setting which must support a wide spectrum of research applications, these instruments are overly costly and complicated for most clinical laboratories. Conversely, many clinical instruments offered in the past were either too restricted in analytical capability to perform all of the desirable clinical tests, or too closely resembled the costly research instruments with large lasers and a sorting capability.

Another consideration in the design of newer models has been the realization that small, air-cooled lasers have many of the advantages and few of the disadvantages of the large water-cooled ion lasers (205). Use of these lasers has permitted the development of smaller, less expensive, easier to install flow cytometers. Large (5 watt) argon ion lasers have been the mainstay for commercial flow cytometers because of their strong blue-green 488 nm line (approximately 200 to 400 mw) which is suitable for exciting many of the popular DNA stains, particularly propidium iodide, and labels for fluorescent antibodies, particularly fluorescein and phycoerythrin (204). Their ability to emit other useful wavelengths, including ultraviolet, has also been important for research applications (145). The air-cooled argon lasers used in the new instruments emit much less energy (15 to 25 mw at 488 nm), but these instruments have been configured for simultaneous analysis of signals from fluorescein combined with either phycoerythrin or propidium iodide, with good sensitivity, using sophisticated light collection optics (202). Three-color analysis using fluorescein, phycoerythrin, and 7-amino-actinomycin D (another DNA stain) is also possible in such a single laser system, although its clinical utility has not been demonstrated (182). Other small air-cooled lasers such as helium-neon, emitting at 633 nm (red), or helium-cadmium emitting at 325 nm (ultraviolet) have been shown to be practical for flow cytometry using antibodies labeled with allophycocyanin (142) and the valuable DNA-specific dye, 4,6-diamindino-2-phenylindole (DAPI) respectively (205). This raises the possibility of multibeam instruments using combinations of air-cooled lasers in place of the argon-krypton or argon ion-dye laser combinations used previously. Multibeam instruments permit much more versatility in combining fluorochromes for multiparameter analysis compared with single beam instruments (203). Using combinations of air-cooled lasers in place of the pairs of water-cooled lasers currently used in multibeam instruments, would significantly reduce their cost. However, the optical complexity and alignment problems associated with multibeam instruments would still pose a formidable obstacle to their use in the average clinical laboratory. Possibly new approaches such as the alignment-free wave guide optics as proposed by Shapiro and Hercher (206) might simplify multibeam instruments and broaden their appeal in the future.

Turning to recent developments in data analysis for FCM, significant progress relevant to clinical laboratories may be imminent. Major manufacturers of FCM instruments are beginning to understand the need for compatibility with commonly available microcomputers. It seems likely that such compatibility will be available with their next generation of instruments. What will be offered by major vendors and how useful it will be is still unclear at this writing, however. To fill the market gap, several systems from small, independent vendors are now available, *e.g.*, the Cellsoft® (Cellsoft Biotechnology, Research Triangle Park, NC) and the 4 Cyte® (Howard Shapiro, West Newton, Massachusetts) systems. These can be retrofitted to older instruments to expand their data analysis capabilities. The systems we have examined bypass the on-board (integral) FCM computer, feeding the analog signals from the signal processor via Y-connectors to an interface containing a separate set of analog to digital converters from which data is transferred to an IBM microcomputer or clone. The systems include IBM compatible analysis software which can be easily customized. This configuration has several advantages, including compatibility with any flow cytometer, the by-passing of the integral FCM computer, and the added capability to use both integral and add-on data acquisition and display systems simultaneously. The independently sold systems are relatively inexpensive compared with stand-alone packages previously offered by major FCM manufacturers and, in addition, they offer a multiparameter list mode capability that expands the range of applications of FCM. Such data systems need to be critically evaluated by additional users. Nevertheless, we anticipate that powerful, portable, and inexpensive FCM data analytical systems will be widely available and in common usage well before the next iteration of this review is published.

Sample Preparation

FCM of Paraffin-Embedded Tissue. One of the most significant developments in clinically oriented FCM has been the demonstration that meaningful FCM analysis of DNA can be performed on nuclear suspensions recovered from thick sections of formalin-fixed, paraffin-embedded tissue blocks of the type routinely prepared and stored in pathology departments (45). Analysis of samples extracted from paraffin-embedded tissue has important practical advantages over analysis of fresh tissue. Obtaining a separate piece of fresh tissue for DNA FCM at the time of surgery is often inconvenient and frequently impossible, for example, when the surgical specimen or biopsy of a solid tumor is very small, or when the need for FCM analysis is not apparent until after all of the tissue has been embedded or discarded. FCM of paraffin blocks can be performed following histopathologic evaluation of tissue sections by conventional light microscopy, a logical time to order special procedures and to select the best area of the specimen for analysis. The approach is uniquely suited to many research applications as well. Because many tumors are sufficiently uncommon in single institutions, assembling a set of patients to determine the value of FCM analysis using fresh tumor tissue obtained prospectively would take several years. Retrospective analysis of paraffin-embedded tissue obviates this obstacle and also allows study of patients whose clinical course is already known. Another problem is that when a block of fresh tissue is dedicated to FCM, the pathologist can never be certain that this particular tissue block contains the cells of diagnostic relevance or is representative of the tumor present on slides made from another piece of tissue. In contrast, a conventional histologic section adjacent to the thick section disaggregated for FCM can conveniently be examined to verify the actual content of the paraffin-embedded tissue block used for FCM. The nuclei recovered in this way exhibit excellent morphological preservation (Fig. 2) offering another means of monitoring the cellular population and allowing correlative morphologic and image analysis studies (174).

On the other hand, FCM of paraffin-embedded tissue also has significant limitations compared with analysis of fresh tissue (45, 104). Formalin fixation produces a significant and unpredictable reduction in the DNA fluorescence of stained nuclei. This precludes the use of external standards, since the absolute DNA fluorescence of diploid populations may vary significantly from block to block. The problem is partially circumvented by using endogenous inflammatory and stromal cells to mark the diploid reference point individually for each specimen block. From a practical standpoint this means that two or more discrete G1G0 peaks should be present to support an interpretation of DNA aneuploidy (108). Notwithstanding these limitations, DNA FCM of paraffin-embedded tissue has been found to correlate quite well with analysis of fresh tissue samples from the same specimen whether analyzed by FCM (104) or cytogenetic procedures (46) (Fig. 2). Generally, coefficients of variation are somewhat larger, and there is more subnuclear debris in deparaffinized specimens than in corresponding fresh specimens (104). Apparently, the downshifting of DNA fluorescence in fixed tissue affects all of the cells in a tissue specimen proportionally, since aneuploidy is not seen in normal tissues or in tumors which have been shown to be diploid by analysis of fresh tissue aliquots (104).

Another important limitation of the paraffin-DNA method is that only bare nuclei can be analyzed at the present time. Cytoplasm, plasma membrane, and stroma are all lost during specimen preparation (Fig. 2). This significantly limits the range of cellular features which can be evaluated. However, several promising reports indicate that measurement of nonDNA nuclear parameters, including biophysical properties (10), oncogene products (238), and proliferation-associated antigens (16) is possible. The development of methods to retain extranuclear cellular components in suspensions obtained from paraffin blocks is a fertile area for future research.

Credit for publishing the first workable method for making nuclear suspensions from paraffin blocks belongs to Dr. David Hedley, and his colleagues in Sydney, Australia (104). The many others who have exploited the idea have closely followed the Hedley protocol, although with some significant refinements. The principal features of the method we used are shown in Figure 3. Hedley's original protocol called for cutting one or more 30-μm sections which were deparaffinized and converted to a nuclear suspension by digestion in 0.5% pepsin, pH 1.5. The nuclear suspension was then stained for DNA quantitation with DAPI. Later, the effect of section thickness on DNA histograms was systematically studied, and 50-μm sections were found to be optimal for most solid tumors (215). Thinner sections tended to increase the proportion of subnuclear fragments from sectioning. Several procedures have been described for selecting precisely circumscribed areas of paraffin-embedded tissue for analysis, such as dissecting small regions or cylindrical cores from the paraffin block (229), or by subdividing the thick sections picked up from a conventional histologic waterbath on microscope slides (174). This is useful where there is only a small region of abnormal epithelium to be studied or to compare a tumor with its adjacent relatively normal appearing epithelium.

Variations of the original pepsin disaggregation pro-

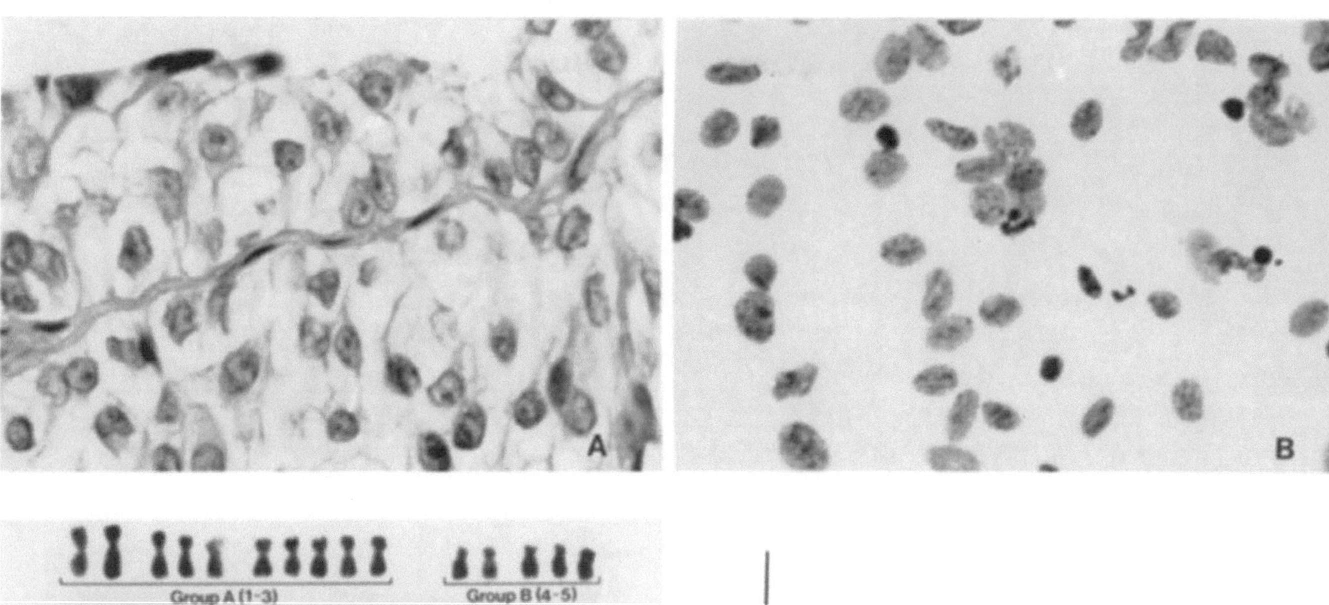

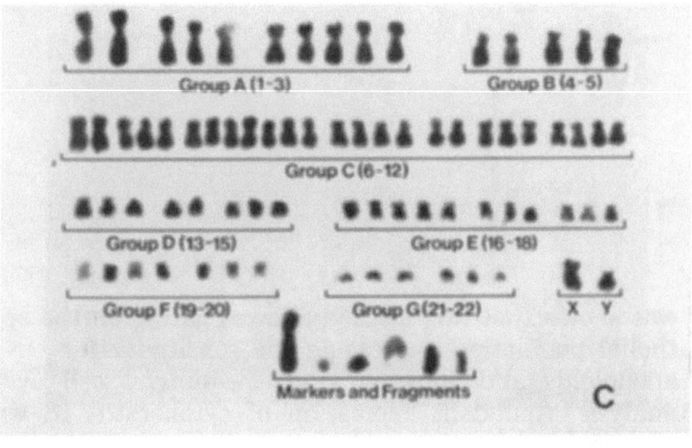

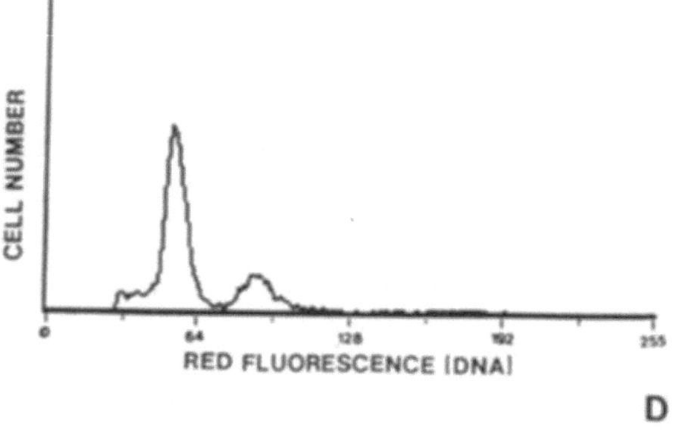

FIG. 2. Multimodality analysis of a human grade II transitional cell carcinoma specimen by light microscopy, FCM of paraffin embedded tissue, and karotyping of adjacent fresh tumor tissue obtained at the time of operation. *A*, Histologic section of tumor. Paraffin embedding, hematoxylin and eosin stain. ×*500*. *B*, Cytocentrifuge preparation of nuclei retrieved from a 50-μm section of a paraffin block from the same tumor. Note the excellent preservation of nuclear morphology. Feulgen stain. ×*500*. *C*, Abnormal hyperdiploid karyotype with several marker chromosomes from the tumor. *D*, DNA histogram derived from FCM of nuclei recovered from the 50-μm section from the paraffin block of the tumor. The largest peak, in channel 50, represents diploid inflammatory cells. The other large peak in channel 80 represents the hyperdiploid tumor cells. DNA abnormality in histogram is consistent with the karyotype shown in 2*C*.

tocol include changing the concentration and the duration of pepsin digestion (239) and substitution of other proteases (229). These modifications may indicate that some laboratories have had difficulty in achieving satisfactory suspensions with the original Hedley protocol (104), at least from some tissues. We have reported that the addition of a detergent-trypsin step, after the pepsin treatment, increases the yield of single nuclei from several tissue types (47). This is a modification of the Vindelov *et al.* (232) procedure for enucleation of fresh tumor tissue. Finally, other dyes besides DAPI have now been widely used, especially propidium iodide after ribonuclease digestion (45).

Multiparameter Analysis of Nonlymphoreticular Cells. Progress has been made in extending multiparameter analysis to cells outside the lymphoreticular compartment. Previously the field of clinical FCM of human cells could be conveniently divided into two realms: (a) quantitative multiparameter analysis of surface antigens in lymphoreticular cells and (b) quantitative DNA analysis of other cell types, principally solid tumor cells. The reasons for the preoccupation with DNA measurement in human solid tumors include the considerable usefulness of DNA analysis for prognosis and detection of malignancy (13, 130), the difficulty of obtaining single cell suspensions of intact solid tumor cells for surface marker analysis (240), and the relative lack of well-defined antigens of biologic importance in solid tumors, at least when compared with the well-established field of cell surface lymphocyte differentiation markers. While the supremacy of DNA in solid tumor analysis seems unlikely to be threatened soon, a number of workers have described multiparameter analysis in which DNA has been combined with another measurement. Table 1 summarizes some of these combinations of parameters.

Several groups have reported simultaneous analysis of DNA and nuclear or cytoplasmic antigens in solid tumor cells. FCM studies of cytoplasmic markers have been described primarily for the few specific solid tumor specimens readily yielding suspensions of intact cells, *e.g.*, bladder barbotage specimens. Nuclear antigens may have wider application because nuclear suspensions can be

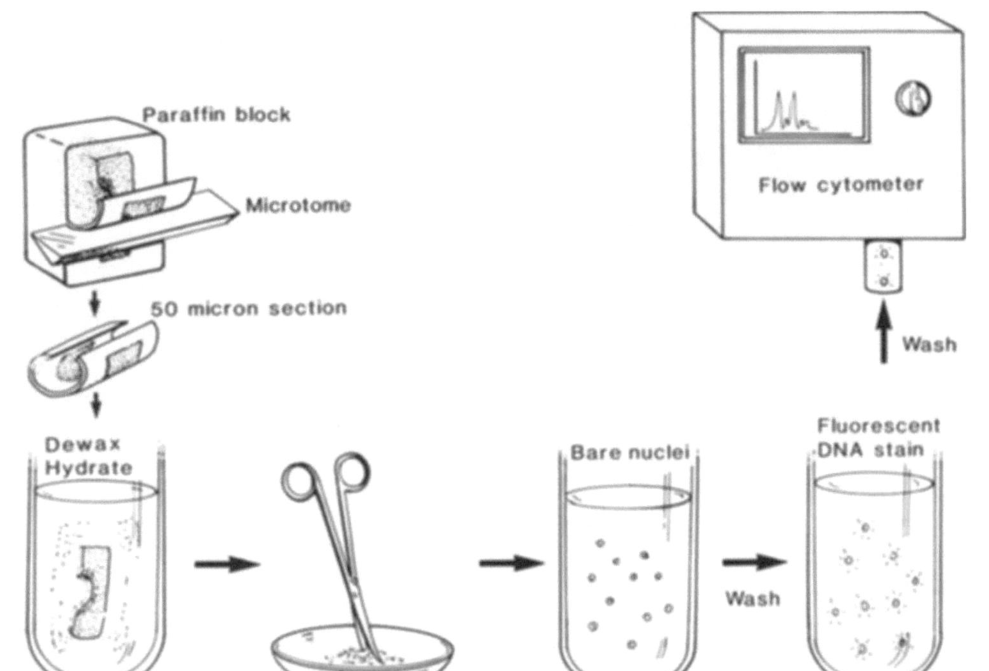

FIG. 3. Method of preparing paraffin-embedded tissue for FCM. See text for details.

TABLE 1. MARKERS COMBINED WITH DNA IN FCM OF SOLID TUMORS

Marker	References
Intrinsic cell properties—light scatter, volume	10, 18, 19, 227
RNA	159
Cytokeratin	67, 175
Oncogene products	51, 239
Proliferation-associated antigens	16
Tumor-associated antigens	52, 227

obtained from almost all tumors. Watson, Sikora, and Evan (239) reported FCM analysis of the c-*myc* nuclear oncoprotein in nuclei recovered from paraffin blocks of a variety of tumors. Czerniac *et al.* (51) studied the cell cycle distribution of the Ha-ras oncogene p21 protein in cultured human tumor cells. Bauer *et al.* (16) described the simultaneous quantitation of a nuclear, proliferation-associated antigen and DNA in nuclei from paraffin-embedded colon carcinomas. The expression of this antigen in colon carcinomas appeared different from the expression in normal colon epithelial cells. Czerniac and Koss (52) found that expression of the "Ca" tumor-associated antigen was low in normal bladder epithelial cells and dipolid transitional cell carcinomas, but high in aneuploid carcinomas. They also studied this antigen for identification of cells in effusions (53). Valet, Russmann and Wirsching (227) showed that simultaneous analysis of carcinoembryonic antigen, cell volume, and DNA allowed identification of colon carcinoma cells in 98% of 170 patients compared with 59% using DNA aneuploidy alone. Feitz *et al.* (67) and Oud *et al.* (175) reported simultaneous analysis of DNA and cytokeratin in urinary bladder carcinoma and endometrial cells, respectively. It was shown that this method allowed gating on the epithelial population, increasing the sensitivity for DNA aneuploidy and allowing more meaningful cell cycle analysis. Abundant expression of cytokeratin 18 was associated with unfavorable prognosis in urinary bladder carcinoma (67).

Although DNA FCM is very powerful for measuring DNA content of resting and dividing cells, it has significant shortcomings for measuring cells actually engaged in DNA synthesis. Measurement of uptake of the thymidine analog, bromodeoxyuridine, using monoclonal antibodies to the altered nucleic acid and FCM have been reported by several investigators (93, 112, 184). This technique gives data comparable to tritiated thymidine uptake (93). It requires pulsing living cells *in vitro* or *in vivo* with bromodeoxyuridine, which significantly limits the applicability of the technique in the clinical arena. However studies of human tumors after *in vivo* infusion of bromodeoxyuridine have been reported (112, 184).

Biophysical parameters of solid tumor cells can be measured to advantage by flow cytometry. Benson, McDougal and Coffey (18) showed that orthogonal light scatter was proportional to nuclear surface area in rat prostate carcinoma cells, and that forward and orthogonal scatter could be used to distinguish tumor cell line variants with different biologic potential. This work was subsequently extended to human prostate carcinoma samples and showed a correlation between scatter parameters and tumor stage (19). Forward and orthogonal light scatter of bare nucleus preparations can be used to partially exclude inflammatory cells and sometimes other irrelevant cells from analysis of epithelial tumors, thus revealing minor aneuploid populations that might otherwise be inapparent (10) (Fig. 4).

Immunocytochemistry of Surface Markers in Hemato-

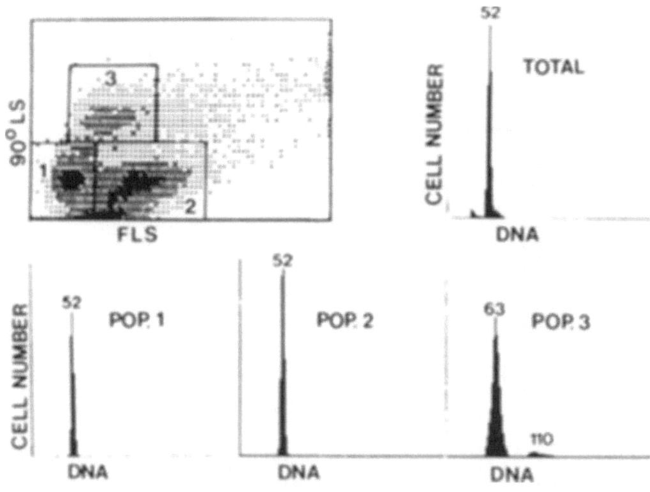

FIG. 4. Use of nuclear scatter gating to detect a minor aneuploid (tumor) population in a urinary bladder barbotage specimen. Starting at *upper left* and moving clockwise: two-dimensional histogram of forward light scatter (*FLS*) *versus* orthogonal light scatter (*90°LS*) reveals 3 distinct populations; total (ungated) DNA histogram shows a large diploid peak in channel 52 with a nondiagnostic shoulder to right; DNA histogram of nuclei in scatter population 3 shows a definitely abnormal (aneuploid) peak in channel 63; diploid DNA histograms of scatter populations 1 and 2 representing inflammatory and other normal cells. Cytology showed many inflammatory cells and rare transitional cell carcinoma cells of intermediate grade.

lymphoid Cells. Surface marker analysis by multicolor immunofluorescence FCM has become the method of choice for discrimination of specific lymphoid, monocytic, and myeloid cells in heterogeneous populations. Identification of specific cell populations within a mixture of many different cells has been used to study functional subpopulations of lymphocytes involved in the immune response, to distinguish between different lineages of other leukocytes, to identify and classify leukemia and lymphomas, to characterize patients with immunodeficiency syndromes, and to monitor shifts in cell populations with patients during the posttransplant period (see below). As the complexity of these heterogeneous systems increases, the requirement for better discrimination among different cells also increases. In theory, one way to enhance discrimination is to use more specific monoclonal antibodies that can uniquely identify a particular subset of cells. There is, however, no assurance that such exquisitely specific antibodies can be prepared, since a direct correlation between level of differentiation, cell function, and cell surface antigen expression may not always exist. An alternative strategy is to apply multiple antibodies to a heterogeneous population with the goal of identifying unique cell populations based on the correlated expression of multiple cell surface markers. This requires the availability of multiple fluorophores with compatible excitation and emission spectra and an instrument able to quantitate two or more fluorophores on a single cell.

Several different techniques have been used to detect multicolor staining of cells in flow systems. Two-color immunofluorescence can be quantified using a single laser system with fluorescein and rhodamine as the fluorophores (144); however, the fluorescence of the cells must be relatively bright for both stains. Sensitivity is lost with this method, since rhodamine is not excited at its optimum by the 488 nm wavelength of the commonly used argon laser system. Also, the emission spectra of fluorescein and rhodamine are close enough to produce considerable interference or "crosstalk." Recently, another group of dyes, the phycobiliproteins, have found widespread usage with multiparameter flow analysis (170) (Table 2). The phycobiliproteins are constituents of blue-green algae. In nature, they are involved in energy transfer steps that enable algae to capture light that is not absorbed efficiently by chlorophyll (89).

There are three major proteins in this group: phycoerythrin (PE), R-phycocyanin, and allophycocyanin (90). PE is especially useful because of its absorption and emission spectra. PE is excited at a wavelength of 488 nm, as is fluorescein, but its emission spectrum is sufficiently different to allow for the simultaneous analysis of cell-surface marker-linked monoclonal antibodies tagged with both fluorophores. Three-color immunofluorescent flow analysis has been demonstrated, but requires a dual laser (so-called "multistation") system. Loken and Lanier (143) have described a method to quantitate three different immunofluorescent labels on a single sample. The three dyes, fluorescein, PE, and Texas red are excited by two lasers (an argon laser and dye laser). Currently, work is underway to do three-color analysis with a single laser system by tandem phycobiliprotein conjugation where PE is covalently linked to allophycocyanin (91). In this tandem phycobiliprotein conjugate, energy is transferred from PE to allophycocyanin with an efficiency of 90%. Excitation of this conjugate occurs at 488 nm and leads to an emission spectrum around 660 nm. This approach should make it possible to simultaneously analyize three surface markers using a relatively inexpensive, bench top air-cooled laser instrument.

CLINICAL SIGNIFICANCE OF FCM—RECENT DEVELOPMENTS

ANALYSIS OF SOLID TUMORS

Table 3 lists the major proposed clinical indications for DNA FCM analysis. In most solid tumor applications, FCM is an adjunct, rather than a replacement for conventional morphology. There are situations in which detection of malignancy by cytopathology is relatively insensitive, and its identification by FCM may be advantageous (113). A correlation between FCM and prognosis

TABLE 2. SPECTRAL CHARACTERISTICS OF SELECTED FLUOROCHROMES USED FOR MULTICOLOR IMMUNOFLUORESCENCE

Dye	Excitation max	Emission max
Fluorescein	494 nm	517 nm
R-Phycoerythrin	495 nm	576 nm
Phycoerythrin-allophycocyanin tandem conjugate	488 nm	660 nm
Rhodamine	545 nm	575 nm
Phycocyanin	620 nm	655 nm
Allophycocyanin	620 nm	660 nm

TABLE 3. PROPOSED CLINICAL USES OF FCM IN SOLID TUMORS

1. Diagnose malignancy where morphology equivocal.
2. Prognosis independent of grade and stage.
3. Subclassify lesions of borderline malignancy.
4. Monitor response to therapy.
5. Establish origin of synchronous or metachronous tumors.

would be of greatest practical importance if its predictive value, sensitivity, and specificity with respect to clinical progression exceeds that of conventional grading and staging. It has been suggested that the combination of DNA FCM and morphologic parameters is more powerful than either applied alone in some clinical settings (165). The value of DNA FCM to subclassify lesions of so-called borderline malignancy is unclear. The issue is clouded by observations that DNA aneuploidy is unequivocally, though uncommonly detected in some benign tumors such as colonic (10) and thyroid adenomas (116), and cutaneous nevi (236), whereas clearly malignant neoplasms of the same cell type do not invariably have DNA abnormalities detectable by FCM (13). Therefore, DNA aneuploidy cannot be considered to be pathognomonic of biological malignancy across the board for all human tumor types.

DNA FCM has been used to probe the interrelatedness of synchronous or metachronous tumors thought to represent separate primaries in patients with multiple tumors (199) (Fig. 5). This application rests on the assumption that the detection of identical or nearly identical aneuploid DNA indices in two or more tumors in the same patient is evidence that one of the lesions represents a metastasis rather than a separate primary. If the tumors have different DNA indices, this suggests an independent origin, although this does not provide definitive proof, since metastases, or even different parts of the same primary tumor, occasionally can have different DNA indices (13). If both or all tumors are diploid, the results are also inconclusive, since a substantial minority of most types of solid tumors are diploid (13).

The clinical significance of FCM of solid tumors has been established primarily for DNA analysis. A general observation is that for many organs, DNA aneuploidy is strongly suggestive of malignancy, and that for specific tumor types, the aneuploid tumors have a more aggressive potential than diploid tumors with similar histopathology (107, 153, 181). The term "DNA aneuploid" rather than "aneuploid" is preferred for data derived from quantitative DNA analysis, as opposed to karyotype studies, where chromosomes are counted (108). Cell cycle analysis may also be of value in that rapid proliferation in the absence of aneuploidy may suggest a tumor, and rapid proliferation may have unfavorable prognostic significance (107, 153, 181).

Although tumor DNA measurements have been extensively discussed in the literature, comments on some practical aspects of histogram interpretation may be helpful (Fig. 6). First is the controversy concerning the definition of DNA aneuploidy. The definition is straightforward for karyotype interpretation but cannot be directly extrapolated to the interpretation of FCM histo-

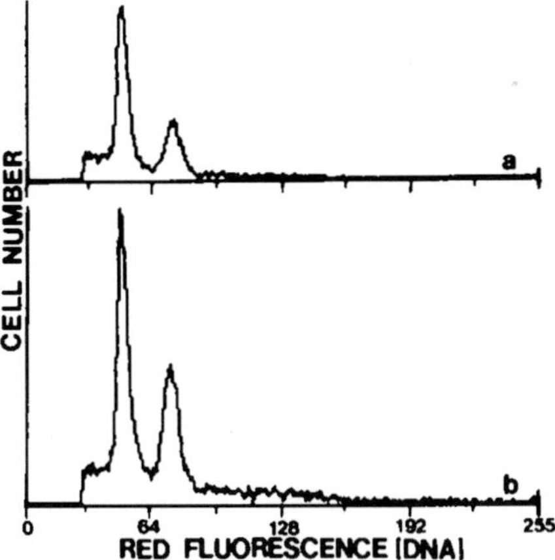

FIG. 5. DNA histograms from two anatomically separate, apparently primary carcinomas from the same colon. The largest peaks, in channel 50, are diploid inflammatory cells. Identical position of the smaller aneuploid peaks from the two specimens suggest that one tumor represents a metastasis from the other (199).

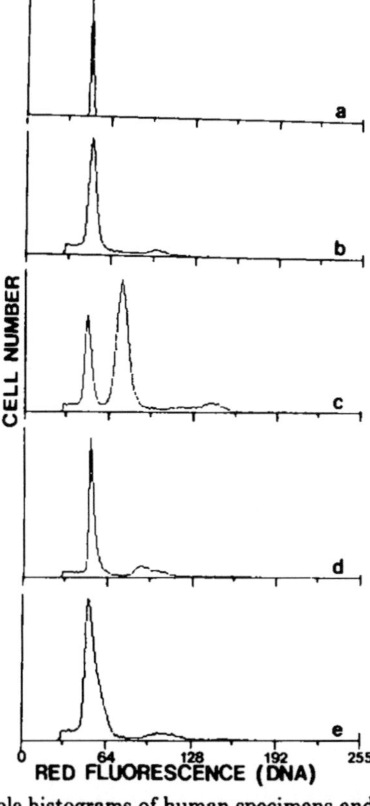

FIG. 6. Sample histograms of human specimens and their interpretation. All material was derived from paraffin blocks. Diploid peaks are in channel 50. *a*, Diploid histogram from resting lymph node with very few dividing cells. *b*, Diploid histogram from breast carcinoma with moderate proliferative activity. *c*, Obvious aneuploid histogram from breast carcinoma with relatively large tumor population and relatively few normal cells. Proliferative fraction of the tumor cells could be readily measured from this specimen. *d*, Aneuploid histogram from breast carcinoma (hypotetraploid) with relatively few tumor cells and many dividing diploid cells. Measurement of proliferative fraction of tumor cells would be virtually impossible in this case. *e*, Suspicious histogram from breast carcinoma in which the diploid peak is severely skewed to the right. A positive interpretation of aneuploidy should not be made from this histogram. Nuclear scatter gating allowed clear separation of peridiploid (aneuploid) peak (see Figure 4 for a similar example illustrating gating).

grams in many cases. Some authors have considered FCM histograms to be aneuploid if they contain an arbitrarily selected percentage of cells outside the diploid range, or if the diploid peak is skewed or broad, even if no discrete, definite abnormal G1 peak is apparent. This is unjustified, since it obscures the distinction between a rapidly dividing diploid population and a clearly aneuploid one (108). Both patterns may indicate the presence of tumor, but may have very different implications with respect to the specificity of the interpretation of malignancy and of the biologic potential of the malignant dyscrasia. The ability to detect DNA aneuploidy by FCM is dependent upon the resolution of the DNA measurements, usually assessed by the coefficient of variation (CV) of the peaks. For this reason, the CVs should be reported both in research and clinical studies (108). While the quest for lower CVs is worthwhile, it is noteworthy that the range of CVs is highly dependent upon the tissue type and the way it is prepared (204). Thus, for example, the low CVs routinely obtained from fresh, uniform suspensions of leukemia cells could not be expected from paraffin blocks of colon cancer. Cell cycle analysis to determine proliferative fraction is also considerably more difficult for most carcinoma specimens than for leukemias. Most solid tumor specimens contain a complex and highly variable mixture of tumor cells, inflammatory cells, and benign stromal cells. The histograms observed may therefore represent a complex composite of overlapping patterns. This problem is accentuated when the CVs of the peaks increase and the relative proportion of tumor cells to contaminating normal cells decreases (155). Even if one uses cytokeratin staining to discriminate epithelial cells, the histogram may be complicated by the presence of benign adjacent epithelial cells. The amount of debris can also affect the apparent S-phase fraction (100). Computerized subtraction of debris may yield improved results (100). Most computer modeling routines currently available for cell cycle analysis were not designed to be applied to complex mixtures of cells (155). In most cases, therefore, cell cycle analysis of solid tumors must be interpreted empirically, and with caution, realizing that the analysis is subject to substantial systematic and random errors.

Having discussed general aspects at FCM of solid tumors, we will outline some specific clinically relevant applications. Table 4 is a listing of FCM studies on a broad spectrum of human tumors. In the text, we have made no effort to be all-inclusive but have focused our attention on recent data on the more common human malignancies and on other selected tumors for which the utility of FCM analysis has been most convincingly demonstrated.

Urinary Bladder Carcinoma. Cells in voided urine and bladder washings were regarded as specimens of choice for early studies on clinical oncology applications of FCM. Here we will attempt to summarize present views on the usefulness of FCM in urologic practice. Applications of FCM to bladder cancer fall into three distinct fields: assessment of prognosis, detection of recurrent tumors, and monitoring response to therapy. Transitional cell carcinoma (TCC) is the most common bladder malignancy in America, and has been most intensively studied (241).

TABLE 4. DNA FCM STUDIES IN SELECTED HUMAN TUMORS

Tumor	Selected recent references
Lung carcinoma	161, 234, 235
Colorectol carcinoma	11, 33, 68, 126, 127, 157, 158, 200, 244, 245
Breast carcinoma	24, 49, 105, 222
Prostate carcinoma	71, 75, 156
Uterine carcinoma	87, 114
Ovarian carcinoma	79, 80, 195
Urinary bladder carcinoma	6, 35, 40, 44, 47, 57, 66, 73, 123, 124, 159, 164, 165, 219, 241
Head and neck carcinoma (Squamous cell)	22, 117, 120
Gastric carcinoma	151
Melanoma	27, 43, 76, 211, 236
Renal cell carcinoma	7, 36
Adrenal carcinoma	25, 125
Thyroid carcinoma	38, 96
Testicular tumors	72, 171
Leukemia	109, 185, 218
Myeloma	12
Lymphoma	17, 37
Brain tumors	112, 212
Sarcomas	106, 132, 152, 160, 226
Neuroblastoma	82
Wilm's tumor	59

With respect to prognostic value, it has long been known that DNA aneuploidy correlates with unfavorable prognosis in TCC (reviewed in Ref. 47). DNA aneuploidy also correlates strongly with tumor grade and stage (66, 73), raising the question whether FCM, at least confined to DNA analysis, provides additional prognostic information independent of histologic assessment, since grade and stage are both reasonably predictive of prognosis in bladder carcinoma (241). Some studies suggest that the demonstration of aneuploidy is useful additional information in patients with grade 2, noninvasive tumors (219). However, Murphy, Chandler, and Trafford (164) reported that FCM DNA analysis offered no independent prognostic information to what could be learned from the assessment of histologic grade alone in an analysis of 63 bladder tumors.

FCM of exfoliated urinary bladder cells is a potentially important technique for monitoring patients who have been conservatively treated for carcinoma. This importance stems from the limitations of conventional techniques, including the high cost, patient inconvenience, and expert personnel required for cystoscopy (65) and the relative subjectivity, unreliability and limited availability of high quality bladder cytology (47). However, controversy exists concerning the sensitivity and specificity of FCM for surveillance of patients at risk for developing recurrent TCC. The Sloan-Kettering experience of Melamed and Klein (159) with over 500 patients is particularly impressive. They found that FCM was positive in 100% of patients with flat carcinoma *in situ*,

TABLE 5. RUSH BLADDER WASHING FCM EXPERIENCE (93 PATIENTS)

True positives[a]	38%
False positives	0%
Predictive positive[b]	2%
True negative	39%
False negative	7%
Unsatisfactory	11%
Suspicious[c]	3%

[a] Positive, aneuploid, or tetraploid, or > 20% of cells hyperdiploid.
[b] Predictive positive = FCM positive with negative cytology and histology but patient later developed obvious recurrence.
[c] Suspicious, 15 to 20% hyperdiploid without aneuploid peak.

92% of patients with invasive TCC, 80% of noninvasive TCC (excluding grade I tumors), and 46% of lesions the Sloan-Kettering pathologists diagnosed as papillomas. The false-positive rate was estimated to be between 2 and 10%, with no patient without urologic neoplasia having a true aneuploid histogram. All false-positive histograms were diploid and were judged abnormal on the basis of high proliferative fraction (defined as more than 15% of cells hyperdiploid). In the Sloan-Kettering series, use of abnormal proliferative fraction as a marker of neoplasia strongly influenced the statistics, since only 42% of noninvasive TCCs (excluding grade I) were aneuploid and 67% of invasive TCCs were aneuploid. Other authors' experiences have generally been somewhat less favorable. Murphy *et al.* (165) reported that FCM was positive in 78% of patients with TCC compared with 75% by cytology. The false-positive rate was approximately 24%, although none had a true aneuploid histogram. deVere White, Olsson, and Deitch (57) reported that FCM was positive in 64% of patients with TCC, and that FCM abnormalities preceded abnormal cystoscopy or cytology in one-third of patients who developed recurrent TCC. However, their false-positive rate was 38%. Their criteria for abnormality appear to have been similar to that of Melamed and Klein (159) *i.e.*, aneuploidy, tetraploidy, or more than 15% hyperdiploid. Chin *et al.* (35) reported that the hyperdiploid fraction was similar in patients with diploid tumors and patients with cystitis. Exclusion of this criterion would lead to a large false-negative rate in their hands, since all grade I, 30 % of grade II, and 23% of grade III tumors were diploid. Our own experience with analysis of bladder washings is summarized in Table 5.

The discrepancies among the laboratories are probably partly due to differences in methods, *i.e.*, Melamed's acridine orange technique allows superior exclusion of irrelevant cells from analysis (40), thus making measurement of proliferative fraction more meaningful, but gives lower resolution DNA analysis (77), making some aneuploid populations harder to detect. Nevertheless, most workers agree that the sensitivity of FCM for detecting all forms of TCC in barbotage specimens is at least as good as expertly interpreted cytomorphology, and probably better than the performance of a cytologist who infrequently sees bladder specimens (159). Sensitivity for the detection of carcinoma *in situ* approaches 100% (124). Also the sensitivity of cytology plus FCM is significantly better than either technique alone (165). An important technical innovation is that FCM analysis of voided urine may yield results similar to barbotage specimens, suggesting the possibility of surveillance of some TCC patients without catheterization (57).

Enthusiasm for the clinical use of FCM of bladder cells must be tempered by a realization that there are some important limitations of the technique at its present stage of development. It is relatively insensitive for detection of diploid tumor cells (159). The criterion of malignancy usually used in the absence of aneuploidy, namely, high replicating fraction, is insensitive and also nonspecific, especially if there is significant bladder inflammation (35). This limitation, plus the desire to better predict the clinical course of individual patients is driving the search for additional markers which could be added to DNA analysis. FCM of bladder cells is critically dependent upon proper specimen collection, and best results have been reported in settings with close cooperation between urologists and the laboratory (159). The eventual usefulness of this technique will not be known until it is tested on a much wider scale by laboratories which are highly competent but which are not directed by pioneers in the development of FCM of bladder cells. In order to assess the clinical value of the technique, and to facilitate its transfer to a wider laboratory community, the National Cancer Institute is currently supporting a FCM Network of five institutions with experience in FCM and urologic pathology (44). They have exchanged "unknown" replicate samples of paraffin-embedded bladder tumors and achieved close agreement in appearance of histograms and their interpretation (44). This indicates that a consensus probably exists within the network regarding acceptable cytochemistry, instrument performance, and histogram interpretation (44), and represents an important first step toward standardization of the technology.

The idea that FCM could be useful for monitoring response to therapy in certain forms of TCC is based upon the unusual clinical aspects of bladder carcinoma that the cancer-bearing organ is resected only as a last resort, and that exfoliated tumor cells can be easily recovered from the bladder lumen. An earlier report suggested that FCM could be used to detect a favorable response of advanced TCC to radiotherapy preceding cystectomy (123). A recent report suggested that FCM was more sensitive, though less specific than cytology for monitoring persistent tumor in patients with superficial TCC treated with Bacillus Calmette-Guerin (6).

Colon Carcinoma. FCM analysis of adenocarcinomas of the colon was found to be of potential clinical value by several authors. Banner *et al.* (11) reported a strong correlation between DNA aneuploidy and advanced Duke's stage disease, raising the possibility that one could predict the extent of disease before definitive surgery rather than retrospectively by examination of the resected surgical specimen. The relationship between aneuploidy and advanced Duke's stage has subsequently been confirmed in another series of 77 patients (126).

Others have shown that DNA analysis may be performed from colonoscopic biopsies (157), and that DNA analysis of superficial parts of the tumor is representative of the tumor as a whole in most cases (200). This could have practical application for tailoring appropriate surgical or adjuvant therapy, *e.g.*, intraoperative radiotherapy for advanced disease (244). However, others have found the relationship between DNA aneuploidy and Duke's stage to be less impressive (158).

Many laboratories have found a strong relationship between DNA aneuploidy and prognosis as reflected in survival rates. Wolley *et al.* (245) reported that, in a series of 33 patients followed more than 3 years, all 13 patients with aneuploid tumors had died or had extensive metastases, whereas only 6 of 20 patients with diploid tumors had died. Also, Kokal *et al.* (126) reported that, in a series of 77 patients analyzed retrospectively from paraffin blocks, DNA aneuploidy was the best predictor of recurrence and short survival in a multivariate analysis of clinical and pathologic parameters. Tetraploidy had a favorable prognostic significance. Chang, Enker, and Melamed (33) found that aneuploidy was prognostically significant for early rectal tumors treated by local excision. On the other hand, Melamed *et al.* (158) observed no correlation between DNA aneuploidy and survival in 22 patients followed prospectively for 3 to 4 years. Apart from the small size of the series, a possible reason for the disagreement with other workers by Melamed *et al.* (158), is use of the DNA/RNA stain, acridine orange, which tends to have lower resolution of DNA abnormalities than the more commonly used propidium iodide or DAPI (77). DNA aneuploidy is not significant for predicting survival in patients who already have hepatic metastases (68, 127).

Several authors have studied DNA FCM of premalignant lesions of the colon. We and others have found that DNA aneuploidy may occur in histologically benign colonic adenomas, and even more frequently in villous adenomas (10, 92, 238, 242). The clinical significance of this is unknown. Also, aneuploidy has been found in mucosal biopsies of diverse histology in patients with inflammatory bowel disease with prevalence increasing with duration of disease (74, 101). Whether such analysis could be used to assess imminent risk of developing carcinoma is a matter for speculation. The finding that aneuploidy seemed equally frequent in hyperplastic and dysplastic areas of colons resected for inflammatory bowel disease, with or without coexisting carcinoma is evidence against a close relationship between the presence of aneuploid cells and the development of clinically significant colonic neoplasia (74).

Prostate Carcinoma. Several laboratories have recently examined the value of DNA FCM in adenocarcinoma of the prostate. In a retrospective analysis of 39 patients with low stage prostate carcinoma, discovered incidentally in transurethral resection chips, with follow-up period of 18 to 20 years, McIntire *et al.* (156) showed that DNA FCM added significant additional prognostic information. Progression occurred in 67% of aneuploid stage A2 cancers, but none of the diploid stage A1 tumors.

In patient series containing a wider spectrum of tumor types, aneuploidy has been found to be more frequent in tumors of advanced stage, and DNA analysis was found to be of additional value to histologic grading for predicting prognosis (71, 75). For example, Fordam *et al.* (71) found that patients with poorly differentiated aneuploid tumors survived an average of 22.4 months after diagnosis *versus* 104.5 months for well-differentiated diploid tumors (71).

Cutaneous Melanoma. Patients presenting with stage I cutaneous melanoma have a highly variable clinical course. This problem has resulted in the description of numerous histologic and clinical prognostic factors, of which tumor thickness appears to be the most significant (9). Clinical course is most difficult to predict in patients with tumors of intermediate thickness. Coon *et al.* (43) studied 177 stage I cutaneous melanoma patients retrospectively using paraffin-embedded material. Of 167 evaluable histograms, 124 were diploid, 35 aneuploid, and 3 tetraploid. Overall, aneuploidy was strongly correlated with recurrence and shorter disease-free survival. For tumors stratified by thickness, FCM was the most significant independent prognostic predictor among all commonly recognized parameters (Fig. 7). These findings must be interpreted, however, in view of the significantly higher prevalence of aneuploidy (54 to 85%) in melanoma reported in other studies (27, 76, 211) compared with this one (22%). This discrepancy may be largely due to a difference in the patient populations studied (236). Unlike previous series, the population of Coon *et al.* (43) consisted entirely of primary stage I lesions, many of which were also low micro stage (thickness). It is possible that Coon *et al.* (43) underdetected aneuploidy in the paraffin-embedded samples of small tumors. Nevertheless, it appears that DNA aneuploidy is a highly signifi-

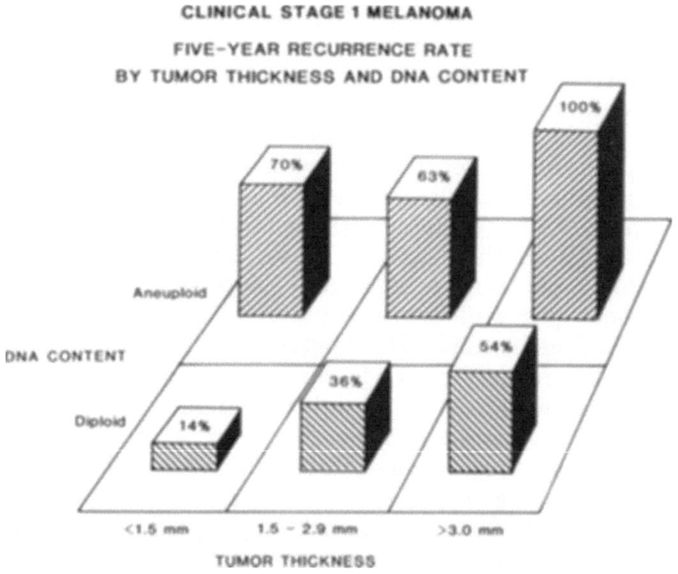

FIG. 7. Three-dimensional graph comparing 5-year recurrence rate, DNA content, and thickness for human cutaneous melanomas. For each thickness, aneuploid tumors had higher recurrence rates than diploid tumors.

cant stratification parameter for patients with stage I cutaneous melanoma.

Ovarian Carcinoma. DNA FCM has been reported to yield important information in ovarian carcinoma. Friedlander *et al.* (80) studied 44 borderline ovarian carcinomas retrospectively, 42 of which were diploid and 2 aneuploid. All patients with diploid tumors did well, but one of the two patients with an aneuploid tumor died from her tumor. More patients with aneuploid borderline ovarian tumors must be studied before the clinical significance of this anecdotal observation can be established. Friedlander *et al.* (79) also reported that DNA aneuploidy was a highly significant prognostic predictor in advanced ovarian carcinoma. In a retrospective analysis of 91 stage III and IV epithelial tumors, the mean survival of the aneuploid tumors was 52 weeks *versus* 123 weeks for the diploid tumors. In a multivariate analysis, DNA aneuploidy was the single best predictor of survival. The prognostic value of DNA FCM in advanced ovarian carcinoma has subsequently been confirmed by another laboratory (195).

Breast Carcinoma. Numerous investigators have performed DNA analysis on breast carcinoma specimens using both FCM and static image analysis. They have looked for correlations with other significant clinical parameters, particularly lymph node status, hormone receptor status, and survival. These studies have been driven by the important clinical need for better prognostic indicators and for accurate predictors of axillary metastases, as guides to appropriate therapy. Earlier studies had shown an overall relationship between DNA aneuploidy and an unfavorable prognosis (24). The majority of breast cancers are aneuploid. Recent studies have examined this relationship in greater detail to determine whether it might have clinical value in managing breast cancer patients. Only FCM studies will be discussed, because the results of static image analysis studies are sufficiently different to make comparison difficult. In perhaps the most optimistic study, Coulson *et al.* (49) prospectively studied 74 patients over a 3-year period. Patients with diploid tumors had an 87% survival during this period, *versus* approximately 50% for the aneuploid groups. Hypodiploid, multiploid, and hypertetraploid groups were particularly unfavorable. There was a strong correlation of aneuploidy with negative estrogen receptor status. In another survival study, Hedley *et al.* (105) studied archival specimens from 105 patients with stage II (node positive) breast cancer. Of these, 32% were diploid. They estimated that patients with diploid tumors were 72% relapse free at 4 years *versus* 43% of patients with aneuploid tumors. However aneuploidy was not an independent prognostic predictor in a multivariate analysis; aneuploidy was highly correlated with a more powerful prognostic predictor, the number of positive axillary nodes. Thorud *et al.* (222) reported no significant difference in relapse rate among aneuploid and diploid tumors in a series of 59 patients. There was also no correlation with clinical node status. McDivitt *et al.* (154) studied 168 consecutive primary breast cancer patients and found 55% aneuploid. There was no correlation between aneuploidy or S-phase fraction *versus* axillary lymph node status or estrogen receptor status. Summarizing these often contradictory studies is difficult, but it seems fair to say that the clinical prognostic value of DNA FCM in breast carcinoma is not well established at present. Difficulty in this area may be related to the often indolent and unpredictable natural history of breast cancer, and the resultant difficulty of designing studies to give clear results. There seems to be little evidence that DNA FCM can predict which patients with clinically localized tumors will be found to have axillary metastases at surgery.

Lung Carcinoma. Considering its great medical importance, lung carcinoma has received relatively little attention by FCM laboratories. This may be partly because of the perception that lung cancer is a rather uniformly lethal disease. Nevertheless some data have been reported. Volm *et al.* (235), in a study of 187 patients, found that 84% were aneuploid. DNA aneuploid tumors had significantly shorter survival times than diploid tumors. Low S-phase fraction was associated with longer survival. The same authors studied 127 patients with advanced (stage III) nonsmall cell tumors, and found no relationship between aneuploidy and survival, but patients with high S-phase fraction treated with adjuvant chemotherapy and radiotherapy had significantly shorter survival (234). Another study found no correlation between aneuploidy and stage, except for adenocarcinomas (161). FCM studies of lung cancer patients could be of greater practical importance as more effective treatment strategies are devised.

Multiparameter Analysis of Normal Lymphoid and Myeloid Cells

The number and functional capacity of circulating peripheral blood leukocytes may reflect the overall state of immune competence of an individual. In recent years, FCM evaluation of lymphocyte subsets has found its place as a useful diagnostic and prognostic tool in several clinical settings, including leukemia and lymphoma, immunodeficiency disorders, autoimmune disease, and transplantation of bone marrow and solid organs. Of particular importance has been the development of monoclonal antibodies which recognize cell surface differentiation antigens, define lymphocyte cell surface phenotypes and facilitate quantitation of T cells, B cells and natural killer (NK) cells, as well as subsets of these populations.

Unfortunately, a complex nomenclature for hematolymphoid cells evolved as a byproduct of the frenetic pace of research in the monoclonal antibody field. This presented many pathologists with a formidable barrier for entry into the diagnostic FCM literature. Early on, an incoherent collection of abbreviations evolved in the research literature. Designations for the commercial equivalents of these reagents were haphazardly created. In order to alleviate problems in nomenclature, the World Health Organization, in conjunction with the International Union of Immunological Societies (IUIS),

Institut National de la Sante et de la Recherche Medicale (INSERM), and the Medical Research Council, sponsored the First International Workshop on Human Leukocyte Differentiation Antigens in November, 1982. Data were collected by 55 research groups from 14 different countries. Statistical methods were used to group antibodies according to reactivities on specific target cells. A method called cluster analysis was used to define groups of antibodies that were statistically similar. These clusters were termed clusters of differentiation (CD). Each antibody in the library was then assigned to a cluster group. Table 6 summarizes the most common CD groups and the commercially available antibodies belonging to each of the groups. Since the first Leukocyte Differentiation Conference, two more have been held, and a total of 45 CD groups have been established (207). Table 7 lists additional leukocyte antigens and their abbreviations commonly analyzed by FCM.

The ability to simultaneously evaluate cells with fluorescein and PE-conjugated antibodies, using the technique of two-color FCM analysis, has led to an even better definition of normal lymphoid subsets. Investigations using this approach have demonstrated the existence of subpopulations with relatively narrow functional repertoires within each of the two major T cell lineages (CD4, T helper/inducer, and CD8, suppressor/cytotoxic) (63, 64, 84, 189). The $CD4^+$ subset can be subdivided by the Leu8 or TQ1 antibodies into two subsets (83, 187). The $Leu8^-$ CD4 cells are the helpers for B cell differentiation in response to pokeweed mitogen (83). The $Leu8^+/CD4^+$ subset contains two additional subsets that function as inducers of suppression ($2H4^+$) (163) and inducers of helper functions ($4B4^+$) (162). The $CD4^+$ $Leu8^+$ subsets also share other functions, including amplifying the development of cytotoxic T cells and proliferation in response to tetanus toxoid and to autologous and allogeneic non-T cells (62, 84). Among the CD8 cells, other subsets have been defined using multiparameter FCM analysis. Reagents are now available that distinguish cytotoxic and suppressor cells. Damle *et al.* (54–56) have described an antigen 9.3, which is present on a $CD8^+$ subset, which mediates HLA class I antigen-restricted cytotoxicity. Landay, Gartland, and Clemant (134) have described an antigen with CD11 antibody specificity, which positively identifies the suppressor subset within the CD8 population. The Leu8 marker has also been used to subdivide the CD8 bearing cells, with both types being required for optimal suppression of B cell responses (119).

Multiparameter FCM analysis has also allowed the phenotypic dissection of a morphologically homogenous population of cells known as large granular lymphocytes (LGL). The phenotypic heterogeneity in this population has resulted in considerable controversy and confusion regarding the lineage of these cells. Using two-color immunofluorescence and FCM, it has been possible to divide the LGL into essentially mutually exclusive subsets based on expression of CD3 or CD16 antigens (136, 172). The relative proportion of $CD16^+$ and $CD3^+$ LGL varies considerably between individuals. In most individuals, the majority of antibody-dependent cellular cytotoxicity and NK activity is contained within the $CD16^+$ fraction of LGLs (177–179, 196). These $CD16^+$ cells lack the CD3 and CD5 pan T cell antigens (177, 196). A proportion of the $CD16^+$ cells do co-express CD8 and CD2 antigens. However, FCM analysis has demonstrated that the expression of CD8 and CD2 on these cells is significantly less than on T cells (137). Essentially all $CD16^+$ NK cells co-express CD11, an antigen associated with complement receptor type 3 (CR3) (5) and the Leu19 (NKH-1) (180) antigen. Although highly variable among individuals, on the average, about 50% of the $CD16^+$ LGL express the Leu7 antigen (137).

Similar to typical T cells, the $CD3^+$ LGL are brightly stained by the CD2 and CD5 antibodies (137, 180). The majority of these cells also express a large quantity of CD8 and the Leu7 antigen structures (137, 180). Unlike the $CD16^+$ cells, only a subset possess CD11. FCM two-color analysis with a newly developed antibody, Leu19/NKH-1, has shown that when this antigen is expressed on $CD3^+$ LGL, it identifies a potent cytotoxic cell that is capable of killing targets irrespective of the major histocompatibility complex restriction characteristic of T cell cytotoxicity (135).

Although human B lymphocytes have not been dissected into distinct subpopulations to the same extent as have T lymphocytes, numerous investigations have revealed diversity within the human B lineage. The impetus for these studies was the immunohistochemical observation that anti-Leu 8, which binds 50 to 70% of peripheral blood B cells, stains nearly all B cells in the mantle zone of lymph nodes and tonsils, but virtually no germinal center B cells (119). Subsequent studies showed that Leu 8^+ B cells activated, *in vitro*, with anti-IgM heavy chain antibody and B cell growth factor lost expression of Leu 8 antigen within 48 to 72 hours (118). The combination of these results suggests that the loss of detectable Leu 8 antigen marks on early stage of antigen-dependent B cell differentiation.

An additional subset of B cells has been identified by two-color FCM using the CD5 (Leu1) marker (81). This surface immunoglobulin bearing $CD5^+$ B cell is consistently present in the peripheral blood and spleen of healthy subjects. When purified $CD5^+$ B cells are transformed by infection with Epstein-Barr virus, autoantibody to the Fc fragment of human IgG and antibody to single-stranded DNA are made. This subset of B cells therefore probably represents that population of cells responsible for autoantibody production in autoimmune diseases such as systemic lupus erythematosus and rheumatoid arthritis (150).

Horan, Slezak, and Poste (110) have further refined the use of two fluorochromes (fluorescein and PE) in a single laser system to identify five lymphocyte subsets. This method permits simultaneous quantitation of T helper cells ($CD4^+$), T suppressor cells ($CD8^+$), B cells ($CD20^+$) monocytes, and NK cells ($CD16^+$). This method offers a significant expansion in the capacity of FCM analysis without the need for new reagents or expensive modifications in instrument design.

TABLE 6. GLOSSARY OF MOST COMMONLY USED MONOCLONAL ANTIBODIES COVERED BY CD NOMENCLATURE

Cluster of differentiation	Antibody (Commercial source)[a]	Specificity
CD 1 (gp 45, 12)[b]	OKT 6 (Ortho); Leu 6 (BD) T 6 (Coulter)	Common thymocyte, langerhans cell
CD 2 (gp 50)	OKT 11 (Ortho); Leu 5 (BD) T 11 (Coulter)	E-rosette receptor
CD 3 (gp 19–29)	OKT 3 (Ortho); Leu 4 (BD) T 3 (Coulter)	Pan T; lymphocyte
CD 4 (gp 56)	OKT 4 (Ortho); Leu 3 (BD) T 4 (Coulter)	Helper/inducer T
CD 5 (gp 67)	OKT 1 (Ortho); Leu 1 (BD) T 1 (Coulter)	T lymphocyte subset B cells
CD 7 (gp 41)	Leu 9 (BD)	T cells, NK cells (95% all T-ALL)
CD 8 (gp 32–33)	OKT 8 (Ortho); Leu 2 (BD) T 8 (Coulter)	Cytotoxic/suppressor T
CD 9 (gp 24)	BA 2 (Hybritech)	Monocytes, non-T, non-B
CD 10 (gp 100)	Anti-CALLA (BD) J 5 (Coulter)	Common acute lymphoblastic leukemia antigen pre-B cells, granulocytes
CD 11b (gp 160)	OKM 1 (Ortho) Leu 15 (BD) Mol (Coulter)	Complement receptor III, monocytes, granulocytes, NK cells, subset T cells
CD 13 (gp 150)	My 7 (Coulter)	Peripheral blood granulocytes and monocytes 5 to 40% normal bone marrow some CFU-C
CD 14 (gp 55)	Leu M 3 (BD) My 4 (Coulter) Mo 2 (Coulter)	90% peripheral blood, monocytes, 5 to 10% normal bone marrow not expressed on myeloid colony forming cells
CD 15	Leu M 1 (BD)	Monocytes and granulocytes
CD 16 (gp 50–60)	Leu 11 (BD)	IgG Fc receptor of natural killer cells, neutrophils, and basophils
CD 19 (gp 95)	Leu 12 (BD) B 4 (Coulter)	Immature B cells, B cells, all B cell malignancies except for myeloma, some non-T-ALL cells
CD 20 (gp 35)	Leu 16 (BD) B 1 (Coulter)	All B cell except for plasma cells B cell tumors except for myeloma, some non-T-ALL cells
CD 21 (gp 140)	CRII (BD) B 2 (Coulter)	C 3d receptor
CD 22 (gp 135)	Leu 14 (BD)	95% circulating B cells; B cells of mantle and germinal center zones of normal lymphoid tissue
CD 24 (gp 45, 55, 65)	BA 1 (Hybritech)	Peripheral blood B cells, reacts weakly granulocytes
CD 25 (gp 55)	IL-2 receptor (BD)	Human IL-2 receptor; T, B, monocytes
CD 33 (gp 67)	MY 9 (Coulter)	Early myeloid
CD 35 (gp 220)	CRI (BD)	B, PMN, Monocyte
CD 38 (gp 45)	Leu 17 (BD) OKT 10 (Coulter)	Immature and activated T cell, NK cells, plasma cells
CD 45 (gp 200)	HLE-1 (BD)	Pan leukocyte
CD 45R (gp 220)	Leu 18 (BD) 2H4 (Coulter)	T suppressor inducer subset, NK, B cells

[a] Coulter, Coulter Immunology (Hialeah, Florida); BD, Becton-Dickinson Immunocytometry Systems (Mountain View, California); Ortho, Ortho Diagnostic Systems (Raritan, New Jersey).

[b] gp, Glycoprotein, molecular weight in kilodaltons.

TABLE 7. GLOSSARY OF ANTIBODIES COMMONLY APPLIED TO HEMATOLYMPHOID CELLS NOT COVERED BY CD NOMENCLATURE

Antibody	Specificity
Leu 7	Large granular lymphocytes within T cell and NK lineages
Leu 19/NKH-1	MHC nonrestricted cytotoxic cells predominantly $CD3^+$ $CD4^-$ $CD8^-$ and express $T\gamma/\delta$ T cell receptor
HLA-DR	Major histocompatability complex class II antigen important in immune interactions, found on B cell monocytes and activated T cells
PCA-1	Plasma cell specific antigen expressed on plasma cells and weakly expressed on granulocytes, monocytes, and activated DR positive T cells
PC-1	Plasma cell antigen
Tdt	Terminal deoxynucleotidyl transferase nuclear enzyme found in immature lymphoid cells

APPLICATION OF MULTIPARAMETER FLOW ANALYSIS FOR LEUKEMIA AND LYMPHOMA PHENOTYPING

As outlined above, multiparameter FCM analysis with the expanding library of monoclonal antibodies has added enormously to the delineation of the differentiation of normal hematolymphoid cells. This has led to an ongoing effort to classify the neoplasms derived from these cells on the basis of the emerging concepts of hematolymphoid cell ontogeny (Figs. 8 and 9).

Acute lymphoblastic leukemia (ALL). ALL is heterogeneous. The first surface markers used to differentiate subclasses of ALL were receptors for sheep erythrocytes, which identify a T cell variant (15 to 25% of all cases), and surface immunoglobulin (SIg), which identifies a B cell variant (5% of cases) (225). Both the T group and this B cell group have a relatively unfavorable prognosis (34). The next important advance in identifying ALL was the development of an antiserum to a common ALL-associated antigen (CALLA) (94). CALLA reactivity identified a non-B, non-T subclass of ALL patients (70% of cases) with a more favorable prognosis than T-ALL, B-ALL, or non-B, non-T-ALL without CALLA (34).

Two important areas of research have prompted a reassessment of non-T-ALL. First, monoclonal antibodies that recognize B cell-associated antigens have been identified; they are present on many non-T-ALL cells, indicating a B cell lineage. The most specific of these antibodies is probably anti-CD19 (Leu12/B4), which reacts with 95% of cases of non-T-ALL (166). Second, clonal rearrangements of immunoglobulin genes provide strong evidence for the B cell lineage of most cases of non-T-ALL (69, 128). Although Ia antigen is present on most non-T-ALL cells, and CALLA is present in 75% of cases of non-T-ALL, these antigens are also identified on approximately 10% of cases of T-ALL. Therefore, B cell-associated antigens which are not identified on T-ALL cells, are the most useful in distinguishing non-T-ALL (167). Another marker that identifies a subset of non-T-ALL is cytoplasmic IgM without SIg. These are considered pre-B cell malignancies (50, 233).

Surface marker data derived from FCM, must sometimes be integrated with information derived from DNA genotyping studies. Virtually all non-T-ALL cells have immunoglobulin heavy chain rearrangement. Not all of them, however, demonstrate light chain rearrangements. Because heavy chain rearrangements also occur in non-B cells (122), immunoglobulin heavy chain rearrangements are insufficient to assign non-T-ALL to the B cell lineage. Nadler *et al.* (167) have proposed that the CD19 antigen provides the most important independent parameter with which to identify B cell-derived non-T cell ALL. More recently, up to 25% of non-T-ALL has been reported to have rearrangements of the T β-receptor (220). The remaining 5% of morphologically and cytochemically defined non-T cell ALLs, which express the Ia but not the CD19 antigen, may represent the earliest stage of pre-B cell differentiation. This hypothetical scheme of early B cell differentiation is further supported by data demonstrating that all of the proposed ALL subgroups can be identified in normal fetal liver and bone marrow and in normal adult bone marrow (167).

T-ALL. T-ALL represents 15 to 25% of cases of ALL. Clinical features associated with T-ALL include a high blast cell count, predominance of older male patients, and a mediastinal mass. The most sensitive marker for T-ALL is probably the pan-T 40 kilodalton (Kd) antigen identified by the anti-Leu-9 antibody (CD7). This antigen is present on most thymocytes and T cells, but not on non-T-ALL or B cell lymphomas or leukemias (139). In a study of 23 patients with T-ALL, all cases expressed the Leu-9 antigen. Although it was previously reported that anti-CD5 is the most sensitive marker for T-ALL (198), three of these 23 patients whose cells were anti-CD7 positive were negative with anti-CD5. However, Anti-CD7 reacts with a small proportion of cases that appear to be myeloid leukemias (32). A high prevalence of CALLA, Ia, and BA-2 expression has been reported in adults with T-ALL (210). Recently, rearrangement of the T β-receptor gene in cases of T-ALL has been reported (193).

The adult lymphoblastic leukemia phenotype has also been evaluated by FCM. In a recent study by Sobol *et al.* (209) it was demonstrated that multiparameter flow analysis revealed a subgroup of patients expressing myeloid antigens in conjunction with B cell or T cell antigens. The patients expressing myeloid antigens with B cell markers were found to have fewer complete remissions and shorter survival than those without myeloid antigens.

Although effective therapy for many patients with ALL has been devised, long-term remission cannot be achieved in about 90% of adults and 30% of children with this disease. Leukemic relapse in these patients cannot be reliably diagnosed by current methods until at least 25% blast cells are present in the bone marrow. Ryan *et al.* (197) have recently reported a FCM method for detection of rare CALLA-positive cells in the peripheral blood. They were able to detect leukemic cells down to the level of 0.001%. Methods such as this may have

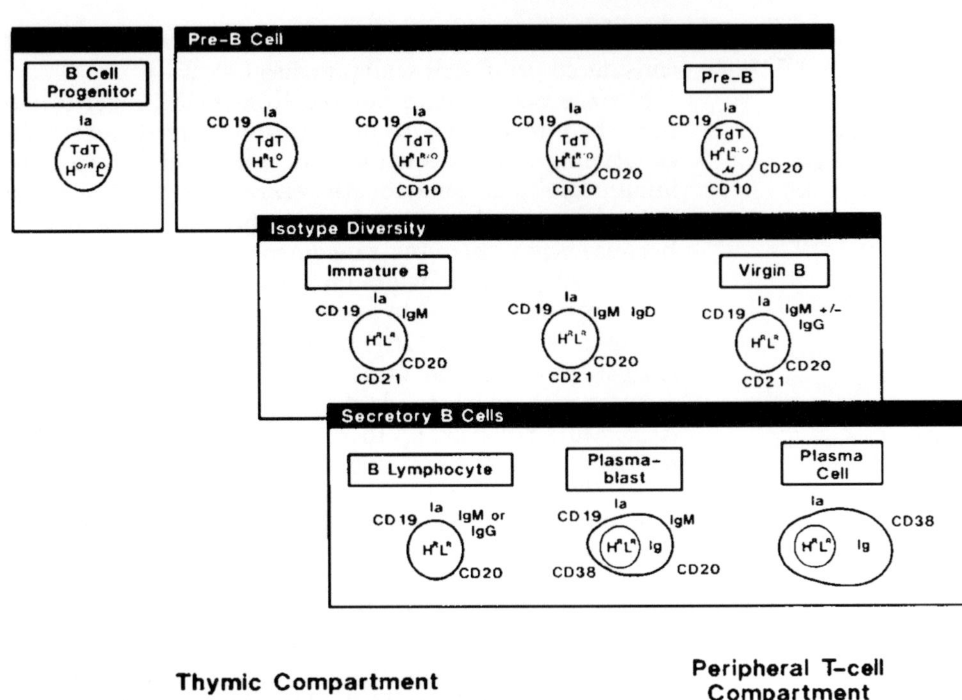

FIG. 8. Schematic representation of human B cell differentiation. *TdT*, terminal deoxnucleotidyl transferase; *H*, heavy chain; *L*, light chain; *O*, germline configuration; *R*, rearranged gene; *n*, cytoplasmic Igm.

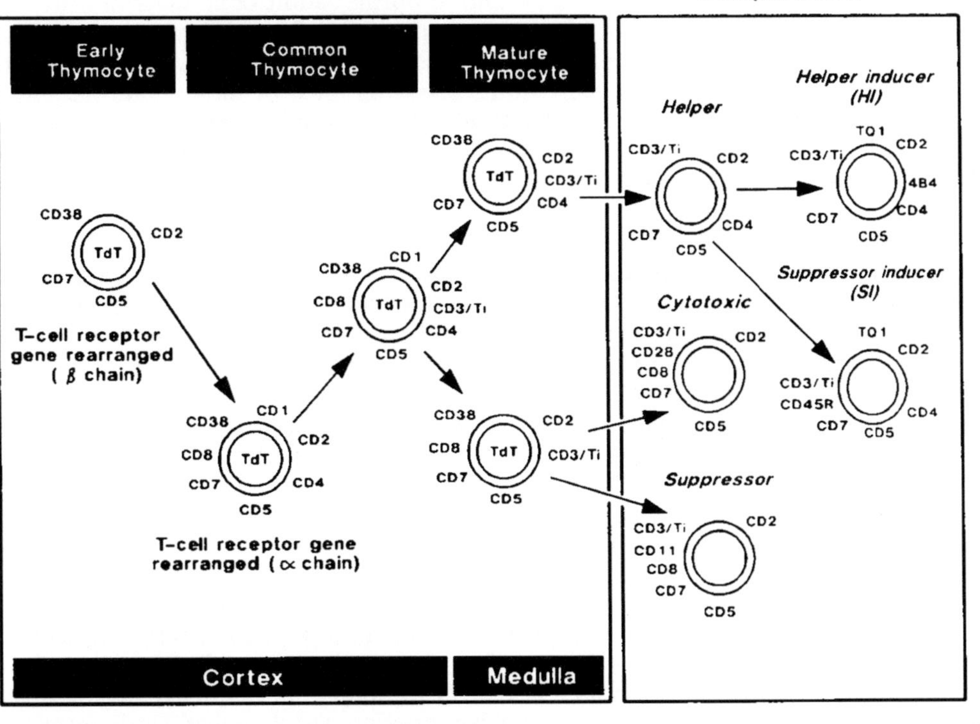

FIG. 9. Schematic representation of human T cell differentiation. *TdT*, terminal deoxnucleotidyl transferase; *Ti*, T cell antigen receptor.

potential for detecting early leukemic relapse which may aid therapy (197).

Non-Hodgkin's Lymphoma. The non-Hodgkin's lymphomas are a diverse group of neoplasms whose pathologic classification is controversial. It is even more difficult to correlate pathologic classification with immunologic classification derived from FCM. Several immunologic patterns have emerged, however, and we will attempt to place them within the non-Hodgkin's lymphoma working classification (169) as well as the Rappaport (13) classification.

Follicular or Nodular Lymphomas. The follicular or nodular lymphomas probably represent neoplastic proliferation of lymph node-derived follicular center B lymphocytes. The cell type may be a small cleaved cell (nodular lymphocytic poorly differentiated lymphocytic lymphoma by the Rappaport classification), mixed small cleaved and large cleaved or noncleaved cells (nodular mixed), or predominately large cell (nodular histiocytic). The first two cell types fall within the working classification as low-grade lymphoma, whereas the latter cell type is classified as an intermediate-grade lymphoma. Although the small cleaved cells will almost always express abundant monoclonal SIg, larger cells may be SIg-negative. However, the small cleaved and large cells will routinely express Ia, CD19, and CD20 antigens, and will often express the CD21 antigen (3). More than half of these cases will also express CD10. Follicular lymphoma cells may be found in the peripheral blood as a "leukemic" phase of the disease (formerly referred to as lymphosarcoma cell leukemia). These cells can usually be differentiated from chronic lymphocytic leukemia (CLL) cells because they may express CD10, which is not expressed on CLL cells (3). Also, they do not express the CD5 pan-T antigen found on CLL cells.

Malignant Lymphoma, Small Lymphocytic. Malignant lymphoma, small lymphocytic (diffuse well-differentiated lymphocytic lymphoma in the Rappaport classification) is a low-grade malignancy, and some cases may be identical to CLL. Also included within this subclassification are the plasmacytoid lymphocytic subgroups with and without an IgM monoclonal gammapathy; some of these cases are similar to Waldenstrom's macroglobulinemia. Surface markers on these small lymphocytic cells include low intensity SIg, receptors for C3 and for the Fc portion of IgG, and Ia, CD20, CD21, CD19, CD24, and other B cell antigens (3).

Malignant Lymphoma, Diffuse Small Cleaved Cell and Diffuse Mixed Small and Large Cell. Malignant lymphoma, diffuse small cleaved cell (diffuse poorly differentiated lymphocytic lymphoma in the Rappaport classification) is an intermediate prognostic group. The cells are B lymphocytes that (similar to follicular lymphoma cells) usually display large amounts of monoclonal SIg. Unlike follicular lymphoma cells, however, they do not usually express CD10. Similar to follicular lymphoma cells, they do not express the CD5 antigen unlike most small lymphocytic lymphomas and CLL which are CD5-positive. However, all these cell types have in common the expression of Ia, CD19, CD20, CD21, and other B cell antigens (3).

Malignant Lymphoma, Diffuse Large Cell and Large Cell Immunoblastic. In the working classification, the diffuse large cell lymphomas are considered within the intermediate prognostic group, whereas large cell immunoblastic lymphoma is a high-grade malignancy. By the Rappaport classification, both of these cell types would be described as histiocytic. This is clearly a misdesignation, since 80 to 90% are B cell tumors. A high percentage of these tumors express transferrin receptor antigens and CD38 (3). Diffuse large cell lymphoma (57 cases) were recently studied and divided into the following subgroups: (a) CD20, CD19, and SIg-positive; CD21-negative (50%); (b) CD20, CD19, SIg, and CD21-positive (30%); (c) CD20 and CD19-positive; SIg and CD21-negative (10%); and (4) CD20 and SIg-positive; and CD21-negative (10%) (78). These data suggest that most of these lymphomas represent the malignant counterpart of B cells at the midstage of differentiation. Ten to 20 percent of cases are T cell lineage; 2% are derived from the monocyte-myeloid lineage.

Tγ Lymphoproliferative Disease. Tγ lymphocytes are a subset of T lymphocytes with receptors for the Fc portion of IgG. A lymphoproliferative disorder made up of predominately Tγ lymphocytes has been described and is referred to as chronic Tγ lymphoproliferative disease. Cells from chronic Tγ lymphoproliferative disease usually contain acid phosphatase and β-glucuronidase and express the pan-T antigens CD3, CD2, the suppressor-associated antigens CD8, and the NK-associated antigen Leu-7 (HNK-1) (190).

Cutaneous T Cell Lymphoma (Mycosis fungoides. Sezary Cell Leukemia). Skin lesions are the most prominent feature of patients with cutaneous T cell lymphoma. In the skin, the malignant cells are referred to as mycosis fungoides cells, and in the peripheral blood as Sezary cells. In most cases, the cells express the phenotype associated with normal helper/inducer T lymphocytes (CD5, CD3, CD4-positive) (133) and function as helper T lymphocytes in *in vitro* assays (26). The 3A1 antibody (CD7), which reacts with 85% of normal circulating T lymphocytes and with mycosis cells in the skin, does not generally react with Sezary cells in the blood (102).

Adult T Cell Leukemia/Lymphoma. Adult T cell leukemia/lymphoma is associated with a human retrovirus designated human T cell leukemia/lymphoma virus-1 (HTLV-1). Common clinical features include a rapid onset of symptoms with rapidly progressive cutaneous lesions and hypercalcemia (28). The malignant circulating cells typically express the phenotype of helper/inducer T lymphocytes and the Tac antigen (CD25) that identifies the IL-2 receptor (224).

(CLL). The B lymphocyte characteristic of CLL displays a relatively small amount of SIg, estimated to be less than 9,000 molecules per cell (221). Relatively weak fluorescence of SIg has been used to distinguish CLL from the leukemic phase of nodular and diffuse lymphocytic lymphomas and from prolymphocytic leukemia in which the cells generally display considerably more SIg (138). Immunoglobulin isotype analyses indicate that most CLL display a single heavy chain class; typically, IgM or IgM and IgD. Less commonly, IgG, IgA or no heavy chain determinant is found. CLL cells display either k or λ light chains but never both. Some data suggest that heavy chain switching can occur in B-CLL, which may indicate increasing maturity of the malignant cell (138). Other studies indicate that CLL cells contain only IgM or IgM and IgD, and that IgG is extrinsic and not synthesized by the leukemic cells (194). B-CLL cells display receptors for mouse erythrocytes, a feature characteristic of immature B lymphocytes (99). The cells also have the receptor for the Fc portion of IgG and complement with a relative increase of C3d receptors (CR2) over C3b receptors (CR1); this is typical of immature B cells (192). B-CLL cells display Ia and human B cell antigens such as CD24, CD20, CD21, and CD19. A curious finding is that B-CLL cells display a 65-kd glycoprotein antigen previously thought to be restricted to T lymphocytes. This antigen was first recognized by using heteroantisera, later, it was recognized with the CD5 monoclonal antibodies (70). The precise meaning of this anomalous expression of a T cell antigen is unclear, although a normal B cell counterpart has been reported in human tonsil and lymph nodes, and stimulation of normal B cells *in vitro* with phorbol ester may induce expression of this antigen (29).

Hairy Cell Leukemia. Hairy cell leukemia (leukemic reticuloendotheliosis) is characterized by invasion of the bone marrow and spleen by morphologically distinct mononuclear cells with "hairy" cytoplasmic projections. Surface markers of hairy cells are most consistent with a monoclonal proliferation of B lymphocytes (115). SIg with a single light chain is frequently identified, as are B cell-associated antigens including Ia, CD20, and CD24 (58). The PCA-1 antigen typically on plasma cells is identified on hairy cells; these data suggest that hairy cells may be pre-plasma cells (2). Perhaps the most convincing evidence for the B cell origin of hairy cells comes from studies of immunoglobulin genes which indicate clonal rearrangement of heavy chain genes and at least one light chain gene. Most cases of hairy cell leukemia demonstrate the 53-kd to 57-kd Tac antigen (CD25) typically identified on certain T cell malignancies and activated T cells (129).

Myeloma and Related Disorders. The malignant B cells of Waldenstrom's macroglobulinemia express SIg and Ia, CD20, and CD19 antigens (131). Unlike CLL cells, however, these cells express the PCA-1 antigen but do not express the CD21 antigen nor do they rosette with mouse erythrocytes (131). The plasma cell and its malignant counterpart, the myeloma cell, represent the most differentiated B lymphocytes. These cells have cytoplasmic immunoglobulin but usually lack SIg and the Ia, CD20, and CD19 antigens. Plasma cells and myeloma cells, like other mature B lymphocytes, usually lack CD10, but a recent study has suggested that rare cases of CD10-positive myeloma represent an aggressive subtype with a poor prognosis (61). Plasma cells and myeloma cells stain intensely with the CD38 monoclonal antibody as well as the anti-PCA-1 and anti-PC-1 antibodies (21).

Acute Myelogenous Leukemia (AML). Because of differences in prognosis and therapy, it is important to distinguish between AML and the lymphoid leukemias. Although differences in morphology and histochemistry often lead to the correct diagnosis, the distinction between immature variants of AML and ALL is not always evident. Monoclonal reagents that identify antigens expressed by myeloid but not lymphoid leukemias (or vice versa) are therefore important. Monoclonal antibodies have been extensively tested for reactivity to myeloid and lymphoid leukemia. Each of the antigenic determinants defined by these antibodies (CD11, CD13, MY8, and CD33) is expressed by more than one-half of patients with AML (53 to 91%), defined as antibody binding by 10 to 20% of malignant cells in each patient. The accuracy of immunologic diagnosis can be extended by using more than one antimyeloid reagent in conjunction with antibodies that detect antigenic determinants uniquely expressed by B or T lymphoid leukemias (CD10, CD20, CD19, and CD3). Occasionally, however, this approach has produced seemingly contradictory results, with the detection of leukemia cells with myeloid and lymphoid differentiation markers. These rare situations may reflect the existence of bipotential clones of malignant cells expressing features of more than one lineage (95).

Chronic myelogenous leukemia (CML). In the chronic phase of the disease, CML is characterized by an overproduction of relatively mature granulocytes. The acute phase (blast crisis) resembles acute leukemia. Approximately one-third of patients with acute-phase CML demonstrate cells with lymphoid features that include the expression of TdT, CD10, Ia, CD20, and rarely cytoplasmic IgM (8). Rearrangements in immunoglobulin heavy and light chain genes have been reported (8). Rare cases of lymphoid acute phase CML with T cell markers have also been reported (97). Acute phase CML involving myeloid cells is heterogeneous; typically, the cells resemble myeloblasts, but erythroblasts, megakaryoblasts, and monoblasts can also be observed (20). Distinction between lymphoid and myeloid acute phase CML is important because of different responsiveness to specific chemotherapeutic agents.

Multiparameter Analysis of Immune Deficiencies

Deficiencies of the immune system can be either congenital or acquired. We will first discuss how cell surface marker analysis has proven useful in the evaluation of suspected congenital deficiencies. The DiGeorge syndrome, which involves developmental abnormalities of structures derived from the third and fourth paryngeal pouches, presents with variable T cell defects. Two-color flow analysis with monoclonal antibodies to T cell subsets has shown a decrease in mature CD3 and CD8 cells. Additional analysis has revealed cells that appear to be frozen at the common thymocyte stage of differentiation (186, 188).

Infants with severe combined immunodeficiency syndrome can be separated into two basic groups; those with genetically determined deficiency of adenosine deaminase and those presenting without the deficiency. The latter group is composed of three phenotypically different subgroups characterized as follows: (a) cells fail to express thymic specific antigens; (b) cells do not show evidence of differentiation beyond the early prothymocyte (transferrin receptor and CD38 positive); and (c) cells express markers of the late thymocyte stage of differentiation ($CD38^+$, $CD4^+$, $CD8^+$, $CD3^+$) (186). This distinction may have implications for therapy.

B cell immunodeficiency consists of a spectrum of diseases. Common variable hypogammaglobulinemia is characterized by recurrent pyogenic infections and a variable age of onset. In most cases, an intrinsic B cell defect is seen, because B cells from such patients fail to proliferate or secrete immunoglobulin after stimulation by Epstein-Barr virus or T cell growth factors. In a minority of cases, B cells are intrinisically normal and there is an excess of T suppressor cells expressing CD8 and HLA-DR antigens (237). The wave of activated suppressor cells may be preceded by a viral infection such as mononucleosis, which may cause elevated suppressor cells. Other B cell defects include X-linked agammaglobulinemia, with a lack of mature B cells but normal T cell populations. The current thinking is that there is a maturational block of pre-B cells (176).

Monoclonal antibodies and immunofluorescence analysis by FCM have provided a highly sensitive and specific approach to phenotypic analysis of cells from individuals with acquired immunodeficiency syndrome (AIDS) and at risk for AIDS. Stites *et al.* (216) have used multiparameter flow analysis to identify previously unrecognized lymphocyte subsets in this disease. Significant changes in helper/inducer (CD4) and suppressor cytotoxic cells (CD8) have been documented by numerous investigators. Nicholson *et al.* (168) have performed two-color analysis of the CD4 subset and have shown that the $CD4^+$, $TQ1^+$ or $CD4^+$ $Leu8^+$ subset, which is involved in induction of suppressor cells is selectively decreased in AIDS-related subjects. Giorgi *et al.* (88) have performed similar studies, but have not shown a selective loss of $CD4^+$ $Leu8^+$ cells. Gupta (98) has also demonstrated that patients exposed to the human immunodeficiency virus, with clinical manifestations of persistent generalized lymphadenopathy have a quantitative deficiency of both $CD4^+$, $4B4^+$ (inducers of help) and $CD4^+$, $2H4^+$ (inducers of suppression) cells.

The CD8 subset is expanded in subjects at risk for AIDS. Virtually all of these cells are $CD8^+/CD11^-$ (cytotoxic T cells). They also have been shown to express Leu7 antigen and HLA-DR. These cells have been characterized as LGLs with cytotoxic activity and may represent an appropriate response to infections or malignancy in AIDS or AIDS-related complex patients. However, Nicholson *et al.* (168) have analyzed the $CD8^+/CD11^-$ subset of cells in human immunodeficiency virus-infected, asymptomatic individuals who progressed to AIDS. They found no significant correlation with elevated $CD8^+/CD11^-$ cell numbers and a more favorable clinical outcome.

Multiparameter Analysis of Cells from Patients with Autoimmune Disease

Systemic lupus erythematosus (SLE) is a disorder characterized by B lymphocyte hyperreactivity resulting in increased immunoglobulin and autoantibody formation. The initial factors responsible for the increased antibody formation are poorly understood. Decreased numbers of T suppressor cells and suppressor function have been proposed as the causes for this defect. However, many SLE patients have relatively increased circulating $CD8^+$ cells, and some workers have found suppressor activity intact. Two-color flow analysis of peripheral blood lymphocytes from SLE patients has demonstrated an increase in $CD8^+$ $Leu7^+$ cells that are capable of suppressing IL-2 production. This defect may be important in the pathogenesis of SLE (140). Additionally, Stohl, Crow, and Kunkel (217) have utilized flow analysis to identify a subgroup of SLE patients who lack the T4 epitope of CD4 on their lymphocytes. This subgroup of predominantly black individuals have a distinct clinical form of SLE, and present with lymphadenopathy. Their cells are capable of responding to mitogenic stimulation but lack the ability to provide help for antibody production.

Two-color flow analysis of cells from rheumatoid arthritis patients has revealed a predominant subset of SIg-positive B cells that also express the CD5 antigen (31). These cells appear to be responsible for rheumatoid factor production and their relative number may be related to disease activity.

Evaluation of Aplastic Anemia by Multiparameter FCM Analysis

Both clinical and laboratory observations have supported an immunologic mechanism for certain disorders of hematopoiesis. Activated suppressor ($CD8^+$) lymphocytes were detected in the circulation of patients with aplastic anemia as defined by the presence of interleukin (IL)-2 receptors and HLA-DR cell surface antigens. These cells were shown to be responsible for interferon production and mediated suppression of normal bone marrow hematopoietic colony formation *in vitro* (247). An understanding of the mechanisms of suppression caused by these cells could aid in designing more effective therapies. It has been shown that antithymocyte globulin treatment of these patients results in reduced interferon and IL-2 production as measured *in vitro*, a lower proportion of circulating lymphocytes expressing IL-2 receptor, and normalizing helper/suppressor lymphocyte ratio.

Multiparameter FCM has also been used in an effort to better define subsets of patients who recover after antithymocyte globulin therapy. However, a study by Torok-Storb *et al.* (223) failed to show a correlation between elimination of activated suppressor cells and clinical recovery. They did demonstrate by FCM, that an elevation of nucleated red cells correlated with clinical recovery.

Functional Cell Studies by FCM

Evaluation of Neutrophil Function. Duque *et al.* (60) have described methods of evaluating neutrophils by FCM. The cells can be examined for a variety of responses including (a) changes in fluorescence intensity of cyanine dyes sensitive to membrane potential; (b) oxidation of 2′7 dichlorofluorescin to 2′7′ dichlorofluorescein; (c) degranulation; and (d) phagocytosis (15, 213). These techniques can elucidate acquired defects in phagocytic cell function in a variety of clinical conditions such as thermal injury and periodontal disease. The loss of cell-associated fluorescence of potentiometric cyanine dyes such as dipentyloxocarbocyanine iodide has been demonstrated to be indicative of cell activation and presumably of a change in the resting transmembrane potential (201). Neutrophils from patients with chronic granulomatous disease are incapable of generating oxygen metabolities and show a decrease in the ability to undergo a change in the fluorescence intensity of dipentyloxocarbocyanine iodide. Bass *et al.* (14) have reported a FCM procedure for the detection of intracellular formation of dichlorofluorescein as an indicator of the activation of the respiratory burst by stimulated neutrophils. Patients with chronic granulomatous disease fail to exhibit significant amounts of dichlorofluorescein formation in neutrophils following stimulation.

Evaluation of Cytotoxic Cells. Interaction of cytotoxic lymphocytes and target cells resulting in conjugate formation is an early step in the multistage process of target cell lysis. The standard method for evaluating lymphocyte target cell conjugates is by cocentrifuging the populations containing the effector and target cells followed by resuspension of the cell pellet under carefully controlled conditions. The number of conjugates is then measured microscopically. This method has obvious limitations, including tediousness and subjective interpretation of results. More recently FCM methods have been developed using fluorescein labeled effector lymphocytes and rhodamine labeled target cells. This method allows for the more accurate quantitation of conjugate formation (148). The cytolytic phase follows the formation of effector cell-target cell conjugates. The assays to measure cell killing have usually employed ^{51}Cr-labeled targets. More recently, Zarcone *et al.* (246) have shown one can use FCM to measure cell killing by counting targets stained with the dye propidium iodide. Viable targets exclude the dye, whereas dead cells do not and become fluorescent.

FCM Evaluation of the Mixed Lymphocyte Culture. The mixed lymphocyte culture is an *in vitro* method for studying HLA disparity between individuals. It is important in organ transplantation. Lymphocytes become activated and proliferate in the presence of lymphocytes from another, non HLA-identical patient. By the use of cell activation markers and cell cycle analysis, Williams *et al.* (243) have adapted this assay for FCM. Dual parameter flow analysis involved analysis of CD4 and CD8 subsets for the expression of the activation markers 4F2 and the IL-2 receptor. Additionally, DNA content analysis was performed to assess cell proliferation by measuring the percentage of cycling cells (% S phase) (243).

Transplantation

FCM has been used to perform postoperative immunophenotypic monitoring of peripheral blood mononuclear leukocytes from transplant recipients. The correlation of an elevated or normal CD4:CD8 ratio with rejection has been noted (23, 41, 48, 214). Other studies, although failing to find such a correlation (30, 173, 208, 231), noted a correlation between depressed CD4 and CD8 cell counts and rejection (208) or between depressed CD4:CD8 ratio and poor prognosis for reversible rejection (30). Elevated CD4 and CD8 cell counts have been used to distinguish cyclosporin nephrotoxicity from renal allograft rejection (208). Inversion of the CD4:CD8 ratio has been shown to correlate with cytomegalovirus infection in cardiac allograft recipients (173).

Activation antigen monitoring has been utilized to strengthen the correlative findings from immunophenotypic monitoring. Increases in the percentage of late differentiation antigen (149), transferrin receptor (111, 149), and IL-2 receptor (39) positive cells correlates with rejection episodes. Using dual fluorescence FCM techniques, the percentage of CD8 positive cells which express HLA-DR was shown to increase 2 to 6 days before clinical symptoms of rejection (230). Another study found that an elevated percentage or absolute number of CD4-positive cells expressing IL-2 receptor correlates with rejection episodes or infection in cardiac transplant recipients (191).

Recent studies have combined immunophenotypic, activation antigen, and functional analysis to monitor hepatic and renal transplant recipients postoperatively. The percentage of CD8-positive lymphocytes which express IL-2 receptors after phytohemagglutinin stimulation is significantly elevated in patients up to 7 days before and during rejection episodes, when compared with stable patients or normal controls (1, 121). Further refinement of this type of multiparameter analysis by FCM will facilitate monitoring the immunoregulatory capability of the transplant patient's immune system postoperatively.

Lymphocyte subsets with different functions often display the same cell-surface antigens (Fig. 10). For example, CD8 is found on both T suppressor/cytotoxic and NK cells. It was recently reported that because CD8 is expressed on both cell types, the T helper/suppressor ratio, as currently performed, is inaccurate (85). If all $CD8^+$ cells are used to calculate this ratio, it will be artificially low, since some $CD8^+$ cells are NK cells. Interestingly, the $CD8^+$ NK cells have a low surface density of CD8 ($CD8^{dim}$), while $CD8^+$ T cells have a high density of this molecule ($CD8^{bright}$). Thus, subcategorizing lymphocytes according to the density of a particular cell-surface molecule may help delineate both function and phenotype of the cells being studied. Another method is to perform two-color FCM analysis to determine whether two different markers are simultaneously expressed. Recently, Ault, Antin, and Ginsburg (4) performed two-color FCM of cells isolated from bone marrow transplant recipients with 25 different pairs of monoclonal antibodies; they defined 6 distinct lymphocyte subsets, accounting for nearly 100% of the total circulating lymphoid cells. These cells included: (a) T helper cells ($CD4^+$) that coexpressed other markers, including CD2, CD3, CD4, CD5, and CD7; (b) T-suppressor cells ($CD8^{bright}$) coexpressing the same markers as the helper T cells; (c) routine B cells expressing CD19 (and no T cell markers); (d) an unusual type of B cells expressing CD19 that coexpressed CD5; (e) NK cells coexpressing CD2, CD11, and CD16; and, finally, (f) NK cells that expressed CD8. The frequencies of the cells described by Ault, Antin, and Ginsburg (4) were quite variable. Using the similar strategy of two-color immunofluorescence, Gebel, Kaizer, and Landay (86) described a dramatic expansion of $CD8^+/CD11^+$ lymphocytes in all bone marrow transplant recipients. Initially, these investigators did not distinguish between $CD8^{bright}$ and $CD8^{dim}$. Functionally, the cells they described inhibited IL-2 production. Based on previous data, these $CD8^+/11^+$ cells were thought to be an expanded population of T suppressor lymphocytes. Upon further study, however, it became apparent that there were at least two populations of $CD8^+/11^+$ cells: one population consisted of $CD8^{dim}/11^+$ cells, while the second contained $CD8^{bright}/11^+$ cells. Patients who had $CD8^{dim}/11^+$ cells could produce IL-2 after mitogen stimulation and, furthermore, had normal NK

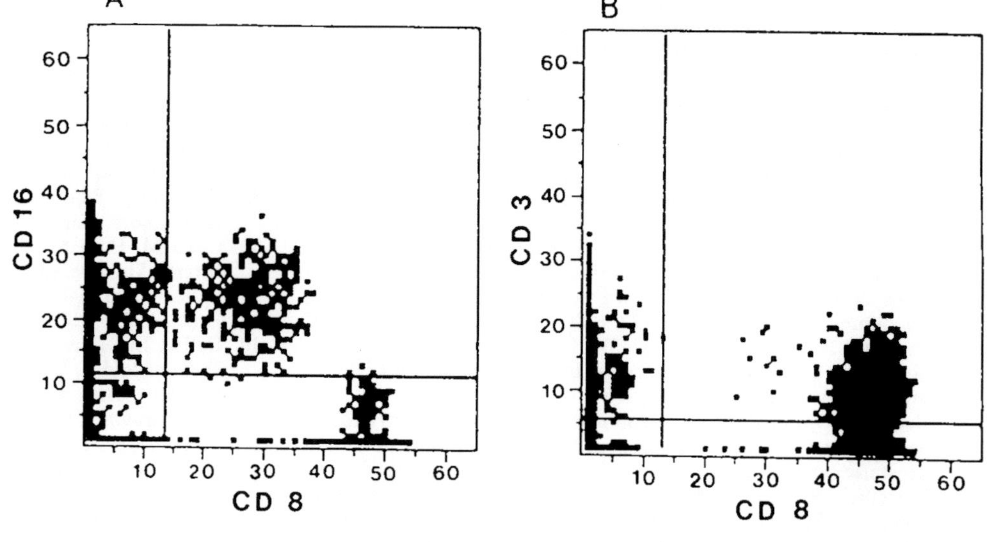

FIG. 10. Dual-fluorescence, flow cytometric analysis of $CD8^+$ cells. Green fluorescence is shown on the X-axis, as detected by fluorescein isothiocyanate (FITC)-labeled CD8. Red fluorescence is shown on the Y-axis, as detected by PE-labeled CD16 and CD3. *A*, Flow histogram showing that $CD8^{dim}$ cells coexpress CD16. *B*, Flow histogram showing the overlap of $CD8^{bright}$ cells with CD3.

function. In contrast, patients with $CD8^{bright}$ cells did not produce IL-2 or have normal NK function.

SUMMARY OF THE SIGNIFICANCE OF FCM TO DIAGNOSTIC PATHOLOGY

FCM may yield clinically useful information in solid tumor patients in carefully specified contexts. Nevertheless the technique has significant limitations at the present time. These include the difficulty in obtaining representative monodisperse cell suspensions for analysis, the fact that histogram interpretation is subjective and controversial, and that cytochemistry, instrumentation, and data analysis vary greatly from laboratory to laboratory. Criteria of laboratory competence and quality control are only partially established. Nevertheless, at least most of these obstacles seem surmountable. Pathologists should play a leading role in integrating FCM data into interpretive surgical pathology reports.

FCM analysis of markers on hematolymphoid cells has proven useful in classifying neoplasms derived from these cells in defining and monitoring immunodeficiency and autoimmune disease, and in organ transplantation. The principal difficulty in this field stems from the limited specificity of the rapidly proliferating reagents and/or the uncertain significance of the markers they detect, leading occasionally to confusing and seemingly contradictory information. FCM assays of cellular function will become increasingly important in the future. Pathologists will need to be increasingly familiar with FCM technology as it moves from the research laboratory to the clinic, and from the academic medical center to a more general clinical laboratory role.

Acknowledgments: We thank Dr. Howard M. Shapiro for helpful discussions, Dr. Seng-jaw Soong for statistical support, Mrs. Mary Meus and Ms. Denise Wiler for help in preparing the illustrations, and Mrs. Sandra Velasco, Mrs. Christine Spano and Ms. Alice Ras for editorial assistance.

This work was supported by National Cancer Institute Grant CA 41040, the Otho Sprague Fund, and the Rayman Research Fund.

Address reprint requests to: Dr. John S. Coon, Department of Pathology, Rush-Presbyterian-St. Luke's Medical Center, 1653 W. Congress Parkway, Chicago, IL 60612-3865.

REFERENCES

1. Anderson J, Kelly M, Economou S, Jensik S, Williams J, Gebel H: Rejection of transplanted organs: a new method of detection. Fed Proc 46:1357, 1987
2. Anderson KC, Boyd AW, Fisher DC, Leslie D, Schlossman SF, Nadler LM: Hairy cell leukemia: a tumor of preplasma cells. Blood 65:620, 1985
3. Anderson KL, Bates MP, Slaugherhopt, Pinkus GS, Schlossman SF, Nadler LM: Expression of human B cell associated antigens on leukemia and lymphomas: a model of human B cell differentiation. Blood 63:1424, 1984
4. Ault K, Antin J, Ginsburg D: Phenotype of recovering lymphoid cell population after bone marrow transplantation. J Exp Med 161:1483, 1985
5. Ault KA, Springer TA: Cross-reaction of a rat-anti-mouse phagocyte-specific monoclonal antibody (anti-mac-1) with human monocytes and natural killer cells. J Immunol 126:359, 1981
6. Badalament RA, Gay H, Whitmore WF, Herr HW, Fair WR, Oettgen HF, Melamed MR: Monitoring intravesical Bacillus Calmette-Guerin treatment of superficial bladder carcinoma by serial flow cytometry. Cancer 58:2751, 1986
7. Baisch HB, Otto U, Kloppel G: Malignancy index based on flow cytometry and histology for renal cell carcinomas and its correlation to prognosis. Cytometry 7:200, 1986
8. Bakhshi A, Minowada J, Anndd A, Cossman J, Jensen JP, Whang Peng J, Waldman TA, Korsmeyer SJ: Lymphoid blast crisis of chronic myelogenous leukemia represent stages in the development of B cell precursors. N Engl J Med 309:826, 1983
9. Balch CM, Murad TM, Soong SJ, Ingalls AL, Halper NB, Maddox WA: A multifactorial analysis of melanoma: prognostic histopathological features comparing Clark's and Breslow's staging methods. Ann Surg 188:732, 1978
10. Banner BF, Chacho MS, Roseman DL, Coon JS: Multiparameter flow cytometric analysis of colon polyps. Am J Clin Pathol 87:313, 1987
11. Banner BF, Tomas-de la Vega JE, Roseman DL, Coon JS: Should flow cytometric DNA analysis precede definitive surgery for colon carcinoma? Ann Surg 202:740, 1985
12. Barlogie B, Alexanian R, Dixon D, Smith L, Smallwood L, Delasalle K: Prognostic implications of tumor cell DNA and RNA content in multiple myeloma. Blood 66:338, 1985
13. Barlogie B, Raber MN, Schumann J, Johnson TS, Drewinko B, Swartzendruber DE, Gohde W, Andreeff M, Freireich EJ: Flow cytometry in clinical cancer research. Cancer Res 43:3982, 1983

14. Bass DA, Pancre JW, DeChatelet LR, Szeda P, Seeds MC, Thomas MT: Flow cytometric studies of oxidative product formation by neutrophils. J Immunol 130:190, 1983
15. Bassoe CF, Solsvik J, Laerum OD: Quantitation of single cell phagocytic capacity by flow cytometry. Flow Cytometry 4:170, 1980
16. Bauer KD, Clevenger CV, Endow RK, Murad T, Epstein AL, Scarpelli DG: Simultaneous nuclear antigen and DNA content quantitation using paraffin-embedded colonic tissue and multiparameter flow cytometry. Cancer Res 46:2428, 1986
17. Bauer KD, Merkel DE, Winter JN, Marder RJ, Hauck WW, Wallemark CB, Williams TJ, Variakojis D: Prognostic implications of ploidy and proliferative activity in diffuse large cell lymphomas. Cancer Res 46:3173, 1986
18. Benson MC, McDougal DC, Coffey DS: The application of perpendicular and forward light scatter to assess nuclear and cellular morphology. Cytometry 5:515, 1984
19. Benson MC, Walsh PC: The application of flow cytometry to the assessment of tumor cell heterogeneity and the grading of human prostatic cancer: preliminary results. J Urol 135:1194, 1986
20. Bettelhein P, Lutz D, Majdin O, Paietta E, Haas O, Linkesch W, Neumann E, Lechner K, Krapp W: Cell lineage heterogeneity in blast crisis of chronic myeloid leukemia. Br J Haematol 59:395, 1985
21. Bhan AK, Nadler LM, Stashenko P, McCluskey RT, Schlossman SF: Stages of B cell differentiation in human lymphoid tissue. J Exp Med 154:757, 1981
22. Bijman JT, Wagener DJT, Wessels JMC, van den Broek P, Ramaekers FCS: Cell size, DNA, and cytokeratin analysis of human head and neck tumors by flow cytometry. Cytometry 7:76, 1986
23. Binkley WF, Valenzuela R, Braun WE, Deodhar SD, Novick AC, Steinmuller DR: Flow cytometry quantitation of peripheral blood T-cell subsets in human renal allograft recipients. Transplant Proc 15:1163, 1983
24. Boon ME, Auer GU, van Kaamnn H, Schwinghammer H: Classifying breast carcinomas with DNA measurements and morphometry. Cytometry 5:469, 1984
25. Bowlby LS, DeBault LE, Abraham SR: Flow cytometric analysis of adrenal cortical tumor DNA: relationship between cellular DNA and histopathologic classification. Cancer 58:1499, 1986
26. Broder J, Edelson RL, Lutzman MA, Nelson DL, MacDermott RP, Dunn ME, Goldman CK, Meade BD, Waldmann TA: The Sezary-syndrome: a malignant proliferation of helper T cells. J Clin Invest 58:1297, 1976
27. Bruchner T, Hiddeman W, Nomann B, Kleinemeir B, Schumann J, Gohde W, Ritter J, Muller KM, von Bassewitz DB, Dressner A, Grundmann E: Differential pattern of DNA-aneuploidy in human malignancies. Pathol Res Pract 179:310, 1985
28. Bunn PA, Schechter GP, Jaffe E, Blayney D, Young RC, Matthews MS, Blattner W, Broder S, Robert-Guroff M, Gallo RC: Clinical course of retrovirus associated adult T cell lymphoma in the United States. N Engl J Med 309:257, 1983
29. Caligaris CF, Gobbi M, Boyill M, Janossy G: Infrequent normal B lymphocytes express features of B chronic lymphocytic leukemia. J Exp Med 155:623, 1982
30. Carter NP, Cullen PR, Thompson JF, Bewick ALT, Wood RFM, Morris PJ: Monitoring lymphocyte subpopulations in renal allograft recipients. Transplant Proc 15:1157, 1983
31. Casali P, Burastero SE, Nakamura M, Inghirani G, Notkins AL: Human lymphocytes making rheumatoid factor and antibody to single stranded DNA belong to Leu 1+ B cell subset. Science 236:77, 1987
32. Chan LC, Pegram SM, Greaves MF: Contribution of immunophenotype to the classification and differential diagnosis of acute leukemia. Lancet 1:475, 1985
33. Chang K, Enker WE, Melamed M: Influence of tumor cell DNA ploidy on the natural history of rectal cancer. Am J Surg 153:184, 1987
34. Chessels JM, Hardisty RM, Rapson NT, Greaves MF: Acute lymphoblastic leukemia in children: classification and prognosis. Lancet 2:1307, 1977
35. Chin JL, Huben RP, Nava E, Rustum YM, Greco JM, Pontes JE, Frankfurt OS: Flow cytometric analysis of DNA content in human bladder tumors and irrigation fluids. Cancer 56:1677, 1985
36. Chin JL, Pontes JE, Frankfurt OS: Flow cytometric deoxyribonucleic acid analysis of primary and metastatic human renal cell carcinoma. J Urol 133:582, 1985
37. Christensson B, Tribukait B, Linder IL, Ullman B, Biberfeld P: Cell proliferation and DNA content in non-Hodgkin's lymphoma. Flow cytometry in relation to lymphoma classification. Cancer 58:1295, 1986
38. Christov K: Flow cytometric DNA measurements in human thyroid tumors. Virchows Arch [B] 51:255, 1986
39. Coles M, Rose M, Yacoub M: Appearance of cells bearing the Interleukin-2 receptor in peripheral blood of cardiac transplant patients and their correlation with rejection episodes. Transplant Proc 19:2546, 1987
40. Collste LG, Darzynkiewicz Z, Traganos F, Sharpless TK, Sogani P, Grabstald H, Whitmore WF, Melamed MR: Flow cytometry in bladder cancer detection and evaluation using acridine orange metachromatic nucleic acid staining of irrigation cytology specimens. J Urol 123:478, 1980
41. Colvin RB, Cosimi AB, Burton RC, Delmonico FL, Jaffers G, Rubin RH, Tolkoff-Rubin WE, Giorgi JV, McCluskey R, Russel PJ: Circulating T-cell subsets in 72 human renal allograft recipients: the OKT4+/OKT8+ cell ratio correlates with reversibility of graft injury and glomerulopathy. Transplant Proc 15:1166, 1983
42. Colvin RB, Preffer FI: New technologies in cell analysis by flow cytometry. Arch Pathol Lab Med 111:628, 1987
43. Coon JS, Bines S, Kheir S, Soong S: DNA flow cytometry in stage I cutaneous melanoma. Cytometry 1 (Suppl):55, 1987
44. Coon JS, Deitch AD, deVere White RW, Koss LG, Melamed MR, Reeder JF, Weinstein RS: Interinstitutional variability in DNA flow cytometric analysis of tumors—the National Cancer Institute's Flow Cytometry Network (NCI-FCN) experience. Cancer, in press
45. Coon JS, Landay AL, Weinstein RS: Flow cytometric analysis of paraffin embedded tumors. Implications for diagnostic pathology. Human Pathol 117:435, 1986
46. Coon JS, Schwartz D, Summers JL, Miller AW, Weinstein RS: Flow cytometry of deparaffinized nuclei in urinary bladder carcinoma. Comparison with cytogenetic analysis. Cancer 57:1594, 1986
47. Coon JS, Schwartz D, Weinstein RS: Markers in the analyses of human urinary bladder carcinoma. Adv Pathol, in press
48. Cosimi AB, Colvin RB, Burton RC, Rubin RH, Goldstein G, Kung PC, Hanson WP, Delmonico FL, Russell P: Use of monoclonal antibodies to T-cell subsets for immunologic monitoring and treatment in recipients of renal alografts. N Engl J Med 305:308, 1981
49. Coulson PB, Thornthwaite JT, Wooley TW, Sugarbaker EV, Seckinger D: Prognostic indicators including DNA histogram type, receptor content, and staging related to human breast cancer patient survival. Cancer Res 44:4187, 1984
50. Crist W, Boyett J, Roper M, Pullen J, Metzgar R, Van Eys J, Ragab A, Starling K, Viotti T, Cooper M: Pre B cell leukemia responds poorly to treatment: a pediatric oncology study group. Blood 63:707, 1984
51. Czerniak B, Herz F, Wersto RP, Koss LG: Expression of Ha-ras oncogene p21 protein in relation to the cell cycle of cultured human tumor cells. Am J Pathol 126:411, 1987
52. Czerniak B, Koss LG: Expression of Ca antigen on human urinary bladder tumors. Cancer 55:2380, 1985
53. Czerniak B, Papenhausen PR, Herz F, Koss LG: Flow cytometric identification of cancer cells in effusions with Cal monoclonal antibody. Cancer 55:2783, 1985
54. Damle NK, Engleman EG: Immunoregulatory T cells circuits in man: alloantigen-primed T cells activate alloantigen-specific suppressor T cells in the absence of the initial antigen stimulus. J Exp Med 158:159, 1983
55. Damle NK, Mohagheghpour N, Engleman EG: Soluble antigen-primed inducer T cells activate antigen-specific suppressor T cells in the absence of antigen-pulsed accessory cells: phenotypic definition of suppressor-inducer and suppressor-effector cells. J Immunol 132:644, 1984
56. Damle NK, Mohagheghpour N, Hansen JA, Engleman EG: Alloantigen-specific cytotoxic and suppressor T lymphocytes are

derived from phenotypically distinct precursors. J Immunol 131:2296, 1983
57. deVere White RW, Olsson CA, Deitch AD: Flow cytometry: role in monitoring transitional cell carcinoma of bladder. Urology 28:15, 1986
58. Divine M, Farcet JP, Gourdin MF, Tabilio A, Vasconcelos A, Andre C, Jouoult D, Bouguet J, Reyes F: Phenotype studies of fresh and cultured hairy cells with the use of immunologic markers and electron microscopy. Blood 64:547, 1984
59. Douglass EC, Look AT, Webber B, Parham D, Wilimas JA, Green AA, Roberson PK: Hyperdiploidy and chromosomal rearrangements define the anaplastic variant of Wilms' tumor. J Clin Oncol 6:975, 1986
60. Duque RE, Phan SH, Hudson JL, Till GO, Ward PA: Functional defects in phagocytic cells following thermal injury. Applications of flow cytometricanalysis. Am J Pathol 118:116, 1985
61. Durie BGM, Grogan TM: CALLA-positive myeloma: An agressive subtype with poor survival. Blood 66:229, 1985
62. Engleman EG, Berike C, Grumet FC, Evans RL: Activation of human T lymphocyte subsets: helper and suppressor/cytotoxic T cells recognize and respond to distinct histocompatability antigens. J Immunol 127:2124, 1981
63. Engleman EG, Warnke R, Fox RI, Dilley J, Beniko CJ, Levy R: Studies of a human T lymphocyte antigen recognized by a monoclonal antibody. Proc Natl Acad Sci USA 78:1791, 1981
64. Evans RL, Wall DW, Platsoucas CD, Siegal FP, Fikrig SM, Testa CM, Good RA: Thymus-dependent membrane antigens in man: inhibition of cell-mediated lympholysis by monoclona I antibodies to TH2 antigen. Proc Natl Acad Sci USA 78:544, 1981
65. Farrow GM: Pathologist's role in bladder cancer. Semin Oncol 6:198, 1979
66. Farsund T, Hostmark JG, Laerum OD: Relation between flow cytometric DNA distribution and pathology in human bladder cancer. Cancer 54:1771, 1984
67. Feitz WFJ, Beck HLM, Smeets AWGB, Debruyne FMJ, Vooijs GP, Herman CJ, Ramaekers FCS: Tissue-specific markers in flow cytometry of urological cancers: cytokeratins in bladder carcinoma. Int J Cancer 36:349, 1985
68. Finan PJ, Quirke P, Dixon MF, Dyson JED, Giles GR, Bird CC: Is DNA aneuploidy a good prognostic indicator in patients with advanced colorectal cancer? Br J Cancer 54:327, 1986
69. Foon KA, Billing RJ, Terasaki P, Cline MJ: Immunologic classification of acute lymphoblastic leukemmia: implications for normal lymphoid maturation. Blood 56:1120, 1980
70. Foon KA, Billing RJ, Terasaki PI: Dual B and T markers in acute and chronic lymphocytic leukemia. Blood 55:16, 1980
71. Fordham MVP, Burdge AH, Matthews J, Williams G, Cooke T: Prostatic carcinoma cell DNA content measured by flow cytometry and its relation to clinical outcome. Br J Surg 73:400, 1986
72. Fossa SD, Pettersen EO, Thorud E, Melvik JE, Ous A: DNA flow cytometry in human testicular cancer. Cancer Lett 28:55, 1985
73. Fossa SD, Thorud E, Pettersen EO, Shoaib MC, Scott-Knudsen O, Ous S: DNA flow cytometry in human bladder carcinoma. Pathol Res Pract 181:291, 1986
74. Fozard JB, Quirke P, Dixon MF, Giles GR, Bird CC: DNA aneuploidy in ulcerative colitis. Gut 27:1414, 1986
75. Frankfurt OS, Arbuck SG, Chin JL, Greco WR, Pavelic ZP, Slocum HK, Mittelman A, Piver SM, Pontes EJ, Rustum YM: Prognostic applications of DNA flow cytometry for human solid tumors. Ann NY Acad Sci 468:276, 1986
76. Frankfurt OS, Greco WR, Slocum HK, Arbuck SG, Gamarra M, Pavelic ZP, Rustum YM: Proliferative characteristics of primary and metastatic human solid tumors by DNA flow cytometry. Cytometry 5:6701, 1984
77. Frankfurt OS, Huben RP: Clinical applications of DNA flow cytometry for bladder tumors. Urology 23 (Suppl):29, 1984
78. Freedman AS, Boyd AW, Anderson KC, Fisher DL, Pinkus GS, Schlossman SF, Nadler LM: Immunologic heterogeneity of diffuse large cell lymphomas. Blood 65:630, 1985
79. Friedlander ML, Hedley DW, Taylor IW, Russell P, Coates AS, Tattersall MHN: Influence of cellular DNA content on survival in advanced ovarian cancer. Cancer Res 44:397, 1984
80. Friedlander ML, Russell P, Taylor IW, Hedley DW, Tattersall MHN: Flow cytometric analysis of cellular DNA content as an adjunct to the diagnosis of ovarian tumours of borderline malignancy. Pathology 16:301, 1984
81. Gadol N, Ault KA: Phenotypic and functional characterization of human Leu1 (CD5) B cells. Immunol Rev 93:24, 1986
82. Gansler T, Chatten J, Varello M, Bunin GR, Atkinson B: Flow cytometric DNA analysis of neuroblastoma. Cancer 58:2453, 1986
83. Gatenby PA, Kansas GS, Xian C, Evans R, Englemann EG: Dissection of immunoregulating subpopulations of T lymphocytes within the helper and suppressor sublineages in man. J Immunol 129:1997, 1982
84. Gatenby PA, Kotzin BL, Engleman EG: Induction of immunoglobulin secreting cells in the human autologous mixed leukocyte reaction: regulation by helper suppressor lymphocyte subsets defined by monoclonal antibodies. J Immunol 127:2130, 1981
85. Gebel HM, Anderson JE, Gottschalk L, Bray RA: Determination of helper:suppressor T cell ratios. N Engl J Med 316:113, 1987
86. Gebel HJ, Kaizer H, Landay AL: Characterization of circulating suppressor T lymphocytes in bone marrow transplant recipients. Transplantation 43:258, 1987
87. Geisinger KR, Homesley HD, Morgan TM, Kute TE, Marshall RB: Endometrial adenocarcinoma: a multiparameter clinicopathologic analysis including the DNA profile and the sex steroid hormone receptors. Cancer 58:1518, 1986
88. Giorgi JV, Nishanian PG, Schmid I, Hultin LE, Cheng H, Detels R: Selective alterations in immunoregulatory lymphocyte subsets in early HIV (Human T-lymphotropic virus type III/Lymphadenopathy associated-virus) infection. J Clin Immunol 7:140, 1987
89. Glazer AN: Light harvesting by phycobilisomes. Ann Rev Biophys Chem 14:4, 1985
90. Glazer AW: Phycobilisomes: structure and dynamics. Ann Rev Microbiol 36:173, 1982
91. Glazer AW, Stryer L: Fluorescence tandem phycobiliprotein conjugates emission wavelength: shifting by energy transfer. Biophys J 43:383, 1983
92. Goh HS, Jass JR: DNA content and the adenoma-carcinoma sequence in the colorectum. J Clin Pathol 39:387, 1986
93. Gray JW: Monoclonal antibodies against bromodeoxyuridine. Cytometry 6:499, 1985
94. Greaves MF, Brown G, Rapson NT, Lister TA: Antisera to acute lymphoblastic leukemia cells. Clin Immunol Immunopathol 4:67, 1975
95. Greaves MF, Chan LC, Furley AJW, Watt SM, Molgaard HV: Lineage promiscuity in hemopoietic differentiation and leukemia. Blood 67:1, 1986
96. Greenebaum E, Koss LG, Elequin F, Silver CE: The diagnostic value of flow cytometric DNA measurements in follicular tumors of the thyroid gland. Cancer 56:2011, 1985
97. Griffin JD, Tantravahi R, Canellos GP, Wisch SS, Reinherz EL, Sherwood G, Beveridge RP, Daley JF, Lane H, Schlossman SF: T cell surface antigen in a patient with blast crisis of chronic myeloid leukemia. Blood 61:640, 1985
98. Gupta S: Subpopulations of CD4+ (T4+) cells in homosexual/bisexual men with persistant generalized lymphadenopathy. Clin Exp Immunol 68:1, 1987
99. Gupta S, Pahwa R, O'Reilly R, Good RA, Siegel FP: Ontogeny of lymphocyte subpopulations in human fetal liver. Proc Natl Acad Sci USA 73:919, 1976
100. Haas D, Feichter G, Gaerttler K, Kaufman M: Influence of systematic errors on the evaluation of the S phase portions from DNA distributions at solid tumors as shown for 328 breast carcinomas. Cytometry 8:377, 1987
101. Hammarberg C, Slezak P, Tribukait B: Early detection of malignancy in ulcerative colitis. Cancer 53:291, 1984
102. Haynes BF, Hersley LL, Jeyasothy BU: Phenotypic characterization of skin infiltrates T cells in cutaneous T cell lymphoma: Comparison with benign T cell infiltrates. Blood 60:463, 1982
103. Hedley DW, Friedlander ML, Taylor IW: Application of DNA flow cytometry to paraffin-embedded archival material for the study of aneuploidy and its clinical significance. Cytometry 6:327, 1985
104. Hedley DW, Friedlander ML, Taylor JW, Rugg CA, Musgrove EA: Method for analysis of cellular DNA content of paraffin-embedded pathological material using flow cytometry. J Histochem Cytochem 31:1333, 1983

105. Hedley DW, Rugg CA, Ng AB, Taylor IW: Influence of cellular DNA content on disease-free survival of stage II breast cancer patients. Cancer Res 44:5395, 1984
106. Helio H, Karaharju E, Nordling S: Flow cytometric determination of DNA content in malignant and benign bone tumours. Cytometry 6:165, 1985
107. Herman CJ, McGraw TP, Marder RJ, Bauer KD: Recent progress in clinical quantitative cytology. Arch Pathol Lab Med 111:505, 1987
108. Hiddemann W, Schumann J, Andreeff M, Barlogie B, Herman CJ, Leif RC, Mayall BH, Murphy RF, Sandberg AA: Convention on nomenclature for DNA cytometry. Cytometry 5:445, 1984
109. Hiddemann W, Wormann B, Ritter J, Thiel E, Gohde W, Lahme B, Henze G, Schellong G, Riehm, Buchner T: Frequency and clinical significance of DNA aneuploidy in acute leukemia. Ann NY Acad Sci 468:227, 1986
110. Horan PK, Slezak S, Poste G: Improved flow cytometric analysis of leukocyte subsets: simultaneous identification of five cell subsets using two-color immunofluorescence. Proc Natl Acad Sci USA 83:8361, 1986
111. Hoshinaga K, Mohanakumar T, Wood NL, Szentpetery S, Lower RR: Increase in transferrin receptors as a marker for rejection and infection in human cardiac transplantation. Transplant Proc 19:2534, 1987
112. Hoshino T, Nagashima T, Murovic J, Levin EM, Levin VA, Rupp SM: Cell kinetic studies of in situ human brain tumors with bromodeoxyuridine. Cytometry 6:627, 1985
113. Hostmark J, Vigander T, Skaarland E: Characterization of pleural effusions by flow-cytometric DNA analysis. Eur J Respir Dis 66:315, 1985
114. Iversen OE: Flow cytometric deoxyribonucleic acid index: A prognostic factor in endometrial carcinoma. Am J Obstet Gynecol 155:770, 1986
115. Jansen J, LeBien TW, Kersey JH: The phenotype of the neoplastic cells of hairy cell leukemia: studies with monoclonal antibodies. Blood 59:609, 1982
116. Joensuu HI, Klemi P, Eerola L: DNA aneuploidy in follicular adenomas of the thyroid gland. Am J Pathol 124:373, 1986
117. Johnson TS, Williamson KD, Cramer MM, Peters LJ: Flow cytometric analysis of head and neck carcinoma. DNA index and S-fraction from paraffin-embedded sections: comparison with malignancy grading. Cytometry 6:461, 1985
118. Kansas GS, Wood GS, Engleman EG: Maturational and functional diversity of human B lymphocytes delineated with anti-Leu-8. J Immunol 134:3003, 1985
119. Kansas GS, Wood GS, Fishwild DM, Engleman EG: Functional characterization of human T lymphocyte subsets distinguished by monoclonal anti-Leu-8. J Immunol 134:2995, 1985
120. Kaplan AS, Caldarelli DD, Cacho M, Bruce DR, Hutchinson J, Conway S, Coon JS: Retrospective DNA analysis of head and neck squamous cell carcinoma. Arch Otolaryngol Head Neck Surg 112:1159, 1986
121. Kelly M, Gebel H, Williams J, Jensik S, Economou S, Anderson J: Immunologic rejection of a renal allograft: prediction with a new peripheral blood assay. Fed Proc 46:1356, 1987
122. Kitchingham GR, Rovigatti U, Mauer AM, Melvin S, Murphy SB, Stass S: Rearrangement of immunoglobulin chain genes in T cell acute lymphoblastic leukemia. Blood 65:725, 1985
123. Klein F, Whitmore W, Wolf R, Herr HW, Sogani P, Staiano-Coico L, Melamed MR: Presumptive down staging from preoperative irradiation for bladder cancer as determined by flow cytometry: a preliminary report. Int J Radiat Oncol Biol Phys 9:487, 1983
124. Klein FA, Herr HW, Whitmore WF, Sogani PC, Melamed MR: An evaluation of automatic flow cytometry (FCM) in detection of carcinoma in situ of the urinary bladder. Cancer 50:1003, 1982
125. Klein FA, Kay S, Ratliff JE, White FK, Newsome HH: Flow cytometric determinations of ploidy and proliferation patterns of adrenal neoplasms: an adjunct to histological classification. J Urol 134:862, 1985
126. Kokal W, Sheibani K, Terz JJ, Harada JR: Tumor DNA content in the prognosis of colorectal carcinoma. J Am Med Assoc 255:3123, 1986
127. Kokal WA, Duda RB, Azumi N, Sheibani K, Kemeny MM, Terz JJ, Harada JR: Tumor DNA content in primary and metastatic colorectal carcinoma. Arch Surg 121:1434, 1986
128. Korsmeyer SJ, Arnold A, Bakhshi A, Ravetch JV, Sieberlist U, Hieter PA, Sharrow SO, LeBien TW, Kersey JH, Podlack DG, Leder P, Waldmann TA: Immunoglobulin gene rearrangement and cell surface antigen expression in acute lymphocytic leukemias of T cell and B cell precursor origins. J Clin Invest 71:301, 1983
129. Korsmeyer SJ, Greene MC, Cossman J, Hsu SM, Jensen JP, Neckers LM, Marshall JL, Bakhshi A, Depper SM, Leonard WJ, Jaffe ES, Waldman TA: Rearrangement and expression of immunoglobulin genes and expression of TAC antigen in hairy cell leukemia. Proc Natl Acad Sci USA 80:4522, 1983
130. Koss LG, Greenbaum E: Measuring DNA in human cancer. JAMA 255:3158, 1986
131. Koziner B, Kempin S, Passe G, Gee T, Good RA, Clarkson BD: Characterization of B cell leukemias: a tentative immunomorphological scheme. Blood 56:815, 1980
132. Kreichbergs A, Tribukait B, Willems J, Bauer HCF: DNA flow cytometry of soft tissue tumors. Cancer 59:128, 1987
133. Kung PC, Berger CL, Goldstein G, Longento P, Edelson RL: Cutaneous T cell lymphoma: characterization by monoclonal antibodies. Blood 57:261, 1981
134. Landay A, Gartland GL, Clemant L: Characterization of a phenotypically distinct subpopulation of Leu 2+ cells which suppress T cell proliferative responses. J Immunol 131:2757, 1983
135. Lanier LL, Le AM, Civin CI, Loken MR, Phillips JH: The relationship of CD16 (Leu11) and Leu19 (NKH-1) antigen expression on human peripheral blood NK cells and cytotoxic T lymphocytes. J Immunol 136:4480, 1986
136. Lanier LL, Le AM, Phillips JH, Warner NL, Babcock GF, Kay HD, Smith DL, Sullivan G, Mandell GL, Donowitz GR: Subpopulations of human natural killer cells defined by expression of the Leu7 (HNK-1) and Leu-11 (NK-15) antigens. J Immunol 131:1789, 1983
137. Lanier LL, Philips JH: A map of the cell surface antigens expressed on resting and activated human natural killer cells. In Leukocyte Typing II, edited by Reinherz RL, Haynes BF, Nadler LM, Bernstein ID, p 57. New York, Springer Verlag, 1985
138. Ligler FS, Kettman JR, Smith G, Frenkel EP: Immunoglobulin phenotype on B cells correlates with clinical stage of chronic lymphocytic leukemia. Blood 62:256, 1983
139. Link M, Warnke R, Finlay D, Amylon M, Miller R, Dilley J, Levy R: A single monoclonal antibody identifies T cell lineage of childhood lymphoid malignancies. Blood 2:722, 1983
140. Linker-Israeli M, Bakke A, Quismonio F, Horwitz D: Correction of interluekin 2 production in patients with systemic lupus erythematosus by removal of spontaneously activated suppressor cells. J Clinical Invest 75:762, 1985
141. Loken MR: Simultaneous quantitation of Hoechst 33342 and immunofluorescence on viable cells using a fluorescence activated cell sorter. Cytometry 1:136, 1980
142. Loken MR, Keij JF, Kelley KA: Comparison of helium-neon and dye lasers for the excitation of allophycocyanin. Cytometry 8:96, 1987
143. Loken MR, Lanier L: Three-color immunofluorescence analysis of Leu antigens on human peripheral blood using two lasers on a fluorescence activated cell sorter. Cytometry 5:151, 1984
144. Loken MR, Parks DR, Herzenberg LA: Two-color immunofluorescence using a fluorescence activated cell sorter. J Histochem Cytochem 25:899, 1977
145. Loken MR, Stall AM: Flow cytometry as an analytical and preparative tool in immunology. J Immunol Methods 50:R85, 1982
146. Look AT, Melvin SL, Williams DL, Brodeur GM, Dahl GV, Kalwinsky DK, Murphy SB, Mauer AM: Aneuploidy and percentage of S-phase cells determined by flow cytometry correlate with cell phenotype in childhood acute leukemia. Blood 60:959, 1982
147. Lovett EJ, Schnitzer B, Keren DF, Flint A, Hudson JL, McClatchey KD: Application of flow cytometry to diagnostic pathology. Lab Invest 50:115, 1984
148. Luce G, Sharrow S, Shaw S, Gallop P: Enumeration of cytotoxic cell target cell conjugates by flow cytometry using internal fluorescent stains. Biofeedback Self Regul 3:370, 1985

149. Lungu O, Reed E, Smith C, Rose E, Marboe C, Hardy M, Reemtsma K, Fenoglio J, Suciu-Foca N: Immunologic monitoring of heart allograft recipients. Transplant Proc 19:2548, 1987
150. Lydyard PM, Youinou PY, Cooke A: CD5 positive B cells in rheumatoid arthritis and chronic lymphocytic leukemia. Immunol Today 8:371, 1986
151. Macartney JC, Camplejohn RS, Powell G: DNA flow cytometry of histological material from human gastric cancer. J Pathol 148:273, 1986
152. Mankin HJ, Connor JF, Schiller AL, Perlmutter N, Alho A, McGuire M: Grading of bone tumors by analysis of nuclear DNA content using flow cytometry. J Bone Joint Surg 67:404, 1985
153. Mauro F, Teodori L, Schumann J, Gohde W: Flow cytometry as a tool for the prognostic assessment of human neoplasa. Int J Radiat Oncol Biol Phys 12:625, 1986
154. McDivitt RW, Stone KR, Craig RB, Palmer JO, Meyer JS, Bauer WC: A proposed classification of breast cancer based on kinetic information. Cancer 57:269, 1986
155. McGuire WL, Meyer JS, Barlosie B, Kute TE: Impact of flow cytometry on predicting recurrence and survival in breast cancer patients. Breast Cancer Res Treat 5:117, 1985
156. McIntire TL, Murphy WM, Coon JS, Chandler RW, Schwartz D, Conway S, Weinstein RS: The prognostic value of DNA ploidy combined with histologic substaging for incidental carcinoma of the prostate gland. Am J Clin Pathol, in press
157. McKinley M, Budman D, Caccese W, Weissman G, Scheidt N, Kahn E, Bronzo R: Evaluation of colonic neoplasia by flow cytometry of endoscopic biopsies. Am J Gastroenterol 80:47, 1985
158. Melamed MR, Enker WE, Banner P, Janor AJ, Kessler G, DarzynKiewicz Z: Flow cytometry of colorectal carcinoma with three-year follow-up. Dis Colon Rectum 29:184, 1986
159. Melamed MR, Klein FA. Flow cytometry of urinary bladder irrigation specimens. Human Pathol 15:302, 1984
160. Mellin W, Roessner A, Grundmann E, Wormann B, Hiddemann W, Immenkamp M: Biological characterization of human bone tumors. VII. Detection of malignancy in a giant cell tumor of bone by flow cytometric DNA analysis. Pathol Res Pract 180:619, 1985
161. Moran RE, Melamed MR: Flow cytometric analysis of human lung cancer; correlation with histologic type and stage. Analyt Quant Cytol 6:99, 1984
162. Morimoto C, Letvin N, Boyd A, Hagan M, Brown H, Kornacki M, Schlossman SF: The isolation and characterization of the human helper inducer cell subset. J Immunol 134:3762, 1985
163. Morimoto C, Letvin N, Distaso J, Aldrich W, Schlossman SF: The isolation and characterization of the human suppressor inducer T cells subset. J Immunol 134:1508, 1985
164. Murphy WM, Chandler RW, Trafford RM: Flow cytometry of deparaffinized nuclei compared to histological grading for the pathological evaluation of transitional cell carcinomas. J Urol 135:694, 1986
165. Murphy WM, Emerson LD, Chandler RW, Moinuddin SM, Soloway MS: Flow cytometry versus urinary cytology in the evaluation of patients with bladder cancer. J Urol 136:815, 1986
166. Nadler LM, Anderson KC, Marti G, Bates M, Park E, Daley JF, Schlossman SF: B4, a human B lymphocyte associated antigen expressed on normal mitogen activate and malignant B lymphocytes. J Immunol 134:2228, 1985
167. Nadler LM, Korsmeyer SJ, Anderson KC, Boyd AU, Slaugherhaupt B, Park E, Jenson J, Coral F, Meyer FJ, Sallar SE, Ritz J, Schlossman SF: B cell origin of non-T cell acute lymphoblastic leukemia: a model for discrete stages of neoplastic and normal pre B cell differentiation. J Clin Invest 74:332, 1984
168. Nicholson JKA, Jones BM, Echenberg DN, Spira TJ, McDougal S: Phenotypic distribution of T cells of patients who have subsequently developed AIDS. Clin Immunol Immunopathol 43:82, 1987
169. The non-Hodgkin's lymphoma pathologic classification project, National Cancer Institute sponsored study of the classification of non-Hodgkin's lymphoma survey and description of a working formalization for clinical usage. Cancer 49:2112, 1982
170. Oi VT, Glaser AW, Stryer L: Fluorescent phycobiliprotein conjugates for analyses of cells and molecules. J Cell Biol 93:981, 1982
171. Oosterhuis JW, deJong B, Cornelisse CJ, Molenaar IM, Meiring A, Idenburg V, Koops HS, Sleijfer DT: Karyotyping and DNA flow cytometry of mature residual teratoma after intensive chemotherapy of disseminated nonseminomatous germ cell tumor of the testis: a report of two cases. Cancer Genet Cytogent 22:149, 1986
172. Ortaldo JR, Sharrow SO, Timonen T, Herberman RB: Determination of surface antigens on highly purified human NK cells by flow cytometry with monoclonal antibodies. J Immunol 127:2401, 1981
173. O'Tolle CM, Maber P, Spiegelhalter DJ, Walker JR, Stovin P, Wallwork J, English TAH: "Rejection of Infection" predictive value of T-cell subset ratio, before and after heart transplantation. Heart Transplant 4:518, 1985
174. Oud PS, Hanselaar TGJM, Reubsaet-Veldhuizen JAM, Meijer JWR, Gemmink AH, Pahlplatz MMM, Beck HVM, Vooijs GP: Extraction of nuclei from selected regions in paraffin embedded tissue. Cytometry 7:595, 1986
175. Oud PS, Henderik JBJ, Beck HLM, Veldhuizen JAM, Vooijs GP, Herman CJ, Ramaekers FCS: Flow cytometric analysis and sorting of human endometrial cells after immunocytochemical labeling for cytokeratin using a monoclonal antibody. Cytometry 6:159, 1985
176. Pearl ER, Vogler LB, Okos AJ, Crist WM, Lawton AR III, Cooper MD: B lymphocyte precursors in human bone marrow: an analysis of normal individuals and patients with antibody deficient states. J Immunol 120:1169, 1978
177. Perussia B, Stann S, Abraham S, Fanning V, Trinchieri G: Human natural killer cells analyzed by B73.1, A monoclonal antibody blocking Fc receptor function. J Immunol 130:2133, 1983
178. Perussia B, Trinchieri G: Antibody 3G8, specific for the human neutrophil Fc receptor reacts with natural killer cells. J Immunol 132:1410, 1984
179. Perussia B, Trinchieri G, Jackson A, Warner NL, Faust J, Rumpold H, Kraft D, Lanier LL: The Fc receptor for IgG on human natural killer cells: phenotypic, functional, and comparative studies with monoclonal antibodies. J Immunol 133:180, 1984
180. Phillips JH, Warner W, Lanier LL: Correlation of biophysical properties and cell surface antigenic profile of percoll gradient-separated human natural killer cells. Nat Immun Cell Growth Regul 3:73, 1984
181. Quirke P, Dyson JED: Flow cytometry: Methodology and applications in pathology. J Pathol 149:79, 1986
182. Robinovitch PS, Torres RM, Engel D: Simultaneous cell cycle analysis and two-color surface immunofluorescences using 7 amino-actinomycin D and single laser excitation: applications to study of cell activation and the cell cycle of murine LY-1 B cells. Immunology 136:2769, 1986
183. Rappaport H: Tumors of the hematopoeitic system. In Atlas of Tumor Pathology, Section B fascile 8, Washington DC, US Armed Forces Institute of Pathology, 1966
184. Raza A, Ucar K, Preisler HD: Double labeling and in vitro vs in vitro incorporation of bromodeoxyuridine in patients with acute nonlymphocytic leukemia. Cytometry 6:633, 1985
185. Redner A, Melamed MR, Andreeff M: Detection of central nervous system relapse in acute leukemia by multiparameter flow cytometry of DNA, RNA, and CALLA. Ann NY Acad Sci 468:241, 1986
186. Reinherz EL, Cooper MD, Schlossman SF, Rosen FS: Abnormalities of T cell maturation and regulation in human beings with immunodeficiency disorders. J Clin Invest 68:699, 1981
187. Reinherz EL, Morimoto C, Fitzgerald K, Hussey RE, Daley J, Schlossman SF: Heterogeneity of human T4+ inducer T cells defined by a monoclonal antibody that delineates two functional subpopulations. J Immunol 128:463, 1982
188. Reinherz EL, Rubenstein AJ, Geha RS, Stel Kaukas AJ, Rosen FS, Schlossman SF: Abnormalities of immunoregulatory T cells in disorders of immune function. N Engl J Med 301:1018, 1979
189. Reinherz EL, Schlossman SF: The differentiation and function of human T lymphocytes. Cell 19:821, 1980
190. Reynolds CW, Foon KA: Tγ lymphoproliferative disease and related disorders in man and experimental animals: a review of the clinical cellular and functional characterization. Blood 64:1146, 1984
191. Roodman ST, Miller LW, Tsai C, Pennington DG, Kanter K, McBride L: Interleukin-2 receptors (IL2R) on T4 cells in cardiac

transplantation. Fed Proc 46:1356, 1987
192. Ross GD, Polky MS: Specificity of human lymphocyte complement receptors. J Exp Med 141:1163, 1975
193. Royer HD, Acuto O, Fabbi M, Tizard R, Ramachardrin K, Smart JE, Reinherz EL: Genes encoding the Tiβ subunit of the antigen MHC receptor undergo rearrangement during intrathymic ontogeny prior to surface T3-Ti expression. Cell 39:266, 1984
194. Rubartelli A, Sitia R, Zicca A, Grossi CE, Ferrarini M: Differentiation of chronic lymphocytic leukemia cells: Correlation between the synthesis and secretion of immunoglobulins and the ultrastructure of the malignant cells. Blood 62:495, 1983
195. Rudenburg CJ, Cornelisse CJ, Heintz PAM, Hermans J, Fleuren GJ: Tumor ploidy as a major prognostic factor in advanced ovarian cancer. Cancer 59:317, 1987
196. Rumpold H, Kraft D, Obexer G, Bock G, Gebhart W: A monoclonal antibody against a surface antigen shared by human large granular lymphocytes and granulocytes. J Immunol 129:1458, 1982
197. Ryan DH, Mitchell SJ, Hennessy LA, Bauer KD, Horan PK, Cohen HJ: Improved detection of rare CALLA-positive cells in peripheral blood using multiparameter flow cytometry. J Immunol Methods 74:115, 1984
198. Schrott RW, Foon KA, Billing RJ, Fahey JL: Immunologic classification of lymphocytic leukemia based on monoclonal antibody defined cell surface antigens. Blood 59:207, 1982
199. Schwartz D, Banner BF, Roseman DL, Coon JS: Multiple "primary" colon carcinomas: A retrospective flow cytometric study. Cancer 58:2082, 1986
200. Scott NA, Grande JP, Weiland LH, Pemberton JH, Beart RW, Lieber MM: Flow cytometric DNA patterns from colorectal cancer—how reproducible are they? Mayo Clin Proc 62:331, 1987
201. Seligmann B, Gallin JO: Use of lipophilic probes of membrane potential to assess human neutrophil activation: abnormality in chronic granulomatrous disease. J Clin Invest 66:493, 1980
202. Shapiro HM: Laser noise and news. Cytometry 8:248, 1987
203. Shapiro HM: Multistation multiparameter flow cytometry: a critical review and rationale. Cytometry 3:227, 1983
204. Shapiro HM: Practical Flow Cytometry. New York, Alan R. Liss, 1985
205. Shapiro HM: Technical developments in flow cytometry. Hum Pathol 17:649, 1986
206. Shapiro HM, Hercher M: Flow cytometers using optical waveguides in place of lenses for specimen illumination and light collection. Cytometry 7:221, 1986
207. Shaw S: Characterization of human leukocyte differentiation antigens. Immunol Today 167:1, 1987
208. Shen SY, Weir MR, Kosenko A, Revie DR, Ordonez JV, Dagher FJ, Chretien P, Sadler JH: Reevaluation of T cell subset monitoring in cyclosporine-treated renal allograft recipients. Transplantation 40:620, 1985
209. Sobol RE, Mick R, Royston I, Davey FR, Ellison RR, Newman R, Cuttner J, Griffin JD, Collins H, Nelson DA, Bloomfield CD: Clinical importance of myeloid antigen expression in adult acute lymphoblastic leukemia. N Engl J Med 316:1111, 1987
210. Sobol RE, Royston I, LeBien TW, Minowada J, Anderson C, Ellison RR, Bloomfield CD: Adult acute lymphoblastic leukemia phenotypes defined by monoclonal antibodies. Blood 65:730, 1985
211. Sondergaard K, Larsen JK, Muller U, Christiansen IJ, Hou-Jensen K: DNA ploidy characteristics of human malignant melanoma analyzed by flow cytometry and compared with the clinical course. Virchows Arch [B] 42:43, 1983
212. Spaar FW, Ahyai A, Spaar U, Gazso L, Zimmermann A: Flow cytophotometry of nuclear DNA in biopsies of 45 human gliomas and after primary culture in vitro. Clin Neuropathol 5:157, 1986
213. Steinkamp JA, Wilson JS, Saunders GC, Stewart CC: Phagocytosis: flow cytometric quantitation with fluorescent microspheres. Science 215:64, 1982
214. Stelzer GT, McLeish KR, Londen RE, Watson SL: Alterations in T lymphocyte subpopulations associated with renal allograft rejection. Transplantation 37:261, 1984
215. Stephenson RA, Gay H, Fair WR, Melamed MR: Effect of section thickness on quality of flow cytometric DNA content determinations in paraffin-embedded tissues. Cytometry 7:41, 1986
216. Stites DP, Casavant CH, McHugh TM, Moss AR, Beal JL, Ziegler JL, Saunders AM, Warner NL: Flow cytometric analysis of lymphocyte phenotypes in AIDS using monoclonal antibodies and simultaneous dual immunofluorescence. Clinical Immunol Immunopathol 38:161, 1986
217. Stohl W, Crow MK, Kunkel HG: Systemic lupus erythematosus with deficiency of the T4 epitope on T helper/inducer cells. N Engl J Med 312:1671, 1985
218. Suarez C, Miller DR, Steinherz PG, Melamed MR, Andreeff M: DNA and RNA determination in 111 cases of childhood acute lymphoblastic leukaemia (ALL) by flow cytometry: correlation of FAB classification with DNA stemline and proliferation. Br J Haematol 60:677–86, 1985
219. Summers JL, Coon JS, Ward RM, Weinstein RS: Prognosis in carcinoma of the urinary bladder based upon tissue ABH and T antigen status and karyotype of the initial tumor. Cancer Res 43:934, 1983
220. Tawa A, Hozumi N, Mindor M, Mak TW, Gelfand EW: Rearrangement of the T cell receptor β chain gene in non-T cell non-B cell acute lymphoblastic leukemia of childhood. N Engl J Med 313:1033, 1985
221. Terynck T, Dighiero G, Follezou J, Binet JL: Comparison of normal and CLL lymphocyte surface Ig determinants using peroxidase labeled antibodies. I. Detection and quantitation of light chain determinant. Blood 43:79, 1974
222. Thorud E, Fossa SD, Vaage S, Kaalhus O, Knudson OS, Bormer O, Shoaib MC: Primary breast cancer: Flow cytometric DNA pattern in relation to clinical and histopathologic characteristics. Cancer 57:808, 1986
223. Torok-Storb B, Doney K, Sale G, Thomas ED, Storb R: Subsets of patients with aplastic anemia identified by flow microfluorometry. N Engl J Med 312:1015, 1985
224. Tsudo M, Uchiyama T, Uchino H, Yodoid J: Failure of regulation of TAC antigen TCGF receptor in adult T cell leukemia cells by the anti TAC monoclonal antibody. Blood 62:1014, 1983
225. Tsukimoto I, Wong KY, Lumpkin BC: Surface markers as prognostic factors in childhood acute leukemia. N Engl J Med 292:828, 1975
226. Tsushima K, Rainwater LM, Goellner JR, Heerden JA, Lieber MM: Leiomyosarcomas and benign smooth muscle tumors of the stomach: nuclear DNA patterns studied by flow cytometry. Mayo Clin Proc 62:275, 1987
227. Valet G, Russmann L, Wirsching R: Automated flow-cytometric identification of colo-rectal tumour cells by simultaneous DNA, CEA-antibody, and cell volume measurements. J Clin Chem Clin Biochem 22:935, 1984
228. van den Ingh HF, Griffioen G, Cornelisse CJ: Flow cytometric detection of aneuploidy in colorectal adenomas. Cancer Res 45:3392, 1985
229. van Driel-Kulker AMJ, Eysackers MJ, Dessing MTM, Ploem JS: A simple method to select specific tumor areas in paraffin blocks using incident fluorescence microscopy. Cytometry 7:601, 1986
230. van Es A, Baldwin WM, Oljans PJ, Tanke HJ, Ploem JS, van Es LA: Expression of HLA-DR on T lymphocytes following renal transplantation, and association with graft rejection episodes and cytomegalovirus infection. Transplantation 37:65, 1984
231. van Es A, Tanke HJ, Baldwin WM, Oljans PJ, Ploem JS, van Es LA: Ratios of T lymphocyte subpopulations predict survival of cadaveric renal allografts in adult patients on low dose corticosteroid therapy. Clin Exp Immunol 52:13, 1983
232. Vindelov LL, Christensen IJ, Nissen NI: A detergent-trypsin method for the preparation of nuclei for flow cytometric DNA analysis. Cytometry 3:323, 1983
233. Vogler LB, Christ WM, Bockman DE, Pearl ER, Lawton AR, Cooper MD: Pre B cell leukemia. A new phenotype of childhood lymphoblastic leukemia. N Engl J Med 298:972, 1978
234. Volm M, Drings P, Mattern J, Sonka J, Vogt-Moykopf I, Wayss K: Relevance of DNA-fluorimetry and short-term resistance testing for adjuvant treatment of non-small cell lung carcinoma. Anticancer Res 6:931, 1986
235. Volm M, Mattern J, Sonka J, Vogt-Schaden M, Wayss K: DNA distribution in non-small-cell lung carcinomas and its relationship to clinical behavior. Cytometry 6:348, 1985
236. Von Roenn J, Kheir S, Wolter J, Coon JS: Significance of DNA abnormalities in primary malignant melanoma and nevi, a retro-

spective flow cytometric study. Cancer Res 46:3192, 1986

237. Waldmann TA, Durm M, Brador J, Blackman M, Blaese RM, Strober W: Role of suppressor T cells in the pathogensis of common variable hypogammaglobulimenia. Lancet ii:609, 1974
238. Watson JV: Oncogenes, cancer, and analytical cytology. Cytometry 7:400, 1986
239. Watson JV, Sikora K, Evan GI: A simultaneous flow cytometric assay for c-*myc* oncoprotein and DNA in nuclei from paraffin embedded material. J Immunol Methods 83:179, 1985
240. Waymouth C: Methods for obtaining cells in suspension from animal tissues. In Cell Separation Methods and Selected Application, edited by Pretlow TG, Pretlow TP, pp 1–29. New York, Academic Press, 1982
241. Weinstein RS, Schwartz D, Coon JS: Blood group antigens and ploidy as prognostic factors in urinary bladder carcinoma. In New Concepts in Neoplasm as Applied to Diagnostic Pathology, edited by Fenoglio-Preiser CM, Weinstein RS, Kaufman N, pp 225–241. Baltimore, Williams & Wilkins, 1986
242. Weiss H, Wildner GP, Jacobasch KH, Heinz U, Schaelicke W: Characterization of human adenomatous polyps of the colorectal bowel by means of DNA distribution patterns. Oncology 42:33, 1985
243. Williams JM, Loeutscher R, Cotner T, Reddish M, Shapiro HM, Carpenter CB, Strominger JL, Strom TB: Dual parameter flow cytometric analysis of DNA content activation antigen expression and T cell subset proliferation in the human mixed lymphocyte reaction. J Immunol 132:2330, 1984
244. Williams NS, Durdey P, Quirke P, Robinson PJ, Dyson JED, Dixon MF, Bird CC: Preoperative staging of rectal neoplasm and its impact on clinical management. Br J Surg 72:868, 1985
245. Wolly RC, Schreiber K, Koss LG, Karas M, Sherman A: DNA distribution in human colon carcinomas and its relationship to clinical behavior. J Natl Cancer Inst 69:15, 1982
246. Zarcone D, Tilden A, Cloud JG, Friedman H, Landay A, Grossi C: Flow cytometry evaluation of cell mediated cytotoxicity. J Immunol Methods 94:747, 1986
247. Zoumbos NC, Gascon P, Djeu J, Trost S, Young N: Circulating activated suppressor T lymphocytes in aplastic anemia. N Engl J Med 312:257, 1985

Biology of Disease

Transgenic Mice—A Gold Mine for Furthering Knowledge in Pathobiology

R. Andrew Cuthbertson and Gordon K. Klintworth

Howard Florey Institute of Experimental Physiology and Medicine, University of Melbourne, Melbourne, Australia, and Departments of Pathology and Ophthalmology, Duke University Medical Center, Durham, North Carolina

INTRODUCTION

"Transgenic" animals, a term introduced by Gordon and Ruddle in 1981 (57), may be defined as those that have integrated foreign DNA in their somatic cells and perhaps their germ line as a consequence of the experimental introduction of DNA (151). Transgenic mice provide a means of exploring the complex molecular biologic effects of a gene in a living animal. The introduction of foreign DNA into both somatic and germ cells of mammals has made it possible to study the molecular basis of tissue-specific and stage-specific gene expression during development, and the phenotypic effects of altered gene expression.

Transgenic mice breed like any other mice and may be created with a gene whose normal function is known, or with newly identified genes whose function is under investigation. Even foreign genes, not normally part of the mouse genome, or mutant forms of normal mouse genes, can be inserted. The inserted genes are stable and can become integrated into the genome of a host at many chromosomal sites. Many newly introduced genes are transcribed appropriately, but the levels of transcription of inserted genes are unpredictable.

Investigators may take advantage of either the overproduction of a normal gene product, or its synthesis in a cell type that does not normally express it, by putting the transgenic structural gene under the direction of abnormal regulatory sequences. The effect of foreign DNA as an insertional mutagen, that may act as a marker for the site of mutation, may also be studied. Ultimately, it may be possible to inhibit the activation of an endogenous gene in a developing mouse, by introducing a gene coding for a messenger RNA (mRNA) that is complementary to the native mRNA (antisense mRNA), thus forming a double-strand and blocking translation (87).

Although most recent publications on transgenic animals have dealt with mice, DNA integration has also been achieved in pigs, sheep and rabbits (70, 71, 173). In addition, transgenic techniques have proved useful in plant breeding and one application is to confer them with resistance to certain diseases. For example, transgenic *Nicotiana tabacum* plants that synthesize the coat proteins for alfalfa mosaic virus develop fewer primary infections, and slower systemic infections after inoculation with two strains of this virus, than plants that do not express the coat protein of alfalfa mosaic virus (118). Transgenic tobacco plants that express modified genes for insecticidal proteins produced by the Gram-positive Bacillus thuringiensis protect the plants from feeding damage by larvae of the tobacco hornworm (209). For further information on transgenic plants the reader is referred to recent publications on the subject (48, 180).

MOLECULAR BIOLOGIC TECHNIQUES

One of the principle uses of DNA cloning technology is to isolate specific genes from the genome. Since an individual mammalian gene represents only a minuscule portion of the organism's total genomic DNA (estimated at about 0.00005%), the isolation of such a tiny fraction of the DNA depends on having a probe that is specific for the gene in question. A number of strategies are available for probe selection or production (116).

The procedure of Southern blotting (195) provides a means of identifying a small region of DNA which bears the gene of interest. The DNA of the genome may be cleaved into fragments of manageable size using restriction endonuclease digestion. The fragments generated are separated according to size by electrophoresis on an agarose gel, and subsequently transferred to a nitrocellulose filter on which they are immobilized. Thereafter the genomic DNA is exposed *in situ* to a specific radiolabeled probe. Nucleotide sequences complementary to the sequence of the gene of interest which have been labeled with a radioactive isotope serve as probes. Specific hybridization between the probe and the related fragment of genomic DNA will occur and can be detected by autoradiography. A comparable technique may also be used for the analysis of RNA (Northern blotting) (126).

The cloning of a fragment of DNA with a suitable vector allows unlimited amounts of it to be produced in a highly enriched form. Cloning vectors include bacterial plasmids (circular, double-standard molecules of extrachromosomal DNA that can replicate autonomously within a bacterial cell) and bacteriophages (viruses that infect bacterial cells) to continue their usual lifestyle after additional sequences of DNA have been inserted into their genome (126). These elements replicate in bacteria just like the original plasmid or bacteriophage and can be obtained in large numbers along with multiple copies of the original foreign DNA fragment. The supercoiled plasmids or bacteriophages are isolated from the bacterial cultures or cell lysates, respectively and from them the cloned molecules of DNA are recovered by digestion with appropriate restriction endonucleases (30).

Fusion transgenes are made *in vitro* by linking the regulatory region of one gene with a structural protein coding region of another gene. The partners in the fusion may be active in separate tissues in normal mice, or may be derived from different species. In the regulatory region, the promoter which controls initiation of transcription, partially dictates whether a cell type will transcribe the transgene. Promoters that have been used in the production of transgenic mice include those for murine α A-crystallin (147, 219), α 2 type 1 collagen (99), murine metallothionein I (68), murine globin (83), and the mouse mammary tumor virus (112). Tissue-specific expression is dictated by some promoters, such as those of metallothionein (liver) (149), elastase-1 (acinar cells of pancreas) (145, 146, 206), globin (erythrocytes) (29), immunoglobulin κ light chains (B lymphocytes) (199) and insulin-genes (islet cells of pancreas) (25). Certain promoters are inducible under specific conditions, such as the murine metallothionein I promoter which is induced by a variety of environmental stimuli including heavy metals and glucocorticosteroids (162). An introduced structural gene fused to the metallothionein promoter may therefore be activated in transgenic mice by including zinc or cadmium in the diet.

Enhancer elements were originally described as viral sequences that increase the utilization of an adjacent promoter, but that can function upstream (towards the 5′ end) or downstream (towards the 3′ end) of a promoter and over some distance. Enhancers have since been identified in the regulatory regions of many eukaryotic genes. Enhancers used in genetic constructs to produce transgenic mice include those of Simian virus 40 (155), the immunoglobulin heavy chain enhancer (2), and the Moloney murine leukemia virus (*i.e.*, the enhancer sequence from that virus) (110).

METHODS USED TO MAKE TRANSGENIC MICE

The production of transgenic mice relies on (a) isolating a particular gene by using DNA technology, (b) converting the gene to a form suitable for insertion into the developing mouse embryo so that it will subsequently be transcribed, (c) implanting and growing the developing transgenic embryo in pseudopregnant female mice and (d) selecting those mice that carry the transgene. Several techniques have been developed for introducing foreign DNA into mammalian cells. We will discuss those relevant to the production of transgenic mice: microinjection techniques, the use of retroviral infection of embryos and transplantation of embryonic or teratocarcinoma cells.

Excellent reviews on the technical aspects of the molecular biology of DNA integration and of the subsequent expression of genes introduced into mice have recently been published (45, 59, 79, 151, 152, 184, 212). A wide variety of genetic constructs have been inserted in transgenic mice (Table 1). These have not necessarily produced disease and this review will concentrate on those transgenic mice where pathologic states have emerged.

Microinjection of DNA into Mouse Eggs

After the first successful production of transgenic mice by the microinjection of cloned DNA into the pronucleus of single cell mouse embryos in 1980 (60) several investigators have had success with this method (18, 19, 36, 213, 215). The method is an adaptation of a technique for injecting nucleic acid into amphibian eggs (65). A cloned DNA sequence up to at least 50 kilobases (kb) could be introduced directly into the mouse genome with this technique (36), which is the most popular for producing transgenic mice.

The method of microinjection is described in detail elsewhere (20, 58, 79). Large numbers of preimplantation embryos are obtained by administering gonadotrophins to females before mating. This hormonal treatment increases the number of eggs that the ovary releases. On the day after these "superovulated" mice are mated, single cell embryos at the pronuclear stage are harvested from the oviducts. After the removal of the cells that surround the ovum (cumulus cells) by hyaluronidase digestion, the eggs are washed free of debris and enzyme and then inoculated with 1 to 2 picoliters of the appropriate plasmid solution (containing about 1 or more μg/ml of linear DNA), using micromanipulators and an inverted microscope. The plasmid solution is slowly injected into one of the pronuclei of fertilized one-cell embryos with a Hamilton syringe connected to a micrometer in the presence of cytochalasin B. This is done while the egg is maintained in position with a blunt pipette. After the introduction of the DNA, the eggs are washed free of cytochalasin B. As an assay for successful pronuclear microinjection, plasmids containing a transcriptionally active gene or fusion gene (such as metallothionein/thymidine kinase or metallothionein/β-galactosidase) can be injected and its expression can be assayed after incubation for 16 to 24 hours (20).

Vasectomized male mice are mated with females to induce a pseudopregnancy, and the microinjected eggs are implanted into the oviduct of the pseudopregnant mouse. Of the microinjected eggs, 50 to 75% survive and a stable chromosomal integration of the foreign DNA occurs in 10 to 40% of the surviving embryos (19, 79, 109, 213, 215). However, in most cases, the integration appears to take place at the single cell stage, as the

Table 1. Some of the Genes Inserted into Transgenic Mice

Promotor/gene[a]	Species	References
Hematopoietic		
Globins		
β	h	29, 83, 101, 124, 196, 208, 215
	m	29, 83
	ra	36, 109, 213
γ	h	101
δ	h	83
Hybrid γ-β	h	101
Hybrid δ-β	h	83
Fetal γ	h	28
Endocrine		
Insulin	h	25, 26, 183, 210
mMT-1/hGH	h	156
r Elastase 1/hGH	h	72, 145, 146
mMT-1/rGH	r	153, 205
GH-releasing factor	h	67
Gonadotropin-releasing factor	m	130
Exocrine		
Pancreatic elastase I	r	206
Muscle		
Myosin light chain 2	r	185
Immunologic		
Immunoglobulin		
μ Heavy chain	m	64, 76
κ Light chain	m	143, 199
λ Light chain		24
μ and κ chains	m	175
Heavy chain μ (γ1)	h	229
Major histocompatibility complexes		
Class 1 (HLA-A2)	h	131
Class 1	p	50
Class II (Eα)	m	113, 161
Eye		
mα A crystallin chloramphenicol acetyl transferase	b	147, 219
γ2 crystallin/lac Z	b	61
mαA crystallin/T-antigen	v	125
σ crystallin	c	102
Serum proteins		
Transferrin	c	54, 134
α-Fetoprotein	m	104, 105
α 1-Antitrypsin	h	178
Bacterial genes		
Neomycin resistant	b	84
Guanine phosphoribosyltransferase	b	92
Hepatitis B virus		
Hepatitis B surface antigens	v	8, 32
Simian virus 40		
mMT-1/T-antigen	v	17
Early region	v	211
Insulin/early region	v	42, 73
Other viruses		
mMT-1/thymidine kinase	v	154
Retrovirus (δ Mo + Py Mo-MLV)	v	210
Human papovavirus JC fragment	v	190, 191
mMTV/v thymidine kinase	v	174
Oncogenes		
mMTV/c-*myc*	m	112, 197
lg(μ)/c-*myc*	m	1, 2
Enzymes		
mMT-1/HPRT	h	201
Other genes		
mMT-1/Somatostatin	r	119, 121
P element	d	98

Abbreviations: b, bacterial; c, chicken; d, drosophila; GH, growth hormone; h, human; HLA, human leukocyte antigen; HPRT, hypoxanthine-guanine phosphoribosyltransferase; *lac* Z, β-galactosidase gene; m, mouse; Mo-MLV, Moloney murine leukemia virus; mMT-1, murine metallothionein-1; mMTV, murine mammary tumor virus; p, pig; r, rat; ra, rabbit; v, virus.

[a] Promoters are given if a specific foreign or abnormal promoter was included as a fusion gene and are preceded by /. When not listed the natural promoter was included in the construct.

foreign DNA is present in every cell of the transgenic animal. In about a fifth of the transgenic mice produced by microinjection of the primitive embryo, integration into the recipient's DNA takes place later, resulting in animals with foreign DNA in only some cells (*i.e.*, mosaics) (36). When two different linear DNA molecules are coinjected, they integrate together (20).

The original transgenic mice are designated "founder" mice and their offspring often continue to carry the gene, indicating that incorporation is into the germ line as well as the somatic cells (36, 57, 154, 196), the foreign gene usually being inherited as a Mendelian trait. This pattern of inheritance after DNA integration does not always occur, as extrachromosomal DNA may persist as autonomously replicating genetic elements in transgenic mice, giving rise to bizzare patterns of inheritance (114, 164).

The site of integration within the host genome appears to be random (109). From one to several hundred copies of the transgene, primarily arranged in a head to tail tandem array (19, 36, 154), normally integrate at a single site (109). The efficiency of introducing foreign DNA into the eggs of mice has been studied by Brinster *et al.* (20) who found that the optimal conditions for integration involve the injection of several hundred molecules into the male pronucleus of fertilized one-cell embryos. They also noted that linear DNA is integrated more efficiently than circular DNA. Furthermore, the efficiency of transgenic mouse production is influenced by the strain of mouse used. For example, mice that carry foreign growth hormones genes can be more easily produced with C57/BL6 × SJL F1 hybrid mice than with inbred C57/BL6 mice (20).

From an analysis of 262 transgenic mouse pedigrees Wilkie, Brinster, and Palmiter (220) found that 30% of mice produced by microinjection of plasmids into pronucleic are mosaic in the germ line. This implies that in these lines integration of the foreign DNA occurred after the first round of chromosomal DNA replication. In adult transgenic mice, the authors always observed uniform distribution of transgenic cells in the nongerm line tissues, but in some of these mice transgenic cells were excluded from the germ line. Thus the germ line and somatic precursor cell pools are distinct from each other apparently being determined before the primary germ layers form, or initially being composed of fewer cells.

Other Methods

While transgenic mice are now most often produced by the microinjection of DNA into fertilized, mouse egg pronuclei, they were first produced in 1974 by microinjecting Simian virus 40 DNA into the blastocoel cavity of early mouse embryos (91). Subsequently other investigators created transgenic mice by exposing early embryos to retroviruses (88, 90, 192).

Embryonic stem cells, like teratocarcinoma cells, retain a pluripotential capability after growth in culture (44). Transgenic mice can also by produced by injecting the genetic construct into embryonic stem cells (171), or teratocarcinoma cells (15, 132, 136, 137) which are then transferred to 3.5-day-old blastocysts of mice. The blastocysts may then be implanted into pseudopregnant foster mothers which eventually give birth to chimeric offspring (15, 80). Transferred pluripotential cells can differentiate into a variety of tissues, and this method enables the investigator to create transgenic animals with cells that may be first subjected to somatic cell mutations in culture. This method of producing transgenic mice may result in animals with both germ cells and somatic cells of different genetic composition (mosaics) (13, 231), and only single copies of the proviral DNA integrate at random sites in the host genome (84).

After the infection of pre-implantation mouse embryos with retroviruses, the primitive cells acquire a genetic marker and their progeny can be followed during subsequent embryogenesis, because the retrovirus does not infect other cells in the embryo after its initial incorporation into nuclear DNA (194).

Another alternative to DNA microinjection into mouse eggs is nuclear transplantation into fertilized mouse eggs from which the pronuclei have been extracted (81, 203). The advantages and disadvantages of these techniques have recently been reviewed (79).

DETERMINING WHICH MICE ARE TRANSGENIC

The presence of the inserted foreign gene can be confirmed by Southern analysis (195) which involves hybridization of an appropriate probe to restriction enzyme cut and electrophoresed DNA samples prepared from extracts of tissue from the mice (154). In the adult, a piece of tail provides enough DNA for analysis, allowing identification of live transgenic mice. The fetal mouse only contains sufficient DNA for analyses after 13 days of gestation, so the incorporation of foreign genes cannot be determined by Southern analysis in mice that are more immature. Transgene transcription may be distinguished from transcription of the endogeneous gene by either marking the transgene with a bacteriophage DNA sequence, or by inserting a gene foreign to the recipient's genome. If the probe is to a bacteriophage marker sequence it should, of course, only exist in the genome of the transgenics, and not in that of the littermates. If a native gene is inserted, it is necessary to compare the transgenic mice with their normal littermates as the transgene will be in a different site and therefore on a different fragment of DNA after endonuclease digestion and electrophoresis.

Transgene expression can be determined by assays of tissue extracts for the relevant messenger RNA (mRNA) and for the protein. The total cellular RNA is extracted from tissues of interest and subjected to Northern blot analysis with a probe complementary to the relevant mRNA sequence.

It is possible to evaluate the relative expression of the gene insert in different tissues with solution hybridization techniques (95, 133) and to establish the site of transgene transcription in tissue with hybridization histochemistry (82). In the latter technique, labeled probes are used to detect the mRNA coding for the proteins of interest in appropriately prepared tissue sections (158).

SPECIFICITY AND REGULATION OF TRANSGENE EXPRESSION

Experiments in transgenic mice are producing insight into two broad areas of gene regulation by studying the site of gene expression (tissue-specific regulation) and the timing of gene expression during development (developmental regulation).

Tissue-Specific Expression

Normal development involves the differential activation of numerous genes in the different cells that make up the organism (127). By generating transgenic mice by inserting genes that are normally transcribed in a tissue-specific manner one may investigate the regulatory effect of adjacent DNA sequences attached to the gene on its 5′ side (*cis*-acting regulatory sequences) on the tissue specificity of gene expression. Mutant genes may then be used to help define the sequences required for accurate tissue-specific transcription.

Usually, tissue specificity has been studied by injecting DNA containing the gene of interest and then harvesting various tissues and assaying for the specific mRNA or its protein product. The degree of confidence that one can make about the preservation of tissue specificity of course depends on the level of gene expression and the sensitivity of the assay system.

The first step in the transcription of DNA involves the binding of RNA polymerase to a specific sequence on it, called a promoter. Hybrid genes may be constructed in which a native structural gene has its level of expression and/or tissue distribution altered by being driven by a foreign promoter, or where the control elements of the gene of interest are used to direct the transcription of a gene whose functional expression can be readily detected ("receptor gene"). Reporter genes may produce tumors in tissues where the gene is activated (22), encode for enzymes, whose activity can be detected by a color reaction in tissues where the gene is expressed (147), synthesize hormones that may be assayed or have functional effects in the animal (66, 67), or produce a peptide that may be detected by using radioimmunoassay (165). One limitation of the use of oncogenes as reporter genes is that neoplasms do not necessarily develop in all tissues in which the gene is activated (112). An example of the usefulness of β-galactosidase hybrid gene constructs for monitoring the activity of gene regulatory elements in transgenic mice has been demonstrated in the crystalline lenses of transgenic mice by Goring *et al.* (61).

Studies of tissue-specific gene expression may be divided into those where genes are transcribed predominantly in one-cell type (*e.g.*, elastase I gene in exocrine pancreas (123, 206) and the κ Ig gene in B-lymphocytes (23, 199)), in several cell types (148), or in many cell types (152). Genes normally expressed in several cell types in transgenic mice include the transferrin gene, where mRNA is found in liver, testis (Sertoli cells), and brain (134), and the α-fetoprotein gene that is induced in fetal liver, the yolk sac, and gastrointestinal cells (104, 105). Palmiter and Brinster (152) have suggested that the analysis of the DNA sequences involved in the regulation of expression of adjacent genes (enhancers), that direct the tissue specificity of these genes, might be more complex for genes expressed in a variety of tissues, than where the expression was more restricted.

As a rule, tissue-specific genes are transcribed appropriately, despite being integrated at an abnormal chromosomal location (152, 186, 187). The level of transcription, however, varies widely among founder animals, which have different chromosomal sites of DNA insertion (29, 145, 146, 154, 208), and for some transgenes the level exceeds that of the native gene. The latter suggests that the maximal expression of a particular gene does not depend on its native chromosomal site.

Variability in gene activation between offspring of a founder transgenic mouse may be due to varying DNA methylation (154), whereas variation between a founder animal and its offspring may be explained by mosaicism of the founder (134), probably caused by the occurrence of several cell divisions before integration of the foreign DNA. The number of DNA sequences inserted correlates poorly with the degree of gene expression (29, 145, 146, 206, 208).

Many human genes are transcribed in transgenic mice (25, 69, 85, 183, 208) apparently in a tissue-specific fashion, suggesting that the signals for tissue-specific expression and their recognition, are conserved throughout evolution (152). Some transgenes contain sequences necessary for tissue-specific transcription and a few kb of flanking sequence. These include the mouse κ and μ immunoglobulin genes (64, 169, 175), mouse and human β-globin genes (29), the rat myosin gene (185) and a major histocompatability complex class II gene (161).

The endogenous murine metallothionein (MT)-1 promoter, isolated from an ubiquitous gene that is continuously transcribed in most cells ('house-keeping' gene), is regulated by a variety of environmental stimuli (96). Heavy metals, such as zinc, provide one such class of stimuli. They are thought to associate with regulatory proteins that bind to promoter sequences on the 5′ side of the transcription start site on the DNA (21). The MT-1 gene is widely transcribed in murine tissues, although at markedly different levels. MT-1 gene expression is maximal in liver, kidney, and intestine (213). As a rule, when used to drive a structural gene the MT-1 promoter expresses the fusion gene in the same tissues as the native gene (156), as long as the regulatory DNA sequences on its own molecule effect is activity. Thus, the MT-growth hormone genes stimulate production of growth hormone in the liver (153, 156). These so-called *cis*-acting regulatory DNA elements that contribute to tissue-specific gene transcription, without usually coding for proteins, may be effectively localized by studying transgenic mice.

Genes whose activation is directed by collagen and viral promoters tend to have wide tissue expression. An example is the gene for murine granulocyte-macrophage colony-stimulating factor, driven by the Moloney murine leukemia virus promoter (110). In this case, the transcription of the hemopoietic growth factor gene, which is normally restricted to specific cell types in bone marrow, is expressed more widely, resulting in expansion and activation of macrophage populations and subsequent tissue damage.

A recent report by Crenshaw *et al.* (40) using a construct containing the rat calcitonin gene-related peptide structural gene, driven by the MT promoter, suggests that specific regulatory machinery processes calcitonin gene related peptide transcripts, and that these regulatory molecules are restricted primarily to neurons.

Developmental Specificity

Developmental timing and tissue-specific gene expression appear to be controlled by the same elements, and transgenes are generally activated at the appropriate developmental time (28). The globin gene family has been an attractive system for the study of gene regulation during mammalian development, as their expression is subject to both tissue-specific and temporal regulation (29, 37, 108). Thus, a hybrid mouse/human β-globin gene is expressed predominantly in erythroid tissues. The regulatory sequences closely linked to the β-globin gene specify a correct pattern of tissue-specific transcription during murine embryogenesis even when the gene is integrated in foreign chromosomal positions (29).

Transgenic mice may be used to address fundamental questions in normal development. For example, during the development of mature spermatozoa, small, highly basic proteins (protamines) replace other testicular basic proteins and histones. In transgenic mice harboring the genes for one of these protamines (mPi) the transgene is only transcribed in round spermatids (159).

Another powerful technique for dissecting developmental molecular events deletes specific cell lineages by microinjecting fertilized eggs with a cells-specific promoter/enhancer used to direct the expression of a cytotoxic gene product. Transgenic mice produced with the elastase 1 promoter fused to the diphtheria toxin A polypeptide structural gene lack a normal pancreas at birth because of expression of the toxic gene in pancreatic acinar cells (150). Using a similar technique with γ^2-crystallin/diphtheria toxin fusion genes transgenic mice have been produced with defective fiber development in the crystallin lens and microphthalmos (16). This ablative technique permits lineage relationships and interactions to be analyzed during development by selectively destroying cohorts of cells activating particular gene.

It is noteworthy that all the information needed for the correct developmental activation of the myelin basic protein (MBP) gene must be included in the 37 kb of DNA that contains the MBP gene and modest amounts of sequences adjacent to it (165).

Regulation of Transgene Expression by Environmental Influences

Transgene expression may be modulated by external influences like heavy metals (149, 202), lipopolysaccharide (41), glucose and amino acids (183), gamma-interferon (161) or hormones such as glucocorticoids (157, 227) and estrogen (68). From an analysis of eukaryotic promoter sequences Maniatis, Goodbourn, and Fischer (127) propose that modified regulatory proteins may play a central role in eukaryotic gene regulation. Glucocorticoid regulation of MT gene expression may contribute to normal murine embryogenesis, and several lines of evidence suggest that corticosterone is the primary inducer of fetal MT-1 mRNA (162).

INACTIVATION OF X-LINKED GENES

Transgenic mice are also useful in studying the inactivation of physically linked genes in the mammalian X-chromosome (54). Despite the fact that the cells of female mammals contain twice the number of X-linked genes than males, they have equivalent amounts of most X-linked gene products. This dosage compensation of X-linked genes results from their inactivation of one of the x-chromosomes in female mammals for reasons that remain incompletely understood. DNA methylation in cytosine-plus-guanine-rich regions near ubiquitous genes that are continuously transcribed in most cells seem to be involved (51, 62, 97, 115, 117, 138, 168, 224, 230), and transgenic mice with foreign genes inserted into the X-chromosome have proved useful in studies related to the inactivation of X-linked genes (54, 104). Several proposed models of X-chromosome inactivation require the presence of specific sequences near genes to permit the spread of inactivation into these regions. Goldman *et al.* (54) predicted and confirmed that a chicken transferrin transgene inserted into the X-chromosome would lack those appropriate signal sequences and thus escape inactivation.

PARENTAL IMPRINTING

Both the paternal and maternal genomes appear to be necessary for normal mammalian development. Available evidence indicates that this is due to the selective expression of autosomal genes that are inherited from each parent. Studies in mice indicate that the transcription of certain genes is preordained by the parent from whom the gene is inherited and that the pattern of transcription correlates with a parentally imprinted methylation of the gene. Transgenic mouse strains containing different genetic inserts support this concept of heritable molecular differences between maternally and paternally derived alleles on mouse chromosomes (166, 177, 204). Swain, Stewart, and Leder (204) noted that the RSV LTR/c-*myc* gene, located on an autosome, is inherited from the male parent, it is expressed in the heart and no other tissue. However, if it is inherited from the female parent, the gene is not expressed at all. During passage through the female parent the transgene became methylated and in the male this methylated state was eliminated during gametogenesis.

IMMUNOLOGIC CONSTRUCTS

Transgenic mice expressing immunoglobulin transgenes have been used to analyze the expression of immunoglobulin genes *in vivo*. Because the expression of the *transgenic* immunoglobulin (Ig) gene predominates in the B lymphocyte pool of such animals (53), this system partially alleviates the experimental difficulties imposed by the massive heterogeneity of antibodies produced in the normal animal, and the limitations imposed by using malignant cell lines frozen in a specific stage of differentiation.

The regulation of Ig gene expression involves genomic rearrangement and splicing, and differential cleavage of mRNA precursors. This control is exerted primarily at the level of transcription, as the transcriptional machinery increases the accessibility of Ig gene sequences to enzymes (recombinases) that catalyze their rearrangements. These changes often involve both parental sets of antibody genes, but only one allele eventually directs the synthesis of a functional immunoglobulin in a given cell. This mechanism of "allelic exclusion" is essential to the process of clonal selection.

The elements that regulate Ig gene transcription, the Ig promoters and enhancers, combine to limit Ig gene expression to B lymphocytes, exclusively. In general, transgenic Ig genes faithfully mimic this pattern of expression, regardless of the site of chromosomal insertion, provided these regulatory sequences are included in a given construct. Ig transgene constructs have recently been extensively reviewed (5, 10, 11, 76, 198, 200).

Ig heavy chains are synthesized in two molecular forms, secreted and membrane-bound, from two differentially spliced mRNAs. The membrane-bound form of the γ-heavy chain is sufficient to mediate allelic exclusion (142). There is good evidence that allelic exclusion at the light chain loci is mediated by intact Ig molecules (169).

Expression of the Ig transgene generally inhibits rearrangement of endogenous Ig genes (142, 169, 216). Hybridomas created from spleen cells of transgenic mice containing a rearranged κ light chain gene that produced the encoded polypeptide (productively rearranged gene), expresses this transgene normally, and this complete Ig molecule turns off light chain gene rearrangement (169). However, in transgenic mice where κ light chain transgenes are not transcribed, or where the level of transcription is low, the endogenous κ genes undergo rearrangement. Bucchini *et al.* (24) have shown that a chicken immunoglobulin transgene can itself be rearranged in the lymphoid lineage of transgenic mice. By introducing a productively rearranged IgM heavy chain gene, Herzenberg *et al.* (76) produced mice with a developmental defect in the B cell pool. The lymphoid tissues of these mice lacked virtually all conventional bone marrow-derived B-cells, indicating a serious defect in B-cell lymphogenesis. In contrast, Ly-1 positive B-cells, which are derived from separate precursors, were unaffected. Apparently, the presence of the transgene interfered with normal B-cell development at an early stage, as abnormalities in endogenous Ig heavy chain gene rearrangements were detected in pre-B cells of these animals.

Thy-1 is a cell surface glycoprotein that is coded for by the immunoglobulin supergene family and mice possess two alleles for the Thy-1 gene (Thy-1.1 and 1.2). The expression of Thy-1 differs markedly amongst various tissues in different species and a model for investigating the mechanisms that regulate the tissue distribution of the Thy-1 gene has been developed by introducing the human Thy-1 and the murine gene Thy-1.1 into the germ line of mice homozygous for Thy 1.2. In such transgenic mice the inserted genes are transcribed in different tissues (56). The human Thy-1 gene is not induced in murine cells, such as thymocytes, that express the equivalent murine mouse gene but is expressed in those tissues that normally express the gene in man, such as kidney tubules, blood vessel endothelium and peripheral nerves (nerve fibers and Schwann cells) despite the fact that murine Thy-1 remains inactive in those tissues. Moreover, the human gene is not induced in cells that express mouse but not human Thy-1 (*e.g.*, thymocytes).

PATHOLOGIC STATES PRODUCED IN TRANSGENIC MICE

The insertion of genes into a normal mouse strain may result in transgenic mice that develop pathologic states (Table 2). On the other hand the introduction of foreign genes into a mutant strain manifesting a pathologic state may cure the naturally occuring disorder. By fusing unusual promoters with native structural genes, researchers may modulate the amount of a product, express it prematurely during development or redirect its expression to cells that do not normally transcribe the gene. The synthesis of selected proteins that are secreted into the circulation may be redirected to larger organs such as the liver resulting in massively increased levels in the plasma. Also, regulatory proteins may be induced in cell types that do not normally do so.

Alterations in Growth Regulation

Normal murine growth depends on the physiologic interplay between hypothalamic releasing factors (growth hormone releasing factor and somatostatin), pituitary production of growth hormone and hepatic production of insulin-like growth factor 1 (IGF-1) (also called somatomedin C). Each of the structural genes in this cascade have been put under the control of heterologous promoters (usually metallothionein) to study the effect of elevated and prolonged production of these peptides.

One of the most evocative examples of transgenesis has been the production of 'giant mice' (139, 153, 156). This has been achieved by introducing either rat (153) or human (139, 156) growth hormone (GH) genes or the human growth hormone-releasing factor (hGRF) (66), driven by abnormal promoters, into the murine genome. Using the pronucleus microinjection technique Palmiter *et al.* (153) introduced a construct (MrGH) consisting of the rat GH structural gene driven by the mouse metallothionein-1 promoter MT-(1), into fertilized mouse eggs. After weaning, the mice were given drinking water containing sufficient $ZnSo_4$ (5,000 ppm), to induce almost maximal levels of MT-1 mRNA in the liver without impairing the breeding potential of mice. Six of the seven resultant mice that carried MrGH the fusion gene gained substantially more weight (up to 1.8 times) than their nontransgenic littermates, and several of these transgenic mice had extraordinarily high fusion mRNA levels in their livers (between 800 and 3,000 GH mRNA molecules/liver cell) and growth hormone in their serum. The consequences of excessive GH production are well documented (167) and are believed mainly to follow from increased somatomedin production in the liver (103). Somatomedin production may explain the excessive size of those transgenic animals that have only slightly higher GH levels than normal.

Animals with several copies of the MrGH gene may have produced excess growth hormone constitutively, without heavy metal induction as the effect of the zinc introduction was equivocal in them (153). Use of the MT-1/rat GH fusion gene ensured that the hormone was produced in tissues expressing the MT-1 promoter (in-

TABLE 2. PATHOLOGIC CHANGES PRODUCED IN TRANSGENIC MICE

Pathologic state[a]	Construct	References
Lesions of pancreas		
β-Cell hyperplasia	r Insulin II/SV40 T antigen	3, 73
β-Cell tumors (not defined)	r Insulin II/SV40 T antigen	3, 73
Fetal exocrine pancreatic tumors	r Elastase I/c-H-*ras*	163
Islet cell adenoma	mMT-1/hGH minus SV40 enhancer	135
Pancreatic carcinoma	r Elastase I/SV40 T antigen	144, 146
Pancreatic agenesis	r Elastase I/diphtheria toxin A	150
Disorders of lymphoid tissue		
B-cell lymphoma	Ig(Eμ)/c-*myc*	2
Lymphoid hyperplasia	Ig (Eμ)/Thy 1.2	31
Lymphomas	Ig(Eμ and Ek)/c-*myc*	1
Lymphocytic (T and B) tumors	mMTV LTR/c-*myc*[b]	112
Perturbed B lymphocyte development	Ig(Eμ)/c-*myc*	111
Thymic hyperplasia	hGHR/SV40 T antigen	14
Thymic depletion	tat Gene of h T-lymphotropic virus type I	140
Renal disorders		
Kidney tumors (type not specified)	JC and BK viruses[b]	190
Glomerular segmental sclerosis	mThy-1.1/hThy-1	100
Tumors of breast		
Mammary gland tumors (type not specified)	m Whey acidic protein promoter/Ha-*ras*[b]	7
Mammary adenocarcinoma	mMTV LTR/c-*myc*[b]	112, 197
Disorders of development		
Abnormal long bone development	mMT-I/c-*fos*	176
Early postimplantation embryonic death	hGH (insertional mutagenic effect)	38, 214
Early postimplantation embryonic death	Retrovirus (insertional mutagenic effect)	193
Limb deformity	mMTV LTR-c-*myc* (insertional mutagenic effect)	225
Ocular abnormalities		
Tumors of crystalline lens	α-A-crystalline/SV40 large T antigen	125
Intraocular macrophages and numerous ocular abnormalities	Mo MLV LTR/mGM-CSF	110
Defective lens formation and microphthalmos	γ-Crystalline/diphtheria toxin A	16
Defective lens development	Mo MLV LTR/c-*mos*	97a
Tumors of liver		
Hepatocellular carcinoma	mMT-1/hGH minus SV40 enhancer	135
Hepatocellular carcinoma	JC and BK viruses	190
Disorders of nervous system		
Peripheral neuropathy with abnormal myelination	mMT-1/hGH minus SV40 enhancer	135
Demyelination of central nervous system	JC virus early region	191
Choroid plexus papillomas	mMT-I/SV40 large T antigen	17, 155
Tumors of peripheral nerves	tat Gene of h T-lymphotropic virus type I	77
Miscellaneous lesions		
Mast cell tumors	mMTV LTR/c-*myc*[b]	112
Salivary gland adenocarcinoma	m whey acidic protein promoter/v-Ha-ras*	7
Mesenchymal tumors	tat gene of h T-lymphotropic virus type I	140
Sertoli cell testicular tumors	mMTV LTR/c-*myc*[b]	112
Skin fibropapillomas	Bovine papillomavirus	107
Adrenal neuroblastomas	JC and BK viruses[b]	190
Cardiac atrial hyperplasia	ANF/TAG	47a
Growth disorders		
Increased somatic growth	mMT-1/rGH	153
Increased somatic growth	mMT-1/hGH-releasing factor	67
Lesions of pituitary gland		
Pituitary hyperplasia	mMT-1/hGH-releasing factor	67
Enzyme disorders		
Lesch-Nyhan model	Cells deficient in HPRT	80
Synergistic Acceleration of Tumor Formation (i.e. happen earlier if both oncogenes present)	Co-expression of mMTV/v-Ha-*ras* and mMTV/c-*myc*	189
Viral diseases		
HBsAg in serum	HBsAg	8
HBsAG regulated by sex steroid	HBsAg	47
Gene therapy		
Correction of murine beta-thalassemia	m and h beta globin	35
Correction of lit dwarf mouse growth	mMT-1/r GH	69
Correction of Eα-deficiency	$E^k\alpha$	113
Correction of hypogonadal mouse	gonadotropin-releasing hormone	130
Correction of shiverer mouse	Myelin basic protein	165
Altered protein products		
Abnormal milk proteins	Sheep beta-lactoglobulin	188

Abbreviations: ANF, atrial natriuretic factor; GH, growth hormone; GHR, growth hormone-releasing factor; GM-CSF, granulocyte macrophage colony stimulating factor; h, human; Ha, Harvey; HBsAg, hepatitis B surface antigen; HPRT, hypoxanthine-guanine phosphoribosyltransferase; Ig, immunoglobin; LTR, long terminal repeat; m, mouse; mMT-1, murine metallothionein promoter-1; mMTV, murine mammary tumor virus; Mo MLV, Moloney murine leukemia virus; MT, metallothionein; r, rat; SV40, Simian virus 40; TAG, SV40 T antigen oncogene Thy, thymocyte.

[a] The pathologic state in most transgenic mice has not been fully characterized by pathologists.

[b] Transgenic mice develop more than one type of neoplasms.

cluding liver, kidney and intestine), instead of the pituitary. The lack of physiologic regulation and the ectopic production of GH in these transgenic mice probably accounted for their accelerated growth. In another study, mice expressing a MT-1 human GH (MhGH) fusion gene were larger than their littermates at weaning, and then grew at 2 to 3 times the normal rate until 11 to 13 weeks (156). Of 33 mice, 22 were 18% or more larger than their littermates at 13 weeks. Growth did not correlate with the number of incorporated copies of the MT/hGH construct in the transgenic mice. Transgenic animals had elevated insulin like growth factors (IGF-1) levels, that were inversely related to circulating hGH, perhaps explaining the poor correlation between circulating hGH levels and rate of growth.

Light microscopy of appropriately stained sections of the pituitary gland in the MhGH transgenic mice (156) disclosed a marked reduction in the number of acidophilic cells (cells making somatostatin and prolactin), presumably due to feedback inhibition by the increased concentrations of hGH or IGF-1. The histologic appearance of the pituitary glands of these transgenic mice resemble those of mice with a genetic deficiency in GH production (*lit/lit* mice) (9).

Because transgenic mice containing the MT-1/rGH fusion gene are expected to express rGH in their islets of Langerhans, Welsh *et al.* (218) studied the translational regulation of GH in islets and found that in β cells, GH follows the normal regulated pathway of secretory granule transport and exocytosis.

Enhanced growth does not depend on a highly homologous peptide because rat and human GH differ in 67 out of 191 amino acids (182) and the experiments by Palmiter *et al.* (153, 156) confirmed the importance of the role of IGF-1 in stimulating the abnormal rate of growth. The mice were normally proportioned rather than acromegalic because the growth activity occurred before closure of epiphyses. The effects of excess production of IGF-1 driven from MT-1 or albumin promoters are currently being studied (152).

The gene for the "major urinary protein" is induced in high levels in the liver of male mice after puberty, due perhaps to the male pulsatile secretion of GH, and its presence has been used as a indication of sexual differentiation in the liver. In male transgenic mice containing either the MT1/rGH or MT1/hGH transgenes, this sex-specific production of the "major urinary protein" by the liver is suppressed (141), presumably as a consequence of the chronic constant production of excessive amounts of growth hormone, which also (141) allegedly stimulates premature aging (152).

Hammer *et al.* (66) examined the consequences of abnormal hGRF gene expression by establishing strains of transgenic mice containing the promoter/regulatory region of MT-1 and the coding region of the human GRF gene. The hGRF promoter protein produced in these animals resulted in measurable amounts of hGRF and increased levels of mouse GH in plasma, as well as accelerated growth rates relative to control littermates. The pituitary glands of these animals were markedly hyperplastic and at least three times normal size. The animals were analogous to humans suffering from a growth disorder associated with elevated serum GH levels, pituitary hyperplasia, and sometimes a GRF-secreting tumor of the pancreas or bronchus (170).

The production of somatostatin in ectopic sites in transgenic mice has not affected growth, in spite of high circulating levels of somatostatin-like immunoreactivity (119). Possible explanations for this normal growth include the fact that most circulating immunoreactive "somatostatin" was neither somatostatin-14, nor somatostatin-28, but rather a 6 kilodalton peptide that may have no biologic activity. Furthermore, the prolonged elevation in circulating somatostatin may have produced desensitization of somatostatin receptors (119).

Both the MT-1/somatostatin and the MT-1/human growth hormone constructs are selectively transcribed in gonadotroph cells of the anterior pituitary (119, 120) and sequences common to both these fusion genes may be responsible for their abnormal gonadotroph-specific expression (121). Somatostatin secretion from these gonadotropic cells can be stimulated by luteinizing hormone releasing factor indicating that a neurosecretory peptide encoded by a foreign gene can enter the regulated secretory pathway of pituitary cells from transgenic mice (121).

Aside from the aforementioned transgenic mice with excessive growth, some transgenic mice manifest retarded growth. For example, when folate metabolism is perturbed by the introduction of foreign dihydofolate reductase genes the resultant mice are smaller than normal and have skeletal, pigmentation and fertility defects (55).

Neoplasms

A recent detailed review of oncogenesis in transgenic mice has been published (74). In many reports, oncogenes have been used in the transgenic constructs, such as the large T antigen of Simian virus 40 (SV40). In some cases the oncogene has been used as a "receptor gene" to study different promoters, whereas other studies have analyzed the role of these genes in development and oncogenesis.

Early experimental systems designed to study the effects of SV40 gene products in oncogenesis did not produce tumors. For example, injection of SV40 into the blastocoel cavity of murine embryos resulted in transgenic mice containing the SV40 genome, but tumors were not noted in these animals (91). A decade later Brinster *et al.* (17) placed the SV40 genes in a plasmid containing the metallothionein fusion gene known to be induced in transgenic animals, to develop an experimental system that would maximize SV40 gene expression. Using this approach, mice containing the SV40 enhancers and genes induced early in the cycle of infection that code for large and small T antigen (207) consistently develop choroid plexus papillomas or carcinomas (17, 155). SV40 large T antigen proteins and mRNA were always present in affected tissues in much greater concentration than unaffected tissues (155). By making mice with constructs consisting of reduced forms of the original transgene, Palmiter *et al.* (155) found that in directing tumors to the choroid plexus the large T antigen was sufficient, the MT fusion gene was dispensable, and that the SV40 enhancer (72 base pair repeat region) played an important role. These choroid plexus tumors exhibit the highest density of serotonin receptors (6,600 fmol/mg protein) found in any tissue (226). The immune system of the transgenic mice that develop choroid plexus tumors to not recognize SV40 antigen, which is part of their transgene, as foreign (46), but most mice that remain tumor-free generate a normal cellular immune response to SV40 after immunization with the virus (46).

When the enhancer sequence is deleted from an SV40 transgene that also contains the methallothionein promoter and the human growth hormone structural gene, different pathologic states ensue, implying a change in the pattern of large T antigen expression. These transgenic mice develop a dysmyelinating peripheral neuropathy and sometimes hepatocellular carcinomas and islet cell adenomas of the pancreas, probably of β-cell origin (135). Nerves from severely affected mice contain a marked paucity of myelin and numerous large and irregular-shaped Schwann cell nuclei. Some Schwann cells have mitotic figures and neurones in the ventral horns of the spinal cord or peripheral ganglia manifest degenerative changes. The peripheral neuropathy is reminescent of Dejerine-Sottas neuropathy in man (232) and the peripheral nerve lesions of trembler mouse mutants (122).

Adams *et al.* (1, 2) investigated the tumorogenic effects of particular constructs by using dysregulated induction of the c-*myc* protooncogene to study the genesis of lymphomas *in vivo*. Using mice bearing the c-*myc* oncogene subjugated to the lymphoid-specific immunoglobulin heavy chain enhancer (Eμ) they showed that the c-*myc* oncogene is a potent inducer of lymphomas (1, 2). No tumors arise within the first year of life in mice carrying either the normal c-*myc* gene and its 5′ flanking region (*i.e.*, the section of DNA to the left or "upstream" of the gene) or the truncated form lacking the noncoding first exon. Therefore, the efficacy and specificity of the Eμ/c-*myc* constructs used to create these transgenic mice are almost certainly due to the immunoglobulin enhancers. The construct bearing Eμ upstream of c-*myc* exon 1, analogous to that found in the mouse plasmacytoma ABPC17 (34) is particularly potent, frequently eliciting a disseminated monoclonal or oligoclonal lymphoma/leukemia with massively enlarged lymph nodes, splenomegaly and an enlarged thymus. The blood almost always contains numerous lymphoblast-like cells (2). The c-*myc* oncogene perturbs B lymphocyte development in the Eμ-*myc* line of transgenic mice (111).

Transgenic mice containing the *tat* gene of human T-lymphotropic virus type I under the control of its own long terminal repeat produces two phenotypes in the absence of other virus genes. One phenotype develops multiple tumors of the nerve sheaths of peripheral nerves and in this regard resembles von Recklinghausen's multiple neurofibromatosis of man (77).

The induction of a variety of oncogenes has been shown to induce neoplasms in transgenic mice, but the mere presence of specific oncogenes does not result in tumor formation, as neoplasms do not develop in all tissues that transcribe the transgene (112). Expression of the *ras* oncogene in acinar cells of the pancreas in transgenic mice induces pancreatic neoplasms (163). Pancreatic adenomas and insulinomas have been produced with promoter/enhancer elements from elastase-1 or insulin genes respectively fused to SV40 T antigen genes (22, 73, 135). Several separate strains of transgenic mice that carry either the v-Ha-*ras* or the c-*myc* gene driven by the mouse mammary tumor virus (MMTV) promoter/enhancer have been produced (189). MMTV/v-Ha-*ras* transgenic mice manifest a diffuse hyperplasia of the Harderian gland, or focal malignant neoplasms of the mammary, salivary and lymphoid tissue. The Harderian gland hyperplasia seems to need only the abnormal action of the v-Ha-*ras* gene, whereas the focal malignancies probably require additional somatic events. When the MMTV/v-Ha-*ras* and MMTV/c-*myc* strains are crossed to yield hybrid mice, their joint action causes a dramatic and synergistic acceleration of oncogenesis. Since these neoplasms arise stochastically and are apparently monoclonal in origin, additional somatic events appear necessary for their full malignant progression, even in the presence of activated v-Ha-*ras* and c-*myc* transgenes. Other examples of oncogene constructs that elicit neoplasms with or without other pathologic changes are summarized in Table 2.

Ocular Manifestations in Transgenic Mice

A naturally occurring tumor of the ocular lens has never been reported suggesting that there is something special about the crystalline lens that prevents malignancy. Mahon *et al.* (125) directed the transcription of an oncogene, the SV40 T-antigen, to the lens in transgenic mice by using the murine α A-crystallin promoter, to determine whether the crystalline lens could be transformed *in vivo*. In these animals large T antigen was detected early in lens development and elicited morphologic abnormalities and specificity interferred with differentiation of lens fiber cells. The affected animals developed neoplasms of the lens epithelium which obliterated the eye and invaded surrounding tissues. Both α- and β-crystallins persisted in many of the neoplastic lens cells, with γ-crystallin was selectively reduced. Light microscopy of tissue sections of the eyes of these transgenic mice disclosed that the lens was replaced by a mass of small, mitotically active anaplastic cells that had grown outside the lens capsule and was infiltrated with blood vessels. An abnormal, multilayered lens epithelium was observed in many areas. Cells from the lens of two founder animals grew rapidly in culture and lacked contact inhibition.

The alpha A crystallin promoter has been used to study lens-specific expression and developmental regulation of the bacterial chloramphenicol acetyl transferase gene (147, 219). Goring *et al.* (61) used the γ_2 crystallin promoter fused to the coding region of the bacterial *lac*Z gene as the transgene construct. An *in situ* assay technique disclosed high levels of β-galactosidase activity exclusively in the central nuclear fiber cells of the crystalline lens of offspring from the three founder mice. Since the δ-crystallin gene of the chicken is not present in the mouse (160) it served as a convenient structural gene marker in a study by Kondoh *et al.* (102). They used the microinjection technique to introduce the δ-crystallin gene into transgenic mice, finding, to their surprise gene induction not only in the lens, but also in pyramidal neurons of the pyriform cortex. If EK mouse carcinoma cells transferred with δ-crystallin gene are injected into mouse blastocyst and then implanted in a foster mother the gene is expressed the crystallin lens of the eye and the brain (102).

Transgenic mice in which the murine granulocyte-macrophage colony stimulating factor structural gene is driven by the Moloney murine leukemia virus promoter (110) develop a striking ocular abnormality. Transgene activation causes retinal degeneration and detachment, cataracts and a marked intraocular accumulation of macrophages mediated by indiscriminant macrophage activation.

Transgenic mice produced with a construct containing the γ-crystallin promoter and diphtheria toxin A polypeptide structural genes, develop microphthalmos secondary to defective lens fiber development (16). Mice homozygous for this foreign gene insert apparently manifest anophthalmos.

Developmental Anomalies

After the startling success with which molecular embryologists studying Drosophila have mapped the genes responsible for pattern formation during development (52), mammalian embryologists have been frustrated by the difficulties of making molecular connections between the phenotype of a dysmorphic mutation and the specific gene in which the mutation occurs. The analysis of mechanisms that control mammalian embryogenesis is hampered by the lack of mutants that affect developmental processes that are understood at a molecular level. In transgenic mice, the foreign DNA occasionally inserts within an endogenous gene. When such an insertional mutation occurs, it disrupts the function of the normal gene and produces inherited developmental anomalies. For example, spontaneous coat-color mutations have resulted from the insertion of a retrovirus in mice (93). With insertional mutagenesis the site of insertion of the foreign DNA is important in the production of the mutation rather than the nature of the inserted construct. The possibility of disrupting a native gene by the insertion of a transgene offers a potential and powerful strategy to study developmental abnormalities. In transgenic mice of this type it is possible to probe the inserted DNA of known sequence, and hence to clone and identify the native gene.

Foreign DNA probably inserts into the host chromosome at a random site, although there may be some bias (152). Disruption of the function of an endogenous gene, or activation of a gene by providing a foreign promoter/enhancer after insertion of foreign DNA would seem possible and even likely. The overall frequency of insertional mutation appears from published data to be about 7% (152). This is, however, almost certainly an underestimate as some mutations will be lethal (38, 75, 128, 181, 214), whereas others may not be morphologically obvious. In mammals, both the insertion of retroviruses into the germline by viral infections of mouse embryos (88) and of recombinant DNA by microinjection into the zygote (152) have been successful at creating transgenic mouse strains that carry mutations that are lethal to early embryos (89, 128, 214) or express the mutation later in embryogenesis causing limb defects, for example (225).

Insertional mutagenesis has been produced in transgenic mice after the injection of plasmid DNA containing the human growth hormone gene into a fertilized egg. Because the gene insertion was lethal at the egg cylinder stage on days 4 and 5 of gestation, shortly after implantation Covarrubias *et al.* (39), proposed that many genes are recruited to activity at about the time of embryonic implantation presenting a large target of vulnerability to mutagenesis.

Most insertional mutations are probably transmitted in a mendelian recessive manner and thus only become apparent after inbreeding of the transgenic offspring. One embryologically lethal mutant results from an insertional mutation in the α-1 collagen gene (75, 181). Transgenic mice containing the exogenous Moloney murine leukemia virus (Mo-MLV) develop normally when the mice are homozygous for the inserted gene at certain loci (Mov1 to Mov12), but when the gene is in certain other loci (Mov 13) the insertion is lethal and associated with embryonic degeneration in the homozygous state by date 15 of gestation (89). An insertion at the Mov 34 locus is also lethal in the homozygous state but when at this locus the embryos die shortly after implantation. By cloning and mapping the integrated provirus and the flanking sequences of this lethal transgenic mouse line (Mov 34), Soriano, Gridley, and Jaenisch (193) demonstrated that proviral integration interferes with the expression of this yet uncharacterized developmentally vital adjacent gene, which is ubiquitously transcribed in normal embryos.

Another transgenic insertional mutation leads to a severe defect in limb formation with fusion of several bones (radius and ulna; tibia and fibula; bones of the feet) and missing bones of the feet (225). This recessive mutation is phenotypically identical to other spontaneous mutations that cause limb deformities (63) and the insertion site is closely linked on chromosome 2 to a dominant mutation (49) that gives rise to a related limb dysmorphism. Thus in this case, the inserted element provides a molecular genetic link to the control of limb morphogenesis in the mammalian embryo.

Transgenic Mice Relevant to Human Viral Diseases

Transgenic inserts of viral genomic material can be used to study the tropism and pathogenicity of viruses. Thus far, this approach has proved useful with hepatitis B virus and the human papovavirus, designated JC virus.

Hepatitis B Virus. The hepatitis B virus (HBV) causes a wide range of manifestations in humans. These manifestations vary from individuals with no apparent disease, acute hepatitis, fulminant hepatitis and, especially in endemic areas, hepatocellular carcinoma. Why specific individuals are affected differently remains poorly understood, but such questions can, and are being addressed in studies on transgenic mice containing inserts of the hepatitis B virus genome.

Chisari *et al.* (32) have produced a chronic hepatitis B surface antigen carrier state in transgenic mice by microinjecting DNA fragments containing the coding regions for the HBV surface antigen (HbsAg), pre-S and X antigens. The normal HBV and inducible promoters were used and gene expression, which was not tissue-specific, was probably influenced by the insertion site and cellular factors. Both HBsAg and pre-S antigens were detectable within the cytoplasm of hepatocytes and renal tubular epithelium. Whereas high serum levels of

HBsAg were detectable and appeared authentic as assessed by antigenicity, polypeptide composition, mean particle diameter and density as well as morphology, tissue damage was not apparent in these transgenic animals, supporting the hypothesis that cellular injury is not a direct consequence of expression of the HBsAg or pre-S regions of the HBV genome.

JC Virus Transgenic Mice. The human papovavirus, designated JC virus, a virus related to BK virus and SV40, contains several genes: genes for the early and late region of the virus and genes for T antigen and viral structural proteins. In humans, this ubiquitous virus causes neurological tumors and a chronic demyelinating disease (progressive multifocal leukoencephalopathy) that usually occur in immunosuppressed individuals (4, 94). JC virus does not produce a detectable abnormality when innoculated directly into mice (206), but a demyelinating disease develops in transgenic mice that contain part of the JC virus (the early region) under the control of JC virus promoter/enhancer elements (191). Half of the founder transgenic mice with this insert were stillborn and four of the others died from tumors of the adrenal medulla early in life. The offspring of two surviving male founders developed a severe tremor on movement and seizures by 3 weeks of age, before succumbing at 4 to 6 weeks. Such affected transgenic mice lack normal myelin sheaths in the central, but not the peripheral, nervous system and this correlates with the expression of JC virus T-antigen in the brain. Phagocytosis of myelin by macrophages is a prominant feature.

Attempts to Produce Transgenic Mice with Specific Disorders

Lesch-Nyhan Syndrome. Hypoxanthine-guanine phosphoribosyltransferase (HPRT) catalyzes the formation of inosinate and guanylate in the metabolism of purine. The gene for this enzyme, which is located on the X-chromosome, has been characterized and cloned. A severe deficiency of HPRT in man results in a neurologic disorder characterized by an excessive production of uric acid, mental retardation, choreoathetosis and a compulsive tendency to self-mutilation. An animal model of this so-called Lesch-Nyhan syndrome would be valuable in studying the disease, as well as in evaluating the potential of treating it by gene replacement. This has been attempted by injecting murine embryonal stem cell lines that are deficient in HPRT into blastocysts of mouse embryos (80) and then implanting the blastocysts into pseudopregnant foster mothers. The resulting female offspring were heterozygous for HPRT-deficiency, but male transgenic mice with the HPRT insert do not develop the clinical phenotype of the human disease.

Kuehn *et al.* (106) have proposed a further potential animal model for Lesch-Nyhan syndrome. They used cultured mouse embryonal cells, mutated by retroviral insertion and selected for loss of HPRT activity to construct chimeric mice. Breeding from the animals has resulted in mutant strains having the same biochemical defects as Lesch-Nyhan syndrome. Transgenic mice containing an MT-1/human HPRT structural gene express HPRT on induction by cadmium and manifest increased levels of human HPRT in the brain (201).

Amyloidosis. Type 1 familial amyloidotic polyneuropathy is characterized by the systemic deposition of a variant of the normal plasma protein transthyretin (formerly designated pre-albumen). In an attempt to establish a model of this disease, Sasaki *et al.* (179) created transgenic mice that produced the variant transthyretin by microinjecting a MT-1/transthyretin variant structural gene construct. Five transgenic mice producing detectable levels of human transthyretin were obtained and three of these showed relatively high serum concentrations (between 0.67 and 1.40 mg/dl). While their levels are still several fold lower than in patients with certain types of familial amyloidotic polyneuropathy, breeding of homozygous mice may manifest these high levels in the animal model.

Autoimmune Diseases. The ability to regulate and direct the expression of genes coding for histocompatibility antigens on various tissues (12) opens up the possibility for exploring the cause and pathogenesis of autoimmune diseases in transgenic mice.

RESISTANCE TO CHEMOTHERAPEUTIC AGENTS

Genes conferring resistance to chemotherapeutic agents can produce resistance to drug toxicity in transgenic animals. For example, a mutant dihydrofolate reductase (DHFR) that is 270 times more resistant to methotrexate (MTX) than the wild-type enzyme was obtained from a mouse fibroblast line grown in high concentrations of MTX. The structural gene for this mutant enzyme has been cloned and transgenic mice containing a construct consisting of it and the SV40 early promoter have been produced (86). Such transgenic animals are relatively resistant to the gastrointestinal side effects of MTX that kills control mice. This murine DHFR gene has also been shown to produce MTX resistance in petunias! (43)

TOLERANCE OF ANTIGENS IN TRANSGENIC MICE

The question of whether transgenic mice will or will not develop tolerance to antigens coded for by the inserted construct depends on the timing of gene expression. For instance, Adams *et al.* (3) produced transgenic mice using the SV40 virus T antigen under the control of the insulin gene regulatory region. Each lineage of the transgenic mice was either tolerant or nontolerant to T antigen. In the nontolerant lines, autoantibodies arose with high frequency and were accompanied by lymphocytic infiltration and disruption of the islets of Langerhans. One might expect the immunologic response to a protein produced by an integrated transgene to be similar to that of other self-antigens, but a high level of serum autoantibodies to T antigen were observed in three of the four transgenic mouse lineages. In these transgenic mice both nontolerance and the autoimmune response appear to be a consequence of the delayed onset of T antigen expression during β-cell development. Thus, the transgenic experiment provides a model of both self-tolerance and autoimmunity.

Correction of Genetic Defects in Transgenic Mice: "Gene Therapy"

The possibility of treating certain inherited diseases by "gene replacement therapy" is under current investigation and details about the potential procedures have recently been reviewed (6, 222).

Bone marrow cells can be readily isolated and cultured in the laboratory and can be efficiently infected with retroviruses. Transfected bone marrow cells may be used, therefore, to deliver genes to animals with genetic diseases characterized by an absence or deficiency of a specific protein. To achieve this mouse bone marrow cells can be transformed with genes fused to promoter genes of retroviruses, and subsequently transplanted into lethally irradiated mice (78, 221, 223). This technique has several disadvantages: (a) the inserted retroviral genes may activate endogenous retroviral genomes in the recipient (78), (b) because numerous random retroviral integrations follow the transfection of multiple marrow cells, some integration may be detrimental to the recipient, (c) the activation of genes in retroviral vectors has proved difficult, especially in human bone marrow cells (172), and (d) bone marrow is probably not an acceptable site for the production of certain proteins.

Another approach for delivering genes in the treatment of certain genetic diseases is by the implantation of fibroblasts transfected with a gene that is defective in the host. Using this method Selden *et al.* (184) found that implants of murine fibroblasts transfected with a human growth hormone fusion gene synthesize and secrete human growth hormone which is detectable in the serum. Such implants of transfected fibroblasts survive for 3 months and their function depends on the location and size of the implant, as well as the histocompatibility of the donor cells with the recipient. The production of human growth hormone by such implants can be modified by regulatory effectors and with appropriate immunosuppression. The transfected cells can be tested for the expression and proper regulation of the transfected gene and for the absence of adverse integration events.

Several experimental studies on "gene therapy" have employed known genetic mutations in mice.

Dwarfism. The primary defect in dwarf mice homozygous for the mutation *little* (*lit/lit*) seems to involve receptors for growth hormone-releasing factor with the result that the somatotroph cells do not produce adequate quantities of growth hormone. This mutant mouse is an experimental model for the human hereditary disorder, isolated GH deficiency type 1, and as in its human counterpart exogenous growth hormone corrects male infertility and stimulates body growth. In one of the first examples of gene therapy for a genetic disorder Hammer, Palmiter, and Brinster (69) restored growth to near normal levels in this *lit/lit* mutant strain by inserting an MT/rGH fusion gene. Attempts to use the human and rat growth hormone genes with their own promoters were unsuccessful. The 'cured' mice containing the fusion gene had massively elevated serum levels of GH and the females were sterile.

Defects in Immune Response. A genetic defect in the immune response has also been corrected by genetic engineering (113, 161, 228). Mutant mice, incapable of expressing endogenous E^d_α genes and thus having macrophages with a restricted ability to present certain antigens to T cells, have been treated by the introduction of a cloned E^d_α gene (113). Transgenic animals containing this insert are able to present a synthetic antigen to T cells, unlike their mutant littermates.

Hypogonadism. Reproductive competence in mammals is dependent upon the correct expression of a gene that encodes the precursor protein for the decapeptide gonadotropin-releasing hormone (GnRH) and the 56-amino acid-containing peptide (GnRH-associated peptide) in hypothalamic neurons. These peptides are released into the circulation where they stimulate the pulsatile release of gonadotropins and suppress prolactin secretion from the anterior pituitary gland. Failure of this system leads to hypogonadism often associated with hyperprolactinemia. The hypogonadal mouse has a deficiency in gonadotropin secretion leading to a failure of postnatal development of the testes and ovaries and consequence sterility. The primary genetic defect in this autosomal recessive condition involves a deletional mutation of at least 33.5 kb encompassing the distal half of the structural gene for the common biosynthetic precursor of GnRH and GnRH-associated peptide (129). This deletion, which removes the two exons that encode for most of the GnRH-associated peptide, results in a transcriptionally active, but translationally incompetent truncated gene. Mason *et al.* (130) introduced a DNA fragment containing the mouse GnRH gene into wild-type mice, and by a series of matings with *hgp*/+ heterozygotes, the transgene was introduced onto a *hpg/hpg* homogygote background. Transgenic *hpg/hpg* homozygotes display tissue-specific induction of the GnRH transgene, reach full sexual maturity, and are capable of mating and raising healthy litters. Pituitary and serum concentrations of lutenizing hormone, follicle-stimulating hormone and prolactin are restored to those of normal controls. Hybridization histochemistry and immunocytochemical studies have disclosed that GnRH expression is restored in appropriate hypothalamic neurons of the transgenic hpg animals, showing neural specific expression of the transgene.

Demyelinatng Disorders. 'Shiverer' mice, which have an autosomal recessive mode of inheritance, manifest characteristic abnormalities including tremor, convulsions and early death. Myelin is deficient in their central nervous system, but the myelin sheaths are only slightly thinner than normal in the peripheral nervous system. Very little myelin is observed around the axons in their central nervous system, including the optic nerves, which lacks myelin basic protein (MBP). Mice homozygous for the 'shiverer' state have been successfully treated by introducing the wild-type MBP gene into their genome (165). In shiverer mice homozygous for the transgene normal appearing myelin with major dense and interperiod lines surrounds most axons. These transgenic mice support the hypothesis that the phenotypic changes in the shiverer mice result from a deletion of the MBP gene.

Thalassemias. The thalassemias are characterized by anemia and morphologically abnormal erythrocytes (hypochromia, microcytosis, target cells and poikilocytosis), and are due to structurally normal hemoglobin that is synthesized at a decreased rate. Murine β-thalassemia (mutant $Hbt^{th\text{-}1}$) can be reversed by the introduction of the natural human β-globin gene which codes for functional β-globin chains, into their genome (35) and such, transgenic mice with the inserted human β-globin gene are larger than the β-thalassemic mutant.

SYNTHESIS OF IMPORTANT PROTEINS

The feasibility of "genetic farming" of complex heterologous proteins that are extensively modified after genetic translation, has been demonstrated in transgenic mice that synthesize human factor IX, the substance that is deficient in human hemophilia B (33). Such mice transcribe high levels of human factor IX mRNA and produce a γ-carboxylated glycosylated protein that is indistinguishable from normal human plasma factor IX, even from the standpoint of biological clotting activity. Insertion of exogenously rearranged Ig genes into transgenic mice has been suggested as a new strategy for making human monoclonal antibodies (27). These observations support the belief that larger transgenic livestock could be used for future production of certain medically important compounds.

Transgenic mice also illustrate the potential for improving the milk composition of cattle by gene transfer. The mammary glands of transgenic mice carrying the sheep beta-lactoglobulin gene (not present in normal mice), synthesize abundant quantities of β-lactoglobulin during lactation (188).

VALUE OF TRANSGENIC MICE: PROSPECTIVE

As we have emphasized in this review, it is possible to use gene transfer to (a) study the molecular basis of tissue-specific and stage-specific gene expression during animal development; (b) investigate the phenotypic effects of altered gene expression, and (c) explore the effects of insertional mutagenesis. These approaches allow new experimental strategies for answering basic questions in many areas of mammalian biology, and will continue to provide new animal models for human diseases. Transgenic mice are also useful in assessing the feasibility of gene replacement therapy in genetic diseases in which a specific protein is absent or defective. The effect of gene replacement can be evaluated in spontaneously occurring inherited disorders in mice.

By studying transgenic mice with genes coding for growth, disease resistance, or for proteins of medical or scientific value the feasibility of having such genes expressed in domestic farm animals can be evaluated. Improvements in understanding the phenotypic activation of gene expression, the development of effective nucleotide constructs that are complementary to the native DNA (antisense constructs) (87), and the understanding of inducible promoters that will provide the tight control of gene expression, will make transgenic mice even more powerful and versatile in exploring questions in pathobiology. Using these tools transgenic animals will furnish opportunities for answering basic questions in areas such as oncogenesis, as well as on the pathogenesis of diseases produced by viruses.

The daunting fact that the production of a single transgenic mouse line potentially creates hundreds or even thousands of hours of subsequent work for biologists emphasizes the importance of asking the right questions of this new and bountiful technique. Undoubtedly the impact of transgenic technology on basic studies in pathobiology, neurobiology, immunology and normal as well as perturbed development will be immense.

Acknowledgments: The authors would like to thank Drs. Lynn Corcoran and F. Stephen Vogel for constructively criticizing this manuscript.

This work was supported in part by grants-in-aid from the National Health and Medical Research Council of Australia, the Meyer Family Trusts, the Ian Potter Foundation, and the Howard Florey Biomedical Foundation, and by grants from the National Eye Institute (RO1-EY-00146 and P30-EY-05722).

R. A. C. is an Australian Post-Doctoral Fellow of the Australian National Health and Medical Research Council.

Address reprint requests to: Gordon K. Klintworth, M.D., Ph.D., Department of Pathology, Duke University Medical Center, Durham, NC 27710.

REFERENCES

1. Adams JM, Harris AW, Langdon WY, Pinkert CA, Brinster RL, Palmiter RD, Corcoran LM, Alexander WS, Graham MW and Cory S: c-*Myc*-induced lymphomagenesis in transgenic mice and the role of the Fr-1 locus in lymphoid neoplasia. Curr Trop Micro Immunol 132:1, 1986
2. Adams JM, Harris AW, Pinkert CA, Corcoran LM, Alexander WS, Cory S, Palmiter RD, Brinster RL: The c-*myc* oncogene driven by immunoglobulin enhancers induces lymphoid malignancy in transgenic mice. Nature 318:533, 1985
3. Adams TE, Alpert S, Hanahan D: Non-tolerance and autoantibodies to a transgenic self antigen expressed in pancreatic beta cells. Nature 325:223, 1987
4. Aksamit AJ, Major EO, Ghatak NR, Sidhu GS, Paraisi JE, Guccion JG: Diagnosis of progressive multifocal leukoencephalopathy by brain biopsy with biotin labelled DNA: DNA *in situ* hybridization. J Neuropathol Exp Neurol 46:556, 1987
5. Alt F, Blackwell TK, Yancopoulos GD: Immunoglobulin genes in transgenic mice. Trends Genet 1:231, 1985
6. Anderson WF: Prospects for human gene therapy. Science 226:401, 1984
7. Andres A-C, Schönenberger C-A, Groner B, Henninghausen L, LeMeur M, Gerlinger P: Ha-*ras* oncogene expression directed by a milk protein gene promotion tissue specificity, hormonal regulation, and tumor induction in transgenic mice. Proc Natl Acad Sci USA 84:1299, 1987
8. Babinet C, Farza H, Morello D, Hadchouel M, Pourcel C: Specific expression of hepatitis B surface antigen (HBsAg) in transgenic mice. Science 230:1160, 1985
9. Beamer WG, Eicher EM: Stimulation of growth in the little mouse. J Endocrinol 71:37, 1976
10. Benoist C, Gerlinger P, LeMeur M, Mathis D: Transgenic mice: new wave immunogenetics. Immunology Today 7:138, 1986
11. Bieberich C, Scangos G: Transgenic mice in the study of immunology. Bioassays 4:245, 1986
12. Bieberich C, Scangos G, Tanaka K, Jay G: Regulated expression of a murine class I gene in transgenic mice. Ann NY Acad Sci 478:255, 1986
13. Botteri FM, van der Putten H, Miller AD, Fran H, Verma IM: Recombinant retroviruses in transgenic mice. Ann NY Acad Sci 478:255, 1986
14. Botteri FM, van der Putten H, Wong DF, Sauvage CA, Evans RM: Unexpected thymic hyperplasia in transgenic mice harboring a neuronal promoter fused with simian virus 40 large T antigen. Mol Cell Biol 7:3178, 1987
15. Bradley A, Evans M, Kaufman MH, Robertson E: Formation of germ-line chimera from embryo-derived teratocarcinoma cells. Nature 309:255, 1984

16. Breitman ML, Clapoff S, Rossant J, Tsui L-C, Glode LM, Maxwell IH, Bernstein A: Genetic ablation: targeted expression of a toxin gene causes microphthalmia in transgenic mice. Science 238: 1563,1987
17. Brinster RL, Chen HY, Messing A, Van Dyke T, Levine AJ, Palmiter RD: Transgenic mice harboring SV40 T-antigen genes develop characteristic brain tumors. Cell 327:367, 1984
18. Brinster RL, Chen HY, Trumbauer ME, Avarbock MR: Translation of globin messenger RNA by the mouse ovum. Nature 283:499, 1980
19. Brinster RL, Chen HY, Trumbauer ME, Senear AW, Warren R, Palmiter RD: Somatic expression of herpes thymidine kinase in mice following injection of a fusion gene into eggs. Cell 277:223, 1981
20. Brinster RL, Chen HY, Trumbauer ME, Yagle MK, Palmiter RD: Factors affecting the efficiency of introducing foreign DNA into mice by microinjecting eggs. Proc Natl Acad Sci USA 84:4438, 1985
21. Brinster RL, Chen HY, Warren R, Sarthy A, Palmiter RD: Regulation of metallothionein-thymidine kinase fusion plasmids injected into mouse eggs. Nature 296:39, 1982
22. Brinster RL, Palmiter RD: Production of tumors following the introduction of T-antigen genes into mice. In Genetic Manipulation of the Mammalian Ovum and Early Embryo, edited by Costantini F, Jaenisch R, New York, Cold Spring Harbor Laboratory Press, 1985
23. Brinster RL, Richie KA, Hammer RE, O'Brien RL, Arp B, Storb U: Expression of a microinjected immunoglobulin gene in the spleen of transgenic mice. Nature 306:332, 1983
24. Bucchini D, Reynaud CA, Ripoche MA, Grimal H, Jami J, Weill JC: Rearrangement of a chicken immunoglobulin gene occurs in the lymphoid lineage of transgenic mice. Nature 326:409, 1987
25. Bucchini D, Ripoche MA, Stinnakre MG, Desbois P, Lores P, Monthioux E, Absil J, Lepesant JA, Pictet R, Jami J: Pancreatic expression of human insulin gene in transgenic mice. Proc Natl Acad Sci USA 83:2511, 1986
26. Burki K, Ullrich A: High efficiency transformation of the human insulin gene into fertilized mouse eggs. EMBO J 1:127, 1982
27. Buttin G: Exogenous Ig gene rearrangement in transgenic mice: a new strategy for human monoclonal antibody production? Trends Genet 3:205, 1987
28. Chada K, Magram J, Costantini F: An embryonic pattern of expression of a human fetal globin gene in transgenic mice. Nature 319:685, 1986
29. Chada K, Magram J, Raphael K, Radice G, Lacy E, Costantini F: Specific expression of a foreign beta-globin gene in erythroid cells of transgenic mice. Nature 314:377, 1985
30. Chen CW, Thomas CA Jr: Recovery of DNA segments from agarose gels. Anal Biochem 101:339, 1980
31. Chen S, Botteri F, Van der Putten H, Landel CP, Evans GA: A lymphoproliferative abnormality associated with inappropriate expression of the Thy-1 antigen in transgenic mice. Cell 51:7, 1987.
32. Chisari FV, Pinkert CA, Millich DR, Filippi P, McLachlan A, Palmiter RD, Brinster RL: A transgenic mouse model of the chronic hepatitis B surface antigen carrier state. Science 6:1157, 1985
33. Choo KH, Raphael K, McAdam W, Peterson MG: Expression of active human blood clotting factor IX in transgenic mice: use of a cDNA with complete mRNA sequence. Nucleic Acids Res 15:871, 1987
34. Corcoran LM, Cory S and Adams JM: Transposition of the immunoglobin heavy chain enhancer to the *myc* oncogene in a murine plasmacytoma. Cell 40:71, 1985
35. Costantini F, Chada K, Magram J: Correction of murine β-thalassemia by gene transfer into the germ line. Science 233:1192, 1986
36. Costantini F, Lacy E: Introduction of a rabbit β-globulin gene into the mouse germ line. Nature 294:92, 1981
37. Costantini F, Radice G, Magram J, Stamatoyannopoulos G, Papayannopoulou T, Chada K: Developmental regulation of human globin genes in transgenic mice. Cold Spring Harbor Symp Quant Biol 50:361, 1985
38. Covarrubias L, Nishida Y, Mintz B: Early postimplantation embryo lethality due to DNA rearrangements in a transgenic mouse strain. Proc Natl Acad Sci USA 83:6020, 1986
39. Covarrubias L, Nishida Y, Terao M, D'Eustachio P, Mintz B: Cellular DNA rearrangements and early developmental arrest caused by DNA insertion in transgenic mouse embryos. Mol Cell Biol 7:2243, 1987
40. Crenshaw EB III, Russo AF, Swanson LW, Rosenfeld MG: Neuron-specific alternative RNA processing in transgenic mice expressing a metallothionein-calcitonin fusion gene. Cell 49:389, 1987
41. Durnam DM, Hoffman JS, Quaife CJ, Benditt EP, Chen HY, Brinster RL, Palmiter RD: Induction of mouse metallothionein-1 mRNA by bacterial endotoxin is independent of metals and glucocorticoid hormones. Proc Natl Acad Sci USA 81:1053, 1984
42. Efrat S, Baekkeshor S, Lane D, Hanahan D. Coordinate expression of the endogenous p53 gene in β cells of transgenic mice expressing hybrid insulin-SV40 transgenic genes. EMBO J 6:2699, 1987
43. Eichholtz DA, Rogers SG, Horsch RB, Klee HJ, Hayford M, Hoffman NL, Braford SB, Fink C, Flick J, O'Connell KM, Fraley RT: Expression of mouse dihydrofolate reductase gene confers methotrexate resistance in transgenic petunia plants. Somatic Cell Mol Genet 13:67, 1987
44. Evans MJ, Kaufman MH: Establishment on culture of pluripotential cells from mouse embryos. Nature 292:154, 1981
45. Evans RM, Swanson L, Rosenfeld MG: Creation of transgenic animals to study development and as models of human disease. Recent Progr Hormone Res 41:317, 1985
46. Faas SJ, Pan S, Pinkert CA, Brinster RL, Knowles BB: Simian virus 40 (SV40)-transgenic mice that develop tumors are specifically tolerant to SV40 T antigen. J Exp Med 165:417, 1987
47. Farza H, Salmon AM, Hadchouel M, Moreau JL, Babinet C, Tiollais P, Pourcel C: Hepatitis B surface antigen gene expression is regulated by sex steroids and glucocorticoids in transgenic mice. Proc Natl Acad Sci USA 84:1187, 1987
47a Field LJ: Atrail natriuretic factor-SV40 T antigen transgenes produce tumors and cardiac arrhythmias in mice. Science 239:1029, 1988
48. Fischoff DA, Bowdish KS, Perlak FJ, Marrone PG, McCormick SM, Niedermeyer JG, Dean DA, Kusano-Kretzmer K, Mayer EJ, Rochester DE, Rogers SG, Fraley RT: Insect tolerant transgenic tomatoe plants. Biotechnology 5:807, 1987
49. Forsthoefel PF: Genetics and manifold effects of Strong's luxoid gene in the mouse, including its interactions with Greens' luxoid and Carter's luxate genes. J Morphol 110:391, 1962
50. Frels WI, Bluestone JA, Hodes RJ, Capecchi MR, Singer DS: Expression of a microinjected porcine class I major histocompatibility complex gene in transgenic mice. Science 228:577, 1985
51. Gartler SM, Riggs AD: Mammalian X-chromosome inactivation. Annu Rev Genet 17:155, 1983
52. Gehring WJ: Homeoboxes in the study of development. Science 236:1245, 1987
53. Gerlinger P, LeMeur M, Irrmann C, Renard P, Wasylyk C, Wasylyk B: B-lymphocyte targeting of gene expression in transgenic mice with the immunoglobulin heavy-chain enhancer. Nucleic Acids Res 14:6565, 1986
54. Goldman MA, Stokes KR, Idzerda RL, McKnight GS, Hammer RE, Brinster RL, Gartler SM: A chicken transferrin gene in transgenic mice escapes X-chromosome inactivation. Science 236:593, 1987
55. Gordon JW: A foreign dihydrofolate reductase gene in transgenic mice acts as a dominant mutation. Mol Cell Biol 6:2158, 1986
56. Gordon JW, Chesa PG, Nishimura H, Rettig WJ, Maccari JE, Endo T, Seravalli E, Seki T, Silver J: Regulation of Thy-1 gene expression in transgenic mice. Cell 50:445, 1987
57. Gordon JW, Ruddle RH: Integration and stable germ line transmission of genes injected into mouse pronuclei. Science 214:1244, 1981
58. Gordon JW, Ruddle RH: Gene transfer into mouse embryos: production of transgenic mice by pronuclear injection. Methods Enzymol 101:411, 1983
59. Gordon JW, Ruddle RH: DNA-mediated genetic transformation of mouse embryos and bone marrow—a review. Gene 33:121, 1985
60. Gordon JW, Scangos GA, Plotkin DJ, Barbosa JA, Ruddle RH: Genetic transformation of mouse embryos by microinjection of purified DNA. Proc Natl Acad Sci USA 77:7380, 1980
61. Goring DR, Rossant J, Clapoff S, Breitman ML, Tsui L-C: *In situ* detection of beta-galactosidase in lenses of transgenic mice with

a gamma-crystallin/*lac* Z gene. Science 235:456, 1987

62. Graves JAM: 5-Azactyidine induced re-expression of alleles on the inactivate X-chromosome in a hybrid mouse cell line. Exp Cell Res 141:99, 1982
63. Green MC: Mutant genes and linkages. In Biology of the Laboratory Mouse, Ed 2, edited by Green EL, pp 87–150. New York, McGraw Hill, 1966
64. Grosschedl R, Weaver D, Baltimore D, Costantini F: Introduction of mu immunoglobulin gene into the mouse germ line: specific expression in lymphoid cells and synthesis of functional antibody. Cell 38:647, 1984
65. Gurdon JB, Melton DA: Gene transfer in amphibian eggs and oocytes. Ann Rev Genet 15:189, 1981
66. Hammer RE, Brinster RL, Palmiter RD: Use of gene transfer to increase animal growth. Cold Spring Harbor Symp Quant Biol 50:379, 1985
67. Hammer RE, Brinster RL, Rosenfeld MG, Evans RM, Mayo KE: Expression of human growth hormone-releasing factor in transgenic mice results in increased somatic growth. Nature 315:413, 1985
68. Hammer RE, Idzerda RL, Brinster RL, McKnight S: Estrogen regulation of the avian transferrin gene in transgenic mice. Mol Cell Biol 6:1010, 1986
69. Hammer RE, Palmiter RD, Brinster RL: Partial correction of murine hereditary growth disorder by germ-line incorporation of a new gene. Nature 311:65, 1984
70. Hammer RE, Pursel VG, Rexroad CE Jr, Wall RJ, Bolt DJ, Ebert KM, Palmiter RD, Brinster RL: Production of transgenic rabbits, sheep and pigs by microinjection. Nature 315:680, 1985
71. Hammer RE, Pursel VG, Rexroad CE Jr, Wall RJ, Bolt DJ, Palmiter RD, Brinster RL: Genetic engineering of mammalian embryos. J Anim Sci 63:269, 1986
72. Hammer RE, Swift GH, Ornitz DM, Quaife CJ, Palmiter RD, Brinster RL, MacDonald RJ: The rat elastase-I regulatory element is an enhancer that directs correct cell specificity and developmental onset of expression in transgenic mice. Mol Cell Biol 7:2956, 1987
73. Hanahan D: Heritable formation of pancreatic beta-cell tumours in transgenic mice expressing recombinant insulin/simian virus 40 oncogenes. Nature 315:115, 1985
74. Hanahan D: Oncogenesis in transgenic mice. In Oncogenes and Growth Control, edited by Graf, T, Kahn P, pp 349–363. Heidelberg, Springer-Verlag, 1986
75. Harbers K, Kuehn M, Delius H, Jaenisch R: Insertion of retrovirus into the first intron of a α collagen gene leads to embryonic lethal mutation in mice. Proc Natl Acad Sci USA 81:1504, 1984
76. Herzenberg LA, Stall AM, Braun J, Weaver D, Baltimore D, Herzenberg LA, Grosschedl R: Depletion of the predominant B-cell population in immunoglobulin μ heavy chain transgenic mice. Nature 329:71, 1987
77. Hinrichs SH, Nerenberg M, Reynolds PK, Khoury G, Jay G: A transgenic mouse model for human neurofibromatosis. Science 237:1340, 1987
78. Hock RA, Miller AD: Retrovirus-mediated transfer and expression of drug resistance genes in human haematopoietic progenitor cells. Nature (London) 320:275, 1986
79. Hogan BLM, Costantini F, Lacy E: Manipulation of the Mouse Embryo: A Laboratory Manual. New York, Cold Spring Harbor Laboratory Press, 1986
80. Hooper M, Hardy K, Handyside A, Hunter S, Monk M: HPRT-deficient (Lesch-Nyhan) mouse embryos derived from germline colonization by cultured cells. Nature 326:292, 1987
81. Hoppe PC, Illmensee K: Microsurgically produced homozygous-diploid uniparental mice. Proc Natl Acad Sci USA 74:5657, 1977
82. Hudson P, Penschow J, Shine J, Ryan G, Niall H, Coghlan J: Hybridization histochemistry: Use of recombinant DNA as a "homing probe" for tissue localization of specific mRNA populations. Endocrinology 108:353, 1981
83. Humphries RK, Berg P, DiPietro J, Bernstein S, Baur A, Nienhuis AW, Anderson WF: Transfer of human and murine globin-gene sequences into transgenic mice. Am J Hum Genet 37:295, 1985
84. Huszar D, Balling R, Kothary R, Magli MC, Hozumi N, Rossant, J, Bernstein A: Insertion of a bacterial gene into the mouse germ line using an infectious retrovirus vector. Proc Natl Acad Sci USA 82:8587, 1985
85. Isobe K, Kollias G, Kolsto AB, Grosveld F: T cell independent Thy-1 alloantibody response with the use of transgenic mice. J Immunol 137:2089, 1986
86. Isola LM, Gordon JW: Systemic resistance to methotrexate in transgenic mice carrying a mutant dihydrofolate reductase gene. Proc Natl Acad Sci USA 83:9621, 1986
87. Izant JE, Weintraub H.: Constitutive and conditional suppression of exogenous and endogenous genes by anti-sense RNA. Science 229:345, 1985
88. Jaenisch R: Germ line integration and Mendelian transmission of the exogenous Moloney leukemia virus. Proc Natl Acad Sci USA 73:1260, 1976
89. Jaenisch R, Harbers K, Schnieke A, Löhler J, Chumakov I, Jähner D, Grotkopp D, Hoffman E.: Germline integration of Moloney murine leukemia virus at the Mov 13 locus leads to recessive lethal mutation and early embryonic death. Cell 32:209, 1983
90. Jaenisch R, Jahner D, Nobis P, Simon T, Lohler J, Harbers K, Grotkopp D: Chromosomal position and advance of retroviral genomes inserted into germ line of mice. Cell 24:519, 1981
91. Jaenisch R, Mintz B: Simian virus 40 DNA sequences in DNA of healthy adult mice derived from preimplantation blastocysts injected with viral DNA. Proc Natl Acad Sci USA 71:1250, 1974
92. Jahner D, Haase K, Mulligan R, Jaenisch R: Insertion of the bacterial *gpt* gene into the germ of mice by retroviral infection. Proc Natl Acad Sci USA 82:6927, 1985
93. Jenkins NA, Copeland NG, Taylor BA, Lee BK: Dilute (*d*) coat color mutation of DBA/2J mice is associated with the site of integration of an ectroopic MuLV genome. Nature 293:370, 1981
94. Johnson RT: Evidence for polyomaviruses in human neurological diseases. In Polyomaviruses and Human Neurological Disease: Proceedings of a Conference held at the Fogarty International Center, National Institutes of Health, Bethesda Maryland, June 14-16, 1982, edited by Sever JL, Madden DL, p 183. New York, Alan R. Liss, 1983
95. Kafatos FC, Jones WC, Efstratiadis A: Determination of nucleic acid sequence homologies and relative concentrations by a dot hybridization procedure. Nucleic Acids Res 7:1541, 1979
96. Kägi JHR, Nordberg M (Editors:) Metallothionein, Birhäuser Verlag, Basel, 1979
97. Keith DH, Singer-Sam J, Riggs AD: Active X-chromosome DNA is unmethylated at eight CCGG sites clustered in a guanine-plus-cytosine-rich island at the 5′ end of the gene for phosphoglycerate kinase. Mol Cell Biol 6:4122, 1986

97a Khillan JS, Oskarsson MK, Propst F, Kuwabara T, Vande Woude GF, Westphal H: Defects in lens fiber differentiation are linked to *c-mos* overexpression in transgenic mice. Gene Dev 1:1327, 1987

98. Khillan JS, Overbeek PA, Westphal H: Drosophila P element integration in the mouse. Dev Biol 109:247, 1985
99. Khillan JS, Schmidt A, Overbeek PA, de Crombrugghe B, Westphal H: Developmental and tissue-specific expression directed by the alpha$_2$ type 1 collagen promoter in transgenic mice. Proc Natl Acad Sci USA 83:725, 1986.
100. Kollias G, Evans DJ, Ritter M, Beech J, Morris R, Grosveld F: Ectopic expression of Thy-1 in the kidneys of transgenic mice induce functional and proliferative abnormalities. Cell 51:21, 1987
101. Kollias G, Wrighton N, Hurst J, Grosveld F: Regulated expression of human A gamma-, beta-, and hybrid gamma beta-globulin genes in transgenic mice: manipulation of gamma developmental expression patterns. Cell 46:89, 1986
102. Kondoh H, Katoh K, Takahashi Y, Fujisawa H, Yokoyama M, Kimura S, Katsuki M, Saito M, Nomura T, Hiramoto Y, Okada TS: Specific expression of the chicken δ-crystallin gene in the lens and the pyramidal neurons of the piriform cortex in transgenic mice. Dev Biol 120:177, 1987
103. Kostyo JL, Isaksson O: Growth hormone and the regulation of somatic growth. Int Rev Physiol 13:255, 1977
104. Krumlauf R, Chapman VM, Hammer RE, Brinster RL, Tilghman SM: Differential expression of alpha-fetoprotein genes on the inactive X chromosome in extraembyronic and somatic tissues of a transgenic mouse line. Nature 319:224, 1986
105. Krumlauf R, Hammer RE, Tilghmam SM, Brinster RL: Developmental regulation of alpha-fetoprotein genes in transgenic mice. Mol Cell Biol 5:1639, 1985
106. Kuehn MR, Bradley A, Robertson EJ, Evans MJ: A potential animal model for Lesch-Nyhan syndrome through introduction of HPRT mutations into mice. Nature 326:295, 1987

107. Lacy M, Alpert S, Hanahan D: Bovine papillomavirus genome elicits skin tumors in transgenic mice. Nature 322:609, 1986
108. Lacy E, Costantini FD: Structure and expression of foreign globin genes in transgenic mice. Prog Clin Biol Res 134:13, 1983
109. Lacy E, Roberts S, Evans EP, Burtenshaw MD, Costantini RE: A foreign beta-globin gene in transgenic mice: integration at abnormal chromosomal positions and expression in inappropriate tissues. Cell 34:343, 1983
110. Lang RA, Metcalf D, Cuthbertson RA, Lyons I, Stanley E, Kelso A, Kannourakis G, Williamson J, Klintworth GK, Gonda TJ, Dunn AR: Transgenic mice expressing a hemopoietic growth factor gene (GM-CSF) develop accumulations of macrophages, blindness and a fatal syndrome of tissue damage. Cell 51:675, 1987
111. Langdon WY, Harris AW, Cory S, Adams JM: The *c-myc* oncogene perturbs B lymphocyte development in Eμ-*myc* transgenic mice. Cell 47:11, 1986
112. Leder A, Pattengale PK, Kuo A, Stewart TA, Leder P: Consequences of widespread deregulation of the *c-myc* gene in transgenic mice: multiple neoplasms and normal development. Cell 23:485, 1986
113. Le Meur M, Gerlinger P, Benoist C, Mathis D: Correcting an immune-response deficiency by creating E alpha gene transgenic mice. Nature 316:38, 1985
114. Léopold P, Vailly J, Cuzin F, Rassoulzadegan M: Maintenance of autonomous genetic elements in twelve transgenic mouse strains established after transfer of pPyLT1 DNA. Biochem Biophys Res Commun 141:1162, 1986
115. Lester SC, Korn NJ, DeMars R: Derepression of genes on the human inactive X chromosome: evidence for differences in locus-specific rates of derepression and rates of transfer of active and inactive genes after DNA-mediated transformation. Somatic Cell Genet 8:265, 1982
116. Lewin B: Genes III, Ed 3, New York, John Wiley & Sons, 1987
117. Lock LF, Melton DW, Caskey CT, Martin GR: Methylation of the mouse *hprt* gene differs on the active and inactive chromosomes. Mol Cell Biol 6:914, 1986
118. Loesch-Fries LS, Merlo D, Zinnen T, Burhop L, Hill K, Krahn K, Jarvis N, Nelson S, Halk E: Expression of alfalfa mosaic virus RNA 4 in transgenic plants confers virus resistance. EMBO J 6:1845, 1987
119. Low MJ, Hammer RE, Goodman RH, Habener JF, Palmiter RD, Brinster RL: Tissue-specific post-translational processing of pre-prosomatostatin encoded by a metallothionein-somatostatin fusion gene in transgenic mice. Cell 41:211, 1985
120. Low MJ, Lechan RM, Hammer RE, Bristner RL, Habener JF, Mandel G, Goodman RH: Gonadotroph-specific expression of metallothionein fusion genes in pituitaries of transgenic mice. Science 231:1002, 1986
121. Low MJ, Stork PJ, Hammer RE, Brinster RL, Warhol MJ, Mandel G, Goodman RH: Somatostatin is targeted to the regulated secretory pathway of gonadotrophs in transgenic mice expressing a metallothionein-somatostatin gene. J Biol Chem 261:6260, 1986
122. Low PA, McCloud JG: Hereditary demyelinating neuropathy in the trembler mouse. J Neurol Sci 26:565, 1975
123. MacDonald RJ, Hammer RE, Swift GH, Davis BP, Brinster RL: Transgenic progeny inherit tissue-specific expression of rat elastase I genes. DNA 5:393, 1986
124. Magram J, Chada K, Costantini F: Development regulation of a cloned adult beta-globin gene in transgenic mice. Nature 315:338, 1985
125. Mahon KA, Chepelinsky AB, Khillan JS, Overbeek PA, Piatigorsky J, Westphal H: Oncogenesis of the lens in transgenic mice. Science 235:1622, 1987
126. Maniatis T, Fritsch EF, Sambrook J: Molecular Cloning: A Laboratory Manual. Cold Spring Harbor Laboratory, Cold Spring Harbor, NY, 1982
127. Maniatis T, Goodbourn S, Fischer JA: Regulation of inducible and tissue-specific gene expression. Science 236:1237, 1987
128. Mark WH, Signorelli K, Lacy E: An insertional mutation in a transgenic mouse line results in developmental arrest at day 5 of gestation. Cold Spring Harbor Symp Quant Biol 50:453, 1985
129. Mason AJ, Hayflick JS, Zoeller RT, Young WS III, Phillips HS, Nikolics K, Seeburg PH: A deletion truncating the gonadotropin-releasing hormone gene is responsible for hypogonadism in the *hpg* mouse. Science 234:1366, 1987
130. Mason AJ, Pitts SL, Nikolics K, Szonyi, Wilson JN, Seeburg PH, Stewart TA: The hypogonadal mouse: reproductive functions restored by gene therapy. Science 234:1372, 1986
131. Matsunaga T, Cabilly-Horesh O, Terz D, Lee A, Chirstian L, Ohno S, Biro AP: Use of transgenic mice with human MHC class 1 gene (HLA-A2). Adv Exp Med Biol 186:341, 1985
132. McGrath J, Solter D: Nuclear transplantation in the mouse embryo by microsurgery and cell fusion. Science 220:1300, 1983
133. McKnight GS: The induction of ovalbumin and conalbumin mRNA by estrogen and progesterone in chick oviduct explant cultures. Cell 14:403, 1978
134. McKnight GS, Hammer RE, Kuenzel EA, Brinster RL: Expression of the chicken transferrin gene in transgenic mice. Cell 34:335, 1983
135. Messing A, Chen HY, Palmiter RD, Brinster RL: Peripheral neuropathies, hepatocellular carcinomas and islet cell adenomas in transgenic mice. Nature 316:461, 1985
136. Mintz B, Cronmiller C: METT-1: a karyotypically normal *in vitro* line of developmentally totipotent mouse teratocarcinoma cells. Som Cell Genet 7:485, 1981
137. Mintz B, Illmensee K: Normal genetically mosaic mice produced from malignant teratocarcinoma cells. Proc Natl Acad Sci USA 72:3585, 1975
138. Mohandas T, Sparkes RS, Shapiro LJ: Reactivation of an inactive human X chromosomes: evidence of X inactivation by DNA methylation. Science 211:393, 1981
139. Morello D, Moore G, Salmon AM, Yaniv M, Babinet C: Studies on the expression of an H-2K/human growth hormone fusion gene in giant transgenic mice. EMBO J 5:1877, 1986
140. Nerenberg M, Hinrichs SH, Reynolds RK, Khoury G, Jay G: The *tat* gene of human T-lymphotropic virus type I induces mesenchymal tumors in transgenic mice. Science 237:1324, 1987
141. Norstedt G, Palmiter RD: Secretory rhythm of growth hormone regulates sexual differentiation of mouse liver. Cell 36:805, 1984
142. Nussenzweig MC, Shaw AC, Sinn E, Danner DB, Holmes KL, Morse HC 3d, Leder P: Allelic exclusion in transgenic mice that express the membrane form of immunoglobulin mu. Science 236:816, 1987
143. O'Brien RL, Brinster RL, Storb U: Somatic hypermutation of an immunoglobulin transgene in kappa transgenic mice. Nature 326:405, 1987
144. Ornitz DM, Hammer RE, Messing A, Palmiter RD, Brinster RL: Pancreatic neoplasia induced by SV40 T-antigen expression in acinar cells of transgenic mice. Science 238:188, 1987
145. Ornitz DM, Palmiter RD, Hammer RE, Brinster RL, Swift GH, MacDonald RJ: Specific expression of an elastase-human growth hormone fusion gene in pancreatic acinar cells of transgenic mice. Nature 313:600, 1985
146. Ornitz DM, Palmiter RD, Messing A, Hammer RE, Pinkert CA, Brinster RL: Elastase I promoter directs expression of human growth hormone and SV40 T-antigen genes to pancreatic acinar cells in transgenic mice. Cold Spring Harbor Symp Quant Biol 50:399, 1985
147. Overbeek PA, Chepelinsky AB, Khillan JS, Piatigorsky J, Westphal H: Lens-specific expression and developmental regulation of the bacterial chloramphenicol acetyltransferase gene driven by the murine alpha A-crystallin promoter in transgenic mice. Proc Natl Acad Sci USA 82:7815, 1985
148. Overbeek OA, Lai SP, Van Quill KR, Westphal H: Tissue-specific expression in transgenic mice of a fused gene containing RSV terminal sequences. Science 231:1574, 1986
149. Palmiter RD: Molecular biology of metallothionein gene expression. In Mctallothionein II: Proceedings of the Second International Meeting on Metallothionein and Other Low Molecular Weight Usual-Binding Proteins, edited by Kagi JHK, Kojima, Y, Basel Birkhauser-Verlag, 1987
150. Palmiter RD, Behringer RR, Quaife CJ, Maxwell F, Maxwell IH, Brinster RL: Cell lineage ablation in transgenic mice by cell-specific expression of a toxin gene. Cell 50:435, 1987
151. Palmiter RD, Brinster RL: Transgenic mice. Cell 41:343, 1985
152. Palmiter RD, Brinster RL: Germ line transformation of mice. Ann Rev Genet 20:465, 1986
153. Palmiter RD, Brinster RL, Hammer RE, Trumbauer ME, Rosenfeld MG, Birnberg NC, Evans RM: Dramatic growth of mice that develop from eggs microinjected with metallothionein-growth hor-

mone fusion genes. Nature 300:611, 1982
154. Palmiter RD, Chen HY, Brinster RL: Differential regulation of metallothionein-thymidine kinase fusion genes in transgenic mice and their offspring. Cell 29:701, 1982
155. Palmiter RD, Chen HY, Messing A, Brinster RL: SV40 enhancer and large-T antigen are instrumental in development of choroid plexus tumours in transgenic mice. Nature 316:457, 1985
156. Palmiter RD, Norstedt G, Gelinas RE, Hammer RE, Brinster RL: Metallothionein-human GH fusion genes stimulate growth of mice. Science 222:809, 1983
157. Payvar F, DeFranco D, Firestone G, Edgar B, Wrange O, Okret S, Gustafsson JA, Yamamoto KR: Sequence specific binding of glucocorticoid receptor of MTV DNA at sites within and upstream of the transcribed region. Cell 35:381, 1983
158. Penschow JD, Haralambidis J, Aldred P, Tregear GW, Coghlan JP: Localization of gene expression in CNS using hybridization histochemistry. Methods Enzymol 124:534, 1986
159. Peschon JJ, Behringer RR, Brinster RL, Palmiter RD: Spermatid-specific expression of protamine 1 in transgenic mice. Proc Natl Acad Sci USA 84:5316, 1987
160. Piatigorsky J: Lens crystallins and their gene families. Cell 38:620, 1984
161. Pinkert CA, Widera G, Cowing C, Heber-Katz E, Palmiter RD, Flavell RD, Brinster RL: Tissue-specific inducible and functional expression of the E alpha d MHC class II gene in trangenic mice. EMBO J 4:2225, 1985
162. Quaife C, Hammer RE, Mottet NK, Palmiter RD: Glucocorticoid regulation of metallothionein during murine development. Dev Biol 118:549, 1986
163. Quaife CJ, Pinkert CA, Ornitz DM, Palmiter RD, Brinster RL: Pancreatic neoplasia induced by *ras* expression in acinar cells of transgenic mice. Cell 48:1023, 1987
164. Rassoulzadegan M, Leopold P, Vailly J, Cuzin F: Germ line transmission of autonomous genetic elements in transgenic mouse strains. Cell 46:513, 1986
165. Readhead C, Popko B, Takahashi N, Shine HD, Saavedra RA, Sidman RL, Hood L: Expression of a myelin basic protein gene in transgenic shiverer mice: correction of the dysmyelinating phenotype. Cell 48:703, 1987
166. Reik W, Collick A, Norris ML, Barton SC and Surani MA: Genomic imprinting determines methylation of parental alleles in transgenic mice. Nature 328:248, 1987
167. Richmond IL, Wilson CB: Pituitary adenomas in childhood and adolescence. J Neurosurg 49:163, 1978
168. Riggs AD, Singer-Sam J, Keith DH: Methylation of the PGK promoter region and an enhancer way-station model for X-chromosome inactivation. Prog Clin Biol Res. 198:211, 1985
169. Ritchie KA, Brinster RL, Storb U: Allelic exclusion and control of endogenous immunoglobulin gene rearrangement in kappa transgenic mice. Nature 312:517, 1984
170. Rivier J, Spiess J, Thorner M, Vale W: Characterization of growth hormone-releasing factor from a human pancreatic islet tumor. Nature 300:276, 1982
171. Robertson E, Bradley A, Kuehn M, Evans M: Germ-line transmission of genes introduced into cultured pluripotential cells by retroviral vector. Nature 323:445, 1986
172. Robertson M: Gene therapy: desperate appliances. Nature (London) 320:213, 1986
173. Robl JM, First NL: Manipulation of gametes and embryos in the pig. J Reprod Fertil 33 (Suppl) 101, 1985
174. Ross SR, Solter D: Glucocorticoid regulation of mouse mammary tumor virus sequences in transgenic mice. Proc Natl Acad Sci USA 82:5880, 1985
175. Rusconi S, Kohler G: Transmission and expression of a specific pair of rearranged immunoglobulin μ and κ genes in a transgenic mouse line. Nature 314:330, 1985
176. Rüther U, Garber C, Komitowski D, Müller R, Wagner EF: Deregulated *c-fos* expression interferes with normal bone development in transgenic mice. Nature 325:412, 1987
177. Sapienza C, Peterson AC, Rossant J, and Balling R: Degree of methylation of transgenes is dependent on gamete of origin. Nature 328:251, 1987
178. Rüther U, Tripodi M, Cortese R, Wagner EF: The human alpha-1-antitrypsin gene is efficiently expressed from two tissue-specific promoters in transgenic mice. Nucleic Acids Res 15:751, 1987
179. Sasaki H, Shigenobu T, Nakazato M, Yoshioka K, Matsuo H, Kato Y, Sakaki Y: Generation of transgenic mice producing a human transthyretin variant: a possible mouse model for familial amyoidotic polyneuropathy. Biochem Biophys Res Comm 139:794, 1986
180. Schell JS: Transgenic plants as tools to study the molecular organization of plant genes. Science 237:1176, 1987
181. Schnieke A, Harbers K, Jaenisch R: Embryonic lethal mutation in mice induced by retrovirus insertion into the $\alpha 1(1)$ collagen gene. Nature 304:315, 1983
182. Seeburg PH, Shine J, Martial JA, Baxter JD, Goodman HM: Nucleotide sequence and amplification in bacteria of structural gene for rat growth hormone. Nature 270:486, 1977
183. Selden RF, Skoskiewicz MJ, Howie KB, Russell PS, Goodman HM: Regulation of human insulin gene expression in transgenic mice. Nature 321:525, 1986
184. Selden RF, Skoskiewicz MJ, Howie KB, Russell PS, Goodman HM: Implantation of genetically engineered fibroblasts into mice: implications for gene therapy. Science 236:714, 1987
185. Shani M: Tissue-specific expression of rat myosin light-chain 2 gene in transgenic mice. Nature 314:283, 1985
186. Shani M: Tissue-specific and developmentally regulated expression of a chimeric actin-globin gene in transgenic mice. Mol Cell Biol 6:2624, 1986
187. Sifers RN, Carlson JA, Clift SM, DeMayo FJ, Bullock DW, Woo SLC: Tissue specific expression of the human alpha-1 antitrypsin gene in transgenic mice. Nucleic Acids Res 15:1459, 1987
188. Simons JP, McClenaghan M, Clark AJ: Alteration of the quality of milk by expression of sheep beta-lactoglobulin in transgenic mice. Nature 328:530, 1987
189. Sinn E, Müller W, Pattengale P, Tepler I, Wallace R, Leder P: Coexpression of MMTV/v-Ha-ras and MMTV/c-*myc* genes in transgenic mice: synergistic action of oncogenes in vivo. Cell 49:465, 1987
190. Small JA, Khoury G, Jay G, Howley PM, Scangos GA: Early regions of JC virus and BK virus induce distinct and tissue-specific tumors in transgenic mice. Proc Natl Acad Sci USA 83:8288, 1986
191. Small JA, Scangos GA, Cork L, Jay G, Khoury G: The early region of human papovavirus JC induces dysmyelination in transgenic mice. Cell 4:13, 1986
192. Soriano P, Cone RD, Mulligan RC, Jaenisch R: Tissue-specific and ectopic expression of genes introduced into transgenic mice by retroviruses. Science 234:1409, 1986
193. Soriano P, Gridley T, Jaenisch R: Retroviruses and insertional mutagenesis in mice: proviral integration at the *Moy* 34 locus leads to early embryonic death. Genes Dev. 1:366, 1987
194. Soriano P, Jaenisch R: Retroviruses as probes for mammalian development: allocation of cells to the somatic and germ lineages. Cell 46:19, 1986
195. Southern E: Detection of specific sequences among DNA fragments separated by gel electrophoresis. J Mol Biol 98:503, 1975
196. Stewart TA, Wagner EF, Mintz B: Human beta globin sequences injected into mouse eggs, retained in adults and transmitted to progeny. Science 217:1046, 1982
197. Stewart TA, Pattengale PK, Leder P: Spontaneous mammary adenocarcinomas in transgenic mice that carry and express MTV/myc fusion genes. Cell 38:627, 1984
198. Storb U: Immunoglobulin transgenic mice. Ann Rev Immunol 5:151, 1987
199. Storb U, O'Brien RL, McMullen MD, Gollahon KA, Brinster RL: High expression of cloned immunoglobulin kappa gene in transgenic mice is restricted to B lymphocytes. Nature 310:238, 1984
200. Storb U, Pinkert C, Arp B, Engler P, Gollahon K, Manz J, Brady W, Brinster RL: Transgenic mice with mu and kappa genes encoding antiphosphorylcholine antibodies. J Exp Med 164:627, 1986
201. Stout JT, Chen HY, Brennard J, Caskey CT, Brinster RL: Expression of human HPRT in the central nervous system of transgenic mice. Nature 317:250, 1985
202. Stuart GW, Searle PF, Palmiter RD: Identification of multiple metal regulatory elements in mouse metallothionein I promoter by assaying synthetic sequences. Nature 317:828, 1985
203. Surani MAH, Barton SC, Norris ML: Development of reconstituted mouse eggs suggest imprinting of the genome during gametogenesis. Nature 308:548, 1984
204. Swain JL, Stewart TA, Leder P: Parental legacy determines

methylation and expression of an autosomal transgene: a molecular mechanism for parental imprinting. Cell 50:719, 1987
205. Swanson LW, Simmons DM, Arriza J, Hammer R, Brinster R, Rosenfeld MG, Evans RM: Novel developmental specificity in the nervous system of transgenic animals expressing growth hormone fusion genes. Nature 317:363, 1985
206. Swift GH, Hammer RE, MacDonald RJ, Brinster RL: Tissue-specific expression of the rat pancreatic elastase I gene in transgenic mice. Cell 38:639, 1984
207. Tooze J (ed): The Molecular Biology of Tumor Viruses, New York, Cold Spring Harbor Laboratory, 1981
208. Townes TM, Lingrel JB, Chen HY, Brinster RL, Palmiter RD: Erythroid-specific expression of human beta-globin genes in transgenic mice. EMBO J 4:1715, 1985
209. Vaeck M, Reynaerts A, Höfte H, Jansens S, De Beuckeleer M, Dean C, Zabeau M, Van Montagu M, Leemans J: Transgenic plants protected from insect attack. Nature 328:33, 1987
210. van der Putten H, Botteri FM, Miller AD, Rosenfeld MG, Fan H, Evans RM, Verma IM: Efficient insertion of genes into the germ line via retroviral vectors. Proc Natl Acad Sci USA 82:6148, 1985
211. van Dyke T, Finlay C, Levine AJ: A comparison of several lines of transgenic mice containing the SV40 early genes. Cold Spring Harbor Symp Quant Biol 50:671, 1985
212. Wagner EF, Stewart CL: Integration and expression of genes introduced into mouse embryos. In: Experimental Approaches to Mammalian Embryonic Development. Rossant J, and Petersen R (Eds), Cambridge University Press, Cambridge, 1986.
213. Wagner TE, Hoppe PC, Jollick JD, Scholl DR, Hodinka RL, Gault JB: Microinjection of a rabbit β-globulin gene in zygotes and its subsequent expression in adult mice and their offspring. Proc Natl Acad Sci USA 78:6376, 1981
214. Wagner EF, Covarrubias L, Stewart TA, Mintz B: Prenatal lethalities in mice homozygous for human growth hormone gene sequences integrated in the germ line. Cell 35:647, 1983
215. Wagner EF, Stewart TA, Mintz B: The human β-globulin gene and a functional viral thymidine gene in developing mice. Proc Natl Acad Sci USA 78:5016, 1981
216. Weaver D, Costantini F, Imanishi-Kari T, Baltimore D: A transgenic immunoglobulin mu gene prevents rearrangement of endogenous genes. Cell 42:117, 1985
217. Weaver D, Reis MH, Albanese C, Costantini F, Baltimore D, Imanishi-Kari T: Altered repertoire of endogenous immunoglobulin gene expression in transgenic mice containing a rearranged Mu heavy chain gene. Cell 45:247, 1986
218. Welsh M, Hammer RE, Brinster RL, Steiner DF: Stimulation of growth hormone synthesis by glucose in islets of Langerhans isolated from transgenic mice. J Biol Chem 261:12915, 1986
219. Westphal H. Overbeek PA, Khillan JS, Chepelinsky AB, Schmidt A, Mahon KA, Bernstein KE, Piatigrosky J, de Crombrugghe B: Promoter sequences of murine alpha A crystallin, murine alpha 2(1) collagen or of avian sarcoma virus genes linked to the bacterial chloramphenicol acetyltransferase gene direct tissue-specific patterns of chloramphenicol acetyltransferase expression in transgenic mice. Cold Spring Harbor Symp Quant Biol 50:411, 1985
220. Wilkie TM, Brinster RL, Palmiter RD: Germline and somatic mosaicism in transgenic mice. Dev Biol 118:9, 1986
221. Williams DA, Lemischka IR, Nathan DG, Mulligan RC: Introduction of new genetic material into pluripotent haematopoietic stem cells of the mouse. Nature (London) 310:476, 1984
222. Williams DA, Orkin SH: Somatic gene therapy: current status and future prospects. J Clin Invest 77:1053, 1986
223. Williams DA, Orkin SH, Mulligan RC: Retrovirus-mediated transfer of human adenosine deaminase gene sequences into cells in culture and into murine hematopoietic cell in vivo. Proc Natl Acad Sci USA 83:2566, 1986
224. Wolf SF, Jolly DJ, Lunnen KD, Friedmann T, Migeon BR: Methylation of the hypoxanthine phosphoribosyltransferase locus on the human X chromosome: implications for X-chromosome inactivation. Proc Natl Acad Sci USA 81:2806, 1984
225. Woychik RP, Stewart TA, Davis LG, D'Eustachio P, Leder P: An inherited limb deformity created by insertional mutagenesis in a transgenic mouse. Nature 318:36, 1985.
226. Yagaloff KA, Lozano G, van Dyke T, Levine AJ, Hartig PR: Serotonin 5-HT_{1c} receptors are expressed at high density on choroid plexus tumors from transgenic mice. Brain Res 385:389, 1986
227. Yamamoto KR: Steroid receptor regulated transcription of specific genes and gene networks. Ann Rev Genet 19:209, 1985
228. Yamamura K, Kitutani H, Folsom V, Clayton LK, Kimoto M, Akira S, Kashiwamura S, Tonegawa S, Kishimoto T: Functional expression of a microinjected Ed alpha gene in C57BL/6 transgenic mice. Nature 216:67, 1985
229. Yamamura K, Kudo A, Ebihara T, Kamino K, Araki K, Kumahara Y, Watanabe T: Cell-type-specific and regulated expression of a human gamma 1 heavy-chain immunoglobulin gene in transgenic mice. Proc Natl Acad Sci USA 83:2152, 1986
230. Yen PH, Patel P, Chanault AC, Mohandas T, Shapiro LJ: Differential methylation of hypoxanthine phosphoribosyltransferase genes on active and inactive human X chromosomes. Proc Natl Acad Sci USA 81:1759, 1984
231. Yu, S-F, Ruden IV, Kantoff PW, Garber C, Seibers M, Ruther U, Anderson WF, Wagner EF, Gilboa E: Self-inactivating retroviral vectors designed for transfer of whole genes into mammalian cells. Proc Natl Acad Sci USA 83:3194, 1986
232. Zu Rhein GM, Chou S: Particles resembling papova viruses in human demyelinating disease. Science 148:1477, 1965

Index

FSC
www.fsc.org
MIX
Papier aus verantwortungsvollen Quellen
Paper from responsible sources
FSC® C105338

If you have any concerns about our products, you can contact us on
ProductSafety@springernature.com

In case Publisher is established outside the EU, the EU authorized representative is:
Springer Nature Customer Service Center GmbH
Europaplatz 3, 69115 Heidelberg, Germany

Printed by Libri Plureos GmbH
in Hamburg, Germany